Diagnostic Criteria in Autoimmune

Diagnostic Criteria in Autoimmune Diseases

Yehuda Shoenfeld
Tel-Aviv University, Tel-Aviv, Israel

Ricard Cervera
University of Barcelona, Barcelona, Catalonia, Spain

M. Eric Gershwin
University of California at Davis, Davis, CA, USA

Editors

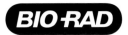
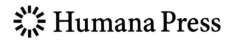

Editors

Prof. Yehuda Shoenfeld
Sheba Med. Center
Dept. Medicine "B"
52 621 Tel-Hashomer
Israel
shoenfeld@post.tau.ac.il

Prof. Ricard Cervera
Hospital Clinic
Servei de Malalties
Autoimmunes
Villarroel, 170
08036 Barcelona
Catalonia, Spain
rcervera@clinic.ub.es

Prof. M. Eric Gershwin
University of California at Davis
School of Medicine
Division of Rheumatology,
Allergy, and Clinical Immunology
Davis, CA 95616
USA
megershwin@ucdavis.edu

ISBN: 978-1-60327-284-1 (softcover)   e-ISBN: 978-1-60327-285-8

ISBN: 978-1-60327-427-2 (hardcover)

DOI: 10.1007/978-1-60327-285-8

Library of Congress Control Number: 2008933364

Printed on acid-free paper

9 8 7 6 5 4 3 2 1

springer.com

Preface

Autoimmune diseases are a family of more than 100 illnesses that develop when underlying defects in the immune system lead the body to attack its own organs, tissues, and cells. While many of these diseases are rare, collectively they affect, according to the Autoimmune Diseases Coordinating Committee (ADCC) of the U.S. National Institutes of Health, between 14.7 and 23.5 million people in the USA – up to 8% of the population – and their prevalence is rising. Because a complete cure is not available for nearly every one of these 100 autoimmune diseases, patients face a lifetime of illness and treatment. And, because most of these diseases disproportionately afflict women, and are among the leading causes of death for young and middle-aged women, they impose a heavy burden on patients' families and on society.

For these reasons, major efforts in autoimmune disease research and development must be directed toward reducing the impact of these conditions. These efforts should include, among other goals and again according to the ADCC, the generation of more accurate epidemiologic profiles of autoimmune diseases, the development of a greater understanding of the fundamental biologic principles underlying disease onset and progression, the provision of improved diagnostic tools to permit preclinical or presymptomatic diagnosis, the creation of more effective interventions, and the production of public and professional education and training programs.

For instance, the development of biomarkers can enable earlier diagnosis as well as aid physicians in selecting and monitoring treatment. New technologies, such as genomics and proteomics, can provide scientists with the tools to study gene and protein patterns in tissue samples, providing vital insights into the onset and progression of disease. However, we also need to gain a better understanding of the distribution of these diseases through epidemiologic studies, and of the environmental triggers that contribute to their onset. As we learn more about the genetic and environmental factors contributing to these diseases, we will be able to develop effective prevention strategies that arrest the autoimmune process before it can irreversibly damage the body, as also the ADCC points out.

But the first and most essential step in the management of autoimmune diseases is, no doubt, the recognition of the autoimmune disease itself by the attending physician. Autoimmune diseases can affect any part of the body, and have a myriad of clinical manifestations that make diagnosis an extremely difficult task. At the same time, autoimmune diseases share many features both at their onset and during follow-up. In addition, overlapping genetic traits enhance susceptibility to many of the diseases, so that a patient may suffer from more than one autoimmune disorder, or multiple autoimmune diseases may occur in the same family.

Conversely, despite the diversity in their presentation and natural history, autoimmune diseases share a number of underlying mechanisms, and thus have the potential to respond to treatment with the same or related therapies. More selective and less toxic immunosuppressive and immunomodulatory agents are currently being used to treat these disorders, and promising immune tolerance approaches are emerging. However, several factors limit our ability to conduct the most efficient clinical trials. For example, we lack standardized classification and diagnostic criteria for many autoimmune diseases.

These problems have prompted us to gather in a comprehensive book a critical review of 103 autoimmune diseases, dividing them into two main groups, namely systemic and organ-specific autoimmune diseases. We hope to offer a contemporary overview of these conditions with special emphasis on diagnosis. Each chapter contains the essential information required by attending physicians as well as bench scientists to understand the definition of a specific autoimmune disease, the diagnostic criteria, and the treatment. Moreover, established classification and diagnostic criteria have been quoted when available and, if not, authors have been asked to propose such criteria. *Diagnostic Criteria in Autoimmune Diseases* was conceived for publication and debut on the occasion of the Sixth International Congress of Autoimmunity to be held in Porto, Portugal, on September 2008.

We have tried to produce a book of considerable intellectual caliber and this would not have occurred without the enthusiastic support of the authors. We wish to thank Richard Lansing and his staff at Springer for their hard work. The editors and all the contributors also extend special thanks to Kathy Wisdom for her devotion and zeal in helping us to put this volume together.

Finally, and most importantly, this text is dedicated to the sufferers of autoimmune diseases in the hope that they some day will be cured.

Yehuda Shoenfeld
Ricard Cervera
M. Eric Gershwin

Contents

II. SYSTEMIC VASCULITIS

III. IDIOPATHIC INFLAMMATORY MYOPATHIES

VI. HEPATOBILIARY AND PANCREATIC AUTOIMMUNE DISEASES

VII. GASTROINTESTINAL AUTOIMMUNE DISEASES

VIII. CUTANEOUS AUTOIMMUNE DISEASES

IX. CARDIOVASCULAR AND PULMONARY AUTOIMMUNE DISEASES

Contributors

ALFREDO ADAN, MD, PHD, Department of Ophthalmology, Institut Clinic d'Oftalmologia, Hospital Clinic Universidad de Barcelona, Barcelona, Catalonia, Spain

RAPHAEL ADAR, MD, Department of Medicine C and the Rheumatic Disease Unit and the Department of Vascular Surgery, Chaim Sheba Medical Center, Tel-Hashomer, Israel, and the Tel-Aviv University Tel-Aviv, Israel

FRANK ALDERUCCIO, BSC HONS, PHD, Department of Immunology, Monash University, Australia

DANIELA AMITAL, MD, Department of Psychiatry B, Ness-Ziona Mental Health Center, Ness-Ziona, Israel

HOWARD AMITAL, MD, MHA, Head of Department of Medicine D, Meir Medical Center, Kfar-Saba, Israel, Affiliated to Sackler Faculty of Medicine, Tel-Aviv University, Tel-Aviv, Israel

JUAN-MANUEL ANAYA, MD, Professor of Medicine, Cellular Biology and Immunogenetics Unit, Corporation for Biological Research, Medellín-Colombia, and, Universidad del Rosario, Bogotá, Colombia

JORDI ARA, MD, Nephrology Department, Hospital Germans Trias, Badalona, Barcelona, Catalonia, Spain

FRANCISCO DE ASSIS ANDRADE, Hospital do Olho and Centro Oftalmológico de Botafogo, Rio de Janeiro, Brasil

AFTAB A. ANSARI, PHD, Professor, Department of Pathology, Emory University School of Medicine, Atlanta, Georgia, USA

JORDI ANTON, MD, Associate Professor, Pediatric Rheumatology Unit, Hospital Sant Joan de Déu, University of Barcelona, Barcelona, Catalonia, Spain

YOLANDA ARCE, MD, Nephrology Department, Puigvert Foundation, Universidad Autónoma de Barcelona, Barcelona, Catalonia, Spain

GOWTHAMI M. AREPALLY, MD, Division of Hematology, Duke University Medical Center, Durham, North Carolina

PILAR ARRIZABALAGA CLEMENTE, MD, PHD, Nephrology and Renal Transplant Service, Hospital Clinic, Biomedicial Investigation Institute August Pi I Sunyer, Barcelona, Catalonia, Spain

YOAV ARNSON, Department of Medicine D, MD, Meir Medical Center, Kfar-Saba, Israel, Affiliated to the Sackler Faculty of Medicine, Tel-Aviv University, Tel-Aviv, Israel

RONALD A. ASHERSON, Division of Immunology, School of Pathology, University of the Witwatersrand, Johannesburg, South Africa

YEMIL ATISHA-FREGOSO, MD, Department of Internal Medicine, Instituto Nacional de Cienias Medicas y Nutricion, Salvador Zubiran, Mexico

FRANCESC BALAGUER, MD, Department of Gastroenterology, Institut Clinic de Malalties Digestives i Metabòliques, Hospital Clínic, Barcelona, Catatonia, Spain

JOSÉ BALLARIN, MD, PHD, Nephrology Department, Puigvert Foundation, Universidad Autónoma de Barcelona, Barcelona, Catalonia, Spain

JOAN-ALBERT BARBERÀ, MD, Department of Medicine, University of Barcelona, and, Senior Consultant, Department of Pulmonary Medicine, Thorax Institute, Hospital Clínic, Barcelona, Catalonia, Spain

ELENA BARTOLONI BOCCI, MD, Department of Clinical and Experimental Medicine, Rheumatology Unit, University of Perugia, Perugia, Italy

AVIV BARZILAI, MD, Dermatology Department, Sheba Medical Center (Affiliated to the Sackler Faculty of Medicine), Tel Aviv University, Israel

SHARON BAUM, MD, Dermatology Department, Sheba Medical Center (Affiliated to the Sackler Faculty of Medicine), Tel Aviv University, Israel

YACKOV BERKUN, MD, Lecturer, Sackler Faculty of Medicine, Tel-Aviv University, Rheumatology and Immunology Clinic, Associate Director of Safra Childrens Hospital, Sheba Medical Center, Tel-Hashomer, Israel

CHRISTIAN BERTHOU, MD, PHD, Department of Immunopathology, Brest University Medical School, Brest, France

MARIA LAURA BERTOLACCINI, MD, Lupus Research Unit, The Rayne Institute, King's College London School of Medicine, St. Thomas' Hospital, London, UK

CORRADO BETTERLE, MD, Chair of Clinical Immunologo, Endocrine Unit, Department of Medical and Surgical Sciences, University of Padova, Padova, Italy

NICOLA BIZZARO, MD, Laboratory of Clinical Pathology, Ospedale Civile, Tolmezzo, Italy

ISABEL BLANCO, MD, Servei de Pneumologia, Institut Clínic del Tórax, Hospital Clínic, Universitat de Barcelona, Barcelona, Catalonia, Spain

STEFANO BOMBARDIERI, MD, Rheumatology Unit, Department of Internal Medicine, University of Pisa, Italy

ELOÍSA BONFÁ, MD, Rheumatology Division, University of São Paulo, School of Medicine, São Paulo, Brazil

GISELA BONSMANN, MD, Department of Dermatology, University of Münster, Münster, Germany

RODRIGO ANTONIO BRANDÃO NETO, MD, Emergency Department of São Paulo University, School of Medicine, São Paulo, Brazil

MIQUEL BRUGUERA, MD, Liver Unit, Hospital Clínic, University of Barcelona, Barcelona, Catalonia, Spain

ROSA BOU, MD, Pediatric Rheumatology Unit, Hospital Parc Tauli, Sabadell, Barcelona, Catalonia, Spain

ALBERT BOVÉ, MD, Laboratory of Autoimmune Diseases "Josep Font", IDIBAPS, Department of Autoimmune Diseases, School of Medicine, University of Barcelona, Hospital Clinic, Barcelona, Catalonia, Spain

CHRISTOPHER L. BOWLUS, MD, Division of Gastroenterology and Hepatology, University of California at Davis Medical Center, Sacramento, California, USA

CHIARA BRIANI, MD, Department of Neurosciences, University of Padova, Padova, Italy

PILAR BRITO-ZERÓN, MD, Laboratory of Autoimmune Diseases "Josep Font", IDIBAPS, Department of Autoimmune Diseases, Hospital Clinic, Barcelona, Catalonia, Spain

CRISTINA CABRERA, MD, Nephrology Department, Puigvert Foundation, Universitat Autonoma de Barcelona, Barcelona, Catalonia, Spain

MARIO H. CARDIEL, MSC, Unidad de Investigación "Dr. Mario Alvizouri Muño", Hospital General "Dr. Miguel Silva, Morelia, Michoacán, Mexico

FRANCISCO CARMONA, MD, Head of the Service of Gynaecology, Hospital Clínic, Barcelona, Catalonia, Spain

PATRIZIO CATUREGLI, MD, Departments of Pathology and, Molecular Microbiology and Immunology, The Hohns Hopkins University, Baltimore, Maryland, USA

JOHN CASTIBLANCO, MD, Cellular Biology and Immunogenetics Unit, Corporation for Biological Research, Medellín, Colombia

ILARIA CAVAZZANA, MD, Rheumatology and Clinical Immunology, University and Spedali Civili of Brescia, Italy

ANGELA CERIBELLI, MD, Rheumatology and Clinical Immunology, University and Spedali Civili of Brescia, Italy

RICARD CERVERA, MD, PHD, FRCP, Department of Autoimmune Diseases, Hospital Clínic, Associate Professor, Department of Medicine, University of Barcelona, Catalonia, Spain

JOAB CHAPMAN, MD, Department of Neurology, Sheba Medical Center and Sackler Faculty of Medicine, Tel Aviv University, Israel.

MARIA C. CID, MD, Vasculitis Research Unit, Department of Autoimmune Diseases, Institute of Medicine and Dermatology, Hospital Clinic, University of Barcelona, Institut d'Investigacions, Biomèdiques August Pi i Sunyer (IDIBAPS), Barcelona, Catalonia, Spain

ROLANDO CIMAZ, MD, Rheumatology, Meyer Hospital, Firenze, Italy

DOUGLAS B. CINES, MD, Vice Chair, Pathology and Laboratory Medicine, University of Pennsylvania School of Medicine, Philadelphia, Pennsylvania, USA

KARSTEN CONRAD, MD, Institute of Immunology, Medical Faculty of the Technical University Dresden, Dresden, Germany

ELENA CSERNOK, MD, Department of Rheumatology, University Hospital Schleswig-Holstein, Campus Lübeck, Lübeck Germany

MAURIZIO CUTOLO, MD, Research Laboratory and Clinical Academic Unit of Rheumatology, Department of Internal Medicine, University of Genova, Italy

MICHAEL DAVID, MD, Dermatology Department, Rabin Medical Center, Beilinson Campus, Petah Tiqwa, Israel, Affiliated to Tel-Aviv University, Sackler Faculty of Medicine, Tel-Aviv, Israel

VALÉRIE DEVAUCHELLE-PENSEC, MD, PHD, Department of Immunopathology, Brest University Medical School, Brest, France

MONTSERRAT M. DÍAZ, MD, Clinical Nephrology Department, Puigvert Foundation, Universidad Autónoma de Barcelona, Barcelona, Catalonia, Spain

ANDREA DORIA, MD, Division of Rheumatology, University of Padova, Padova, Italy

ZAMIR DVORISH, MD, Department of Medicine D, Meir Medical Center, Kfar-Saba, Israel, Affiliated to the Sackler Faculty of Medicine, Tel-Aviv University, Tel-Aviv, Israel

MICHAEL EHRENFELD, MD, Department of Medicine C and the Rheumatic Disease Unit and, the department of Vascular Surgery, Chaim Sheba Medical Center, Tel-Hashomer, Israel, and, the Tel-Aviv University, Tel-Aviv, Israel

YULIA EINAV, PHD, Mathematical Biology Unit, Faculti of Sciences, Holon Institute of Technology, Israel

ALON EISEN, MD, Department of Medicine D, Meir Medical Center, Kfar-Saba, Israel, Affiliated to Sackler Faculty of Medicine, Tel-Aviv University Tel-Aviv, Israel

URS. ENYDEGGER, MD, Consultant Octapharma Switzerland, Transfusion Therapy Consultancy TTC, Emeritus Medical Faculty University of Bern, Switzerland

RICARDO O. ESCÁRCEGA, MD, Internal Medicine, Temple University Hospital Philadelphia, Philadelphia, Pennsylvania, USA

GEORGINA ESPÍGOL, MD, Department of Autoimmune Diseases, Medicine and Dermatology Institute, Hospital Clinic, University of Barcelona, Barcelona, Catalonia, Spain

GERARD ESPINOSA, MD, PHD, Department of Autoimmune Diseases, Hospital Clínic, Barcelona, Catalonia, Spain

IVET ETCHEGARAY-MORALES, MD, Systemic Autoimmune Diseases Research Unit, HGR #36, CMN Manuel Ávila Camacho, IMSS, Puebla, México

ALBERTO FALORNI, MD, PHD, Department of Internal Medicine, Section of Internal Medicine and Endocrine and Metabolic Sciences, University of Perugia, Perugia, Italy

EDUARDO FERREIRA BORBA, MD, PHD, Division of Rheumatology, University of Sao Paulo, São Paulo, Brazil

SIMONE FERRERO, MD, Department of Obstetrics and Gynecology, San Martino Hospital and, University of Genoa, Italy

CAROLINA FIGUEROA, MD, Department of Gastroenterology, Hospital Clínic/IDIBAPS, CIBER EHD, Barcelona, Catalonia, Spain

IVAN FOELDVARI, MD, Hamburger Zentrum fuer Kinder- and Jungerrheumatologie, Am Klinikum Eilbek Hamburg, Germany

FRANCO FRANCESCHINI, MD, Rheumatology and Clinical Immunology, University and Spedali Civili of Brescia, Italy

Jozélio Freire De Carvalho, MD, PHD, Assistant Professor, Faculdade de Medicina e Hospital das Clínicas da Faculdade de Medicina da Universidade de São Paulo, São Paulo-SP, Brazil

Marvin J. Fritzler, MD, PHD, University of Calgary, Calgary, Alberta, Canada

Salvador Fuentes-Alexandro, MD, Internal Medicine CMN siglo XXI, Instituto Mexicano del Seguro Social, DF, Mexico

Claudio Galarza-Maldonado, MD, Unidad de Enfermedades Reumaticas y Autoinmunes (UNERA), Hospital Monte Sinaí, Cuenca, Ecuador

Mauro Galeazzi, MD, Unità Operativa Complessa di Rheumatologia, University of Siena, Siena, Italy

Mario Garcia-Carrasco, MD, PHD, Systemic Autoimmune Diseases Research Unit, HGR #36, CMN Manuel Ávila Camacho, IMSS, Puebla, México, and, Rheumatology Department, Benemerita Universidad Autonoma de Puebla, School of Medicine, Puebla, México

Pedram Gerami, MD, Northwestern University Medical Center, Chicago, Illinois

Roberto Gerli, MD, Rheumatology Unit, Department of Clinical and Experimental Medicine, University of Perugia, Perugia, Italy

M. Eric Gershwin, MD, Division of Rheumatology, Allergy and Clinical Immunology, University of California at Davis, School of Medicine, Davis, California, USA

Ibtissem Ghedira, PHARMD, PHD, Laboratory of Immunology, Faculty of Pharmacia, Monastir, Tunisia

Anna Ghirardello, MD, Division of Rheumatology, University of Padova, Padova, Italy

Joan Giralt, MD, Institut Clinic d'Oftalmologia, Hospital Clinic. Universidad de Barcelona, Barcelona, Catalonia, Spain

Ramon Gomis, MD, PHD, Department of Endocrinology, Hospital Clínic, Barcelona, Catalonia, Spain

Alexander Gorshtein, MD, Department of Internal Medicine E, Meir Hospital, Kfar Saba, Israel

Josep M. Grau, MD, PHD, Department of Internal Medicine, Muscular Research Group, Hospital Clínic, Professor of Medicine, University of Barcelona, Barcelona, Catalonia, Spain

Francesc Graus, MD, Service of Neurology, Hospital Clinic, Universitat de Barcelona and, Institut d' Investigació Biomèdica August Pi i Sunyer (IDIBAPS), Barcelona, Catalonia, Spain

Wolfgang L. Gross, MD, Department of Rheumatology, University Hospital Schleswig-Holstein, Campus Lübeck, Lübeck Germany

Loïc Guilleven, MD, Department of Internal Medicine and, Referral Center for Necrotizing Vasculitides and Systemic Sclerosis, Cochin Hospital, Paris, France, and, Systemic Diseases Study Group, University Paris 5 – René Descartes, Paris, France

Philippe Guilpain, MD, Department of Internal Medicine and, Referral Center for Necrotizing Vasculitides and Systemic Sclerosis, Cochin Hospital, Paris, France, and, Systemic Diseases Study Group, University Paris 5 – René Descartes, Paris, France

Felicia A. Hanzu, MD, Diabetes and Obesity Laboratory, Institut d'Investigaciones Biomediques August Pi I Sunyer (IDIBAPS), University of Barcelona, Barcelona, Catalonia, Spain

Thomas Hellmark, PHD, Department of Clinical Sciences in Lund, Lund University, Sweden

José Hernández-Rodríguez, MD, Vasculitis Research Unit, Department of Autoimmune Diseases, Institute of Medicine and Dermatology, Hospital Clinic, University of Barcelona, Institut d'Investigacions, Biomèdiques August Pi i Sunyer (IDIBAPS), Barcelona, Catalonia, Spain

Sophie Hillion, PHD, Department of Immunopathology, Brest University Medical School, Brest, France

Julia U. Holle, MD, Department of Rheumatology, University Hospital Schleswig-Holstein, Campus Lübeck, Lübeck Germany

Graham R. V. Hughes, MD, Lupus Research Unit, The Rayne Institute, King's College London School of Medicine, St. Thomas' Hospital, London, UK

Sarosh R. Irani, BA, MRCP, Department of Clinical Neurology, University of Oxford, John Radcliffe Hospital, Oxford, UK

Luis J. Jara, MD, Direction of Education and Research, Hospital de Especialidades, Centro Médico, La Raza, Instituto Mexicano del Seguro Social, Mexico City, Mexico

Mario Jiménez-Hernández, MD, Rheumatology Department, School of Medicine, Benemérita Universidad Autónoma de Puebla; Systemic Autoimmune Diseases Research Unit, HGR #36, CMN Manuel Ávila Camacho, IMSS, Puebla, Mexico

Cees G. M. Kallenberg, MD, PHD, Professor of Medicine, Head Department of Clinical Immunology, University Medical Center Groningen, University of Groningen, Groningen, The Netherlands

Martin Kaass, MD, Department of Pediatrics, Medical Faculty of the Technical University of Dresden, Dresden, Germany

Aharon Kessel, MD, Allergy and Clinical Immunology, Bnai-Zion Medical Center, The Bruce Rappaport Faculty of Medicine, Technion Medical School, Haifa, Israel

Munther A. Khamashta, MD, Senior Lecturer/Consultant Physician, Lupus Unit, The Rayne Institute, St. Thomas Hospital, London, UK

Aannegret Kuhn, MD, Department of Dermatology, University of Düesseldorf, Düesseldorf, Germany

Bethan Lang PHD, Neurosciences Group, Department of Clinical Neurology, Weatherall Institute of Molecular Medicine, John Radcliffe Hospital, Oxford University, Oxford, UK

Yair Levy, MD, Department of Internal Medicine E, Meir Hospital, Kfar Saba, Israel

Roger A. Levy, MD, Diagnósticos da América SA and, Discipline of Rheumatology, Faculdade de Ciências Médicas, Universidade do Estado do Rio de Janeiro, Brasil

Maurício Levy-Neto, MD, PHD, Rheumatology Division, University of São Paulo, School of Medicine, São Paulo, Brazil

Baraf Lior, MD, Department of Medicine E, Meir Medical Center, Kfar-Saba, Affiliated to the Sackler Faculty of Medicine, Tel-Aviv University, Tel-Aviv, Israel

Margalit Lorber, MD, Autoimmune Disease Unit, Division of Medicine, Rambam Health Campus, The Rappaport Faculty of Medicine, Technion, Haifa, Isreal

JUAN MAÑÁ, MD, Associate Professor of Medicine, Department of Internal Medicine, Institut d'Investigació Biomèdica de Bellvitge (IDIBELL), Bellvitge University Hospital, University of Barcelona, Barcelona, Catalonia, Spain

AMANI MANKAI, PHD, Department of Immunopathology, Brest University Medical School, Brest, France, and, Laboratory of Immunology, Faculty of Pharmacia, Monastir, Tunisia

LORETO MASSARDO VEGA, MD, Departamento de Immunología Clínica y Reumatología, Facultad de Medicina, Pontificia Universidad Catolica de Chile, Santiago, Chile

GABRIELA MEDINA, MD, MSC, Clinical Research Unit, Hospital de Especialidades, Centro Médico, La Raza, Instituto Mexicano del Seguro Social, Mexico City, Mexico

FRANCESCA MENCONI, MD, Division of Endocrinology, University of Cincinnati College of Medicine, Cincinnati, Ohio, USA

CLAUDIA MENDOZA-PINTO, MD, Systemic Autoimmune Diseases Research Unit, HGR &, CMN Manuel Ávila Camacho, IMSS, Puebla, México

PIER LUIGI MERONI, MD, Department of Internal Medicine, University of Milan and IRCCS Instituto Auxologico Italiano, Italy

ARIEL MILLER, MD, PHD, Multiple Sclerosis and Brain Research Center, Rappaport Facility of Medicine & Research Institute, Technion-Israel Institute of Technology, Department of Neurology, Carmel Medical Center, Haifa, Israel

RON MILO, MD, Department of Neurology, Barzilai Medical Center, Ashkelon, Ben-Gurion University of Negev, Israel

DANIEL MIMOUNI, MD, Dermatology Department, Rabin Medical Center, Beilinson Campus, Petah Tiqwa, Israel, Affiliated to Tel-Aviv University, Sackler Faculty of Medicine, Tel-Aviv Israel

DIMITRIS MITSIAS, MD, Department of Pathophysiology, School of Medicine, National University of Athens, Athens, Greece

MARIA MOLINA-MOLINA, MD, PHD, Departament Investigacions de Patología Experimental, Institut d'Investigacions Biomèdiques de Barcelona, Consejo Superior de Investgaciones Científicas, Institut d'Investigacions Biomèdiques August Pi I Sunyer, Barcelona, Catalonia, Spain

MARTA MOSCA, MD, Rheumatology Unit, Department of Internal Medicine, University of Pisa, Italy

HARALAMPOS M. MOUTSOPOULOS, MD, FACP, FRCP, Department of Pathophysiology, School of Medicine, National University of Athens, Athens, Greece

SALVADOR NAVARRO, MD, PHD, Department of Gastroenterology, Institut Clinic de Malalties Digestives i Metabòliques, Hospital Clínic, Barcelona, Catatonia, Spain

GIDEON NESHER, MD, Department of Internal Medicine A and, The Rheumatology Service, Shaare-Zedek Medical Center, Jerusalem, Israel

LAURA F. NEWELL, MD, Department of Hematology, University of Washington, Seattle, Washington, USA

UDI NUSSINOVITCH, MD, Department of Medicine B, Chaim Sheba Medical Center, Tel-Hashomer, Israel

YAEL L. OPPENHEIM, MD, Endocrinology and Diabetes Associates of Long Island, Rockville Center, NY, USA

HEDI ORBACH, MD, Head of Internal Medicine B Department, Wolfson Medical Center, Holon, Israel

SHAI PADEH, MD, Pediatric Rheumatology, Safra Children Hospital, Chaim Sheba Medical Center, Tel-Hashomer, Israel, and, Sackler School of Medicine, Tel-Aviv University, Tel-Aviv, Israel

ZIV PAZ, MD, MSC, Department of Medicine 'B', Center for Autoimmune Diseases, Chaim Sheba Medical Center, (Affiliated to Tel-Aviv University), Tel-Hashomer, Israel

LARA E. PEREIRA, PHD, Department of Pathology and Laboratory Medicine, Emory University, Atlanta, Georgia, USA

JUAN CARLOS PÉREZ-ALVA, MD, Cardiovascular Institut., Hospital Angeles, Puebla, Mexico

SHIMON POLLACK, MD, Associate Professor of Medicine & Immunology, Rappaport Faculty of Medicine – Technion, Israel Institute of Technology, Director, Institute for Allergy, Immunology & AIDS, Rambam Medical Center, Haifa, Israel

BERNARDO PONS-ESTEL, MD 3, Hospital provincial de Rosario, Universidad Nacional de Rosario, Rosario Argentina

GIOVANNI PORCIELLO, MD, Unità Operativa Medicina Interna, Ospedale Misericordia e Dolce, Prato, Italy

SERGIO PRIETO, MD, Department of Autoimmune Disease, Medicine and Dermatology Institute, Hospital Clínic, University of Barcelona, Barcelona, Catalonia, Spain

CARLOS QUEREDA, MD, Nephrology Department, Hospital Ramón y Cajal, Madrid, Spain

ROBERTO ROCCHI, MD, Institute of Endocrinology, University of Pisa, Italy

ROSA MARIA RODRIGUES PEREIRA, MD, PHD, Rheumatology Division, University of São Paulo, School of Medicine, São Paulo, Brazil

NOEL R. ROSE, MD, PHD, Professor of Pathology, Professor of Molecular Microbiology and Immunology, Director, Johns Hopkins Center for Autoimmune Disease Research, Bloomberg School of Public Health, Baltimore, Maryland, USA

MANUEL RAMOS-CASALS MD, PHD, Department of Autoimmune Diseases, Hospital Clínic, Barcelona, Catalonia, Spain

ADRIANA ROJAS-VILLARRAGA, MD, Cellular Biology and Immunogenetics Unit, Corporation for Biological Research, Medellín-Colombia, and, Universidad del Rosario, Bogotá, Columbia

NICOLETTA RONDA, MD, Department of Clinical Medicine, Nephrology and Health Science, University of Pharma, Italy

RICARDO RONDINONE, MD, Division of Rheumatology, University of Padova, Padova, Italy

NURIT ROSENBERG, PHD, Amalia Biron Research Institute of Thrombosis and Hemostasis, Sheba Medical Center, Tel-Hashomer, Israel

TOMEU ROSSIÑOL, MD, Service of Neurology, Hospital Clinic, Universitat de Barcelona and, Institut d' Investigació Biomèdica August Pi i Sunyer (IDIBAPS), Barcelona, Catalonia, Spain

ALEJANDRO RUIZ-ARGÜELLES, MD, Laboratorios Clínicos de Puebla, Puebla, Mexico

VINCENT RULAND, MD, Department of Dermatology, University of Düesseldorf, Düesseldorf, Germany

OPHIRA SALOMON, MD, Amalia Biron Research Institute of Thrombosis and Hemostasis, Sheba Medical Center, Tel-Hashomer, Israel

SHARONJEET SANGHA, MD, Department of Internal Medicine, University of California at Davis Medical Center, Sacramento, California, USA

LAIA SANS, MD, Nephrology Department, Puigvert Foundation, Universidad Autónoma de Barcelona, Barcelona, Catalonia, Spain

MIQUEL SANS, MD, PHD, Department of Gastroenterology, Hospital Clínic I Provincial/IDIBAPS, CIBER EHD, Barcelona, Catalonia, Spain

ALAIN SARAUX, MD, PHD, Department of Immunopathology, Brest University Medical School, Brest, France

PIERCARLO SARZI-PUTTINI, MD, Department of Rheumatology, Rheumatology Unit, L Sacco University Hospital, Milan, Italy

MÅRTEN SEGELMARK, MD, Department of Nephrology, Clinical Sciences in Lund, Lund University, Sweden

CARLO SELMI, MD, PHD, Division of Rheumatology, Allergy and Clinical Immunology, University of California at Davis, Davis, CA, and, Division of Internal Medicine, Department of Clinical Sciences 'Luigi Sacco', University of Milan, Milan, Italy

ALBERT SELVA-O'CALLAGHAN, MD, PHD, Internal Medicine Department, Hospital Vall d'Hebrón, Universitat Autónoma de Barcelona, Barcelona, Catalonia, Spain

SUK SEO, MD, Pfleger Liver Institute, David Geffen School of Medicine at UCLA, Los Angeles, California, USA

ANNA SERRANO-MOLLAR PHD, Departament de Patología Experimental, Institut d'Investigaciones Científicas, Institut d'Investigaciones Biomèdiques August Pi I Sunyer, Barcelona, Catalonia, Spain

BORIS SHENKMAN, MD, PHD, Amalia Biron Research Institute of Thrombosis and Hemostasis, Sheba Medical Center, Tel-Hashomer, Israel

YANIV SHERER, MD, Department of Medicine B, Center of Autoimmune Diseases, Sheba Medical Center, Tel-Hashomer, and, Sackler Faculty of Medicine, Tel-Aviv University, Israel

YEHUDA SHOENFELD, MD, FRCP (HON.), Department of Medicine B, And Sackler Faculty of Medicine, Tel-Aviv University, Israel, and, Incumbent of the Laura Schwartz Kipp Chair, for Research of Autoimmune Diseases, Tel-Aviv University, Israel

CLOVIS ARTUR A. SILVA, MD, PHD, Pediatric Rheumatology Unit, Department of Pediatric, University of Sao Paulo, Brazil

GLEB SLOBODIN, MD, Department of Internal Medicine A, Bnai-Zion Medical Center, Technion Medical School, Haifa, Israel

RICHARD D. SONTHEIMER, MD, Department of Dermatology, Richard and Adeline Fleischaker Chair in Dermatology Research, University of Oklahoma Health Sciences Center, Adjunct Investigator, Oklahoma Medical Research Foundation, Oklahoma City, Oklahoma, USA

ALEX STAGNARO-GREEN, MD, MHPE, Senior Associate Dean for Academic Affairs, Touro University College of Medicine, Hackensack, New Jersey, USA

ALBERTO SULLI, MD, Research Laboratory and Clinical Academic Unit of Rheumatology, Department of Internal Medicine, University of Genova, Italy

MARTINE SZYPER-KRAVITZ, MD, Center for Autoimmune Diseases and, Department of Medicine B, Chaim Sheba Medical Center Tel-Hashomer, Sackler Faculty of Medicine, Tel Aviv University, Israel

ROSARIA TALARICO, MD, Rheumatology Unit, Department of Internal Medicine, University of Pisa, Italy

IRA N. TARGOFF, MDDepartment of Medicine, University of Oklahoma Health Sciences Center, Veterans Affairs Medical Center, Oklahoma Medical Research Foundation, Oklahoma City, Oklahoma, USA

ANGELA TINCANI, MD, Rheumatology and Clinical Immunology, University and Spedali Civili of Brescia, Italy

BAN-HOCK TOH, MBBS, DSC, Autoimmunity Laboratory, Centre for Inflammatory Diseases, Department of Medicine, Southern Clinical School, Faculty of Medicine, Nursing and Health Services, Monash University, Clayton, Victoria, Australia

YARON TOMER, MD, FACP, Division of Endocrinology, University of Cincinnati College of Medicine, Cincinnati, Ohio, and, Cincinnati VA Medical Center, Cincinnati, Ohio, USA

ELIO TONUTTI, MD, Immunopatologia e Allergologia, Azienda Ospedaliero-Universitaria S. Maria della Misericordia, Udine, Italy

NATALIE J. TOROK, MD, Division of Gastroenterology and Hepatology, University of California Davis Medical Center, Sacramento, California, USA

DARIA LA TORRE, MD, Department of Internal Medicine, Section of Internal Medicine and Endocrine and Metabolic Sciences, University of Perugia, Perugia, Italy

ELIAS TOUBI, MD, Bnai-Zion Medical Center, The Bruce Rappaport Faculty of Medicine, Technion Medical School, Haifa, Israel

HENRI TRAU, MD, Dermatology Department, Sheba Medical Center (Affiliated to the Sackler Faculty of Medicine), Tel Aviv University, Israel

FABIO TUCCI, MD, A. Meyer Children's Hospital, Firenze, Italy

JOSEPH M. TUSCANO, MD, Department of Internal Medicine and, The UC Davis Cancer Center, Division of Hematology and Oncology, University of California, Davis School of Medicine, Sacramento, California, USA

MANUEL FRANCISCO UGARTE, MD, Universidad Nacional Mayor de San Marcos, and, Department of Rheumatology, Hospital Almenara, Lima, Peru

AVRAHAM UNTERMAN, MD, Department of Medicine 'B' and, Center for Autoimmune Disease, Sheba Medical Center, Tel-Hashomer, Israel

OLGA VERA-LASTRA, MD, Internal Medicine Department, Hospital de Especialidades, Centro Médico, La Raza, Instituto Mexicano del Seguro Social, Mexico City, Mexico

JENNY WALKER, MD, University of Calgary, Calgary, Alberta, Canada

HOBART W. WALLING, MD, PHD, Private Practice of Dermatology, Coralville, Iowa, USA

SENGA WHITTINGHAM, MBCHB, PHD, Department of Biochemistry and Molecular Biology, Monash University, Australia

ASHER WINDER, MD, Tel-Aviv University, Israel, And, Hematology Department, Wolfson Medical Center, Holon, Israel

ANTONI XAUBET, MD, PHD, Department of Respiratory Diseases, Hospital Clínic. Barcelona, Associate Professor of Medicine,

University of Barcelona, Servei de Pneumologia, Hospital Clínic, Barcelona, Catalonia, Spain

BERKUN YACKOV, MD, Associate Director, Pediatric Rheumatology, Safra Children Hospital, Chaim Sheba Medical Center, Tel-Hashomer, Israel, and, Sackler School of Medicine, Tel-Aviv University, Tel-Aviv, Israel

LEVY YAIR, MD, Department of Medicine E, Meir Medical Center, Kfar-Saba, Affiliated to the Sackler Faculty of Medicine, Tel-Aviv University, Tel-Aviv, Israel

JOYCEHISAE YAMAMOTO, MD, PHD, University of São Paulo, School of Medicine, São Paulo, Brazil

PIERRE YOUINOU, MD, DSc, Department of Immunopathology, Brest University Medical School, Brest, France

SANDRA ZAMPIERI, MD, Division of Rheumatology, University of Padova, Padova, Italy

GISELE ZANDMAN-GODDARD, Department of Medicine C, Wolfson Medical Center, Holon, Israel, And, Sackler Faculty of Medicine, Tel-Aviv University, Israel

Part I
Classical Systemic Autoimmune Diseases

1
Systemic Lupus Erythematosus

Maria Laura Bertolaccini, Graham R.V. Hughes and Munther A. Khamashta

Abstract Systemic lupus erythematosus (SLE) is the most diverse of the autoimmune diseases, characterised by a wide range of clinical features and the production of multiple autoantibodies. The diagnosis is based on the clinical features and the presence of a wide variety of autoantibodies, most of which are directed to double stranded DNA (ds-DNA), nuclear antigens, ribonucleoproteins and cell surface antigens. The treatment includes the use of antimalarial agents to corticosteroids and/or immunosuppressive agents.

Keywords SLE · autoantibodies · BILAG · renal markers · ds-DNA · CNS

SLE is a chronic multisystem autoimmune disease of unknown aetiology, characterised by the production of predominantly non-organ specific autoantibodies directed to several self molecules found in the nucleous, cytoplasm and cell surface and a wide range of clinical manifestations. The primary pathological findings are those of inflammation, vasculitis, immune complex deposition and vasculopathy.

The course of the disease is characterised by periods of flares and remission. The incidence of SLE varies from 2 to 7.6 cases per 100,000 individuals per year, the highest prevalence being in Afro-Caribbeans, followed by Asians. The sex ratio is 9:1 in favour of females with a disease onset between the ages of 15–55.

Familial aggregation of SLE is well described and twin studies demonstrate high concordance rates in monozygotic twins. Multiple genes, in particular HLA class II genes, have been implicated in the development of the disease. A higher frequency of DR2 and DR3 has been described in Caucasian SLE patients, as well as in black SLE patients. Homozygous deficiency of the complement components may also influence disease susceptibility.

The laboratory hallmark of the disease is the presence of ANA, appearing in more than 95% of individuals with lupus. The commonest pattern is a diffuse or homogeneous nuclear staining. Anti-DNA and anti-Sm antibodies are rarely seen in other conditions and have therefore high specificity for SLE. Whilst anti-DNA titres frequently vary over time and disease activity, anti-Sm titres are usually constant.

SLE can involve any organ or system in the body. Polyarthritis, oral ulcers and skin rashes, including photosensitivity, are the most common features. The most frequent organs involved are the kidneys and the brain. Hematological manifestations, such as haemolytic anemia, lymphopenia and thrombocytopenia are frequent. Nonspecific features like fatigue, fever or anorexia are early frequent features of SLE.

The American College of Rheumatology published in 1982 a revised set of criteria that have been widely used for decades in the classification of the disease (1). These criteria were later updated to include the presence of antiphospholipid antibodies (aPL) as a criterion for SLE (2) (Table 1.1).

The long-term prognosis of patients with SLE has improved from 50% survival in the 1950's to around 90% in the 1990's, likely due to a combination of improved recognition of the disease and better approaches to therapy.

Epidemiology

The incidence of SLE in the general population varies according to the characteristics of the population studied (i.e. age, gender, race, ethnic/national origin or period of time studied) from 3.3 cases per 100,000 persons per year in Iceland (3) and 4.8 cases per 100,000 persons per year in Sweden (4) to 0.7 to 7.2 cases per 100,000 persons per year in the USA (for a review, see ref (5)).

From: Y. Shoenfeld et al. (eds.): *Diagnostic Criteria in Autoimmune Diseases*, DOI: 10.1007/978-1-60327-285-8_1,
© 2008 Humana Press, Totowa, NJ

TABLE 1.1. American College of Rheumatology classification criteria for systemic lupus erythematosus.

Criteria
1. Malar rash
2. Discoid rash
3. Photosensitivity
4. Oral ulcer
5. Arthritis
6. Serositis
– *Pleurisy*
– *Pericarditis*
7. Renal disorder
– *Persistent proteinuria*
– *Cellular casts*
8. Neurologic disorder
– *Psychosis*
– *Seizures*
9. Hematologic disorder
– *Hemolytic anemia*
– *Leukopenia*
– *Lymphopenia*
– *Thrombocytopenia*
10. Immunologic disorder
– *Anti-DNA*
– *Anti-Sm*
– *Antiphospholipid antibodies*
11. Antinuclear antibody

This classification is based on 11 criteria. For the purposes of identifying patients in clinical studies, a person must be classified as having SLE if any four or more of the 11 criteria are present, serially or simultaneously, during any interval of observation (1, 2).

The presentation and course of the disease appear highly variable between patients of different ethnic origins, where African-Americans and Orientals are believed to have a more severe disease than Caucasian whites (6).

It is now known that autoantibodies to DNA may be present on average 2.7 years prior to diagnosis and up to 9.3 years earlier. Anti nuclear antibodies (ANA) may occur earlier than anti-DNA antibodies. Interestingly, anti-Sm and anti-RNP antibodies appear shortly before diagnosis suggesting a crescendo of autoimmunity resulting in clinical illness (7).

Clinical Manifestations

Polyarticular, symmetrical and episodic arthralgia occurs in about 90% of all patients with SLE, usually in the absence of clinically overt arthritis. Tenosynovitis is more common than erosive synovitis and is the cause of the "swan-neck" deformities and ulnar deviation seen in the Jaccoud's arthritis of lupus, seen in around 10% of the patients. Muscle involvement has been reported in 30–50% of SLE patients, usually induced by an adjacent arthralgia but also both corticosteroid and antimalarial therapy may cause a myopathy and this should be considered.

The skin is a common target for the disease and cutaneous lesions occur in up to 85% of SLE patients, being the butterfly rash the most characteristic feature. This rash is erythematous, often blotchy, and found mainly over the malar bones and across the bridge of the nose. In addition to maculopapular and discoid lesions, splinter haemorrhages, dilated capillaries at the nail base, bullous lesions, angioneurotic oedema, *livedo reticularis* and buccal and nasal ulceration can also be present. Vasculitic skin lesions are usually found at the finger tips or on the extensor surface of the forearm, as well as in the malleoli, leading to tender, deep leg ulcers which can be difficult to treat.

The kidneys are frequently involved in patients with lupus. More than 70% of patients with SLE have renal involvement at some stage of their disease. The World Health Organisation (WHO) classification for lupus nephritis has been updated to allow more accurate descriptions of renal histopathology specimens by the International Society of Nephrology (ISN) and the Renal Pathology Society (RPS) (8) (Table 1.2). Of the different pathological classes, diffuse proliferative glomerulonephritis (WHO class IV) has the worst prognosis, resulting in 11–48% of patients with end stage renal disease at 5 years.

The lungs may also be affected. Parenchymal alterations have been described in 18% of patients. These patients had interstitial fibrosis, pulmonary vasculitis and interstitial pneumonitis. However, many non-specific pulmonary lesions previously attributed to SLE, such as alveolar haemorrhage, alveolar wall necrosis, oedema and hyaline membranes, are probably secondary to factors such as intercurrent infection, congestive heart failure, renal failure and oxygen toxicity.

Abnormal pulmonary function tests, diminished total lung capacity and flow rates, poor diaphragmatic movement, basal crepitations and occasionally cyanosis and clubbing are found in up to 50% of SLE patients. A similar proportion of SLE patients may have an acute lupus pneumonitis with a mononuclear cell infiltrate detectable in the alveolar septae. Dyspnoea, pleuritic chest pain and coughs are common complaints in these patients. Haemoptysis is less common and true pulmonary haemorrhage from necrotizing alveolar capillaritis is rare.

Pleural effusions may reflect a generalized disease flare. The effusions are normally small to moderate in size and are usually exudates (i.e. protein content >3 g/100 mL).

The heart can also be targeted by SLE, with abnormalities of the electrocardiogram, notably of the T wave, as the most frequent pericardial manifestation. A pericardial rub is also common. Adhesive chronic pericarditis and very large effusions causing tamponade are very rare.

Whilst true myocardial involvement is less frequent than pericardial disease, prolongation of the PR interval (approximately 10%), fibrinoid degeneration, myocardial infarction and coronary stenosis due to arteritis are occasionally seen. Systolic murmurs are not uncommon

TABLE 1.2. International Society of Nephrology/Renal Pathology Society (ISN/RPS) 2003 classification of lupus nephritis (8).

Class I	
Minimal mesangial lupus nephritis	Normal glomeruli by LM, but mesangial immune deposits by IMF
Class II	
Mesangial proliferative lupus nephritis:	Mesangial hypercellularity or matrix expansion by LM, with mesangial immune deposits. Few isolated subepithelial or subendothelial deposits may be visible by IMF or EM, but not by LM
Class III	
Focal lupus nephritis[a]:	Active or inactive focal, segmental or global endo or extracapillary GMN involving <50% of all glomeruli. Focal subendothelial immune deposits, with or without mesangial alterations
Class III (A)	– *Active lesions*: focal proliferative lupus nephritis
Class III (A/C)	– *Active and chronic lesions*: focal proliferative and sclerosing lupus nephritis
Class III (C)	– *Chronic inactive lesions with glomerular scars*: focal sclerosing lupus nephritis
Class IV	
Diffuse lupus nephritis[b]:	Active or inactive diffuse, segmental or global endo- or extracapillary glomerulonephritis involving ≥50% of all glomeruli, typically with diffuse subendothelial immune deposits, with or without mesangial alterations.
Diffuse segmental(IV-S)	• ≥ 50% of the involved glomeruli have segmental lesions, involving less than half of the glomerular tuft
Diffuse global (IV-G)	• ≥ 50% of the involved glomeruli have global lesions
Class IV-S or G (A)	– *Active lesions*: diffuse segmental or global proliferative lupus nephritis
Class IV-S or G (A/C)	– *Active and chronic lesions*: diffuse segmental or global proliferative and sclerosing lupus nephritis
Class IV-S or G (C)	– *Chronic inactive lesions with scars*: diffuse segmental or global sclerosing lupus nephritis
Class V	
Membranous lupus nephritis[c]:	Global or segmental subepithelial immune deposits or their morphologic sequelae by LM, IMF or EM with or without mesangial alterations
Class VI	
Advanced sclerosis lupus nephritis	≥ 90% of glomeruli globally sclerosed without residual activity

EM: electron microscopy; GMN: glomerulonephritis; IMF: immunofluorescencia; LM: light microscopy.
[a] Indicate the proportion of glomeruli with active and with sclerotic lesions.
[b] Indicate the proportion of glomeruli with fibrinoid necrosis and/or cellular crescents.
[c] Class V lupus nephritis may occur in combination with class III or IV, in which case both will be diagnosed.

and usually reflect the hyperdynamic circulation due to the anaemia seen in these individuals. Diastolic murmurs are very rare.

Libman-Sacks endocarditis is a well known feature of SLE, which rarely causes clinically significant lesions. They are most frequently found adjacent to the edges of the mitral and tricuspid valves.

The brain is another target organ (9). Nervous system manifestations are present in up to 70% of patients with SLE. The spectrum of CNS manifestations varies widely, from those with severe, life-threatening presentation, such as transverse myelitis or stroke, to those with more subtle and subclinical abnormalities in neurocognitive functions, such as memory, intellect and learning. The clinical diversity of the disorder, the difficulty to define outcome measures and the lack of diagnostic criteria has been considered for long the biggest obstacle to study treatment options and compare different therapeutic regimens. Only recently specific criteria for neuropsychiatric lupus (NPSLE) has been formulated by the American College of Rheumatology (ACR) (10). This new nomenclature includes case definitions, reporting standards, and diagnostic testing recommendations for different 19 neuropsychiatric syndromes.

An emerging concept is the distinction between central nervous system manifestations due to lupus and those due to the antiphospholipid syndrome (APS). A wide variety of neuropsychiatric manifestations attributable to APS have been described including strokes, seizures, movement disorders, transverse myelopathy, demyelination syndromes, transient ischaemic attacks, cognitive dysfunction, visual loss and headaches including migraine. Data from our unit applying the ACR nomenclature to assess the prevalence of CNS disorders in a large cohort of SLE patients showed that cerebrovascular disease, headache and seizures are correlated with aPL (11). The differential diagnosis between multiple sclerosis and demyelination associated with APS may be difficult on imaging grounds although electroencephalography may offer some clues suggestive of cerebrovascular insufficiency (12).

Non-specific gastrointestinal clinical features have also been described amongst SLE patients. Abdominal pain due to ileal and colonic perforations and regional enteritis occurs in about 20% of cases. Pathologically, necrotizing vasculitis is usually found when perforation occurs.

A normochromic, normocytic anaemia is usually seen in SLE, along with low levels of both the serum iron and iron binding capacity. This abnormality is due to chronic inflammation and shunting of elemental iron from erythroblasts to macrophages.

Haemolytic anaemia as detected by the Coombs' test is another rare feature of SLE. Autoimmune thrombocytopenia occasionally manifests simultaneously with haemolytic anaemia; condition known as Evan's syndrome.

Thrombocytopenia (platelet count $<100 \times 10^9$/l) and persistent leucopenia ($<4.0 \times 10^9$/l) are also frequent in SLE.

Other non-specific manifestations such as fever, lymphadenopathy, hair loss and Raynaud's phenomenon are all commonly found in SLE patients. Fever in lupus patients may be striking and often requires extensive investigation to exclude concurrent infection.

Lymphadenopathy may also be dramatic in SLE, to such an extent that lymph node biopsy may have to be performed to exclude malignancy.

Serological Features

When there is a strong clinical suspicion that a patient has SLE, the ANA is the best laboratory test to obtain, although these antibodies may also be present in healthy individuals, mainly in old age, and in a multitude of other diseases, such as chronic infection, chronic liver disease and other autoimmune rheumatic diseases (13). In some cases, the ANA may be positive even before the diagnosis of SLE (7). ANA has been detected by immunofluorescence microscopy (IFM) initially on rodent tissues of varying types, such as mouse kidney and rat liver. Currently the most widely described technique is IFM on HEp-2 cells that remains the test of choice. Many patterns of IFM on HEp-2 cells are recognized (Table 1.3), but not all of these patterns occur in SLE. The pattern of staining often reflects the predominant antibody present in the serum. Specific

IFM patterns of ANA, like anti-centromere pattern, are associated with Raynaud's phenomenon and limited scleroderma. Sera with ANA that gives a homogenous nuclear or a speckled staining pattern need to be characterized for specific individual antigens (SS-A/Ro, SS-B/La, Sm, RNP, ds-DNA, etc) in order to obtain clinically useful information. A nuclear homogeneous pattern is typically produced by anti-histone antibodies whilst anti-RNP, anti-Sm, anti-Ro and anti-La antibodies can produce a nuclear speckled pattern. Anti-dsDNA antibodies can give a rim and peripheral pattern and anti-ribosomal P antibodies make a cytoplasmic pattern.

Double stranded DNA antibodies (anti-dsDNA) have been considered useful and valuable in the diagnosis of SLE. Testing for anti ds-DNA is useful in establishing the diagnosis of SLE. In fact, 60 to 80 % of SLE patients have positive tests by the Farr, Chritidia or ELISA assays at some time during their illness. Some studies suggest a strong correlation between increasing levels of anti-dsDNA and a subsequent flare, particularly of renal disease.

Sm antibodies are very specific for SLE and they are considered one of the classification criteria along with ANA and anti ds-DNA (2), however, monitoring their levels is of limited value in the care of lupus patients in clinical practice. Serial determinations have shown limited antibody level variation over time in most patients.

Anti-Ro (SS-A) and anti-La (SS-B) antibodies are associated with the neonatal lupus syndrome and subacute cutaneous lupus and anti-60 kDa Ro antibodies have been reported to be in close association with leucopenia, thrombocytopenia, interstitial pneumonitis and vaculitis.

Numerous studies have shown a strong correlation between anti-C1q and lupus nephritis. Anti-C1q are useful to identify SLE patients at risk for renal disease and monitoring anti-C1q titres is potentially more helpful in the early diagnosis of nephritis or prediction of renal flares than the currently employed parameters of disease activity (14). However, testing for these antibodies is still not routinely done in all centres.

Other autoantibodies such as those directed to chromatin have been shown to be sensitive and specific for SLE and drug-induced lupus. The presence of these antibodies has been related to renal involvement and in less proportion to hematological manifestations, arthritis, malar rash, pleuritis and oral ulcers (15). High titres of antinucleosome antibodies are reported in 60–80% of patients with lupus disease activity and renal involvement. They have also been found in some patients who were negative for anti-dsDNA and suggested to be a better predictor factor than anti-dsDNA antibodies for future flare (16). They are not widely available in routine clinical laboratories, and hence yet their value in daily clinical practice remain unknown.

Although anti-ribosomal P antibodies have been suggested to be specific markers for psychiatric manifestations of SLE, particularly psychosis and depression, data

TABLE 1.3. Patterns of immunofluorescence on HEp-2 cells.

Pattern on IFM	Suggested antigen specificity	Related diseases
Homogeneus	DNA	SLE
Diffuse	Histone	DIL, SLE
Peripheral (rim)	dsDNA	SLE
Speckled-Coarse	Sm, U1-RNP	SLE,SS overlap
Speckled-Fine	Ro, La	SS, SCLE, CHB, NL
Centromere (46 dots)	CENP	CREST
Nucleolar-Speckled	Scl-70, RNA polymerase 1	Scl
Nucleolar-Homogeneus	Pm-Scl, Ku	Scl, PM-Scl-SLE
Cytoplasmic	Ribosomal P Protein	SLE

CHB, Congenital Heart Block; CREST, Limited scleroderma; DIL, Drug Induced Lupus NL, Neonatal Lupus; PM, Polymyositis; Scl, Scleroderma; SCLE, Subacute Cutaneous Lupus; SLE, Systemic Lupus Erythematosus; SS, Sjögren's Syndrome.

available in the literature is controversial. Although some studies have confirmed the association of anti-ribosomal P antibodies with neuropsychiatric manifestations, an international meta-analysis combining standardized data from 1.537 lupus patients from 14 research teams has shown no association at all (17).

aPL are present in around one third of patients with SLE. In clinical practice, anticardiolipin antibodies (aCL) detected by ELISA and the lupus anticoagulant (LA) detected by clotting assays are the most widely used and standardised tests for the detection of aPL. However, the aPL family has expanded and recently, a variety of plasma proteins, also known as phospholipid binding proteins, have been implicated as targets for aPL. These include β_2 glycoprotein I (β_2GPI), prothrombin, protein C, protein S, annexin V, kininogens and factor XII (18). The presence of these antibodies is associated with recurrent arterial and/or venous thrombosis and pregnancy morbidity manifested by early and/or late losses. This will be discussed in detail in another chapter.

Diagnosis of SLE

The clinical diagnosis of SLE hinges on careful and very thorough assessment of the presenting clinical features, examination of all the organ systems and selected investigations. Symptoms often occur intermittently and cumulatively over many months and years. Many non-specific features, such as oral ulcers, arthralgia, hair fall, Raynaud's phenomenon, photosensitive rashes, pleuritic chest pains, headaches, fatigue, fevers and lymphadenopathy, may indicate presenting features of the disease. Thorough clinical examination and routine blood and urine analysis are mandatory. Blood count abnormalities such as anaemia, neutropenia, lymphopenia and thrombocytopenia are also common.

The objective assessment of lupus has depended on a number of disease activity scoring systems which usually give a single numeric value. The British Isles Lupus Assessment Group (BILAG) is emerging as a useful tool in clinical trials as it describes disease activity based on the physician's intention to treat and also gives a clear picture of affected organs and systems. It has recently undergone revision and is being validated (19). Other disease activity scoring systems have also been updated including the SLEDAI 2K and an adjusted mean SLEDAI-AMS that describes disease activity over time.

Damage describes irreversible events resulting from lupus disease activity and its treatment. The Systemic Lupus International Collaborating Clinics/American College of Rheumatology (SLICC/ACR) Damage Index is validated and widely used to describe damage (20). The link between damage and an increased risk of morbidity and mortality is now clear.

Conclusions

SLE is the most diverse of the autoimmune diseases, characterised by a wide range of clinical features and the production of multiple autoantibodies. The diagnosis is based on the clinical features and the presence of a wide variety of autoantibodies. A thorough assessment of the presenting clinical features, examination of all the organ systems and routine blood and urine analysis are mandatory.

Although, the ACR classification criteria have been established, these are specifically designed for research studies and should not be used for diagnosing the disease.

References

1. Tan EM, Cohen AS, Fries JF, Masi AT, McShane DJ, Rothfield NF, Schaller JG, Talal N, Winchester RJ. The 1982 revised criteria for the classification of systemic lupus erythematosus. *Arthritis Rheum* 1982; 25: 1271–7.
2. Hochberg MC. Updating the American College of Rheumatology revised criteria for the classification of systemic lupus erythematosus. *Arthritis Rheum* 1997; 40: 1725.
3. Gudmundsson S, Steinsson K. Systemic lupus erythematosus in Iceland 1975 through 1984. A nationwide epidemiological study in an unselected population. *J Rheumatol* 1990; 17: 1162–7.
4. Nived O, Sturfelt G, Wollheim F. Systemic lupus erythematosus in an adult population in southern Sweden: Incidence, prevalence and validity of ARA revised classification criteria. *Br J Rheumatol* 1985; 24: 147–54.
5. Danchenko N, Satia JA, Anthony MS. Epidemiology of systemic lupus erythematosus: A comparison of worldwide disease burden. *Lupus* 2006; 15: 308–18.
6. Lau CS, Yin G, Mok MY. Ethnic and geographical differences in systemic lupus erythematosus: An overview. *Lupus* 2006; 15: 715–9.
7. Arbuckle MR, McClain MT, Rubertone MV, Scofield RH, Dennis GJ, James JA, Harley JB. Development of autoantibodies before the clinical onset of systemic lupus erythematosus. *N Engl J Med* 2003; 349: 1526–33.
8. Weening JJ, D'Agati VD, Schwartz MM, Seshan SV, Alpers CE, Appel GB, Balow JE, Bruijn JA, Cook T, Ferrario F, Fogo AB, Ginzler EM, Hebert L, Hill G, Hill P, Jennette JC, Kong NC, Lesavre P, Lockshin M, Looi LM, Makino H, Moura LA, Nagata M. The classification of glomerulonephritis in systemic lupus erythematosus revisited. *J Am Soc Nephrol* 2004; 15: 241–50.
9. Sanna G, Bertolaccini ML, Cuadrado MJ, Khamashta MA, Hughes GR. Central nervous system involvement in the antiphospholipid (Hughes) syndrome. *Rheumatology (Oxford)* 2003; 42: 200–13.
10. ACR ad hoc commitee on neuropsychiatric lupus nomenclature. The American College of Rheumatology nomenclature and case definitions for neuropsychiatric lupus syndromes. *Arthritis Rheum* 1999; 42: 599–608.
11. Sanna G, Bertolaccini ML, Cuadrado MJ, Laing H, Khamashta MA, Mathieu A, Hughes GRV. Neuropsychiatric

manifestations in systemic lupus erythematosus: Prevalence and association with antiphospholipid antibodies. *J Rheumatol* 2003; 30: 985–92.

12. Lampropoulos CE, Koutroumanidis M, Reynolds PP, Manidakis I, Hughes GR, D'Cruz DP. Electroencephalography in the assessment of neuropsychiatric manifestations in antiphospholipid syndrome and systemic lupus erythematosus. *Arthritis Rheum* 2005; 52: 841–6.

13. Alba P, Bertolaccini ML, Khamashta MA. The use of laboratory methods in differential diagnosis and treatment of SLE and antiphospholipid syndrome. *Exp Rev Clin Immunol* 2007; 3: 613–22.

14. Marto N, Bertolaccini ML, Calabuig E, Hughes GR, Khamashta MA. Anti-C1q antibodies in nephritis: Correlation between titres and renal disease activity and positive predictive value in systemic lupus erythematosus. *Ann Rheum Dis* 2005; 64: 444–8.

15. Gomez-Puerta JA, Burlingame RW, Cervera R. Anti-chromatin (anti-nucleosome) antibodies. *Lupus* 2006; 15: 408–11.

16. Su Y, Jia RL, Han L, Li ZG. Role of anti-nucleosome antibody in the diagnosis of systemic lupus erythematosus. *Clin Immunol* 2007; 122: 115–20.

17. Karassa FB, Afeltra A, Ambrozic A, Chang DM, De Keyser F, Doria A, Galeazzi M, Hirohata S, Hoffman IE, Inanc M, Massardo L, Mathieu A, Mok CC, Morozzi G, Sanna G, Spindler AJ, Tzioufas AG, Yoshio T, Ioannidis JP. Accuracy of anti-ribosomal P protein antibody testing for the diagnosis of neuropsychiatric systemic lupus erythematosus: An international meta-analysis. *Arthritis Rheum* 2006; 54: 312–24.

18. Bertolaccini ML, Khamashta MA. Laboratory diagnosis and management challenges in the antiphospholipid syndrome. *Lupus* 2006; 15: 172–8.

19. Isenberg DA, Rahman A, Allen E, Farewell V, Akil M, Bruce IN, D'Cruz D, Griffiths B, Khamashta M, Maddison P, McHugh N, Snaith M, Teh LS, Yee CS, Zoma A, Gordon C. BILAG 2004. Development and initial validation of an updated version of the British Isles Lupus Assessment Group's disease activity index for patients with systemic lupus erythematosus. *Rheumatology (Oxford)* 2005; 44: 902–6.

20. Gladman DD, Urowitz MB, Goldsmith CH, Fortin P, Ginzler E, Gordon C, Hanly JG, Isenberg DA, Kalunian K, Nived O, Petri M, Sanchez-Guerrero J, Snaith M, Sturfelt G. The reliability of the Systemic Lupus International Collaborating Clinics/American College of Rheumatology Damage Index in patients with systemic lupus erythematosus. *Arthritis Rheum* 1997; 40: 809–13.

2
Antiphospholipid Syndrome

Ricard Cervera and Ronald A. Asherson

Abstract   The antiphospholipid syndrome (APS) is defined by the occurrence of venous and arterial thromboses, often multiple, and recurrent fetal losses, frequently accompanied by a moderate thrombocytopenia, in the presence of antiphospholipid antibodies (aPL). Some estimates indicate that the incidence of the APS is around 5 new cases per 100,000 persons per year and the prevalence around 40–50 cases per 100,000 persons. The prevalence is higher among patients with systemic lupus erythematosus (around 30%), deep vein thrombosis (30%), stroke in younger than 50 year-old (25%), and recurrent fetal losses (10%).

The original classification criteria for the APS were formulated at a workshop in Sapporo, Japan, in 1998, during the 8th International Congress on aPL. The Sapporo criteria, as they are often called, were revised at another workshop in Sydney, Australia, in 2004, during the 11th International Congress on aPL. At least one clinical (vascular thrombosis or pregnancy morbidity) and one laboratory (anticardiolipin antibodies, lupus anticoagulant or anti-β_2-glycoprotein I antibodies) criterion had to be met for the classification of APS.

Keywords   Antiphospholipid syndrome · anticardiolipin antibodies · lupus anticoagulant · catastrophic antiphospholipid syndrome

The antiphospholipid syndrome (APS) is defined by the occurrence of venous and arterial thromboses, often multiple, and recurrent fetal losses, frequently accompanied by a moderate thrombocytopenia, in the presence of antiphospholipid antibodies (aPL), namely lupus anticoagulant (LA), anticardiolipin antibodies (aCL), or anti-β_2 glycoprotein-I (β_2GPI) antibodies. The APS can be found in patients having neither clinical nor laboratory evidence of another definable condition (primary APS) or it may be associated with other diseases, mainly systemic lupus erythematosus (SLE) (1) (Table 2.1). Rapid chronological occlusive events, occuring over days to weeks, have been termed the catastrophic APS (Asherson's syndrome) (2, 3). The new umbrella term microangiopathic APS (4) should be considered for several groups of patients with aPL-associated microvascular occlusions, e.g. retinal vascular thromboses, dermatological lesions, nailfold splinter hemorrhages or bowel ischemia (proven) as well as hearing loss or osteonecrosis (unproven).

Epidemiology

Prevalence of the aPL in the general population ranges between 1 and 5%. However, only a minority of these individuals develop the APS. Some estimates indicate that the incidence of the APS is around 5 new cases per 100,000 persons per year and the prevalence around 40–50 cases per 100,000 persons. The prevalence is higher among patients with SLE (around 30%), deep vein thrombosis (30%), stroke in younger than 50 year-old (25%), and recurrent fetal losses (10%) (5).

The prevalence of the catastrophic APS is scarce (less than 1% of all cases of APS) (6) but its potentially lethal outcome emphasizes its importance in clinical medicine today. In order to put together all the published case reports as well as the new diagnosed cases from all over the world, an international registry of patients with catastrophic APS ("CAPS Registry") was created in 2000 by the *European Forum on Antiphospholipid Antibodies*. Currently, it documents the entire clinical, laboratory

From: Y. Shoenfeld et al. (eds.): *Diagnostic Criteria in Autoimmune Diseases*, DOI: 10.1007/978-1-60327-285-8_2,
© 2008 Humana Press, Totowa, NJ

TABLE 2.1. Diseases where aPL have been described.

Systemic autoimmune diseases: Systemic lupus erythematosus, rheumatoid arthritis, systemic sclerosis, primary Sjogren's syndrome, dermato- and polymyositis, vasculitis (polyarteritis nodosa, microscopic polyarteritis, giant cell arteritis, Behçet's disease, relapsing polychondritis, leucocytoclastic vasculitis...).

Infections: Viral (HIV infection, mononucleosis, rubella, parvovirus, hepatitis A, B, C, mumps), bacterial (syphilis, Lyme disease, tuberculosis, leprosy, infective endocarditis, rheumatic fever, *Klebsiella*), protozoal (malaria, toxoplasmosis).

Malignancies: Solid tumors (lung, colon, cervix, prostate, liver, kidney, thymus, esophagus, maxilla, ovary, breast), hematologic (myeloid and lymphatic leukemias, polycythemia vera, myelofibrosis), lymphoproliferative diseases (Hodgkin's disease, non-Hodgkin's lymphoma, lymphosarcoma, cutaneous T-cell lymphoma/Sezary syndrome), paraproteinemias (monoclonal gammapathies, Waldenström macroglobulinemia, myeloma).

Non-malignant hematologic conditions: Idiopathic thrombocytopenic purpura, sickle cell disease, pernicious anemia.

Drugs: Procainamide, phenothiazines, ethosuximide, chlorothiazide, quinine, oral contraceptives.

Other conditions: Diabetes mellitus, autoimmune thyroid disease, inflammatory bowel diseases, dialysis, Klinefelter's syndrome, Ehlers-Danlos syndrome.

TABLE 2.2. Possible pathogenic mechanisms of the aPL.

Inhibition of anticoagulant reactions:
   Inhibition of β_2GPI anticoagulant activity
   Inhibition of the protein C pathway
      Inhibition of protein C activation
      Inhibiton of activated protein C
   Inhibition of antithrombin activity
   Displacement of annexin A5

Cell-mediated events:
On endothelial cells:
   Enhanced endothelial cell procoagulant activity
      Expression of tissue factor
      Expression of adhesion molecules
      Impaired fibrinolysis
   Dysregulation of eicosanoids
      Decreased endothelial cell prostacyclin production
      Increased platelet thromboxan A_2 production
On monocytes:
   Expression of tissue factor
On platelets:
   Enhanced platelet activation/aggregation

and therapeutic data of more than 300 patients whose data has been fully registered. This registry can be freely consulted at the Internet (www.med.ub.es/MIMMUN/FORUM/CAPS.HTM) (7).

History

The association of thrombosis, recurrent fetal losses and thrombocytopenia with the LA phenomenon was observed in early publications in the 60's, but it was not until 1983 that Graham R.V. Hughes linked major cerebral disease (e.g. recurrent strokes) with abortions and the LA in an editorial published in the British Medical Journal (8). The original concept of the APS, however, has been expanded over the years and now includes diverse complications as heart valve lesions, adrenal insufficiency and even avascular necrosis of bone, among many others (5).

Pathogenesis

Despite the strong association between aPL and thrombosis, the pathogenic role of aPL in the development of thrombosis has not been fully elucidated. Available data indicate that many of the autoantibodies associated with APS are directed against a number of plasma proteins and proteins expressed on, or bound to, the surface of vascular endothelial cells or platelets. The involvement of aPL in clinically important normal procoagulant and anticoagulant reactions and on certain cells altering the expression

and secretion of various molecules may offer a basis for definitive investigations of possible mechanisms by which aPL may develop thrombotic events in patients with APS (Table 2.2) (9).

Clinical manifestations

The clinical picture of the APS is characterized by venous and arterial thromboses, fetal losses and thrombocytopenia. Single vessel involvement or multiple vascular occlusions may give rise to a wide variety of presentations (Table 2.3) (6). Any combination of vascular occlusive events may occur in the same individual and the time interval between them also varies considerably from weeks to months or even years.

Laboratory abnormalities

A wide variety of laboratory abnormalities can be found in patients with APS, depending on the organ involvement. The most common immunological features are depicted in Table 2.4. Detection of the LA must be performed according to the guidelines of the International Society on Thrombosis and Hemostasis (Scientific Subcommittee on Lupus Anticoagulants/Phospholipid-Dependent Antibodies) (10).

Classification criteria

The original classification criteria for the APS were formulated at a workshop in Sapporo, Japan, in 1998, during the 8th International Congress on aPL. The Sapporo criteria, as

TABLE 2.3. Most common manifestations in the APS, according to the "Euro-Phospholipid Project" that includes 1000 European patients with this syndrome (5).

Manifestations	%
Peripheral thrombosis	
Deep vein thrombosis	38.9
Superficial thrombophlebitis in legs	11.7
Arterial thrombosis in legs	4.3
Venous thrombosis in arms	3.4
Arterial thrombosis in arms	2.7
Subclavian vein thrombosis	1.8
Jugular vein thrombosis	.9
Neurologic manifestations	
Migraine	20.2
Stroke	19.8
Transient ischemic attack	11.1
Epilepsy	7
Multiinfarct dementia	2.5
Chorea	1.3
Acute encephalopathy	1.1
Transient amnesia	.7
Cerebral venous thrombosis	.7
Cerebellar ataxia	.7
Transverse myelopathy	.4
Hemiballismus	.3
Pulmonary manifestations	
Pulmonary embolism	14.1
Pulmonary hypertension	2.2
Pulmonary microthrombosis	1.5
Fibrosant alveolitis	1.2
Other (adult respiratory distress syndrome, pulmonary hemorrhage, pulmonary artery thrombosis)	.7
Cardiac manifestations	
Valve thickening/dysfunction	11.6
Myocardial infarction	5.5
Angina	2.7
Myocardiopathy	2.9
Vegetations	2.7
Coronary by-pass rethrombosis	1.1
Intracardiac thrombus	.4
Intraabdominal manifestations	
Renal manifestations (glomerular thrombosis, renal infarction, renal artery thrombosis, renal vein thrombosis)	2.7
Gastrointestinal manifestations (esophageal or mesenteric ischemia)	1.5
Splenic infaction	1.1
Pancreatic infarction	.5
Addison's syndrome	.4
Hepatic manifestations (Budd-Chiari syndrome, small hepatic vein thrombosis)	.7
Cutaneous manifestations	
Livedo reticularis	24.1
Ulcers	5.5
Pseudovasculitic lesions	3.9
Digital gangrene	3.3
Cutaneous necrosis	2.1
Splinter hemorrhages	.7
Oteo-articular manifestations	
Arthralgia	38.7
Arthritis	27.1
Avascular necrosis of bone	2.4
Ophthalmologic manifestations	
Amaurosis fugax	5.4
Retinal artery thrombosis	1.5

TABLE 2.3. (Continued)

Manifestations	%
Retinal vein thrombosis	.9
Optic neuropathy	1
E.N.T. manifestations	
Nasal septum perforation	.8
Hematological manifestations	
Thrombocytopenia ($<100,000/\mu l$)	29.6
Hemolytic anemia	9.7
Obstetric manifestations (pregnant female = 590)	
Pre-eclampsia	9.5
Eclampsia	4.4
Abruptio placentae	2
Post-partum cardio-pulmonary syndrome	.5
Fetal manifestations (pregnancies = 1580)	
Early fetal losses (<10 weeks)	35.4
Late fetal losses (≥ 10 weeks)	16.9
Live births	47.7
Prematures	10.6

they are often called, were revised at another workshop in Sydney, Australia, in 2004, during the 11th International Congress on aPL, and published as a consensus statement in 2006 (Table 2.5) (11). At least one clinical (vascular thrombosis or pregnancy morbidity) and one laboratory (aCL, LA or anti-β_2GPI antibodies) criterion had to be met for the classification of APS. In addition to these APS classification criteria, the consensus paper provides specific definitions for commonly associated clinical manifestations of APS (namely, *livedo reticularis*, cardiac valve disease, thrombocytopenia and nephropathy) (11).

The preliminary classification criteria for catastrophic APS were formulated at a workshop in Taormina, Italy, in 2002, during the 10th International Congress on aPL, and published as a consensus statement in 2003 (Table 2.6) (12).

TABLE 2.4. Most common immunological findings in the APS, according to the "Euro-Phospholipid Project" (5).

Parameter	%
aCL	87.9
IgG and IgM aCL	32.1
IgG aCL alone	43.6
IgM aCL alone	12.2
LA	53.6
LA alone	12.1
LA and aCL	41.5
ANA	59.7
Anti-dsDNA	29.2
Anti-Ro/SS-A	14
Anti-La/SS-B	5.7
Anti-RNP	5.9
Anti-Sm	5.5
RF	7.8
Cryoglobulins	3.6

TABLE 2.5. Revised classification criteria for the APS.

Clinical criteria

1. Vascular thrombosis[a]

   One or more clinical episodes of arterial, venous, or small vessel thrombosis, in any tissue or organ. Thrombosis must be confirmed by imaging or Doppler studies or histopathology, with the exception of superficial venous thrombosis. For histopathologic confirmation, thrombosis should be present without significant evidence of inflammation in the vessel wall.

2. Pregnancy morbidity

   (a) One or more unexplained deaths of a morphologically normal fetus at or beyond the 10th week of gestation, with normal fetal morphology documented by ultrasound or by direct examination of the fetus, *or*

   (b) One or more premature births of a morphologically normal neonate before the 34th week of gestation because of: (a) eclampsia or severe preeclampsia defined according to standard definitions, or (b) recognised features of placental insufficiency[b], *or*

   (c) Three or more unexplained consecutive spontaneous abortions before the 10th week of gestation, with maternal anatomic or hormonal abnormalities and paternal and maternal chromosomal causes excluded.

   In studies of populations of patients who have more than one type of pregnancy morbidity, investigators are strongly encouraged to stratify groups of subjects according to a, b, or c above.

Laboratory criteria[c]

1. Anticardiolipin antibody of IgG and/or IgM isotype in serum or plasma, present in medium or high titer (i.e. >40 GPL or MPL, or >the 99th percentile, or >mean + 3SD of 40 healthy controls), on 2 or more occasions, at least 12 weeks apart, measured by a standardized enzyme-linked immunosorbent assay.

2. Lupus anticoagulant present in plasma, on 2 or more occasions at least 12 weeks apart, detected according to the guidelines of the International Society on Thrombosis and Hemostasis (Scientific Subcommittee on Lupus Anticoagulants/Phospholipid-Dependent Antibodies).

3. Anti-β_2 glycoprotein-I antibody of IgG and/or IgM isotype in serum or plasma, present on 2 or more occasions, at least 12 weeks apart, measured by a standardized enzyme-linked immunosorbent assay, according to recommended procedures.

   • Definite antiphospholipid antibody syndrome is present if at least one of the clinical criteria and one[c] of the laboratory criteria are met, with the first measurement of the laboratory test performed at least 12 weeks from the clinical manifestation[d].

[a] Coexisting inherited or acquired factors for thrombosis are **not** reason for excluding patients from APS trials. However, two subgroups of APS patients should be recognized, according to: (a) the **presence**, and (b) the **absence** of additional risk factors for thrombosis. Indicative (but not exhaustive) such cases include: age (>55 in men, and >65 in women), and the presence of any of the established risk factors for cardiovascular disease (hypertension, diabetes mellitus, elevated LDL or low HDL cholesterol, cigarette smoking, family history of premature cardiovascular disease, body mass index ≥30 kg/m², microalbuminuria, estimated GFR <60 mL/min), inherited thrombophilias, oral contraceptives, nephrotic syndrome, malignancy, immobilization, surgery. Thus, patients who fulfill criteria should be stratified according to contributing causes of thrombosis.

[b] Generally accepted features of placental insufficiency include: (1) abnormal or non-reassuring fetal surveillance test(s), e.g., a non-reactive non-stress test, suggestive of fetal hypoxemia, (2) abnormal Doppler flow velocimetry waveform analysis suggestive of fetal hypoxemia, e.g., absent end-diastolic flow in the umbilical artery, (3) oligohydramnios, e.g., an amniotic fluid index of 5 centimeters or less, or (4) a post natal birth weight less than the 10th percentile for the gestational age.

[c] Investigators are strongly advised to classify APS patients in studies into one of the following categories:

   I: More than one Laboratory criteria present (any combination)

   II: Anti-cardiolipin antibody present alone

   II: Lupus Anticoagulant present alone

   II: Anti-β_2 glycoprotein-I antibody present alone

[d] Classification of APS should be avoided if less than 12 weeks or more than 5 years separate the positive aPL test and the clinical manifestation.

TABLE 2.6. Preliminary criteria for the classification of catastrophic APS.

1. Evidence of involvement of three or more organs, systems and/or tissues[a]
2. Development of manifestations simultaneously or in less than a week.
3. Confirmation by histopathology of small vessel occlusion in at least one organ or tissue[b].
4. Laboratory confirmation of the presence of antiphospholipid antibodies (lupus anticoagulant and/or anticardiolipin antibodies).[c]

[a] Usually, clinical evidence of vessel occlusions, confirmed by imaging techniques when appropriate. Renal involvement is defined by a 50% rise in serum creatinine, severe systemic hypertension (>180/100 mm Hg) and/or proteinuria (>500 mg/24 h).

[b] For histopathological confirmation, significant evidence of thrombosis must be present, although vasculitis may coexist occasionally.

[c] If the patient had not been previously diagnosed as having an APS, the laboratory confirmation requires that presence of antiphospholipid antibodies must be detected on two or more occasions at least 6 weeks apart (not necessarily at the time of the event), according to the proposed preliminary criteria for the classification of definite APS (9).

Definite catastrophic APS: All 4 criteria

Probable catastrophic APS:

- All 4 criteria, except for only two organs, systems and/or tissues involvement.
- All 4 criteria, except for the absence of laboratory confirmation at least 6 weeks apart due to the early death of a patient never tested for aPL before the catastrophic APS.
- 1, 2 and 4
- 1, 3 and 4 and the development of a third event in more than a week but less than a month, despite anticoagulation.

Assessment of the Classification Criteria

The revised APS classification criteria (11) provide a more uniform basis for selecting patients for APS research by emphasising risk stratification. They strongly recommend investigating coexisting inherited and acquired thrombosis risk factors in patients with APS, especially in those who are included in clinical trials. A recent assessment of the 2006 revised APS classification criteria has shown that only 59% of the patients meeting the 1999 APS Sapporo classification criteria met the revised criteria (13). Therefore, it is expected that these revised criteria will have positive implications in APS research by way of limiting the inclusion of a heterogeneous group of patients and also by providing a risk-stratified approach. Furthermore, although the APS classification criteria are not meant for clinical porpuses, they are the best available tool to avoid overdiagnosis of APS in clinical practice.

Regarding the classification criteria for the catastrophic APS, a recent validation study showed that they have a sensitivity of 90.3%, a specificity of 99.4%, a positive predictive value of 99.4% and a negative predictive value of 91.1% (14).

Therapy

Elimination of aPL may be accomplished by several therapeutic regimens, including high dose steroid administration, immunosuppression (e.g. cyclophosphamide) or plasma exchange. The decrease or elimination is, however, temporary and antibodies rapidly return (within 1–3 weeks) on cessation of therapy. Therefore, therapy should not primarily be directed at effectively reducing the aPL levels and the use of immunotherapy is generally not indicated, unless required for the treatment of the underlying condition, e.g. SLE, or in acute life-threatening situations, such as the catastrophic APS. The risk of recurrence of thrombosis is markedly increased in the first 6 months after discontinuation therapy, suggesting a "rebound" phenomenon. Therefore, for patients who have already experienced thrombotic events, life-long treatment with anticoagulants is essential (15). However, when the initial thrombotic event is "triggered" by a drug (e.g. oral contraceptives) or trauma, long-term anticoagulation may not really be necessary and antiaggregants, as well as avoidance of the triggering factors, may indeed be sufficiently effective for future thromboprophylaxis.

The thrombocytopenia occuring during the course of the APS is usually mild and does not require any active intervention. However, in a minority of cases it can be severe and refractory to prednisone therapy. In these cases, immunosuppressive therapy (e.g. azathioprine), danazol, intravenous immunoglobulins or rituximab may be effective. The presence of moderate to severe thrombocytopenia in patients with on–going thromboses is not a contraindication for anticoagulation.

For the management of the catastrophic APS, an algorithm has been proposed (Figure 2.1), including the prompt use of heparin, high dose steroids, plasma exchange and/or intravenous immunoglobulins (12).

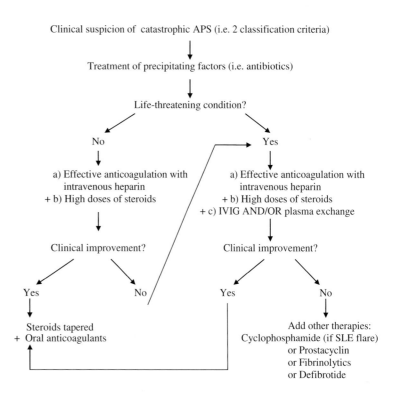

FIGURE 2.1. Treatment algorithm of catastrophic APS.

Prevention

In patients with aPL who have never suffered from a thrombotic event (primary thromboprophylaxis), energetic attempts must be made to avoid or to treat any associated risk factors – e.g. antihypertensives, cholesterol-lowering agents, treatment of active nephritis, avoidance of smoking or sedentarism, etc. Care should be also taken with the administration of oral contraceptives. There may be a case for the prophylactic treatment of individuals with high levels of IgG aCL or persistent LA activity with antiaggregants (aspirin, 75–150 mgr daily), specially in those with added risk factors (16). However, a recently published trial has not confirmed the benefits of aspirin in the APS primary thromboprophylaxis (17). On the other hand, prophylaxis of venous thrombosis is required for patients undergoing surgical procedures (particularly hip surgery), those requiring long stays in bed, or during the puerperium. The use of low-molecular weight subcutaneous heparin is recommended in those circumstances.

Low-dose aspirin (50–100 mg daily) administered from the begining of pregnancy until just prior to delivery is the accepted standard for the prevention of fetal loss today. This may be combined with daily subcutaneous heparin in the face of previous fetal losses using aspirin (18, 19). Warfarin administration should be discontinued as soon as pregnancy is diagnosed, since it is teratogenic. In addition, close monitoring of pregnancy with doppler techniques, in order to detect early placental vascular insufficiency, and delivery with the first signs of fetal distress are mandatory (20).

References

1. Asherson RA, Cervera R, Piette JC, Shoenfeld Y (eds.). *The Antiphospholipid Syndrome II – Autoimmune Thrombosis.* Amsterdam, Elsevier; 2002.
2. Asherson RA. The catastrophic antiphospholipid syndrome. *J Rheumatol* 1992; 19: 508–12.
3. Piette JC, Cervera R, Levy RA, Nasonov EL, Triplett DA, Shoenfeld Y. The catastrophic antiphospholipid syndrome – Asherson's syndrome. *Ann Med Interne* 2003; 154: 195–6.
4. Asherson RA, Pierangeli SS, Cervera R. Is there a microangiopathic antiphospholipid syndrome? *Ann Rheum Dis* 2007; 66: 429–32.
5. Petri M. Epidemiology of the antiphospholipid antibody syndrome. *J Autoimmun* 2000; 15: 145–51.
6. Cervera R, Piette JC, Font J, Khamashta MA, Shoenfeld Y, Camps MT, et al. Antiphospholipid syndrome. Clinical and immunologic manifestations and patterns of disease expression in a cohort of 1000 patients. *Arthritis Rheum* 2002; 46: 1019–27.
7. Bucciarelli S, Espinosa G, Cervera R, Erkan D, Gómez-Puerta JA, Ramos-Casals M, et al. Mortality in the catastrophic antiphospholipid syndrome. Causes of death and prognostic factors in a series of 250 patients. *Arthritis Rheum* 2006; 54: 2568–76.
8. Hughes GRV. Thrombosis, abortion, cerebral disease and the lupus anticoagulant. *Br Med J* 1983; 287: 1088–9.
9. Espinosa G, Cervera R, Font J, Shoenfeld Y. Antiphospholipid syndrome: Pathogenic mechanisms. *Autoimmun Rev* 2003; 2: 86–93.
10. Brandt JT, Triplett DA, Alving B, Scharrer I. Criteria for the diagnosis of lupus anticoagulants: An update. *Thromb Haemost* 1995; 74: 1185–90.
11. Miyakis S, Lockshin MD, Atsumi T, Branch DW, Brey RL, Cervera R, Derksen RHWM, De Groot PG, Koike T, Meroni PL, Reber G, Shoenfeld Y, Tincani A, Vlachoyiannopoulos PG, Krilis SA. International consensus statement on an update of the classification criteria for definite antiphospholipid syndrome (APS). *J Thromb Haemost* 2006; 4: 295–306.
12. Asherson RA, Cervera R, de Groot PG, Erkan D, Boffa MC, Piette JC, Khamashta MA, Shoenfeld Y for the Catastrophic Antiphospholipid Syndrome Registry Project Group. Catastrophic antiphospholipid syndrome: International consensus statement on classification criteria and treatment guidelines. *Lupus* 2003; 12: 530–4.
13. Kaul M, Erkan D, Sammaritano L, Lockshin MD. Assessment of the 2006 revised antiphospholipid syndrome classification criteria. *Ann Rheum Dis* 2007; 66: 927–30.
14. Cervera R, Font J, Gómez-Puerta JA, Espinosa G, Cucho M, Bucciarelli S, Ramos-Casals, M, Ingelmo M, Piette JC, Shoenfeld Y, RA Asherson for the Catastrophic Antiphospholipid Syndrome Registry Project Group. Validation of the preliminary criteria for the classification of catastrophic antiphospholipid syndrome. *Ann Rheum Dis* 2005; 64: 1205–9.
15. Lim W, Crowther MA, Eikelboom JW. Management of antiphospholipid antibody syndrome: A systematic review. *JAMA* 2006; 295: 1050–7.
16. Alarcón-Segovia D, Boffa MC, Branch W, Cervera R, Gharavi A, Khamashta M, Shoenfeld Y, Wilson W, Roubey R. Prophylaxis of the antiphospholipid syndrome: A consensus report. *Lupus* 2003; 12: 499–503.
17. Erkan D, Harrison MJ, Levy R, Peterson M, Petri M, Sammaritano L, Unalp-Arida A, Vilela V, Yazici Y, Lockshin MD. Aspirin for primary thrombosis prevention in the antiphospholipid syndrome: A randomized, double-blind, placebo-controlled trial in asymptomatic antiphospholipid antibody-positive individuals. *Arthritis Rheum* 2007; 56: 2382–91.
18. Tincani A, Branch W, Levy RA, Piette JC, Carp H, Rai RS, Khamashta M, Shoenfeld Y. Treatment of pregnant patients with antiphospholipid syndrome. *Lupus* 2003; 12: 524–9.
19. Carmona F, Font J, Azulay M, Creus M, Fàbregues F, Cervera R, Puerto B, Balasch J. Risk factors associated with fetal losses in treated antiphospholipid syndrome pregnancies: A multivariate analysis. *Am J Reprod Immunol* 2001; 46: 274–279.
20. Cervera R, Balasch J. The management of pregnant patients with antiphospholipid syndrome. *Lupus* 2004; 13: 683–7.

3
Rheumatoid Arthritis

Claudio Galarza-Maldonado, Loreto Massardo, Bernardo Pons–Estel and Mario H. Cardiel

Abstract   Rheumatoid arthritis (RA) is a systemic, chronic inflammatory disease that is manifested in destructive polyarthritis in association with serological evidence of autoreactivity. It is characterized by chronic pain and joint destruction, premature mortality and an elevated risk of disability, with high costs for those suffering from this disease and for society. If this condition is not treated, joint destruction from bone erosion can be expected, as well as progressive inabilities, leading eventually to disability, after a time period that can vary from only a few months to many years, depending on prognostic factors. A serious consequence for those suffering from this disease is the loss of their ability to work, especially in the case of manual workers, since many of them lose their income during the first two years of their illness (1). This situation contrasts with the statement asserting that RA is currently the most common potentially-treatable cause of disability in the western world (2). This might be proven true if treatment would be given to patients during the early stages of the disease – which is recommended in order to change the paradigm of RA therapy toward the immediate application of new effective therapies or schemes combining these therapies.

New agents capable of inducing the remission of this disease have been introduced in clinical practice over the last decade. These include anti-IL1 and anti-IL6 agents, TNFα blockers, B cell depleters and regulators of lymphocyte co-stimulation.

Keywords   Rheumatoid arthritis · early arthritis · biological therapy

Rheumatoid arthritis is clinically recognized as an inflammatory process affecting the joints, however the outstanding number of extra-articular clinical manifestations make this a systemic, autoimmune disease characterized by different clinical patterns. The symptoms accompanying the early stages of this disease may vary from one individual to another, and this frequently makes early diagnosis difficult.

Epidemiology

Rheumatoid arthritis (RA) is distributed universally. There are no reports of areas or ethnic groups in which this disease is not found, and its prevalence does not appear to significantly vary among the groups studied. In Latin America some studies were recently conducted on the prevalence of RA in the population above the age of 15 years. In Mexico (3) a prevalence of 0.3% (95% CI: 0.1–0.6) was found in 2500 subjects. Similarly, the EPISER study conducted in Spain found a prevalence of 0.5% (4).

Incidence

The figures reported are variable. The highest probable, defined annual global incidence rate for RA is 90 cases/100,000 inhabitants in a clinic in Holland. Studies in Finland and Japan demonstrated estimated annual rates of 42 cases/100,000 inhabitants, and 45 cases/100,000 inhabitants, respectively. A decrease in the incidence of RA among women was observed in the last ten years of follow-up (from 92/100,000 between 1960 and 1964, down to 40/100,000 in 1974) (5). The same downward tendency was found between 1970 and 1982 among British females.

It has been stated that this diminishing, selective tendency for females is due to the use and protecting effect from contraceptives, the use of which was disseminated in the mid 1960s. A change in the pattern of illness toward less severity, as suggested in retrospective studies, receives less support in recent literature, which underscores that the long-term clinical course of this disease has changed very little. It is worth commenting that there is consistent information in the literature on cigarette smoking and an

From: Y. Shoenfeld et al. (eds.): *Diagnostic Criteria in Autoimmune Diseases*, DOI: 10.1007/978-1-60327-285-8_3,

increased risk of suffering from rheumatoid arthritis. Mortality: the severity of the disease is associated with shared epitope (SE). All human leukocyte antigen (HLA)-DRB1 alleles associated with rheumatoid arthritis encode a conserved amino acid sequence (QKRAA, QRRAA, or RRRAA) at position 70–74 in the third hypervariable region (HVR3) of the DRbeta(1) chain, which is commonly called the shared epitope.

The global causes of death are similar to the general US population. Some studies mention an excess of deaths from infections, renal and gastrointestinal diseases. Generally, differences are not observed in the frequency of malignant neoplasias in relation to the general population. RA patients die younger than the general population, and this has been observed between the third and tenth years following baseline observation.

Among the factors associated with mortality, the following risk factors for premature death have been identified by different studies and study designs: advanced age, male, greater functional impairment, positive rheumatoid factor, number of swollen joints, co-morbidity and low level of formal education. The economic impact of arthritis is clearly evident. Females with symmetrical polyarthritis earned 26.5% of the wages received by females without arthritis, while males received 47.5% of the wages earned by males without arthritis In Spain the annual average cost was US $10,419.00. Predictors of the high costs were the HAQ disability index, not being able to carry out household tasks, and not being able to work (6).

Pathogenesis

There are different effector pathways and cellular groups involved in the cascade of events leading to the initiation, progression and persistence of the autoinflammatory reaction produced by the irreversible destruction of joint tissue. The perpetuation of the rheumatoid process depends on the involvement of different cellular lines, including synovial cells (such as fibroblast and endothelial and perivascular cells), macrophages, dendritic cells and other immunocompetent cells such as T and B lymphocytes (7).

The inflammatory process and subsequent joint destruction are mediated by the activation of intracellular signaling pathways that stimulate the production of cytokines such as IL-1, TNFα, chemokines, growth factors and adhesion molecules. Adipocytokines are periarticular factors that contribute toward maintaining joint inflammation and that increase the destructive potential of synovial fibroblasts. Adipocytokines such as adiponectin and resistin are found in rheumatoid synovial tissue and may have proinflammatory, destructive effects on the synovial matrix (8).

Elevated concentrations of proinflammatory cytokines such as IL-1 and TNFα are found in both serum and synovial fluid of patients with active disease, in comparison to controls. These cytokines stimulate the release of metalloproteinases by fibroblasts, osteoclasts and condrocytes (9). They also stimulate the expression of adhesion molecules in endothelial cells, increasing the recruitment of neutrophils in joints. These neutrophils release elastases and proteases that degrade proteoglycans in the superficial layer of articular cartilage.

Aside from their local effects, these proinflammatory cytokines manage to enter the bloodstream and are distributed throughout the entire organism, generating both constitutional symptoms and extra-articular manifestations.

Genetic predisposition is significant and is a fundamental determinant in susceptibility to RA. There is concordance between monozygotic twins and a well-defined family predisposition.

Clinical Manifestations

Articular Manifestations

Symmetrical inflammation of large and small articulations accompanied by morning stiffnes are common symptoms of rheumatoid arthritis. Nearly all patients have wrist and hand joints involvement. Compromised metacarpophalangic joints in the initial stages of the disease can lead to an early diagnosis.

In general, any joint can be affected by the disease, and progressive joint damage is accompanied by a diminished quality of life – which can cause varying degrees of functional disability.

Extra-Articular Manifestations

The disease can affect different organs and systems (Table 3.1).

Pathological Features

Early changes in rheumatoid synovial tissue are manifested in hyperplasia of synovial lining cells (SLC), edema, vascular proliferation and lymphocyte infiltration. The pathological changes in asymptomatic articulations include SLC hyperplasia with T CD4+ cell infiltration. B cells are scarce, and vascular proliferation and fibrin deposition are infrequent. In symptomatic joints, the histology of synovial tissue reveals vascular proliferation, polymorphonuclear cell infiltration and fibrin deposition. Vascular proliferation is measured by the production of vascular endothelial growth factors, fibroblastic growth factors, IL-8 and monocyte chemotactic protein (MCP-1) (10).

TABLE 3.1. Extra-articular manifestations.

Type of manifestation	Observations and references
I. Hematopoietic system	
a. Anemic syndrome	50% males, 60–65% females
b. Thrombocytosis	5–10%, Zvaifler et al. (11) May vary according to series, 12–52%; does not predispose to thrombosis
c. Thrombocytopenia	Only exceptional cases
d. Eosinophilia >4%	12.7%. Up to 40% has been observed. More than 5% associated with MEAR and late appearance
e. Leucopenia	Only exceptional cases
II. Reticuloendothelial system	
A. Red cell aplasia	Only exceptional cases
B. Adenomegalia	29%, Zvaifler et al. (11) (118). 82%, non-rigorous studies
III. Subcutaneous nodules	20–30% in seropositive patients, Zvaifler et al. (11) 27%, Massardo et al. (12)
IV. Cardiovascular system	
A. Heart attack	Is rare. Coronary vasculitis Autopsies 15–20%. Anecdotal clinical series
B. Valvular disease	25% with alteration in mitral valve. Autopsies 6–62%. Anecdotal clinical series
C. Mesenteric thrombosis	Only exceptional cases
D. Pericardial effusion	Pericarditis in active RA 10%. Autopsy 40%. Necropsy 11–50%. Clinical series 1.6–2.4%
E. Sinus bradycardia	Conduction disorder. Autopsy: unknown. Clinical series 8–10%.
F. Myocarditis	Diffuse-unspecified endothelial compromise
V. Rheumatoid vasculitis	<1% in most studies. Is more frequent in males, 15 of 50 patients reported by Scott et al. (13) died before 5 years of follow-up. 8% Digital vasculitis. 8% Chilean population, Massardo et al. (12)
VI. Respiratory apparatus	
A. Upper Cricoaritenoides	50% in autopsies. 72.25% in patients with active RA
B. Lower	
1. Pleural effusion	Prevalence <5%, Jurik et al. (14); Joseph et al. (15) More common in males than in females. 21% of 516 patients in the course of evolution. Postmortem, 40–75%
2. Diffuse interstitial fibrosis	1.6% of patients with RA. 41% of 41 patients with alteration in diffusion capacity. 47% with normal thorax X-ray. Zvaifler et al. (11), Anaya et al. (15)
3. Bronchiolitis	Report on cases associated with medication: Metotrexate, D-Penicilin
4. Kaplan Syndrome	2–6%, Shannon et al. (16)
VII. Neurological	
A. Compression neuropathy	
1. Carpal tunnel syndrome	56 cases out of 627 patients. Zvaifler et al. (11) From electromyography (EMG): 50% of patients with RA; 30% are symptomatic
2. Tarsal tunnel syndrome	15–25% from EMG; few are symptomatic
B. Angiopathic neuropathy	4 out of 627 patients. Sensitive-motor neuropathy
C. Autonomic neuropathy	Only exceptional cases
VIII. Eye	
A. Episcleritis	0.17%
B. Scleritis	0.67%
C. Uveitis	Anecdotal. Occurs as a complication of scleritis
D. Brown Syndrome	Only exceptional cases
IX. Sjögren syndrome	14.3%. 29% in Chile, Massardo et al. (12)
Keratoconjunctivitis sicca	11 to 35%
X. Muscular compromise	
A. Muscular weakness	Evident in 80%. Evidence of diminishing I and II fibers in immobilized muscle 25–30%
B. Vasculitis in muscle	Biopsies 9%, Sokoloff.
XI. Renal compromise	7.9% die from non-specific chronic nephritis, Laakso et al. (17) 5.3% die from uremia. Boers et al. (18)
XII. Gastrointestinal compromise	No specific injury. Few cases of amyloidosis. Few reports of arteritis in celiac arteries.
XIII. Felty Syndrome	Variable in published series. 1.89% in Chile by Massardo et al. (12)
XIV. Still Syndrome	Variable in published series. Less than 1%
XV. Amyloidosis	3.3 to 60%, according to autopsy series prior to 1970. Prevalence of 13.3% between 1935 and 1954. Missen et al.

Anaya et al. (19)

Serological Features

Typically, serological markers such as sedimentation rate and reactive C protein are used to measure the disease activity. Reumatoid factor and other autoantibodies that can serve as useful serological markers for establishing the diagnosis and prognosis of the disease.

Until recently, the serum determination of the rheumatoid factor – an immunoglobulin aimed at the constant fraction (cF) of IgG immunoglobulins – was the only test used in the study of this pathology. In fact, the presence of this immunoglobulin is considered as a classification criterion for the illness (20).

Nevertheless, the rheumatoid factor is not highly sensitive or specific (sensitivity 66%, specificity 87%) (21), and can be found in other autoimmune illnesses, neoplasic illnesses, chronic infections, and even in healthy persons (22).

Re-introducing the measurement of antibodies against cyclic citrullinated peptides derived from filagrin (anti-CCP1) (23) has contributed as a valuable instrument which, when used together with the rheumatoid factor (RF), provides important information regarding the prognosis of the disease. The presence of these antibodies has been associated with the development of erosions (24). Ideally, RF and anti-CCP measurements are recommended for patients suspected of having RA. These measurements provide valuable information regarding the risk factors of patients, since those who test serologically positive for one or both of these factors are at greater risk for developing a chronic erosive inflammatory disease.

Diagnostic Criteria

With the objective of distinguishing rheumatoid arthritis from other types of arthritis, the American Rheumatism Association developed classification criteria for this illness (25). The criteria are useful in the case of established RA, providing 91–94% sensitivity and 89% specificity for diagnosing this illness. However, the criteria are not sufficiently reliable when applied to patients with early arthritis. Consequently, the criteria are useful for standardizing patients and for determining their inclusion in clinical studies, however they may be less useful in making decisions regarding a clinical diagnosis.

Prognosis

The objective of RA therapy is to rigorously control inflammation, in order to prevent the illness from advancing, and thus help patients avoid becoming disabled. To reach this objective, it is necessary to diagnosis the illness early, identify patients with the highest probability of rapid progression, and initiate more intensive therapy with patients having this more severe prognosis. The recognized factors indicating a more severe prognosis for patients with early RA are a large number of swollen joints, high PCR or high sedimentation rate levels from the beginning, a positive rheumatoid factor (RF) together with anti-CCP antibodies, the development of erosions discovered early through magnetic resonance images, serious functional disability observed, limited formal education and adverse socioeconomic conditions, plus cigarette smoking (26).

Therapy

"Window of Opportunity" Concept

The "window of opportunity" refers to a very brief period when arthritis begins, and when radiological progression is established. This concept is based on the premise that intense therapeutic intervention at the very beginning of RA was able to "reprogram" the rate at which radiographic damage progressed (18), while a delay of three to nine months in initiating disease-modifying antirheumatic drugs (DMARDS) negatively impacted radiographic progression at the end of two years (27). The "window of opportunity" concept asserts that the use of the most powerful therapies currently available will be more effective, the shorter the duration of RA, and this will eventually lead to a lowered probability of disability. This has sparked hope that in the future affected patients will not require joint replacements or orthopedic surgery and will register a lower rate of mortality caused by premature arteriosclerosis. There has been a notable change since the year 2000 toward an improved RA prognosis for patients receiving therapy during the window of opportunity. Nevertheless, this concept has been challenged and it is not universally accepted.

Treatment of rheumatoid arthritis is aimed at the clinical remission of this condition in patients, and when this is not possible, to at least reduce the progression of the illness (28).

Symptomatic treatment aimed at controlling the pain produced by inflammation includes non-steroid anti-inflammatory drugs, as well as analgesics and corticosteroids. The latter appear to have an impact on the progression of the illness, with a dose of no more than 10 mg daily.

Disease-modifying drugs or DMARDS, which have various immunosuppressing mechanisms, modify the progression of the illness, however unfortunately they have not been able to induce a remission in the conditions of most patients. These drugs continue to be significant in managing these conditions, and this is especially true for methotrexate, particularly in a combined form and with increased effectiveness when administered in the early stages of the illness.

Various scientific groups and associations have reached a consensus that a new type of medication, which is relatively new, should be added to RA treatment, when after eight to twelve weeks, the response to established treatment is minimal or negative. For the moment, the addition of TNFα blocking agents is recommended, for example infliximab, etanercep and adalimumab. Nevertheless, given the degree of effectiveness of other methods for inhibiting inflammation, such as B cell depletion and the inhibition of lymphocyte co-stimulation, other potentially effective agents, specifically rituximab and abatacept, are also currently taken into consideration for controlling the disease in patients who have not responded positively to TNF agents.

References

1. Young, A, et al. How does functional disability in early rheumatoid arthritis (RA) affect patients and their lives? Results of 5 years of follow-up in 732 patients from the Early RA Study (ERAS). *Rheumatology* 2000; 39(6): 603–11.

2. Emery P, M. Salmon, Early rheumatoid arthritis: Time to aim for remission? *Ann Rheum Dis* 1995; 54(12): 944–7.

3. Cardiel MH, Rojas-Serrano J. Community based study to estimate prevalence, burden of illness and help seeking behavior in rheumatic diseases in Mexico City. A COPCORD study. *Clin Exp Rheumatol* 2000; 20: 617–24.

4. Carmona I, Ballina J, Gabriel R, Laffon A. The burden of musculoskeletal diseases in the general population of Spain: Results from a national survey. *Ann Rheum* 2002; 60: 1040–5.

5. Doran MF, Pond GR, Crowson CS, O'Fallon WM, Gabriel SE. Trends in incidence and mortality in rheumatoid arthritis in Rochester, Minnesota, over a forty-year period. *Arthritis Rheum* 2002; 46: 625–61.

6. Lajas C, Abasolo L, Bellajdel B, Hernandez-García C, Carmona L, Vargas E, Lazaro P, Jover JA. Costs and predictors of costs in rheumatoid arthritis: A prevalence – based study. *Arthritis Rheum* 2003; 49: 64–70.

7. Muller-Ladner U, Pap T, Gay RE, et al. Mechanisms of disease: The molecular and cellular basis of joint destruction in rheumatoid arthritis. *Nat Clin Pract Rheumatol* 2005; 1(2): 102–10.

8. Bokarewa M. Resistin, an adipokine with potent proinflammatory properties. *J Immunol* 2005; 174: 5789–95.

9. Smith JB, Haynes MK. Rheumatoid arthritis – a molecular understanding. *Ann Intern Med* 2002; 136: 908–22.

10. Kaiser M, Younge B, Johannes B, et al. Formation of new vasa vasorum in vasculitis production of angiogenic cytokines by multinucleated giant cells. *Am J Pathol* 1999; 155: 765–74.

11. Ustinger PD, Zvaifler NJ, Ehrlich GE. Rheumatoid Arthritis. *J.B. Lippincott company* 1985.

12. Massardo L et al. Clinical expression of rheumatoid arthritis in Chilean patients. *Sem Arthritis Rheum* 1995; 25: 203–213.

13. Scott DGI et al. Systemic rheumatoid vasculitis: A clinical and laboratory study of 50 cases. *Medicine* 1981; 60: 288–295.

14. Jurik AG et al. Prevalence of pulmonary involvement in rheumatoid artritis and its relationship to some caracteristics of the paients. *Scand J Rheumatol* 1982; 11: 217–224.

15. Joseph J et al. Connective tissue disease and the pleura. *Chest* 1993; 104: 262–270.

16. Shannon TM et al. Non-cardiac menifestations of rheumatoid arthritis in the thorax. *J Torca Imagin* 1992; 7: 19–29.

17. Laakso M et al. Mortality from amyloidosis and renal disease in patient with rheumatoid arthritis. *Ann Rheum Dis* 1986; 45: 665–667.

18. Boers M, et al. Randomised comparison of combined step-down prednisolone, methotrexate and sulphasalazine with sulphasalazine alone in early rheumatoid arthritis. *Lancet* 1997; 350(9074): 309–18.

19. Anaya JM, Pineda R, Gomez L, Galarza-Maldonado C, et al. (eds.). Artritis reumatoide, bases moleculares cli' nicas y terape' uticas. CIB, *Medellin*; 2006: 288–9.

20. Arnett FC, Edworthy SM, Bloch DA, et al. The American Rheumatism Association 1987 revised criteria for the classification of rheumatoid arthritis. *Arthritis Rheuma* 1988; 31: 315–24.

21. Golbach-Mansky R, Lee J, McCoy A, et al. Rheumatoid Arthritis associated autoantibodies in patients with sinovitis of recent onset. *Arthritis Res* 2000; 22: 236–43.

22. Correa P, Tobon GJ, Citera G, et al. Anticuerpos anti-CCP en artritis reumatoide: Relación con características clínicas, citocinas Th1/Th2 y HLA-DRB1. *Biomedica* 2004; 24:140–52.

23. Schellekens GA, Visser H, de Jong BAW, et al. The diagnostic properties of rheumatoid arthritis antibodies recognizing a cyclic citrullinaded peptide. *Arthritis Rheum* 2000; 43: 155–63.

24. Symmons DPM. Classification criteria for rheumatoid arthritis-time to abandon rheumatoid factor? *Rheumatology* 2007; 46: 725–6.

25. Arnett FC, Edworthy SM, Bloch DA, et al. The ARA 1987 revised criteria for the classification on rheumatoid arthritis. *Arthritis Rheum* 1988; 31(3): 315–24.

26. Young A. Early rheumatoid arthritis. *Rheum Dis Clin North Am* 2005; 31(4): 659–79.

27. Lard LR, et al. Early versus delayed treatment in patients with recent-onset rheumatoid arthritis: Comparison of two cohorts who received different treatment strategies. *Am J Med* 2001; 111(6): 446–51.

28. Cardiel M, Galarza-Maldonado, Pons-Estel B. First Latin American position paper on the pharmacological treatment of rheumatoid arthritis. *Rheumatology* 2006; 45: ii7–22.

4

Macrophage Activation Syndrome in Juvenile Idiopathic Arthritis

Yackov Berkun and Shai Padeh

Abstract   Macrophage activation syndrome (MAS), life-threatening syndrome of overwhelming inflammation caused by uncontrolled hyperactivation of macrophages, is a rare complication of childhood systemic inflammatory disorders, affecting most often patients with systemic onset juvenile idiopathic arthritis (soJIA). The diagnosis of MAS in soJIA is challenging due to overlapping manifestations of the two diseases. Because MAS is often a fatal condition, prompt diagnosis and immediate therapeutic intervention are important.

Keywords   Hemophagocytic lymphohistiocytosis (HLH) · macrophage activation syndrome (MAS) · juvenile idiopathic arthritis (JIA) · diagnosis · criteria

Introduction

Macrophage activation syndrome (MAS) is a term coined in the past decade to describe a rare, life-threatening syndrome of overwhelming inflammation caused by proliferation and uncontrolled activation of well differentiated macrophages secreting large amounts of inflammatory cytokines. MAS has been reported as a severe complication of childhood systemic inflammatory disorders, affecting most often patients with systemic juvenile idiopathic arthritis (soJIA), but also rarely associated with systemic lupus erythematosus and other rheumatic diseases in children (1). Hyperactivation of macrophages probably driven by T and natural killer (NK) lymphocytes is the cause of the disease. It is characterized by prolonged non remitting fever, pancytopenia, liver disease and hepatosplenomegaly, hemorrhagic diathesis, and neurologic involvement (2). Characteristic biochemical markers include elevated triglycerides, very high serum ferritin and low fibrinogen levels. Low NK cell activity and elevated serum soluble interleukin-2 receptor (sCD25) levels have been recently described (3).

Hemophagocytosis is found in bone marrow, liver, spleen and lymph nodes. MAS usually occurs without any evident trigger, or may follow infection or change in medication regimen in patients with long standing rheumatic diseases, or in some cases, it may herald the rheumatic disease (4). MAS is one of macrophage related disorders, and belongs to a group of acquired, secondary hemophagocytic lymphohistiocytosis (HLH), seen in hematological diseases and different malignancies, viral infections, and autoimmune disorders. It has been suggested to change the term of the disorder to rheumatic disease associated hemophagocytic syndrome, similar to other secondary hemophagocytic syndromes for better uniformity in terminology and medical communication (5). The diagnosis of MAS in soJIA is challenging due to overlapping manifestations of the two diseases. Because MAS is often a fatal condition, prompt diagnosis and immediate therapeutic intervention are important.

Epidemiology

MAS is reported to occur in 7–13% of patients with soJIA (6, 7). Subclinical MAS in soJIA patients is even more common, and it has been suggested that they may be 2 ends of the spectrum of one disease (7, 8). Mortality of 8–22% in MAS has been reported (6, 9), and MAS is responsible significantly to the morbidity and mortality in JIA.

Pathogenesis

Extensive lymphocytes and macrophages activation with overproduction of inflammatory cytokines such as tumor necrosis factor-α, interleukin (IL)-1, and IL-6, account for the clinical and laboratory manifestations. Defective NK cell function has been demonstrated in patients with

From: Y. Shoenfeld et al. (eds.): *Diagnostic Criteria in Autoimmune Diseases*, DOI: 10.1007/978-1-60327-285-8_4,
© 2008 Humana Press, Totowa, NJ

MAS, often with a pattern indistinguishable from other HLH (3, 10). Interestingly, similar NK dysfunction has been demonstrated in soJIA patients, distinguishing it from other JIA subtypes by lower NK cell number and function, and perforin expression (3). The exact mechanism by which deficient NK and cytotoxic T-lymphocyte functions cause the clinical disorder, is unknown. Perforin, antiviral cytotoxic protein secreted by lymphocytes, down-regulates cellular immune response. The deficient NK activity may lead to lymphocyte hyperactivity with secretion of potent macrophage activators. One suggested explanation is that diminished cytotoxic function in MAS patients lead to defective control of infection, persistent antigen stimulation with following escalation of inflammatory process and macrophage overstimulation. Alternative explanation is that deficient cytotoxic function may lead to inefficient apoptosis and removal of overactivated macrophages and lymphocytes (11). These pathogenic findings, common to MAS, HLH and soJIA patients, support the hypothesis that these diseases are different ends of the same spectrum (12).

Clinical and Laboratory Manifestations

The clinical picture of MAS is of acute episode consists of non remitting fever, hepatosplenomegaly, lymphadenopathy, cytopenia, coagulopathy, and central nervous system (CNS) manifestations (headache, disorientation, irritability or lethargy, seizures, coma), (Table 4.1). Other symptoms may include rash (usually fixed), serositis, cardiac and renal involvement. It is often life-threatening, and occasionally fatal (13, 14). Characteristic laboratory findings include a very high serum ferritin, elevated levels of triglycerides, liver enzymes and bilirubin, D-dimers, prolonged prothrombin time with decreased blood cell counts, ESR, fibrinogen and sodium (Table 4.2). Additional markers are low NK cell activity and elevated serum sCD25 levels (3).

A sharp increase in ferritin and decreasing ESR and fibrinogen in face of deteriorating clinical condition of a JIA patient are clues, and should point to the diagnosis of MAS. The pathognomonic histopathological finding is

TABLE 4.1. Symptoms and signs of MAS (2, 13).

	Prevalence (%)
High fever	78–94
Hepatomegaly	61–88
Splenomegaly	45–59
Central nervous system dysfunction	38–53
Hemorrhages	39–44
Lymphoadenopathy	28–41

TABLE 4.2. Laboratory features of MAS (2, 13).

	Prevalence (%)
Hyperferritinemia	87–100
Hypertriglyceridemia	77–100
Abnormal liver function tests	94
Decreased ESR	79–92
Thrombocytopenia	89
Decreased fibrinogen	78–89
Anemia	67–82
Macrophage hemophagocytosis BM	81
Hyponatremia	67–78
Leukopenia	39–56
Hypoalbuminemia	35–54

activated macrophages phagocytosing hematopoietic cells in bone marrow, spleen, or liver.

Diagnostic Criteria

The diagnosis of MAS in soJIA is challenging due to multiple similar manifestations of these diseases, such as fever, hepatosplenomegaly and lymphadenopathy, rash. MAS may be confused with exacerbation of soJIA, a disease with flares and remissions; with infections, which are more common in these patients who are immunosuppressed by their treatment. There is a need for specific diagnostic criteria of the disorder which will take into consideration the similarity to SoJIA.

Previous diagnostic criteria for HLH from 1991 have been used for the diagnosis of MAS (15). They included clinical (fever, splenomegaly), laboratory (cytopenia of two lineages, hypertriglyceridemia and/or hypofibrinogenemia) and histopathological criteria (demonstration of hemophagocytosis in bone marrow or spleen or lymph nodes) (15). For the diagnosis of HLH all criteria are required. In a large series of patients with secondary HLH, elevated levels of ferritin and lactate dehydrogenase were found to be significantly more sensitive than the diagnostic criteria of hypertriglyceridemia and hypofibrogenemia, that were found in only half of patients (16). Another shortcoming of these criteria was the need for tissue confirmation of hemophagocytosis, since biopsy is problematic due to the coagulopathy, and bone marrow aspiration may not always show hemophagocytosis, which may appear later (14). The recent 2004 Revised Diagnostic Guidelines for HLH, includes these five old criteria, and three additional criteria – low or absent NK-cell activity, hyperferritinemia, and high levels of sCD25 (17). For secondary HLH, five of the eight criteria must be fulfilled. In a cohort of familial HLH, the sensitivity of elevated serum ferritin was 0.84, and of high levels of sCD25–0.93 (17). These HLH criteria are been currently used for MAS diagnosis, but are not sufficient to distinguish MAS from SoJIA. As soJIA is characterized by leukocytosis, thrombocytosis, elevated ESR, fibrinogen, ferritin, these tests should be taken into consideration when using criteria for MAS diagnosis.

Recently, Ravelli et al. suggested preliminary diagnostic guidelines for MAS complicating soJIA (13). They compared the frequency of clinical, laboratory, and histopathological features in soJIA patients with MAS to patients with active soJIA. The clinical features analyzed were fever, rash, hepatomegaly, splenomegaly, lymphoadenopathy, hemorrhages, and CNS dysfunction. Laboratory findings included leucopenia, anemia, thrombocytopenia, high ferritin, elevated aspartate and alanine aminotransferase, bilirubin, lactate dehydrogenase, triglycerides, low ESR, albumin, fibrinogen, serum sodium, and bone marrow hemophagocytosis. The ability of each feature to discriminate the episodes of MAS from JIA was evaluated by calculating the sensitivity rate, specificity rate, area under receiver operating characteristic and diagnostic odds ratio (DOR) (Table 4.3). Laboratory and histopathological features, as compared with clinical manifestations, had better discriminating values. Almost all clinical manifestations had higher specificity than sensitivity rate. Hemorrhages and CNS disease, that were present in MAS patients only, had maximal specificity rate and were best clinical discriminators. The strongest laboratory discriminators were decreased platelet count, elevated aspartate aminotransferase, leukopenia, and hypofibrinogenemia, followed by hyponatremia, hyperferritinemia, hypertriglyceridemia, and decreased white blood cell count (13). The combinations of variables that led to best separation between patients and control subjects were identified through "the number of criteria present" method. Only variables available for sufficient number of patients that provided strong discriminating properties and were not duplicative were used.

The best separation between patients and control subjects occurred when any two or more laboratory criteria (DOR = 1309) were simultaneously present; the second best performance was provided by the presence of any 2, 3, or more clinical and/or laboratory criteria (DOR = 765 and 743, respectively). Preliminary diagnostic guidelines for MAS in soJIA, which included 3 clinical and 4 laboratory criteria, were suggested (Table 4.4). Bone marrow

TABLE 4.3. Sensitivity, specificity, diagnostic odds ratio (DOR) of clinical features in MAS patients (13).

	Sensitivity	Specificity	DOR
Fever	0.81	0.04	0.2
Rash	0.45	0.53	0.9
Hepatomegaly	0.61	0.80	6.4
Splenomegaly	0.45	0.71	1.9
Lymphoadenopathy	0.28	0.67	0.8
Hemorrhages	0.39	1	66.8
Central nervous system dysfunction	0.38	1	63.1

TABLE 4.4. Sensitivity, specificity, diagnostic odds ratio (DOR) of laboratory features in MAS patients (13).

	Sensitivity	Specificity	DOR
WBC count < 9.0	0.78	0.88	25.3
Anemia < 10.1	0.94	0.44	13.4
Thrombocytopenia < 262	1.00	0.92	1092
AST > 59	0.92	0.96	248
Fibrinogen < 2.5	0.81	0.97	165
Decreased ESR < 57	0.87	0.76	19.4
Hypertriglyceridemia > 181	0.94	0.88	115
Hyponatremia < 130	0.67	1.00	157
Hypoalbuminemia < 3.2	0.81	0.57	5.6
Hyperferritinemia > 3410	0.88	1.00	115
Macrophage hemophagocytosis in BM	0.81	1.00	45.0

examination for demonstration of macrophage hemophagocytosis was suggested only in cases with doubtful diagnosis (13).

Problems in Current Diagnostics Criteria

Ravelli's guidelines have not been prospectively evaluated. Furthermore, biomarkers such as NK cell activity and sCD25 levels should be considered for incorporation in the criteria. Several new markers, specific for MAS found recently, have not been included in proposed diagnostic criteria. In a recent report of 5 soJIA patients with 9 MAS events, additional laboratory markers, $\beta_2$microglobulin and soluble interleukin-2 receptor were found to be a sensitive indicator of MAS, even when other laboratory markers had not obviously changed, while hypertriglyceridemia, hypoalbuminemia and hyponatremia appeared in 2 patients only (18). The hemoglobin scavenger receptor (CD163), a recently described macrophage differentiation antigen, was found to be useful clinical marker of disorders of macrophages, including HLH (19). Extensive expression of CD163 on hemophagocytic macrophages has been found in MAS patient, suggesting a possible role for CD163 as a specific marker of MAS associated with rheumatic diseases (4). The ability of all these new macrophage specific markers in discriminating between active soJIA and MAS should be further evaluated and incorporated into the criteria.

Treatment

The immediate aim in the treatment of patient with MAS is early and effective suppression of severe hyperinflammation. Intravenous corticosteroids as a first line medication in doses ranging from conventional to pulse methylprednisolone had been proven successful in more than two thirds of MAS patients (9). Cyclosporin A, calcineurin inhibitor of early T-lymphocytes activation, is a preferred second line medication (9). Other second line medications are etoposide and intravenous γ immunoglobulin. Recent HLH 2004 new treatment protocol recommends treating patients with HLH by combination therapy with dexamethasone, etoposide and cyclosporine A (20). In cases of CNS disease, methotrexate is given intrathecally. Serum ferritin level has been recommended for follow up of the treatment response. In patients with severe HLH hematopoietic stem cell transplantation should be considered (20). Considering MAS patients, there are only a few reports of cases treated with etoposide and etanercept.

References

1. Stephan JL, Zeller J, Hubert P, Herbelin C, Dayer JM, Prieur AM. Macrophage activation syndrome and rheumatic disease in childhood: A report of four new cases. *Clin Exp Rheumatol* 1993; 11: 451–6.

2. Ravelli AP, A. Malattia, C. Sala, I, Martini, A. Macrophage activation syndrome in childhood rheumatic diseases. *Curr Rheumatol Rev* 2007; 2: 225–30.

3. Villanueva J, Lee S, Giannini EH, Graham TB, Passo MH, Filipovich A, Grom AA. Natural killer cell dysfunction is a distinguishing feature of systemic onset juvenile rheumatoid arthritis and macrophage activation syndrome. *Arthritis Res Ther* 2005; 7: R30–7.

4. Avcin T, Tse SM, Schneider R, Ngan B, Silverman ED. Macrophage activation syndrome as the presenting manifestation of rheumatic diseases in childhood. *J Pediatr* 2006; 148: 683–6.

5. Athreya BH. Is macrophage activation syndrome a new entity? *Clin Exp Rheumatol* 2002; 20: 121–3.

6. Sawhney S, Woo P, Murray KJ. Macrophage activation syndrome: A potentially fatal complication of rheumatic disorders. *Arch Dis Child* 2001; 85: 421–6.

7. Behrens EM, Beukelman T, Paessler M, Cron RQ. Occult macrophage activation syndrome in patients with systemic juvenile idiopathic arthritis. *J Rheumatol* 2007; 34: 1133–8.

8. Bleesing J, Prada A, Siegel DM, Villanueva J, Olson J, Ilowite NT, Brunner HI, Griffin T, Graham TB, Sherry DD, Passo MH, Ramanan AV, Filipovich A, Grom AA. The diagnostic significance of soluble CD163 and soluble interleukin-2 receptor alpha-chain in macrophage activation syndrome and untreated new-onset systemic juvenile idiopathic arthritis. *Arthritis Rheum* 2007; 56: 965–71.

9. Stephan JL, Kone-Paut I, Galambrun C, Mouy R, Bader-Meunier B, Prieur AM. Reactive haemophagocytic syndrome in children with inflammatory disorders. A retrospective study of 24 patients. *Rheumatology (Oxford)* 2001; 40: 1285–92.

10. Grom AA, Villanueva J, Lee S, Goldmuntz EA, Passo MH, Filipovich A. Natural killer cell dysfunction in patients with systemic-onset juvenile rheumatoid arthritis and macrophage activation syndrome. *J Pediatr* 2003; 142: 292–6.

11. Henter JI. Biology and treatment of familial hemophagocytic lymphohistiocytosis: Importance of perforin in lymphocyte-mediated cytotoxicity and triggering of apoptosis. *Med Pediatr Oncol* 2002; 38: 305–9.

12. Ramanan AV, Grom AA. Does systemic-onset juvenile idiopathic arthritis belong under juvenile idiopathic arthritis? *Rheumatology (Oxford)* 2005; 44: 1350–3.

13. Ravelli A, Magni-Manzoni S, Pistorio A, Besana C, Foti T, Ruperto N, Viola S, Martini A. Preliminary diagnostic guidelines for macrophage activation syndrome complicating systemic juvenile idiopathic arthritis. *J Pediatr* 2005; 146: 598–604.

14. Ramanan AV, Schneider R. Macrophage activation syndrome – what's in a name! *J Rheumatol* 2003; 30: 2513–6.

15. Henter JI, Elinder G, Ost A. Diagnostic guidelines for hemophagocytic lymphohistiocytosis. The FHL Study Group of the Histiocyte Society. *Semin Oncol* 1991; 18: 29–33.

16. Imashuku S, Hlbi S, Todo S. Hemophagocytic lymphohistiocytosis in infancy and childhood. *J Pediatr* 1997; 130: 352–7.

17. Janka GE, Schneider EM. Modern management of children with haemophagocytic lymphohistiocytosis. *Br J Haematol* 2004; 124: 4–14.

18. Kounami S, Yoshiyama M, Nakayama K, Okuda M, Okuda S, Aoyagi N, Yoshikawa N. Macrophage activation syndrome in children with systemic-onset juvenile chronic arthritis. *Acta Haematol* 2005; 113: 124–9.

19. Schaer DJ, Schleiffenbaum B, Kurrer M, Imhof A, Bachli E, Fehr J, Moller HJ, Moestrup SK, Schaffner A. Soluble hemoglobin-haptoglobin scavenger receptor CD163 as a lineage-specific marker in the reactive hemophagocytic syndrome. *Eur J Haematol* 2005; 74: 6–10.

20. Henter JI, Horne A, Arico M, Egeler RM, Filipovich AH, Imashuku S, Ladisch S, McClain K, Webb D, Winiarski J, Janka G. HLH-2004: Diagnostic and therapeutic guidelines for hemophagocytic lymphohistiocytosis. *Pediatr Blood Cancer* 2007; 48: 124–31.

5
Adult Still Disease

Alon Eisen and Howard Amital

Abstract   Adult Still disease (ASD) is a rare systemic inflammatory disorder of unknown etiology chracterized by spiking fever with evanescent rash, arthritis, arthralgia and multiorgan involvenent. It often poses a diagnostic and therapeutic challenge however clear clinical guidelines are lacking. In recent years, few sets of diagnostic criterias have been suggested, based on clinical and laboratorial factors. The emergence of specific diagnostic criteria as well as new strategies treating ASD may all provide the clinician with significant tools in the management of this complex autoimmune disorder.

Keywords   Adult Still disease · arthritis · fever

Introduction

Adult Still disease (ASD) is an inflammatory disorder characterized mainly by spiking high fever, arthritis, rash; and clinical features that resemble juvenile inflammatory arthritis. ASD was first described by Bywaters (1) in 1971 who reported fourteen adult patients with clinical features similar to Still disease. The ASD is a rare condition and found worldwide, with an incidence rate of about 0.16 cases per 100,000 persons per year with an equal gender distribution. The most common age of ASD is between 16 and 35 years, yet it may appear at an older age. Familial aggregation of ASDA has not been identified.

The etiology of ASD is unknown. Several infectious agents have been implicated in the disease pathogenesis and in particularly viruses such as the rubella, echovirus 7, mumps, Epstein-Barr, cytomegalovirus, parainfluenza, parvovirus B19, coxackie, adneno, influenza, herpes, and hepatitis B and C viruses (2). Suspected bacterial pathogens include Yersinia enterocolitica and Mycoplasma pneumoniae. It has also been suggested that ASD may be a form of vasculitis mediated by nonnecrotizing immune complexes. An association has been sought with several HLA loci but no consistent results were recorded (2).

Clinical Manifestations

ASD typically affects several organs as represented in Table 5.1. The typical triad is high-spiking fever, a characteristic rash and arthritis or arthralgia. Fever generally exceeds 39°C appearing in spikes usually in the evening and resolving to normal within few hours. The fever can also be "double-quortitian" with two spikes a day and in 20% of cases, fever is present between the spikes (3). The typical rash is an evanescent, salmon-pink, macular or maculopapular rash, which is observed mostly with the fever spike. It predominantly involves the trunk and proximal extremities with rare involvement of the face and distal limbs. The rash can be pruritic and often can be misdiagnosed as drug related eruption. It can be precipitated by rubbing, a phenomenon known as Koebner phenomenon (3). Arthritis and arthralgia are found in the majority of patients with ASD and increases with intensity in fever spikes. Their presence is less evident at the onset of disease with transient, mild and oligoarticular pattern while later during the course of disease, it may be polyarticular and more severe. The joints affected most frequently are the knees, wrists and ankles although involvement of the elbow, shoulder, proximal and distal interphalangeal, metacarpophalangeal, metatarsophalangeal, temporomandibular and hip

From: Y. Shoenfeld et al. (eds.): *Diagnostic Criteria in Autoimmune Diseases*, DOI: 10.1007/978-1-60327-285-8_5,
© 2008 Humana Press, Totowa, NJ

TABLE 5.1. Clinical manifestations of Adult Still disease.

Clinical manifestation	Frequency (%)
Fever	82–100
Rash	85–87
Arthritis/Arthralgia	69–100
Myalgia	62–84
Sore throat	68–92
Lymphadenpathy	48–74
Splenomegaly	22–65
Pleuritis	15–53
Pericarditis	10–37
Abdominal pain	48
Hepatomegaly	42
Alopecia	24

Data from Pouchot et al. (7), Ohta et al. (5), Masson et al. (18).

TABLE 5.2. Laboratory tests and serological findings in Adult Still disease.

Laboratory finding	Frequency (%)
Elevated ESR/CRP	99
Leukocytosis $\geq$10,000/mm^3	92
$\geq$15,000/mm^3	81
Anemia (hemoglobin $\leq$10 g/dL)	68
Thrombocytosis (platelets $\geq$400,000/mm^3)	62
Coagulation abnormalities	Rare
Elevated liver enzymes (any)	73
Serum Albumin $\leq$ 3.5 g/dL	81
Elevated Ferritin	70
Negative ANA	92
Negative RF	93

ANA: anti nuclear antibody; CRP: C-reactive protein; ESR: Erythrocyte sedimentation rate; RF: rheumatic factor.
Data from Pouchot et al. (7), Ohta et al. (5)

joints have also been described (3). Myalgia is another common manifestation; most often worsens in fever spikes. Liver abnormalities such as hepatomegaly and mild elevated liver enzymes are also common. Abdominal pain is not rare and is usually mild although few cases of severe abdominal pain resembling acute peritonitis have been described (3). Slightly tender, enlarged cervical lymph nodes and splenomegaly occur in about half of the patients (4). Sore throat as non exudative pharyngitis is present in two thirds of the patients usually at the beginning of the illness (4). Cardiac manifestations are less common and include pericarditis, myocarditis and tamponade (4). Pulmonary manifestations include pleuritis, fibrosis, pleural effusions and rarely might deteriorate adult respiratory distress syndrome (3). Renal involvement is rare and includes interstitial nephritis, subacute glomerulitis, mesangial nephritis, renal amyloidosis and rapidly progressive glomerulopathy with renal failure and a poor outcome (3). Hematological manifestations such as thrombotic thrombocytopenic purpura are rare, so is neurological involvement that include cranial nerve palsies, peripheral neuropathy and aseptic meningitis (3).

Laboratory Findings

The laboratory findings in ASD coincide with the systemic inflammation nature of the disease (Table 5.2). The erythrocyte sedimentation rate (ESR) is elevated in all patients and C-reactive protein may also be raised (3). In blood count, the most common finding is leukocytosis which is present in up to 75% of patients, with a predominance of mature and juvenile granulocytes (4). Anemia of chronic disease and reactive thrombocytosis are also common (5). Elevated liver enzymes, particularly transaminases and lactic dehydrogenase are observed in about 70% of patients and frequently occur with concomitance to fever

and arthritis (3). Coagulation abnormalities are rare and include prolongation of prothrombin time or partial thromboplastin time and disseminated intravascular coagulation. Transient mild increase in muscle enzyme can be detected in blood sera (5). ASD is associated with markedly elevated serum ferritin as compared to other autoimmune or inflammatory diseases.

In most studies a serum ferritin level of 1000 ng/ml, five times the upper normal value, has been used to suggest ASD (6). Higher levels of ferritin as up to 30,000 ng/ml has been observed as well. Serum ferritin levels usually correlate with disease activity and subside with remission (6). The glycosylated fraction of ferritin has been found to be more specific than ferritin itself (6). In normal subjects, most of the ferritin is glycosylated whereas in inflammatory diseases and particularly in ASD, the glycosylated fraction of ferritin is low and often below 20% (6). The percentage of glycosylated ferritin in patients with ASD is markedly lower than in other inflammatory diseases (6). Its level remains low in both active disease and in remmision, therefore, can not be used to monitor disease activity or response treatment (3). Use of both total serum ferritin above 1000 ng/ml and a low level of the glycosylated fraction of ferritin (below 20%) may provide a better marker for ASD with a specificity rate as high as 93% (3).

Unlike other rheumatic diseases, ASD is usually **not** associated with a positive rheumatoid factor or with an antinuclear antibody (4). A low titer of either test may appear in up to 10% of patients with ASD and is usually transient. Immunoglobulins and complement concentrations are often normal or elevated in ASD. Furthermore, elevated serum levels of interleukin-6, tumor necrosis factor, interferon gamma and interleukin-18 are observed but these tests are not specific for ASD (4). In most cases of ASD, procalcitonin level is normal (4).

Radiographic Findings

Radiographs during the initial acute phase of ASD are often not specific, being either normal or showing soft tissue swelling or mild joint effusion (3). Characteristic late finding in about 40% of patients is a nonerosive narrowing of the carpometacarpal and intercarpal joint spaces of the wrist, which often progresses to bony ankylosis, most marked in pericapitate region (3). Less common are radiographic intertarsal and tarsometatasal changes and ankylosis of the cervical spine and distal interphalangeal joints. Destruction of the hip joint, and less commonly the knee, has been described as a rare complication that often requires total joint replacement, as opposed to wrist and and ankle involvement which only causes limited disability (3).

Biopsy, Synovial and Serosal Fluids

The findings of biopsy of involved tissue in ASD are not specific, yet it is usually performed in order to exclude other differential diagnosis. The most common biopsy performed is skin biopsy which shows perivascular inflammation of the superficial dermis with lymphocytes and histiocytes. Direct immunofluorescent is ususally negative for immunoglobulins and complement. Other tissues biopsies often reveal non specific inflammatory changes (5). Synovial fluids in ASD are inflammatory with a polymorphonuclear predominance. Pleural and pericardial effusions are often sterile inflammatory exudates (5).

Course of Disease

The clinical course of ASD can be divided into three main patterns, each affecting approximately one-third of patients:

- A self limited or monophasic pattern that lasts up to one year of disease with complete remission and favourable prognosis.
- An intermittent or polycyclic pattern which is characterized by reccurent flares of disease, usually milder than the initial episode (7), with complete remission between exacerbations.
- A chronic pattern characterized by persistently active disease, usually due to chronic articular manifestations, mostly severe destructive arthritis. These patients generally have more disability and the worst prognosis compared to patients who have only systemic symptoms (8). The development of polyarthritis early in the course of ASD, proximal joint arthritis and root joint (shoulder, hip) involvement at disease onset, are predictors of chronic disease course and poor prognosis (3). In addition, the requiremnet of more than two years of systemic corticosteroid treatment are associated with poorer long-term function.

Diagnosis

ASD lacks a test or combination of tests to establish its diagnosis (9). The clinical presentation of ASD is heterogeneous, and the spectrum of differential diagnoses is broad, including infectious, neoplastic, and autoimmune diseases (Table 5.3).

Several classification criteria have been proposed by a number of authors to diagnose ASD, all have been developed from retrospective data analysis (10–14). Six sets of criteria for ASD in well defined patient population studies have been proposed (15). The classification criteria proposed by Cush et al. (10) is the most commonly used with a 80.5% sensitivity rate, yet those of Yamaguchi et al. (11) are more sensitive with 93.5% sensitivity (3, 9). Since, no conrtol group was ever used; no validation of specifity is available. These two classifications include major and minor criteria (Table 5.4) as well as exclusion criteria, mainly systemic, infectious or neoplastic diseases. The exclusion criteria represents a major problem for use in clinical research since only general recommendations are provided and not a precise list of diseases to be excluded nor any lab tests and imaging exams to be performed. As opposed to these two classifications, Fautrel et al. (12) proposed a new set of criteria that does not contain any exclusion criteria and includes the novel marker of serum glycosylated-ferritin as a major criterion. The sensitivity reported in this study was 80.6% and its specificity was 98.5%. Still, the limitation of this diagnostic criterion is that it is not clear what is the

TABLE 5.3. Differential diagnosis of Adult Still disease.

Infectious diseases	Rubella, cytomegalovirus, epstein bar virus, mumps, coxackievirus, adenovirus, hepatitis B, parvovirus, HIV
Neoplasms	Leukemia, lymphoma, angioblastic lymphadenopathy
Granulomatous diseases	Sarcoidosis, Crohn disease, idiopathic granulomatous hepatitis
Vasculitides	Polyarteritis nodosa, Wegener granulomatosis, thrombotic thrombocytopenic purpura, Takayasu arteritis
Connective tissue diseases	Systemic lupus erythematosus, reactive arthritis, spondyloarthropathies, mixed connective tissue disease, Sweet syndrome, dermatomyosis, Schmitzler syndrome
Others	Hemophagocytic syndrome, Kikuchi syndrome, familial mediterranean fever, TNF receptor periodic syndrome

TABLE 5.4. Diagnostic Criteria of Adult Still disease.

Cush et al. (10)	Yamaguchi et al. (11)	Fautrel et al. (12)
2 points each: • Quotidian fever >39°C • Evanescent rash • WBC >12,000 and ESR >40 mm/1 h • Negative ANA and RF • Carpal ankylosis	Major criteria: • Fever >39°C, intermittent, one week or longer • Arthralgia ≥2 weeks • Characteristic rash • WBC >10,000/μL (>80% granulocytes)	Major criteria: • Spiking fever ≥39°C • Arthralgia • Transient erythema • Pharyngitis • PMN ≥80% • Glycosylated ferritin ≤20%
1 point each: • Onset age >35 years • Arthritis • Sore throat • RES involvement or LFT abnormal • Serositis • Cervical or tarsal ankylosis	Minor criteria: • Sore throat • Lymphadenopathy and/or splenomegaly • LFT abnormal • Negative ANA/RF	Minor criteria: • Maculopapular rash • WBC >10,000/μL
Probable ASD: 10 points during 12 weeks observation	Exclusion criteria: • Infections • Malignancies • Rheumatic diseases	4 major criteria or 3 major + 2 minor
Definite ASD: 10 points with 6 months observation	5 criteria, at least 2 major	

ANA: anti nuclear antibody; ESR: Erythrocyte sedimentation rate; LFT: liver function tests; PMN: polymorphonuclear; RF: rheumatic factor; WBC: white blood cells.

value and utility of glycosylated-ferritin as compared to other ASD characteristics. Furthermore, it should be further validated in different population. The comparison of the three most common diagnostic criteria for ASD is presented in Table 5.4.

Treatment

Treatment of ASD is basically empirical, with treatment efficacy data based on case studies and small retrospective trials. The treatment of ASD is based on NSAID's including aspirin, corticosteroids and immunomodulating drugs. An initial use of NSAID's is the first line of treatment generally used, leading to improvement in muscoloskeletal symptoms and fever in 20–25% of cases. In most cases, the response to NSAID's is a good prognostic sign and is frequently characteristic of self limiting disease or intermitent disease (3). The major concern with NSAID therapy are hepatotoxicity, therefore close monitoring of liver function tests, early in the course of the disease is essential.

Unfortunatelly, most patients with ASD will require the use of glucocorticoids at some point during their disease (2). The usual prednisone dose is 0.5 to 1.0 mg/kg per day. Alternative day treatment is of benefit to those with milder disease. Pulse methylprednisolone is used for those requiring long-term use of prednisone or in life threatening disease due to severe hepatic invovlement, cardiac tamponade, disseminated intravascular coagulation or myocarditis. About 76% of patients will favorably respond to glucocorticoids (2).

Disease modifying antirheumatic drugs (DMARDs) are employed when patients do not respond to glucocorticoids or do not tolerate their side effects. DMARDs used are intramuscular gold, D-penicillamine, sulfasalazine, hydroxychloroquine and methotrexate, none of which were investigated in a controlled trial. Methotrexate is used as a steroid sparing agent and has been useful in articular and systemic disease, at a dose of 5–25 mg/week (2). Immunomosupressive agents, including azathioprine, cyclosporine A and cyclophosphamide have been used as well with only modest efficacy. Intravenous immunoglobulins were reported to result in good responses, particularly in induction of remission and control of early disease (16). Anti tumor necrosis factor α have been partially beneficial in several open label trials with Entaracept and Infliximab being the two agents commonly used (17). About 50% of patients will require pharmacologic treatment after 10 years of disease, although the role of treatment in disease remission is not clear.

References

1. Bywaters, EG. Still's disease in the adult. *Ann Rheum Dis* 1971; 30: 121–132.
2. Efthimiou P, Georgy S. Pathogenesis and management of adult-onset still's disease. *Semin Arthritis Rheum* 2006; 36: 144–52.
3. Efthimiou P, Paik PK, Bielory L. Diagnosis and management of adult onset Still's disease. *Ann Rheum Dis* 2006; 65: 564–72.
4. Kadar J, Petrovicz E. Adult-onset still's disease. *Best Pract Res Clin Rheumatol* 2004; 18: 663–76.

5. Ohta A, Yamaguchi M, Kaneoka H, et al. Adult's still's disease: A review of 228 cases from the literature. *J Rheumatol* 1987; 14: 1139–46.

6. Fautrel B, Le Moel G, Saint-Marcoux B, et al. Diagnostic value of ferritin and glycosylated ferritin in adult onset still's disease. *J Rheumatol* 2001; 28: 322–9.

7. Pouchot J, Sampalis JS, Beaudet F, et al. Adult onset Still's disease: Manifestations, disease course and outcome in 62 patients. *Medicine (Baltimore)* 1991; 70: 118–36.

8. Masson C, Le Loet X, Liote F, et al. Adult's still disease: Part II. Management, outcome and prognostic factors. *Rev Rhum (Engl Ed)* 1995; 62: 758–65.

9. Andres E, Ruellan A, Pflumio F, et al. Sensitivity of the criteria used to diagnose adult still's disease in internal medicine practice. A study of 17 cases. *Eur J intern Med* 2002; 13: 136–8.

10. Cush JJ, Medsger TA Jr, Christy WC, et al. Adult-onset Still's disease: Clinical course and outcome. *Arthritis Rheum* 1987; 30: 186–94.

11. Yamaguchi M, Ohta A, Tsunematsu T, et al. Preliminary criteria for classification of adult Still's disease. *J Rheumatol* 1992; 19: 424–30.

12. Fautrel B, Zing E, Golmard JL, et al. Proposal for a new set of classification criteria for adult-onset still disease. *Medicine (Baltimore)* 2002; 81: 194–200.

13. Reginato J, Schumacher HR Jr, Baker DG, et al. Adult onset still's disease: Experience in 23 patients and literature review with emphasis on organ failure. *Semin Arthritis Rheum* 1987; 17: 39–57.

14. Kahn MF, Delaire M. Maladie de Still de l'adulte. In: Kahn, MF, et al. (eds.), *Les maladies Systemiques*. Flammarion, Paris; 1991: 231–8.

15. Masson C, Le Loet X, Liote F, et al. Comparative study of six types of criteria in adult Still's disease. *J Rheumatol* 1996; 23: 495–7.

16. Vignes S, Wechsler B, Amoura Z, et al. Intravenous immunoglobulin in adult Still's disease refractory to non-steroidal anti-inflammatory drugs. *Clin Exp Rheumatol* 1998; 16: 295–8.

17. Fautrel B, Sibilia J, Mariette X, et al. Tumour necrosis factor alpha blocking agents in refractory adult Still's disease: An observational study of 20 cases. *Ann Rheum Dis* 2005; 64: 262–6.

18. Masson C. Le Loet X, Liote F, et al. Adult's still disaese: Part I. Manifestations and complications in sixty-five cases in France. *Rev Rhum (Engl Ed)* 1995; 62: 748–57.

6
Systemic Sclerosis

Jennifer G. Walker and Marvin J. Fritzler

Abstract Systemic sclerosis (SSc) is a chronic disease of unknown etiology, and its classification as a systemic autoimmune rheumatic disease (SARD) is supported by clinical and experimental observations that include the presence of autoantibodies (AAs) and autoreactive T cells. Although some AAs are specific markers for the disease, there has not been widespread adoption of them as specific classification criteria. The application of classification criteria is further hampered by the recognition that diagnosis of SSc encompasses a wide variety of clinical features that prompts the classification of the condition into a number of disease subsets. For practical purposes, most clinicians subclassify the disease as limited cutaneous SSc (lcSSc) or diffuse cutaneous SSc (dcSSc). As diagnostic technologies rapidly evolve and clinicians consider designer therapies for this condition, the development and universal adoption of clinical classification criteria will be a significant challenge.

Keywords Systemic sclerosis · scleroderma · classification · criteria · autoantibodies

Systemic sclerosis (SSc) is a connective tissue disorder characterized by endothelial dysfunction, fibrosis, and the production of autoantibodies (AAs). Excessive collagen deposition results in skin thickening and changes in internal organs that include the lung, vasculature, gastrointestinal tract, and kidney. Endothelial damage leading to vascular dysfunction is manifest as Raynaud's phenomenon, digital ulceration and gangrene, pulmonary arterial hypertension, and renal vascular damage. SSc is usually subclassified as limited or diffuse depending on the extent of skin involvement. The distinction between limited and diffuse SSc varies, but most authorities would concur that patients with truncal and acral involvement have diffuse disease whereas changes distal to the metacarpophalangeal and metatarsophalangeal joints are consistent with limited disease. There is debate over the degree of acral involvement that constitutes limited versus diffuse disease (1). Typically, patients with limited SSc have a more insidious disease onset, and they describe Raynaud's phenomenon for some years prior to the onset of sclerodactyly. In contrast, in those with diffuse SSc the skin thickening tends to more closely coincide with the onset of Raynaud's phenomenon and the disease course is more acute, with most internal organ involvement occurring within 5 years (2). Tables 6.1 and 6.2 summarize clinical features of the disease in the diffuse and limited subsets.

Epidemiology

SSc occurs worldwide, and the incidence and prevalence rates show a wide variation depending on the geographic location, disease definition, classification criteria and methods of case selection. There is evidence that the incidence and prevalence has increased from 2.7 new cases per million to 18.7 and from 138 total cases per million to 660 respectively over a 25-year interval. The higher prevalence rates of approximately 230 cases per million have been reported in the USA and South Australia. The disease occurs more frequently in women than men (4:1), although this ratio is more pronounced in younger patients and less so in adults aged >50 years. The diagnosis of the disease is most commonly made in individuals in the fifth decade but can begin in childhood or septuagenarians. The disease onset is earlier in African-American women than European American women and is more likely to be diffuse disease (reviewed in ref 3). The proportion of (lcSSc) versus (dcSSc) also varies by geographic region and racial group. This is also true of AA markers (discussed below), all giving strong indications that host and environmental factors play a role in disease pathogenesis and expression. Environmental factors of interest associated with an increased risk of

From: Y. Shoenfeld et al. (eds.): *Diagnostic Criteria in Autoimmune Diseases*, DOI: 10.1007/978-1-60327-285-8_6,
© 2008 Humana Press, Totowa, NJ

TABLE 6.1. Clinical features helpful in classification of systemic sclerosis.[a]

Limited cutaneous SSc	Diffuse cutaneous SSc
Raynaud's phenomenon alone for years	Delayed Raynaud's or same as skin
Rare constitutional symptoms	Severe constitutional symptoms
Minimal arthralgias	Arthralgias, carpal tunnel
Puffy fingers	Puffy hands and legs
Telangiectasias and calcinosis (late)	Palpated tendon friction rubs
Skin thickening limited to hands and face	Skin thickening progresses from fingers to trunk rapidly
GI and mild pulmonary fibrosis	GI and pulmonary fibrosis common
Rare heart and kidney	Heart and kidney potentially severe
Anti-centromere antibody	Anti-topoisomerase I (Scl-70)
	Anti-RNA polymerase III
	Anti-fibrillarin

GI, gastrointestinal.
[a] Adapted from ref 2 with permission from Elsevier.

developing the disease include exposure to particulate silica, trichloroethylene and other organic solvents, and heavy metals such as mercury.

TABLE 6.2. Comparison of features in SSc patients with limited cutaneous SSc and diffuse cutaneous SSc.[a]

Feature	Limited cutaneous SSc	Diffuse cutaneous SSc
Demographic		
Age <40 years at onset (%)	50	35
Sex: female (%)	85	75
Duration of symptoms before diagnosis (years)	8.5	2.0
Cumulative survival 10 years after diagnosis (%)	75	65
Organ system involvement (%)		
Skin thickening	95	100
Telangiectasias	80	30
Calcinosis	50	10
Raynaud's phenomenon	95	85
Arthralgias or arthritis	60	80
Tendon friction rubs	3	65
Joint contractures	45	85
Myopathy	10	20
Esophageal hypomotility	75	75
Small intestine hypomotility	25	25
Pulmonary fibrosis	35	45
Pulmonary hypertension	10	<1
Congestive heart failure	5	15
Renal crisis	1	20
Laboratory data		
Antinuclear antibody	95	95
Anti-centromere antibody	50	<5
Anti-topo I	18	30
Anti-RNAP III	2	25
Anti-fibrillarin	<1	12
Anti-PM/Scl	5	15

[a] Adapted from ref 2 with permission from Elsevier.

Genetics

The relative risk of developing SSc, if a first degree relative has it, is a remarkable 13%, although the absolute risk in individual family members is much lower at <1% (3). There is evidence that serological but not clinical subsets of SSc are most highly linked to HLA class II genes (3). A number of other genetic loci have also been identified, and these are thought to be associated with distinct SSc phenotypes based on AA profiles rather than SSc as a single disease entity (3). If these observations are substantiated, they will have implications for design and approach to therapeutic interventions. In the past, there has been considerable interest in SPARC (secreted protein, acidic and rich in cysteine), PTPN22 that (encodes the lymphoid-specific tyrosine phosphatase nonreceptor type 2), and allograft inflammatory factor 1 (AIF1) (reviewed in ref 3). Recent studies have focused on friend leukemia integration 1 (Fli1), a transcription factor that is dysregulated in SSc skin and dermal blood vessels, and appears to play a pathological role in SSc skin fibrosis and vessel degeneration (reviewed in ref 3). Whether these abnormalities are related to genetic polymorphisms in the Fli1 pathway or to epigenetic mechanisms requires clarification.

Laboratory Findings

Laboratory findings vary according to internal organ involvement, but in the absence of acute progressive disease, they may be within the normal range. Elevated erythrocyte sedimentation rates and reduced complement levels have been observed in patients with more active disease (4). Other specific laboratory changes are coincident with organ involvement. For example, acute renal crisis may be marked by an elevated serum creatinine, evidence of hemolysis, and electrolyte disturbance.

Serological Markers

AAs occur in over 95% of patients with SSc, and to date, there are more than 30 AAs associated with SSc (5). The majority of patients have AAs directed to nuclear antigens, and these have specific clinical associations. Anti-centromere (CENP) antibodies occur in 20–40% of patients and are most commonly associated with limited SSc, ischemic digital loss, calcinosis, and pulmonary hypertension. Anti-topoisomerase I antibodies occur in 9–20% of patients and are associated with diffuse SSc, more severe disease, pulmonary fibrosis, and increased mortality. Anti-fibrillarin (U3 ribonucleoprotein) antibodies are reported to be highly specific for SSc, but in most SSc cohorts the prevalence is less than 12%. Although all these antibodies have a high specificity, their low sensitivity means that on their own they are not a useful screen for SSc. Other AAs reported to be relatively specific for SSc and currently available in specialized clinical laboratories include RNA polymerase III (RNAP III), which is identified in 5–25% of SSc sera and has been associated with significant geographic variability and with renal crisis and pulmonary hypertension (reviewed in refs 5 and 6). Antibodies to the polymyositis/scleroderma (PM/Scl) antigens are seen in 14–20% of SSc patients, and most commonly, they identify a subset of patients with overlapping features of SSc and PM (7). There are other, less specific AAs associated with SSc that are also reported to have specific clinical associations, but, at present, they are of limited diagnostic utility.

Recently, a promising new specific AA directed against the platelet-derived growth factor receptor has been identified, and preliminary studies suggest that it is relatively specific for SSc (8 and references therein). However, these studies were based on a functional assay, which is currently not easily adaptable to the clinical setting.

Classification Criteria

There are no universally accepted classification criteria for SSc (reviewed in ref 9). This can be attributed to several factors: (a) rarity of the disease, (b) the absence of a specific diagnostic test, (c) debate regarding subclassification based on the extent of skin involvement, and (d) debate as to whether the limited and diffuse forms of SSc are continuums of one disease or are manifestations of different pathological processes. Despite many clinical similarities, differences in outcome, serology, and genetics support the concept that they may be two separate disease processes.

The two major forms of classification criteria currently in use are those that distinguish SSc from other forms of disease and those that also incorporate some degree of subclassification. Discussion in this chapter will be limited to the American College of Rheumatology (ACR) criteria and more recent classification criteria, as well as a selection of the more influential published subclassification criteria. The ACR classification criteria were designed to differentiate SSc from other forms of disease, and initial external validation recorded high levels of sensitivity and specificity (Table 6.3), (10). Unfortunately, subsequent testing in other disease registries led to the appreciation that these

criteria lacked sensitivity, particularly in identifying patients with limited SSc (1). In addition, diagnostic techniques have advanced since their development, and there is growing support to include specific tests for antinuclear antibodies (ANAs) and nailfold capillaroscopy (reviewed in ref 5). Lonzetti et al. showed that in their cohort of French-Canadian patients the diagnostic value of the ACR criteria could be improved substantially by the addition of ANA and nailfold capillaroscopy evaluations (11). It is widely accepted that the ACR classification criteria are in need of an update, but they remain the most widely cited criteria to receive extensive external validation.

More recently, Nadashkevich et al. proposed an updated classification set that included the presence of AAs but did not include nailfold capillaroscopy (12). These criteria were first derived from the study of a Ukrainian cohort of SSc patients, and other connective tissue diseases (CTDs) were used as comparative groups. The eight criteria derived from the first phase of the study were subsequently tested in a population of 99 Canadian SSc patients and 138 CTD controls. Findings were promising, yielding a 99% sensitivity and 100% specificity (12). However, these criteria have not been widely adopted, possibly because they do not include subclassification of SSc.

Subclassification Criteria

While the need to differentiate SSc from other forms of disease is important, an improved understanding of the disease pathogenesis and the differing outcomes associated with different presentations of the disease has led to the recognition that subclassification of SSc can provide additional crucial information in terms of (a) prognosis in the routine clinical setting, (b) comparison between disease registries, and (c) a guide to emerging therapies. To date, there are 14 published subclassification criteria sets for SSc each proposing two to six separate categories (13), which are generally based on the degree of skin involvement. The majority of survival studies based on the degree of skin involvement suggest that there is no statistically significant differential survival in the three subgroup category, whereas differences in outcome using the two group subclassification set are well recognized (1, 13).

The two subset criteria first proposed by Le Roy in 1988 (14) and later published in modified form in 2001 (Table 6.4) (15) have been the most influential of the subclassification criteria groups. Categories are separated based on the degree of skin involvement, with the later criteria incorporating AAs and nailfold capillaroscopy changes. The 1988 criteria have been widely adopted, but the amended criteria have not been extensively utilized and require further validation. In addition, within these criteria diagnosis requires the presence of Raynaud's phenomenon, something that is not universally present, particularly at the onset of diffuse SSc.

TABLE 6.3. 1980 ACR preliminary classification criteria for systemic sclerosis.[a]

1. Proximal scleroderma, skin involvement extending proximal to metacarpophalangeal joints (major criterion)
2. Sclerodactyly, digital pitting scars of fingertips or loss of substance of the distal fingerpad, and bibasilar pulmonary fibrosis (minor criteria)
3. One major or two or more minor criteria required

[a] Adapted from ref 10.

TABLE 6.4. LeRoy and Medsger revised criteria for the classification of systemic sclerosis (SSc).[a]

Limited SSc	Raynaud's phenomenon (objective documentation)
	Plus any one: SSc-type nailfold capillary pattern or SSc selective autoantibodies
	Or:
	Subjective Raynaud's phenomenon
	Plus both: SSc-type nailfold capillary pattern and SSc selective antibodies
Limited cutaneous SSc	Criteria for limited SSc *plus* distal cutaneous changes
Diffuse cutaneous SSc	Criteria for limited SSc *plus* proximal cutaneous changes
Diffuse fasciitis with eosinophilia	Proximal cutaneous changes without criteria for limited SSc or limited cutaneous SSc

[a] Adapted from ref 15.

Maricq and Valter proposed a more complex subclassification that includes six different categories (16). Once again, the primary separation was based on the degree of skin involvement into three primary categories. Three additional categories are incorporated: (a) Scleroderma sine scleroderma, (b) features of mixed CTDs, and (c) a final group conforming to CREST phenomena but without sufficient changes to be incorporated into the three major skin change groupings. Nailfold capillaroscopy and AAs have been included in these criteria, but the AAs were limited to the presence or absence of CENP as detected by indirect immunofluorescence. As discussed above, CENP antibodies are now known to be one of four or five AAs that have relatively high specificity for SSc. In addition, the advent of multiplexed AA detection has provided a rapid and accurate way of detecting multiple AAs in a single serum sample, a feature which could change current AA paradigms (17). When applied to their database of 165 patients, they were able to show differential clinical outcomes. But in its current form it is difficult to use outside specialized tertiary research settings.

Treatment Options

Treatment options for SSc are still limited to treating specific aspects of organ involvement. Therapies designed to switch off the disease process, such as bone marrow transplantation (18), remain in their infancy. Clinical outcomes with therapies directed against profibrotic mediators, such as connective tissue growth factor and transforming growth factor-β, are in progress. Promising results have been reported with bosentan, a dual endothelin receptor antagonist, which has been shown to improve pulmonary arterial hypertension and digital ulceration (reviewed in ref 19). Proteomic and metabolomic approaches are identifying other common mediators that are potential therapeutic targets, but it is not known if this will result in improved.

Considerations and Future Directions

The wide use and application of classification criteria, particularly the inclusion of AAs into current and future criteria, is met by challenges and issues that must be carefully considered (Table 6.5). First, although classification criteria were clearly devised to standardize the classification of various diseases into uniform groups for research purposes, there appears to be an emerging divergence of clinical diagnostic nomenclature away from current classification criteria. One reason for this is that diagnostic technologies in imaging and serology are moving at such a fast pace and many clinicians are using these new technologies while classification criteria lag behind. It is clear that if classification criteria are to maintain a meaningful role, they will need to be revised and updated more frequently. Second, it is also clear that classification criteria must take into consideration the age of onset of the disease because the onset of SARDs (SARDs) in children or in the elderly often does not follow the clinical picture that is seen in adults. Third, classification criteria need to take into account genetic, racial, and geographic factors. It is becoming clear that the impact of geographic and ethnic variables have a significant impact on the spectrum of features seen in any of the SARDs. Classification criteria must take these variables into consideration to avoid a bias to a particular form of Scl in a given geographic setting. Fourth, diagnostic serology is rapidly moving to array technologies that provide a broad spectrum and wealth of AA, proteomic, genomic, and metabolomic data. In considering which AA might be included in a given classification criteria, it is important to recognize that the majority of SSc patients have more than one AA. While antibodies to CENP, topo I, and fibrillarin tend to be independent variables, the inclusion of other AAs such as PM/Scl or RNAP III will lead to a situation where a patient will have more than one AA. To avoid weighting the classification to serological markers, it will likely be useful to combine AA into a single criterion, an approach taken by Nadashkevich et al. (12). The rapidly emerging

TABLE 6.5. Challenges that must be considered in the inclusion of autoantibodies into classification criteria for systemic sclerosis.

- Divergence of classification criteria from diagnostic practice
- *Age*: Maybe one size (autoantibody) does not fit all
- Genetics/racial/geographic factors
- Early and late antibodies and response to therapy
- Impact of array technologies
  - Most SARD patients have >1 autoantibody
- Impact of the "omics":
  - genomics, ribonomics, proteomics, metabolomics leading to *Theranostics* or designer therapy
- Will disease classification survive as we know it?
- What about: protective, pathogenic, and prognostic autoantibodies
- Standardization

fields of genomics, proteomics, and metabolomics will also bring information to bear that has the potential to markedly improve classification criteria, especially if sub-classification into disease subsets is considered a desirable clinical parameter. The wealth of information provided by these technologies and their application to therapeutics in an expanding field of medicine referred to as "personalized medicine" and "theranostics" (20) raises the possibility that classification criteria may not survive if patients are subdivided into small clinical groups based on single-nucleotide polymorphisms (SNPs) and other genetic markers, cytokine, lymphokine, AA, and metabolite profiles. Last, despite enthusiasm for the potential role for including AA or any of the other biomarkers referred to above in classification criteria of the future, the daunting challenge of standardization looms large. At present, classification criteria of SARD that include AAs are threatened by the lack of standardization of reagents and the assays used to detect them. For example, the sensitivity and specificity of any AA result are highly dependent on the assay used and the reagents used to standardize that assay. Hence, if AAs and other biomarkers are going to become valid biomarkers in classification criteria, there needs to be a stronger and coordinated effort to standardize the reagents and kits used for their detection.

In summary, published classification and subclassification criteria reflect our evolving understanding of SSc pathogenesis. With the available evidence, several conclusions can be drawn regarding the requirements of updated criteria:

1. Differential clinical outcomes within the SSc spectrum emphasize the need for a set that provides some form of subclassification to guide outcome and future treatment options as well as allowing differentiation from other diseases.
2. It is likely that the degree of skin involvement will remain a major differentiating factor and the majority of survival evidence supports a two subset system.
3. AAs have been shown to provide additional important information regarding prognosis and may also guide in the identification of early disease.
4. Nailfold capillaroscopy has some utility in diagnosis and classification, but its application remains highly specialized. This will need careful consideration if it is to be incorporated into future classification criteria.
5. For widespread acceptance, there will need to be international consensus for testing of the criteria and also for standardization of diagnostic assays.

References

1. Walker JG, Pope J, Baron M, Leclercq S, Hudson M, Taillefer S, Edworthy SM, Nadashkevich O, Fritzler MJ. The development of systemic sclerosis classification criteria. *Clin Rheumatol* 2007; 26: 1401–1409.
2. Steen VD. Clinical manifestations of systemic sclerosis. *Semin Cutan Med Surg* 1998; 17: 48–54.
3. Mayes MD, Trojanowska M. Genetic factors in systemic sclerosis. *Arthritis Res Ther* 2007; 9 Suppl 2: S5.
4. Valentini G, Della Rossa A, Bombardieri S, Bencivelli W, Silman AJ, D'Angelo S, Cerinic MM, Belch JF, Black CM, Bruhlmann P, Czirják L, De Luca A, Drosos AA, Ferri C, Gabrielli A, Giacomelli R, Hayem G, Inanc M, McHugh NJ, Nielsen H, Rosada M, Scorza R, Stork J, Sysa A. European multicentre study to define disease activity criteria for systemic sclerosis. II. Identification of disease activity variables and development of preliminary activity indexes. *Ann Rheum Dis* 2001; 60: 592–598.
5. Walker JG, Fritzler MJ. Update on autoantibodies in systemic sclerosis. *Curr Opinion Rheum* 2007; 19: 580–591.
6. Santiago M, Baron M, Hudson M, Burlingame RW, The Canadian Scleroderma Research Group, Fritzler MJ. Antibodies to RNA polymerase III in systemic sclerosis as detected by an ELISA. *J Rheumatol* 2007; 34: 1528–1534.
7. Mahler M, Raijmakers R. Novel aspects of autoantibodies to the PM/Scl complex: clinical, genetic and diagnostic insights. *Autoimmun Rev* 2007; 6: 432–437.
8. Baroni SS, Santillo M, Bevilacqua F, Luchetti M, Spadoni T, Mancini M, Fraticelli P, Sambo P, Funaro A, Kazlauskas A, Avvedimento EV, Gabrielli A. Stimulatory autoantibodies to the PDGF receptor in systemic sclerosis. *N Engl J Med* 354: 2667–2676.
9. Walker JG, Barnabe C, Fritzler MJ. Autoantibodies, classification criteria and diagnosis of systemic autoimmune rheumatic diseases. In: Conrad K, Chan EKL, Fritzler MJ, Sack U, Shoenfeld Y, Wiik A (eds): *From Etiopathogenesis to the Prediction of Autoimmune Diseases: Relevance of Autoantibodies.* Lengerich, Germany, Pabst Science Publishers, 2007, pp. 352–369.
10. Masi AT, Rodnan GP, Medsger T, Jr., Altman RD, D'Angelo WA, Fries JF, LeRoy EC, Kirsner AB, Mackenzie AH, McShane DJ, Myers AR, Sharp GC. Preliminary criteria for the classification of systemic sclerosis (scleroderma). *Arthritis Rheum* 1980; 23: 581–590.
11. Lonzetti LS, Joyal F, Raynauld JP, Roussin A, Goulet JR, Rich E, Choquette D, Raymond Y, Senécal JL. Updating the American College of Rheumatology preliminary classification criteria for systemic sclerosis: addition of severe nailfold capillaroscopy abnormalities markedly increases the sensitivity for limited scleroderma. *Arthritis Rheum* 2001; 44: 735–736.
12. Nadashkevich O, Davis P, Fritzler MJ. A proposal of criteria for the classification of systemic sclerosis. *Medical Science Monitor* 2004; 10: 615–621.
13. Johnson SR, Feldman BM, Hawker GA. Classification criteria for Systemic Sclerosis subsets. *J Rheumatol* 2007; 34: 1855–1863.
14. LeRoy EC, Black C, Fleischmajer R, Jablonska S, Krieg T, Medsger TA, Rowell N, Wollheim F. Scleroderma (systemic sclerosis): classification, subsets and pathogenesis. *J Rheumatol* 1988; 15: 202–205.

15. LeRoy EC, Medsger TA, Jr. Criteria for the classification of early systemic sclerosis. *J Rheumatol* 2001; 28: 1573–1576.

16. Maricq HR, Valter I. A working classification of scleroderma spectrum disorders: A proposal and the results of testing on a sample of patients. *Clin Exp Rheumatol* 2004; 22: S5–S13.

17. Fritzler MJ. Advances and applications of multiplexed diagnostic technologies in autoimmune diseases. *Lupus* 2006; 15: 422–427.

18. Dazzi F, van Laar JM, Cope A, Tyndall A. Cell therapy for autoimmune diseases. *Arthritis Res Ther* 2007; 9: 206.

19. Denton CP. Therapeutic targets in systemic sclerosis. *Arthritis Res Ther* 2007; 9 Suppl. 2: S6.

20. Bissonnette L, Bergeron MG. Next revolution in the molecular theranostics of infectious diseases: microfabricated systems for personalized medicine. *Expert Rev Mol Diagn* 2006; 6: 433–450.

7
Sjögren Syndrome

Dimitris Mitsias and Haralampos M. Moutsopoulos

Abstract   Sjögren syndrome (SS) is a slowly progressive autoimmune disease that affects mainly exocrine glands and extraglandular epithelial tissues (autoimmune epithelitis). It may present alone (primary SS) or in association with another autoimmune disease (mainly systemic lupus erythematosus or rheumatoid arthritis – secondary SS). Criteria have been proposed for the correct classification of patients and are based on the main diagnostic tools for SS diagnosis. Herein, after a brief description of SS pathophysiology, these criteria are extensively discussed.

Keywords   Sjögren syndrome · autoimmune epithelitis · classification criteria · autoantibodies · salivary gland biopsy

Description

Sjögren syndrome (SS) is an ideal model for autoimmunity studies since it combines both organ specific and systemic characteristics. The main targets of autoimmune aggression are the exocrine salivary and lacrimal glands. It presents mainly with xerostomia and keratoconjunctivitis sicca (KCS). It may occur at any age, but it affects mainly women (at a ratio of 9:1) at theirs forty to fifties. It is one of the most common autoimmune diseases with a mean prevalence rate of approximately 1% of the total female population. Genetic predisposition, marked by specific HLA antigens, plus environmental factors (including a probable viral infection, stress and/or other psychological and hormonal factors) interplay in order to make SS clinically evident.

SS is a slowly progressive disease with benign course and minimal mortality. Exception to this rule is the evolution of a well-tolerated lymphoid growth to overt lymphoma (commonly of B cell origin) a development that occurs in approximately 5% of patients. Fortunately, adverse prognostic factors exist and can be early traced upon; these are palpable purpura, hypocomplementemia (low C4) and type II cryoglobulinemia (1) (Table 7.1 and Figure 7.1). The striking difference in the two outcomes has led to the perception of two types of SS – type I with increased probability of lymphoma development and type II without adverse outcomes.

Apart from sicca symptoms, SS manifestations may be extraglandular and non-specific in nature (2) (Figure 7.2).

What should be noted is the fact that the epithelial tissues are the targets of autoaggression irrespective if the organs are the exocrine glands or the kidneys, the lungs, the liver or the thyroid. This has led to coin the term "autoimmune epithelitis" and serves as a valuable guide to the research of SS pathophysiology (3).

The hallmark of SS is the lymphocytic infiltration of tissues. In the majority of cases, T cells predominate (elevated CD4+/CD8+ratio) while in other lesions B cells present in increased numbers. It is those lesions that seem most probable to progress in overt lymphoma in the future. Macrophages and dendritic cells are apparent mainly in lesions with ectopic germinal center formation. Interestingly, interleukin-18, most probably produced by CD68+ macrophages, seems to account for the increase of these cellular populations and a consequent enlargement of the salivary tissue (4). Finally, Foxp3+ T regulatory cells, up to a point follow the autoimmune aggression but in very heavy infiltrates drop in numbers (5). This is an important indication of a probable recession of tolerance mechanisms in heavy, long standing lesions.

B cell hyperactivity is evident by the circulation of increased levels of immunoglobulins and autoantibodies against specific ribonucleoprotein autoantigens, Ro/SS-A and La/SS-B. Anti-La are more specific but less sensitive for SS than anti-Ro since the latter are present in other autoimmune diseases, especially systemic lupus erythematosus (SLE). Other circulating antibodies include rheumatoid factor (RF) and anti-fodrin antibodies. Circulating cryoglobulins type II (monoclonal with rheumatoid

From: Y. Shoenfeld et al. (eds.): *Diagnostic Criteria in Autoimmune Diseases*, DOI: 10.1007/978-1-60327-285-8_7,

TABLE 7.1. Risk factors for lymphoma development in SS (2).

Clinical
   Persistent enlargement of parotid glands
   Splenomegaly
   Lymphadenopathy
   Palpable purpura
   Leg ulcers
Serologic
   Low levels of C4
   Mixed monoclonal (type II) cryoglobulinemia

(a)

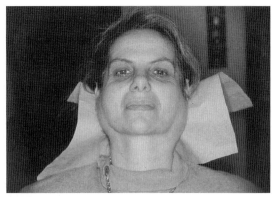

(b)

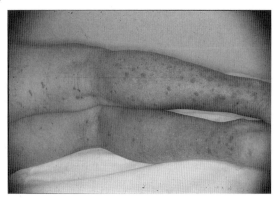

FIGURE 7.1. Persistent parotid gland enlargement (**a**) and palpable purpura (**b**) are two major clinical adverse prognostic factors for future lymphoma formation in SS patients.

factor activity) are observed in approximately 20% of the patients (Table 7.2). The latter, along with hypocomplementemia, is evident in patients with SS and systemic vasculitis, glomerulonephritis and B cell lymphoma. Antimitochondrial antibodies (AMA), along with increased transaminases and alkaline phosphatase, are evident in approximately 7% of SS patients with histologic evidence of primary biliary cirrhosis stage I (6). Circulating anti-thyroglobulin (anti-TG) and anti-thyroid peroxidase (anti-TPO) autoantibodies are present in a considerable

percentage of SS patients with concomitant Hashimoto thyroiditis (7) while the presence of anticentromere antibodies (ACA) correlates with lower incidence of parotid gland enlargement and anti-La antibodies (8). Finally, anti-DNA antibodies are positive in patients with SS-associated SLE, while antiphospholipid (a-PL) and antineutrophil cytoplasmic (ANCA) antibodies are the most frequent atypical antibodies in SS (9, 10).

Classification Criteria

SS may be the sole disease entity (primary SS) or come as sequelae of, or coexist with, another autoimmune disease, mainly SLE and rheumatoid arthritis (RA) (secondary SS). In an attempt to establish criteria for diagnosis that also serve as a common basis for research homogeneity and comparison of the results, after several revisions world's authorities have reached a consensus (11) (Table 7.3).

The first two criteria regard the subjective sicca symptoms, ocular (I) and oral (II), and are detected through the use of detailed questionnaire. A single positive response is sufficient for a criterion to be valid. The other four criteria identify objective signs and need a more detailed discussion.

Objective ocular involvement (III) is evident with the use of either Schirmer's test or Rose Bengal staining. The first quantifies tear secretion with the use of standardized paper strips placed beneath the inferior lid. The wetting of the paper is measured after 5 min and if found less than 5 mm, the test is considered positive. It is performed in unanaesthetized and closed eyes. The Rose Bengal test involves the staining of the corneal epithelium with this aniline, or other ocular, dye. Dry eyes result in KCS and therefore devitalized or damaged epithelium. After slit lamp examination these lesions are revealed and quantified by the van Bijsterveld scoring system; a score ≥ 4 is considered positive.

Objective oral (salivary) involvement (V) is ascertained if at least one of the following three tests is positive. First, whole salivary flow, without stimulation, is reduced in SS patients and if that is less than 1.5 ml in 15 min, the test is positive. The test should be performed with at least two hours avoidance of eating or smoking. Second, parotid sialography (radiographic method) reveals the presence of diffuse sialectasias without evidence of ductal obstruction. Third, salivary scintigraphy with the use of $^{99\,m}$Tc pertechnate is a functional study that estimates uptake and release of the substrate by the salivary glands 60 min after intravenous infusion. The test is positive in case of decreased concentration and/or delayed excretion of the tracer.

The presence of a positive histopathology (IV) and circulating autoantibodies against Ro/SS-A and/or La/SS-B (VI) are the two remaining, and probably most important,

FIGURE 7.2. Clinical manifestations (%) of primary SS, at diagnosis and at 10 years follow up period (1). Kidney involvement includes both interstitial nephritis (mainly) and glomerulonephritis, at a lesser extent. PGE: parotid gland enlargement, PN: peripheral neuropathy.

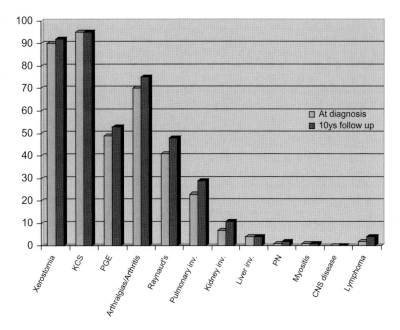

criteria. The minor labial salivary glands (MSG) are easily accessible and biopsies may be obtained with minimal discomfort for the patient. Evaluation of lymphocytic infiltration involves the number of lymphocytic foci (more than 50 cells), adjacent to normal appearing mucous acini, per $4\,mm^2$ of glandular tissue. If the focus score is ≥ 1, the biopsy is positive. However, due to increased discrepancies in the readings of biopsies (12) effort should be taken that expert oral pathologists are involved in the evaluation of the MSG tissues.

The aforementioned criteria were set forward by the European concerted action as early as 1993 (13). In 2002 the American-European consensus group reevaluated the classification for SS patients (11). According to these, a patient without any other potentially associated disease (see below) is classified as primary SS in case 4 out of 6 criteria are positive, *as long as* criteria IV or VI is positive.

TABLE 7.2. Laboratory findings in SS (6–10).

	Approximate %[a]
Anti-Ro/SS-A	>60
Anti-La/SS-B	40
Anti-PL	10–20
ANCA	10–20
ACA	5–10
Anti-DNA	5–10
AMA	7
Anti-TPO	11
Cryoglobulins	15–20

[a] Percentages displayed here are approximate since large variations are evident depending on technical and/or population heterogeneity.
ACA, anti-centromere; AMA, anti-mitochondrial; ANCA, anti-neutrophil cytoplasmic; Anti-PL, anti-phospholipid; Anti-TPO: anti-thyroid peroxidase antibodies.

Alternatively, a patient is also considered as primary SS if he fulfills 3 out of 4 objective (III to VI) criteria. The first set has a sensitivity of 89.5% and a specificity of 95.2%, while the second set has the same specificity and only slightly reduced sensitivity of 84.2%. A slightly lower accuracy was also evident for the second set, that is 90.5% versus 92.7% of the first set. However, any of the two sets can be used to classify primary SS patients.

As far as secondary SS is concerned, a patient with potentially associated disease (e.g. well defined SLE, RA etc.) has secondary SS in case any subjective criterion (I or II) *and* 2 out of III, IV and V are positive.

Of course, not all patients with sicca symptoms have SS and therefore, exclusion criteria are needed to avoid misdiagnosis and incorrect and/or unnecessary treatment. These include conditions like past head and neck irradiation, pre-existing lymphoma, chronic graft versus host disease (GVHD), use of anticholinergic drugs, sarcoidosis and viral infections. In regard to the latter, it is well known that HCV infection may present with chronic lymphocytic sialadenitis that mimics and is histologically hardly distinguishable to SS. The absence of HCV serologic titers and abnormal liver function tests as well as a substantially different target group aids to the distinction of the two entities. HIV infected patients may also present with sicca symptoms and parotid gland enlargement. In this case, the absence of anti-Ro and/or anti-La and the fact that the majority of infiltrating lymphocytes are CD8+ clarify the issue. Other viruses that have been linked to SS, in fact a possible etiopathogenic role is strongly suspected, are herpes viruses, HTLV-1 and most probably coxsackie viruses.

Non-lymphocytic infiltration of salivary glands may also produce clinical pictures resembling SS and include

TABLE 7.3. Revised international Classification criteria for SS (11).

I. Ocular symptoms: a positive response to at least one of the following questions:
  1. Have you had daily, persistent, troublesome dry eyes for more than 3 months?
  2. Do you have a recurrent sensation of sand or gravel in the eyes?
  3. Do you use tear substitutes more than 3 times a day?
II. Oral symptoms: a positive response to at least one of the following questions:
  1. Have you had a daily feeling of dry mouth for more than 3 months?
  2. Have you had recurrently or persistently swollen salivary glands as an adult?
  3. Do you frequently drink liquids to aid in swallowing dry food?
III. Ocular signs: objective evidence of ocular involvement defined as a positive result for at least one of the following two tests:
  1. Schirmer's I test, performed without anesthesia (<5 mm in 5 min)
  2. Rose bengal score or other ocular dye score (≥4 according to van Bijsterveld's scoring system)
IV. Histopathology: in minor salivary glands (obtained through normal-appearing mucosa) focal lymphocytic sialadenitis, evaluated by an expert histopathologist, with a focus score ≥1, defined as a number of lymphocytic foci (which are adjacent to normal-appearing mucous acini and contain more than 50 lymphocytes) per 4 mm^2 of glandular tissue
V. Salivary gland involvement: objective evidence of salivary gland involvement defined by a positive result for at least one of the following diagnostic tests:
  1. Unstimulated whole salivary flow (<1.5 ml in 15 min)
  2. Parotid sialography showing the presence of diffuse sialectasias (punctate, cavitary or destructive pattern), without evidence of obstruction in the major ducts
  3. Salivary scintigraphy showing delayed uptake, reduced concentration and/or delayed excretion of tracer
VI. Autoantibodies: presence in the serum of the following autoantibodies: Antibodies to Ro/SS-A or La/SS-B antigens, or both

Rules of classification
For primary SS
In patients without any potentially associated disease, primary SS may be defined as follows:
a. The presence of any 4 of the 6 items is indicative of primary SS, as long as eitheritem IV (Histopathology) or VI (Serology) is positive
b. The presence of any 3of the 4 objective criteria items (that is, items III, IV, V, VI)
For secondary SS
In patients with a potentially associated disease (for instance, another well defined connective tissue disease), the presence of item I or item II plus any 2 from among items III, IV, and V may be considered as indicative of secondary SS

---

granulomas (sarcoidosis, tuberculosis), amyloid (amyloidosis) and malignant cells (lymphoma, GVHD). Finally, metabolic disorders that may present with sicca symptoms include diabetes mellitus, lipoproteinemias (type II, IV and V) and hemochromatosis. All these entities should in any case be sought and taken into consideration in patients suspected of having SS.

Along with the establishment of the aforementioned criteria, the authors follow a classification tree that reveals with great sensitivity (96.1%) and specificity (94.2%) the SS diagnosis. We propose an algorithm for the workup needed for SS diagnosis (Figure 7.3).

Criticism/Discussion of Criteria

The criteria described are not without criticism. The need for the presence of subjective criteria is strongly argued due to exactly this clearly "subjective" nature of disease perception (14). It is also proposed that positivity of a criterion should lie not only to one diagnostic procedure but two so that specificity is maintained (15).

Herein, a few more points should be made. First, as expected, subjective symptoms and objective findings do not always correlate; in fact there is a wide dichotomy of subjective to objective manifestations especially in patients

over 55 years old (16). Second, apart from whole salivary flow, objective measurement of oral symptoms sparsely involves sialography or scintigraphy that are either invasive or require special instruments to be performed. However, in case one of these methods is needed to establish a firm diagnosis, MR sialography is the preferred imaging modality due to the higher specificity and positive predictive value (PPV) versus scintigraphy (17). The Ro/La antigenic system consists of three different proteins, namely Ro 52 kDa, Ro 60 kDa and La. Anti-La are more specific but less sensitive for SS compared to anti-Ro that are found in many other autoimmune diseases, especially SLE. In addition, the multiplicity of these antigens accounts in part for differences in laboratory methods of their measurement. Counter immuno-electrophoresis (CIE) is the most specific (100%) and sensitive (89%) method but ELISA based techniques are more widely used. The latter also have very high sensitivity and therefore, in order to have good PPV and avoid false positive results, only patients suspected of having SS should be tested (18). What should also be kept in mind is that the antibody levels do not correlate with disease activity and/or treatment due to fluctuation of their levels during disease progress (19). Finally, emphasis is given to the fact that these criteria are "classification" criteria and their purpose is to aid research and communication among scientists and not serve as a diagnostic tool.

FIGURE 7.3. Proposed algorithm for SS diagnosis.

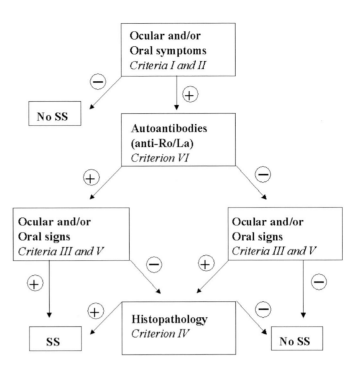

Therapy

There is no definite therapy for SS. The aim is to diminish the discomfort posed by glandular dysfunction, avoid possible complications and increase salivary secretion. To this end, xerostomia is managed with the use of saliva substitutes, intense oral hygiene and prevention of oral infections and periodontal disease. The cholinergic agents pilocarpine hydrochloride and cevimeline are frequently used to augment salivary and lacrimal secretion by the unaffected portions of the glands. Tear substitutes and ophthalmic gels are used on an as-needed basis to minimize KCS symptoms. The use of anticholinergic, diuretic, antihypertensive and antidepressive drugs should be discouraged since it decreases secretions.

The management of extraglandular manifestations needs more aggressive treatment. Arthralgias do well with hydroxychloroquine (200–400 mg/day) while small doses of corticosteroids (<7.5 mg/day of prednisolone) and/or methotrexate (up to 0.2 mg/kg of body weight weekly) can be used if frank arthritis is evident. Systemic vasculitis is managed as the idiopathic forms of vasculitis with cyclophosphamide (2 mg/kg of body weight/day) for 3–6 months followed by mycophenolate mofetil (2–3 gr/day). Finally lymphoma management consists of CHOP regimen (cyclophosphamide, doxorubicin, vincristine and prednisolone) along with anti-CD20 (rituximab) monoclonal antibodies. This combination has increased considerably the survival of SS patients with aggressive types of lymphoma (20).

References

1. Skopouli FN, Dafni U, Ioannidis JP, Moutsopoulos HM. Clinical evolution, and morbidity and mortality of primary Sjogren's syndrome. *Semin Arthritis Rheum* 2000; 29: 296–304.
2. Kassan SS, Moutsopoulos HM. Clinical manifestations and early diagnosis of Sjogren syndrome. *Arch Intern Med* 2004; 164: 1275–84.
3. Moutsopoulos HM. Sjogren's syndrome: autoimmune epithelitis. *Clin Immunol Immunopathol* 1994; 72:162–5.
4. Manoussakis MN, Boiu S, Korkolopoulou P, Kapsogeorgou EK, Kavantzas N, Ziakas P, Patsouris E, Moutsopoulos HM. Rates of infiltration by macrophages and dendritic cells and expression of interleukin-18 and interleukin-12 in the chronic inflammatory lesions of Sjögren's syndrome: correlation with certain features of immune hyperactivity and factors associated with high risk of lymphoma development. *Arthritis Rheum* 2007;56:3977–88.
5. Christodoulou MI, Kapsogeorgou EK, Moutsopoulos NM, Moutsopoulos HM. Foxp3+ T regulatory cells in the autoimmune lesions of Sjögren's syndrome: Correlation with the number of the infiltrating dendtritic cells and macrophages. *Arthritis Rheum* 2007;55:9(suppl)
6. Skopouli FN, Barbatis C, Moutsopoulos HM. Liver involvement in primary Sjogren's syndrome. *Br J Rheumatol* 1994; 33: 745–8.
7. D'Arbonneau F, Ansart S, Le Berre R, Dueymes M, Youinou P, Pennec YL. Thyroid dysfunction in primary Sjogren's syndrome: a long-term followup study. *Arthritis Rheum* 2003; 49: 804–9.
8. Vlachoyiannopoulos PG, Drosos AA, Wiik A, Moutsopoulos HM. Patients with anticentromere antibodies, clinical features, diagnoses and evolution. *Br J Rheumatol*; 32: 297–301.

9. Soliotis FC, Moutsopoulos HM. Sjogren's syndrome. Autoimmunity 2004; 37: 305–7.

10. Ramos-Casals M, Brito-Zeron P, Font J. The overlap of Sjogren's syndrome with other systemic autoimmune diseases. *Semin Arthritis Rheum* 2007; 36: 246–55.

11. Vitali C, Bombardieri S, Jonsson R, Moutsopoulos HM, Alexander EL, Carsons SE, Daniels TE, Fox PC, Fox RI, Kassan SS, Pillemer SR, Talal N, Weisman MH, European Study Group on Classification Criteria for Sjogren's Syndrome. Classification criteria for Sjogren's syndrome: A revised version of the European criteria proposed by the American-European Consensus Group. *Ann Rheum Dis* 2002; 61: 554–8.

12. Vivino FB, Gala I, Hermann GA. Change in final diagnosis on second evaluation of labial minor salivary gland biopsies. *J Rheumatol* 2002; 29: 938–44.

13. Vitali C, Bombardieri S, Moutsopoulos HM, Balestrieri G, Bencivelli W, Bernstein RM, Bjerrum KB, Braga S, Coll J, de Vita S, et al. Preliminary criteria for the classification of Sjogren's syndrome. Results of a prospective concerted action supported by the European Community. *Arthritis Rheum* 1993; 36: 340–7.

14. Fujibayashi T, Sugai S, Miyasaka N, Tojo T, Miyawaki S, Ichikawa Y, et al. Criteria for the diagnosis of Sjögren's syndrome (Japanese criteria III). Supported by the Ministry of Health and Welfare of Japan. In: 1999 Annual reports of research group of autoimmune disease. 1999, 135–8. (In Japanese. English version to be published.)

15. Manthorpe R. Sjogren's syndrome criteria. *Ann Rheum Dis* 2002; 61: 482–4.

16. Hay EM, Thomas E, Pal B, Hajeer A, Chambers H, Silman AJ. Weak association between subjective symptoms or and objective testing for dry eyes and dry mouth: results from a population based study. *Ann Rheum Dis* 1998; 57: 20–4.

17. Tonami H, Higashi K, Matoba M, Yokota H, Yamamoto I, Sugai S. A comparative study between MR sialography and salivary gland scintigraphy in the diagnosis of Sjogren syndrome. *J Comput Assist Tomogr* 2001; 25: 262–8.

18. Franceschini F, Cavazzana I. Anti-Ro/SSA and La/SSB antibodies. *Autoimmunity* 2005; 38: 55–63.

19. Praprotnik S, Bozic B, Kveder T, Rozman B. Fluctuation of anti-Ro/SS-A antibody levels in patients with systemic lupus erythematosus and Sjogren's syndrome: a prospective study. *Clin Exp Rheumatol* 1999; 17: 63–8.

20. Mavragani CP, Moutsopoulos NM, Moutsopoulos HM. The management of Sjogren's syndrome. *Nat Clin Pract Rheumatol* 2006; 2: 252–61.

8
Mixed Connective Tissue Disease

Marta Mosca, Rosaria Talarico and Stefano Bombardieri

Abstract   Mixed connective tissue disease (MCTD) is a condition characterized by the overlap of features of systemic lupus erythematosus (SLE), systemic sclerosis (SSc) and polydermatomyositis (PM/DM) in association with high titers of antibodies against a ribonuclear protein (RNP). Clinical manifestations of MCTD are extremely variable and disease onset may be undifferentiated.

Raynaud phenomenon, swollen fingers, arthritis, myositis, esophageal dysfunction and pulmonary hypertension represent the most frequent clinical manifestations. In the original description, MCTD was described as benign conditions characterized by the absence of renal and neurological manifestations and a good response to corticosteroid therapy. This observation has not been confirmed by studies that have shown that one-third of MCTD patients have a severe disease and require corticosteroid and immunosuppressive therapy. The major cause of death in these patients is pulmonary hypertension, followed by infections.

A debate is still open on whether MCTD represent a distinct clinical entity or rather an overall between different established connective tissue diseases (CTDs). The answer to this question might become clear as more data on disease pathogenesis will be known.

Keywords   Mixed connective tissue disease · classification criteria · anti-U1RNP antibodies

Introduction

Mixed connective tissue disease (MCTD) was first described by Sharp in 1972 as a condition characterized by the overlap of features of systemic lupus erythematosus (SLE), systemic sclerosis (SSc) and polydermatomyositis (PM/DM) in association with high titers of antibodies against a ribonuclear protein (RNP) (1). A debate is still open on whether MCTD constitutes a distinct clinical entity or rather represents the overlap of well-defined conditions or a "bridge" between different connective tissue diseases (CTDs) within the spectrum of systemic autoimmunity (2, 3).

Clinical Manifestations

The clinical manifestations of MCTD at onset and during the follow-up are reported in Table 8.1. The onset of MCTD is variable and is often characterized by the presence of Raynaud phenomenon or arthritis (4, 5, 6, 7).

Raynaud phenomenon is observed in up to 90% of patients and is included in all the different classification criteria. Half of the patients have nailfold capillary changes similar to those found in SSc (8).

Joint involvement is common and is characterized by symmetric arthritis of hands and wrists. In 20% of the patients, an erosive arthritis as well as a tendency to develop Jaccoud arthritis has been observed (4, 5).

Infrequent at disease onset, myositis is observed in up to 70% of the patients during the follow-up. Muscle involvement in MCTD seems less severe than that of PM/DM and more responsive to therapy. Histologically, myositis in MCTD resembles DM more closely. Many patients present with diffuse myalgias, which should be distinguished form myositis (4, 5, 6, 9).

Pulmonary involvement is primarily represented by pulmonary hypertension, which is the primary cause of death in these patients (10, 11, 12). Pulmonary hypertension appears to be correlated with the presence of vasculopathy of pulmonary arteries rather than interstitial lung disease. Interstitial lung disease may also be observed; in a recent study of 144 MCTD patients, chest X rays were abnormal in 91% of patients, of whom 66.6% had active interstitial lung disease detected by high-resolution computed tomography (HRCT) (11).

From: Y. Shoenfeld et al. (eds.): *Diagnostic Criteria in Autoimmune Diseases*, DOI: 10.1007/978-1-60327-285-8_8,
© 2008 Humana Press, Totowa, NJ

TABLE 8.1. Clinical manifestations of mixed connective tissue disease (MCTD) patients at onset and during the disease course.

	At onset (%)	Cumulative (%)
Raynaud's phenomenon	74	90–96
Arthritis/arthralgias	68	95–96; erosions 20
Esophageal dysfunction	9	66–80
Pulmonary dysfunction	0	66–75
Swollen hands	45	66–75
Sclerodactily	11	40–50
Myositis	2	25–51
Skin rash	13	50–53
Leukopenia	9	53
Pleuritis/pericarditis	19	30–43
Pulmonary hypertension	0	23–30
Diffuse sclerosis	0	19
Nervous system disease	2	15–17
Renal disease	0	10–11

Two-thirds of MCTD patients develop swollen hands with sausage fingers, and some patients develop sclerodactily; however, an extensive skin sclerosis seems rare. Other cutaneous manifestations are represented by skin rashes similar to subacute or discoid cutaneous lupus or DM (Gottron papules and heliotrope rash). Some patients may also present livedo reticularis and telangectasias (4, 5, 6).

Esophageal dysfunction has been observed in up to 75% of patients, but may be asymptomatic. Dysphagia has been reported in average 38% of patients (4, 5, 6).

The most frequent form of cardiac involvement is pericarditis, which usually does not cause tamponade. In a study of 16 MCTD patients, noninvasive assessment showed evidence of cardiac abnormalities in 38% of patients and evidence of pericarditis in 25% of patients (13).

Renal involvement is not frequent; renal manifestations include glomerulonephritis, nephrotic syndrome and scleroderma renal crisis. Mesangial and membranoproliferative lesions have been observed. Neurological involvement is rare and is represented by trigeminal nevralgia and vascular headache. Hematological manifestations are represented by cytopenias, particularly leukopenia and thrombocytopenia (4, 5, 6).

Histologically, MCTD is characterized by a widespread vasculopathy that may involve small- and medium-sized vessels. This vasculopathy differs from that observed in SSc as it is less associated with fibrosis and presents immunoglobulin and complement deposits in the vessel walls (4).

Laboratory Abnormalities

MCTD is associated with the presence of high titers of anti-U1RNP antibodies specifically directed against the proteins A, C or 70K complexed with U1RNA (1, 3, 5, 7, 14). Anti-RNP antibodies, however, are not specific for MCTD as they are observed in other CTDs also such as SLE, rheumatoid arthritis (RA) and SSc. Although anti-U1RNP antibodies are crucial for the classification of MCTD, their pathogenetic role in the development of the disease has not been established yet.

Anti-Ro, anti-La and anti-phospholipid antibodies have also been described in MCTD patients with lower frequency.

HLA Type and MCTD

Different studies have shown an association between MCTD and the specific HLA haplotype HLA DR4 (3, 15, 16). In a study comparing MCTD patients, SLE patients and healthy controls, HLA DRw4 was observed in 45% of MCTD patients, 14 of SLE patients and 18% of controls (15). Some authors have suggested the presence of an association between HLA DR4 and the occurrence of erosive arthritis in MCTD patients.

Prognosis

In the original description by Sharp and colleagues, MCTD was described as a rather benign condition characterized by a good response to corticosteroid therapy (1). However, further follow-up of the originally described patients and long-term data on other cohorts of patients have not confirmed this description (4, 5, 17, 18). In a study assessing the long-term outcome of 47 MCTD patients, 38% had continued active disease requiring corticosteroid or immunosuppresive therapy or had died (4). It has been estimated that about one-third of MCTD patients have a favorable outcome, one-third have a more aggressive disease, and the remaining have a good outcome but require continuous therapy with either corticosteroids or immunsuppressive drugs.

The main causes of death in MCTD patients are represented by pulmonary hypertension, respiratory insufficiency, heart failure and infections.

Diagnostic Criteria

Three different sets of classification criteria for MCTD have been validated and are used in the literature (Table 8.2) (1, 19, 20). The original Sharp criteria have been found to have a high sensitivity, but a low specificity. The sensitivity of Alarcon-Segovia criteria varies between 62 and 96% with a high specificity (86–96%), similarto Kasukawa criteria (88% sensitivity and 65.5–87% specificity). Alarcon-Segovia criteria appear the best classification criteria for MCTD (21, 22).

TABLE 8.2. Three different sets of classification criteria for mixed connective tissue disease (MCTD).

Sharp et al. 1972	Alarcon-Segovia et al.	Kasukawa et al.
Major	Serologic	Common symptoms
Myositis, severe	Anti-U1 RNP hemagglutination	Raynaud's phenomenon
Pulmonary involvement	titer ≥ 1:1600	Swollen fingers or hands
Raynaud's phenomenon	Clinical	Anti-RNP antibodies
Swollen hands or sclerodactily	Edema of the hands	Mixed symptoms
Anti-ENA ≥1:10,000 and anti-U1RNP	Synovitis	1. SLE-like features
positive and anti-Sm negative	Myositis	polyarthritis
Minor	Raynaud's phenomenon	lymphadenopathy
Alopecia	acrosclerosis	facial erythema
Leukopenia		pericarditis or pleuritis
Anemia		leuko-thrombocytopenia
Pleuritis		2. SSc-like symptoms
Pericarditis		sclerodactily
Arthritis		pulmonary fibrosis, restrictive changes of lung,
Trigeminal neuropathy		reduced diffusion capacity
Malar rash		hypomotility or dilatation capacity
Thrombocytopenia		3. PM-like findings
Mild myositis		muscle weakness
History of swollen hands		elevated serum levels of muscle enzymes
		Myogenic alterations on EMG
Anti-U1RNP antibodies titer ≥1:4000 AND at least 4 major criteria or anti-U1RNP antibodies titer ≥ 1:1000 AND 2 major criteria among 1,2, 3 AND 2 minor criteria	Serological criteria AND at least 3 clinical criteria, including myositis or synovitis	Anti-U1-RNP AND 1 of the 2 common symptoms AND 1 or more of the mixed symptoms in at least 2 categories

Is MCTD a Distinct Clinical Entity?

Since its description debate still exists on whether MCTD represents a distinct clinical entity or the overlap between other CTDs. Some authors have proposed to consider MCTD as an undifferentiated condition waiting to evolve to more definite CTD (2, 3).

The criticisms to the concept of MCTD are the following: (a) MCTD is not the benign condition initially described, (b) patients may be diagnosed as having other CTD or will develop other CTD during the follow-up, (c) anti-U1RNP antibodies can be observed in other CTD also, (4) the clinical picture of MCTD has been observed in the absence of anti-U1RNP antibodies also, and (5) there are no data suggesting a pathogenetic role for anti-U1RNP antibodies.

Nevertheless, it is certain that MCTDs have peculiar clinical, serological, histological and genetic features. Whether these are sufficient to constitute a distinct clinical entity is difficult to define and probably only a better understanding of pathogenesis and etiology of autoimmune diseases might help in solving this issue (6).

References

1. Sharp GC, Irvin WS, Tan EM, Gould RG, Holman HR. Mixed connective tissue disease – an apparently distinct rheumatic disease syndrome associated with a specific antibody to an extractable nuclear antigen (ENA). *Am J Med* 1972 ; 52: 148–159.

2. Aringer M, Steiner G, Smolen JS. Does mixed connective tissue disease exist? Yes. *Rheum Dis Clin North Am* 2005; 31: 411–420.

3. Swanton J, Isenberg D. Mixed connective tissue disease: still crazy after all these years. *Rheum Dis Clin North Am* 2005; 31: 421–436.

4. Burdt MA, Hoffman RW, Deutscher SL, Wang GS, Johnson JC, Sharp GC. Long term outcome in mixed connective tissue disease. Longitudinal clinical and serologic findings. *Arthritis Rheum* 1999; 42: 899–909.

5. Lundberg I, Hedfors E. Clinical course of patients with anti-RNP antibodies. A prospective study of 32 patients. *J Rheumatol* 1991; 18: 1511–1519.

6. Maddison PJ. Mixed connective tissue disease: overlap syndromes. *Baillieres Clin Rheumatol* 2000; 14: 111–124.

7. Kasukawa R. Mixed connective tissue disease. *Internal Med* 1999; 38: 386–393.

8. Grader-Beck T, Wigley FM. Raynaud's phenomenon in mixed connective tissue disease. *Rheum Dis Clin North Am* 2005; 31: 465–481.

9. Hall S, Hanrahan P. Muscle involvement in mixed connective tissue disease. *Rheum Dis Clin North Am* 2005; 31: 509–517.

10. Bull TM, Fagan KA, Badesch DB. Pulmonary vascular manifestations of mixed connective tissue disease. *Rheum Dis Clin North Am* 2005; 31: 451–464.

11. Bodolay E, Szekanecz Z, Devenyi K, et al. Evaluation of lung disease in mixed connective tissue disease (MCTD). *Rheumatology* 2005; 44: 656–661.

12. Vegh J, Szodoray P, Kappelmayer J, Csipo I, Udvardy M, Lakos G, et al. Clinical and immunoserological characteristics of mixed connective tissue disease associated with pulmonary arterial hypertension. *Scan J Immunol* 2006; 64: 69–76.

13. Oetgen WJ, Mutter ML, Lawless OJ, Davia JE. Cardiac abnormalities in mixed connective tissue disease. *Chest* 1983; 83: 185–188.

14. Greidiger EL, Hoffman RW. Autoantibodies in the pathogenesis of MCTD. *Rheum Dis Clin North Am* 2005; 31: 437–450.

15. Ruuska P, Hameenkorpi R, Forsberg S, et al. Differences in HLA antigens between patients with mixed connective tissue disease and systemic lupus erythematosus. *Ann Rheum Dis* 1992; 51: 52–55.

16. Gendi NST, Welsh KI, Van Venrooij WJ, Vancheeswaran R, Gilroy J, Black CM. HLA type as predictor of mixed connective tissue disease differentiation. *Arthritis Rheum* 1005; 38: 259–266.

17. Nimelstein SH, Brody S, McShane D, Holman NR. Mixed connective tissue disease: a subsequent evaluation of the original 25 patients. *Medicine* 1980; 59: 239–248.

18. Lundberg IE. The prognosis of mixed connective tissue disease. *Rheum Dis Clin North Am* 2005; 31: 535–547.

19. Kasukawa R, Tojo T, Miyawaki S. Preliminary diagnostic criteria for classification of MCTD. Kasukawa R, Sharp GC eds. *Mixed Connective Tissue Diseases*. Amsterdam: Elsevier, 1987: pp. 23–32.

20. Alarcon-Segovia D, Villareal M. Classification and diagnostic criteria for mixed connective tissue diseases. In: Mixed Connective Tissue Diseases and Antinuclear Antibodies. Kasukawa R, Sharp GC. Amsterdam: Elsevier, 1987: pp. 23–32.

21. Amigues JM, Cantagrel A, Abbal M, and Mazieres B. Comparative study of 4 diagnosis sets for mixed connective tissue disease in patients with anti-rnp antibodies. *J Rheumatol* 1998; 25: 2055–2062.

22. Alarcon-Segovia D and Cardiel MH. Comparison between 3 diagnostic criteria for mixed connective tissue disease. *J Rheumatol* 1898; 16: 328–334.

9
Relapsing Polychondritis

Mauro Galeazzi and Giovanni Porciello

Abstract   Relapsing polychondritis (RP) is a systemic autoimmune disorder characterized by episodic and progressive inflammatory disease most commonly presenting as inflammation of the cartilage of the ears, nose, tracheobronchial tree and joints. The course of RP varies from a low-grade, mild condition up to a fulminating and rapidly progressive disease. Spontaneous remissions are common.

This chapter also summarizes important aspects of the disease with a focus on diagnostics criteria. In fact, over the years, three sets of diagnostic criteria for RP have been proposed by McAdam, Damiani and Levine, and Michet, respectively. Although these criteria have not been re-examined by consensus group members and despite the lack of validation, these show high affordability in discriminating patients affected by RP in every day clinical practice.

In conclusion, for achieving reliable classification criteria that would also be useful for the diagnosis of RP, more extensive multicenter studies are needed.

Keywords   Relapsing Polychondritis · classification criteria · diagnosis

Relapsing Polychondritis

Relapsing polychondritis (RP) is an episodic and progressive inflammatory disease most commonly presenting as inflammation of the cartilage of the ears, nose, tracheobronchial tree and joints.

Epidemiology

RP is most commonly reported in whites, begins between the age of 20 and 60 years, with a peak in the 40 s. The annual incidence has been estimated as 3.5 cases per million (1). The male-to-female ratio appears to be equal in some series of cases, but Trentham reported a ratio of 3:1 (2).

History

In 1923, Kaksch-Wartenhorst described the first clinical picture of RP as "polychondropathia" (3). The disease also has been called chondromalacia, diffuse perichondritis, chronic atrophic polychondritis, diffuse chondrolysis and dyschondroplasia. The term *relapsing polychondritis* was first introduced in 1960 by Pearson et al., who described a rare condition characterized by *relapsing* inflammatory disease of cartilagineous structures (4).

Pathogenesis

Although the etiology of RP remains unknown, the pathogenesis seems to be an immunologic reaction to type II collagen present in the cartilage and in the sclera of the eye. Patients with RP have demonstrated both autoantibodies and cellular immune reaction to type II, IX and XI collagen. Immunofluorescence studies of affected cartilage have shown granule deposits of immunoglobulin and complement, suggesting the presence of immune complexes. Most recently, an increase in HLA-DR4 antigen was detected in patients with RP, suggesting a genetic predisposition for the disease (5, 6).

From: Y. Shoenfeld et al. (eds.), *Diagnostic Criteria in Autoimmune Diseases*, DOI: 10.1007/978-1-60327-285-8_9,
© 2008 Humana Press, Totowa, NJ

TABLE 9.1. Clinical features of relapsing polychondritis (7).

Feature	Presenting (%)	Cumulative (%)
Auricular chondritis	43	89
Arthritis	32	72
Nasal chondritis	21	61
Ocular inflammation	18	59
Layngotraceal symptoms	23	55
Reduced hearing	7	40
Vestibular dysfunction	4	28 no study by McAdam
Microhematuria	15	26 only study by Michet
Saddle nose deformity	11	25 no study by McAdam
Cutaneous	4	25 no study by McAdam
Laryngotracheal stricture	15	23 only study by Michet
Vasculitis	2	14 no study by McAdam
Elevated creatinine	7	13 only study by Michet
Aortic or mitral regurgitation	0	12 no study by McAdam
Aneurysm	0	4 only study by Michet

Data derived from three large case series and reviews (2: *n 66*; 10: *n 112*; 11: *n 159* = 337 patients).

Clinical Manifestations

The clinical features of RP are illustrated in Table 9.1 (7).

–   Auricular chondritis and arthritis are the most common presenting signs, characterized respectively by the pain, swelling, redness of the cartilaginous portion of the external ear and oligo or polyarthritis. The arthritis is intermittent, migratory, asymmetric, seronegative and generally nonerosive.

Conductive hearing loss can result from stenosis of the auditory canal, otitis media or Eustachian tube chondritis. Sudden onset of vertigo and hearing loss may occur owing to involvement of the vasculitis of the auditory artery. Chondritis of nasal cartilage, laryngeal and tracheobronchial tract may result in collapse nasal cartilage (saddle nose deformity), choking sensation, cough, stridor, respiratory obstruction with high morbidity and mortality. Secondary infections of the respiratory tract are also common in patients with severe airway involvement.

–   Ocular inflammation occurs in 60% of patients. Common presentations are scleritis, episcleritis, conjunctivitis, iritis, keratitis, optic neuritis, retinopathy and corneal melt. Less common are orbital pseudotumor, extraocular muscle palsy and lid edema.
–   Dermatologic involvement is frequent during the course of the disease. Oral ulcers are the most commonly mucocutaneous lesion, followed by erythema nodosum, purpura, pustules, superficial phlebitis, livedo reticularis and limb ulcerations.
–   Cardiovascular involvement in RP includes aortites, pericarditis, aortic and mitral regurgitation, cardiac ischemia and complete heart block. Vascular involvement of large vessels may present as thoracic and abdominal aneurysm, thrombophlebitis and arterial thrombosis due to vasculitis or coagulopathy.

–   Renal involvement in RP is not frequent and includes mesangial expansion, IgA nephropathy, tubulointerstitial nephritis and segmental necrotizing crescentic glomerulonephritis (2, 8, 9,10, 11).
–   Neurologic manifestations in RP occur in approximately 3% of patients and most commonly involve cranial nerves II, III, IV, VI, VII and VIII. Cerebral vasculitis, headaches, cerebral aneurism, thromboencephalitis, confusion and seizures have been also described.
–   Associated disorders: More than 30% of patients with RP have a rheumatological or hematological disease such as systemic lupus erythematosus, rheumatoid arthritis, systemic sclerosis, Sjögren syndrome, Behçet's disease, Wegener's granulomatosis, Churg–Strauss syndrome, cryoglobulinemia, dysmyelopoietic syndrome, Hodgkins and non-Hodgkins lymphoma and chronic myelomonocytic leukaemia. In most cases, the associated disorders precede the onset of RP by several months or years. Because of the myriad of disease associations, it has been proposed that the RP be thought of as a syndrome, which can be primary or secondary (10, 12, 13, 14, 15).

Biochemical Features

The laboratory tests are nonspecific and helpful only when they serve to exclude other conditions or associated disorders to RP. The findings are only an elevated erythrocyte sedimentation rate during active disease, moderate leukocytosis and mild anemia typical of chronic disease. Antibodies to collagen types II, IX and XI can be detected in one-third of patients, but such antibodies can be found in other rheumatologic conditions and have limited diagnostic value because of relatively low specificity. Anti-collagen type II antibodies are found in the acute phase of RP, and their serum levels seem to correlate with disease severity (5), but Trentham reports that this antibody does not correlate with disease activity or severity (2).

Occasionally, patients may have positive antinuclear antibodies (ANAs), rheumatoid factor, anti-native DNA, anti-neutrophil cytoplasm antibodies, and cryoglobulins, but these patients may have overlaps with other autoimmune disease.

Pathological Features

No biopsy finding is pathognomonic for RP; therefore, biopsy is not necessary because the diagnosis is based on clinical features. Histologically, RP is characterized by perichondrial inflammation that involves mainly lymphocytes, but neutrophils may be predominant in early lesions. Granulation tissue or fibrosis, and calcification or ossification may be found (8). Immunoflorescence studies may show the presence of immunoglobulins and C3 deposits along the chondrofibrous junction and in perichondral vessel walls.

Diagnostic Criteria

Diagnostic criteria (Table 9.2) for RP were described by McAdam et al. in 1976 (8), Damiani and Levine in 1979 (16), and Michet et al. in 1986 (9). These three sets of criteria are currently used by several authors for the diagnosis of RP because they are considered complementary to each other instead of antithetic.

The diagnostic criteria of McAdam et al. require at least three of the six following criteria: bilateral auricular chondritis, nonerosive inflammatory polyarthritis, nasal chondritis, ocular inflammation, respiratory tract chondritis, and cochlear or vestibular dysfunction.

Biopsy is not necessary in the presence of a typical clinical presentation. If the clinical presentation is uncertain, histological examination can exclude other causes of chondritis, such as bacterial infections, syphilis, leprosy, fungal invasion and overlap vasculitis.

The diagnostic criteria of Damiani and Levine require only one of following three criteria:

—   at least three of McAdam's criteria with nonhistological confirmation
—   one or more of McAdam's criteria with histological confirmation
—   chondritis in two or more separate anatomical locations with response to steroids and/or dapsone.

The diagnostic criteria of Michet et al. require only one of following two criteria:

—   inflammatory episodes involving at least two of these sites: auricular, nasal and laryngotracheal cartilages
—   one of the earlier mentioned sites and two other manifestations, including ocular inflammation, hearing loss, vestibular dysfunction or seronegative inflammatory arthritis. These criteria overlap with the prior.

Criticism on the Diagnostics Criteria

The three sets of criteria mentioned earlier are useful for diagnostic purposes, but they have never been officially validated mainly for four reasons:

1) these criteria have been empirically defined on the basis of the personal experience of each author without a larger international consensus of experts;
2) the three studies lack a control group; this is not methodologically correct and does not even allow to build a classification tree or to perform a statistical analysis for the validation of classification criteria;
3) specificity, sensitivity, diagnostic accuracy and positive and negative predictive values have never been calculated for the absence of adequate control groups.

TABLE 9.2. Diagnostic criteria for relapsing polychondritis.

Author	Criteria	Required	Total
McAdam et al. (8)	1) Recurrent chondritis of both auricles	3	6
	2) Nonerosive inflammatory polyarthritis		
	3) Chondritis of nasal cartilage		
	4) Inflammation of ocular structures including conjunctivitis, keratitis, scleritis/episcleritis and uveitis		
	5) Chondritis of the respiratory tract involving laryngeal and tracheal cartilages		
	6) Cochlear or vestibular damage manifested by neurosensory hearing loss, tinnitus and vertigo.		
Damiani and Levine (16)	1) At least three of McAdam's criteria	1	3
	2) One or more of McAdam's criteria and positive histology.		
	3) Chondritis in two or more separate anatomical locations with response to steroids and/or dapsone.		
Michet et al. (9)	1) Inflammatory episodes involving at least two of three sites: auricular, nasal or laryngotracheal cartilage	1	2
	2) One of those sites and two other manifestations, including ocular inflammation, vestibular dysfunction, seronegative arthritis and hearing loss		

Furthermore, the lack of controls does not even allow an "a posteriori" statistical evaluation of these parameters;

4) the criteria proposed by Damiani and Michet are substantially based on those elaborated by McAdam; therefore they have a selection bias determined by both a single author's experience and, again, a lack of control group.

Nevertheless, despite the lack of validation, these criteria show high affordability in discriminating patients affected by RP. In fact, some of criteria such as auricular chondritis, saddle nose deformity and laryngeal chondritis are very frequent in RP while they are absent or not so frequent in other conditions. In fact RP shares several signs and symptoms with other systemic diseases that should be considered in differential diagnosis. Diseases that must be considered in the differential diagnosis include polyarterite nodosa, Cogan's syndrome, Behçet's disease, sarcoidosis, rheumatoid arthritis and Takayasu syndrome where auricular, nasal and laringeal chondritis have never been reported. In any case, and especially in controversial cases, cartilage biopsy has been demonstrated to be a determinant for the differential diagnosis with other forms of chondritis, including infection chondritis sustained by leprosy, Syphilis, Streptococcus, Pseudomonas, traumatic chondritis, neoplastic chondritis such as natural Killer lymphoma and various malignancies and vasculitis chondritis which include those seen in Wegener's granulomatosis where saddle nose deformity is frequent.

Prognosis

The course of RP varies from a low-grade, mild condition up to fulminating and rapidly progressive disease. Spontaneous remissions are common. The survival rate is 74% at 5 years and 55% at 10 years in the study of Michet, but Trentham in 1988 reported a 94% survival rate and average disease duration of 8 years. Common causes of death are pulmonary infection, airway collapse, systemic vasculitis and glomerulonephrits. Factors predictive of the severity of the disease and fatalities are anemia, saddle nose deformity, vasculitis, arthritis, laryngotracheal strictures and hematuria at the time of diagnosis (2, 9).

Therapy

A standardized therapeutic protocol for RP has not been established because the disease is rare.

Nonsteroidal anti-inflammatory drugs, dapsone and/or colchicine have been used in mild polychondritis limited to arthralgia and nasal or auricular chondritis with benefits. Dapsone is often first used for the systemic manifestations of RP in some patients, but 9 of 14 patients in other series did not respond to this drug (2, 8).

Corticosteroids continue to be a mainstay of medical management of RP and decrease the frequency and severity of attacks. Traditional therapy is 10–20 mg/day of prednisone for mild to moderate auricular and nasal chondritis or arthritis. Doses of prednisone 0.75 to 1 mg/kg of body weight per day or pulse methylprednisolone (1 g/day for 3 days) and/or an immunosuppressive agent (azathioprine, cyclophosphamide, methotrexate or cyclosporine) should be initiated in patients with more severe disease, such as acute airway obstruction and cardiovascular and renal involvement.

Other therapies reported in refractory cases are plasmapheresis, anti-CD4 monoclonal antibodies and autologous stem-cell transplantation.

Intravenous infusions of infliximab have been used in resistant RP with good response.

Surgical intervention is indicated for certain respiratory and cardiovascular complications (2, 17, 18, 19).

References

1. Lutthra HS. Relapsing polychondritis. In: Rheumatoloy, Klippel JH, Dieppe PA, eds. Vol 27, St. Louis, Mosby 1998; 1–4.
2. Trentham DE, Le CH. Relapsing polychondritis. *Ann Intern Med* 1998; 129: 114–22.
3. Jaksch-Warnhorst R. Polychondropathia. *Wien Arch Int Med* 1923; 6: 93–100.
4. Pearson MC, Kline MH, NewcomerDV. Relapsing polychondritis. *N Engl J Med* 1960; 263: 51–8.
5. Alsalmeh S, Mollenhauer J, Scheuplein F et al. Preferential cellular and humoral immune reactivities to native and denatured collagen types IX and XI in a patient with fatal relapsing chondritis. *J Rheumatol* 1993; 20: 1419–1424.
6. Lang B, Rothenfusser A, Lanchbury JS, Rauh G et al. Susceptibility to relapsing polychondritis is associated with HLADR4. *Arthritis Rheum* 1993; 36: 660–4.
7. Peter D. Kent, Clement J. Michet, Jr and Harvinder S. Luthra. Relapsing polychondritis. *Current Opinion in Rheumatology* 2004; 16: 56–61.
8. McAdam LP, O Hanlan MA, Bluestone R et al. Relapsing polychondritis: prospective study of 23 patients and review of the literature. *Medicine* (Baltimore) 1967; 55: 193–215.
9. Michet CJ Jr, McKenna CH, Luthra HS et al. Relapsing polychondritis. Survival and predictive role of early disease manifestations. *Ann Int Med* 1986; 104: 74–78.
10. Tillie-Leblond I, Wallaert B, Leblond D et al. Respiratory involvement in relapsing polychondritis. Clinical, functional, endoscopic and radiographic evaluations. *Medicine* (Baltimore) 1998; 77: 168–176.
11. Chang Miller A, Okamura M, Torres VE et al. Renal involvement in relapsing polychondritis. *Medicine* (Baltimore) 1987; 66: 202–217.

12. Sundaram MB, Rajput AH. Nervous system complications of relapsing polychondritis. *Neurology* 1983; 33: 513–515.

13. Strobel ES, Lang B, Schumacher M et al. Cerebral aneurysm in relapsing polychondritis, *J Rheumatol* 1992; 19: 1482–1483.

14. Wasserfallen JB, Schaller MD. Unusual rhombencephalitis in relapsing polychondritis. *Ann Rheum Dis* 1992; 51: 1184.

15. Priori R, Conti F, Pittoni V et al. Relapsing polychondritis : a syndrome rather than a distinct clinical entity? *Clin Exp Rheumatol* 1997; 15: 334–335.

16. Damiani JM, Levine HL. Relapsing polychondritis. *Laryngoscope* 1979; 89: 929–46.

17. Priori R, Paroli MP, Luan FL et al. Cyclosporin A in the treatment of relapsing polychondritis with severe recurrent eye involvement. *Br J Rheumatol* 1993; 32: 352.

18. Rosen O, Thiel A, Massenkeil G et al. Autologous stem-cell transplantation in refractory autoimmune diseases after in vivo immunoablation and ex vivo depletion of mononuclear cells. *Arthritis Research* 2000; 2: 327–36.

19. Cazabon S, Over K, Butcher J. The successful use of infliximab in resistant relapsing polychondritis and associated scleritis. *Eye* 2005; 19: 222–4.

20. Carter JD. Treatment of relapsing polychondritis with a TNF antagonist (letter). *J Rheumatol* 2005; 32: 1413.

10
Raynaud Phenomenon

Mario García-Carrasco, Mario Jiménez-Hernández, Ricardo O. Escárcega,
Ivet Etchegaray-Morales and Juan Carlos Pérez-Alva

Abstract   Raynaud phenomenon is an episodic vasospasm of the peripheral arteries, causing pallor followed by cyanosis and redness with pain and sometimes paresthesia, and, rarely, ulceration of the fingers and toes (and in some cases of the ears or nose). Primary or idiopathic Raynaud phenomenon (Raynaud disease) occurs without an underlying disease. Secondary Raynaud phenomenon (Raynaud syndrome) occurs in association with an underlying disease – usually connective tissue disorders such as scleroderma, systemic lupus erythematosus, rheumatoid arthritis, or polymyositis. The disorder occurs fairly commonly and can have a variety of other presentations, ranging from mild discomfort to severe pain. It can eventually lead to ulcerations, tissue necrosis, and gangrene. Advances in vascular physiology have showed the role of the endothelium as well as endothelium-independent mechanisms in the altered vasoregulation of Raynaud phenomenon. This has opened promising therapeutic avenues, and it is likely that therapies targeted toward specific pathophysiological steps become available in the near future.

Keywords   Raynaud phenomenon · pathophysiology · endothelium · easospasm

Raynaud phenomenon (RP) is characterized by episodic vasospasm of arteries and arterioles, manifested clinically by the sequential development of digital blanching, cyanosis, and rubor of the fingers or toes following cold exposure and subsequent rewarming (1, 2). Reversible vasospasm of the extremities occurs either as an isolated symptom without underlying disorder (primary Raynaud phenomenon) or in association with another disorder or condition (secondary Raynaud phenomenon) (3).

Epidemiology

Raynaud phenomenon has a worldwide distribution and it has been described in adults and in children, although its prevalence is raised in cold climates where the risk of exposure to low ambient temperatures is greatest. The most commonly affected demographic group is women, approximately three to five times more frequently than men. Duration, frequency, and severity of symptoms increase during the colder months (3). Individual population-based survey estimates range from 2.9 to 16.8%, in overall prevalence (2.9–21% in women; 0.5–13.5% in men). The average age of

onset is 31 years; >75% of patients begin having symptoms before 40 years of age (4).

History

In 1862, Auguste-Maurice Raynaud in his thesis "Local asphyxia and symmetrical gangrene of the extremities" described for the first time color changes of the hands and feet triggered by exposure to cold temperature. In his observations, he affirmed that the phenomenon was a local asphyxia of the extremities which was a result of increased irritability of the central parts of the cord presiding over vascular innervations (5). However Raynaud failed to distinguish between transitory episodes of ischemia and fixed arterial obstruction with gangrene. But he corrected his mistake, and he differentiated fixed obstruction and gangrene from what we now know as Raynaud phenomenon. Later, Lewis suggested that the cause of the phenomenon was not central but peripheral, owing to spasm of the digital arteries and that the abnormal element in the reaction to cold is a direct reaction and because of a peculiar condition of the vessel wall locally. Allen and Brown criteria, negative immunological tests are now judged by most investigators to

From: Y. Shoenfeld et al. (eds.): *Diagnostic Criteria in Autoimmune Diseases*, DOI: 10.1007/978-1-60327-285-8_10,
© 2008 Humana Press, Totowa, NJ

be essential to distinguish primary from secondary Raynaud phenomenon.

Classification

In general, RP is classified as either primary (PRP) or secondary (SRP). PRP occurs as an isolated finding in an otherwise healthy individual. In fact, most experts think that the primary form is merely an exaggeration of normal physiological responses to cold environmental temperatures or emotional stress or both, rather than a disease (6). In SRP, there is an associated disorder detected upon assessment; the underlying pathological condition or disease alters regional blood flow by damaging blood vessels, interfering with neural control of the circulation, or changing either the physical properties of the blood or the levels of circulating mediators that regulate the digital and cutaneous circulation (2). The distinction is important, because prognosis, severity, and treatment can all be affected. The causes of SRP are associated with a rheumatic or connective tissue disease, such as systemic sclerosis, systemic lupus erythematosus, Sjögren syndrome (7), or dermatomyositis. Also, certain medications, such as β-blockers and ergotamine, have been associated with SRP, as well occupational exposure to hand-transmitted vibration, trauma, and certain chemotherapeutic agents such as bleomycin, vinblastine, and cisplatin (6). Smoking is not associated with RP in women but is associated with increased risk in men; likewise heavy alcohol consumption in women is associated with increased risk of RP whereas moderate alcohol consumption in men is associated with reduced risk (8).

Pathogenesis

The pathogenesis of RP is not completely understood. Normal regulation of peripheral blood flow depends on several factors, as well as intrinsic vascular tone, sympathetic nervous activity, circulating neurohumoral substances, and blood viscosity (9). Vasomotor control mechanisms can be subdivided into those that are intrinsic to the vessel wall and those that are extrinsic to the vessel. In addition, vasoregulation is mediated by endothelium-dependent and endothelium-independent mechanisms; there is evidence that endothelium-dependent processes might be more important in the exacerbation than in the initiation of Raynaud phenomenon, especially of the secondary form of the disorder. The specific pathophysiological abnormalities that induce the disorder most likely differ for each of the underlying conditions of secondary and primary forms of the disease. The mechanisms postulated to cause Raynaud phenomenon including vascular abnormalities include those of both structure and function,

increased sympathetic nervous system activity, high digital vascular reactivity to vasoconstrictive stimuli, several circulating vasoactive hormones, and decreased intravascular pressure. Intravascular abnormalities include platelet activation, impaired fibrinolysis, increased viscosity, and probably oxidant stress. Neural abnormalities are also involved, including deficiency of the vasodilator calcitonin gene-related peptide (released from sensory afferents), α2-adrenoreceptor activation (possibly with upregulation of the normally "silent" α2C-adrenoreceptor), and a central nervous system component (10). The endothelial injury may be attributable to repeated vasospastic attacks causing ischemic reperfusion injury to the endothelium. This injury causes the release of free radicals and other products that damage the endothelium besides endothelial dysfunction resulting from a decrease in the vasodilator chemical nitric which results in vasospasms. In some cases, locally released or systemically circulating vasoconstrictors may participate, including endothelin, 5-hydroxytryptamine, and thromboxane (11). These interactions are influenced by several factors: physical activity, the ambient temperature, the individual's emotional state, and direct traumatic or inflammatory insults to the vessels. Consequently, the vascular endothelium, smooth muscle cells, and nerve terminals form an integrated unit in which specific interactions and soluble mediators released in the microenvironment contribute together to determine the key issue which is the imbalance between vasoconstriction and vasodilatation.

Clinical Manifestations

In general, RP is associated with three specific stages in response to an individual's exposure to cold stimuli or emotional stress (1). At the start, pallor develops in the fingers or toes, and occasionally the tip of the nose or an earlobe is affected; this is caused by vasospasm of the digital arteries and arterioles and associated reduction in blood flow. Subsequently, cyanosis develops, which is caused by pooling of deoxygenated blood and the flow of this deoxygenated blood through the digital blood vessels. Finally, there is reactive hyperemia and rubor of the fingers or toes, resulting from the refilling of the vasospastic vessels with oxygenated blood. Approximately 60% of patients will exhibit all three color changes (12). Symptoms of RP depend on the severity, frequency, and duration of the blood vessel spasm. Some patients will exhibit only one (10–30%) or two (14–40%) of the color changes (10). In addition to the digital color changes, these patients are frequently are associated with paresthesias-like numbness and tingling that will disappear once the color returns to normal; however these symptoms make patients uncomfortable, they are usually not in pain at this time. But, as the disorder progresses, patients may develop varying degrees of pain because the blood vessel spasms become

TABLE 10.1. Clinical history of PR.

- Primary Raynaud
  - Symmetric attacks
  - Absence of tissue necrosis, ulceration, or gangrene
  - Absence of secondary cause after history and general physical examination
  - If no abnormal clinical or laboratory signs have developed for >2 years, secondary disease highly unlikely
- Secondary Raynaud
  - Onset >35 years of age
  - Asymmetric episodes more intense and painful
  - Inquire regarding arthritis, myalgias, fever, dry membranes, rash, or cardiopulmonary symptoms
  - Inquire about past or current drug use
  - Any exposure to toxic agents
  - Any repetitive trauma

more sustained and the sensory nerves become irritated by the lack of oxygen (10). Most patients with mild disease notice skin discoloration only upon cold exposure. In some cases, poor oxygen supply to the tissue can cause the tips of the digits to ulcerate which can become infected (11). With continued lack of oxygen, gangrene of the digits can occur. Patients with secondary RP can also have symptoms related to their underlying diseases. RP is the initial symptom in 70% of patients with scleroderma and other rheumatic diseases (13). (see also Table 10.1)

Pathological Features

Histological study includes various methods such as nailfold capillary microscopy, which has an impressive cost/effectiveness ratio: it is simple, non-invasive, and inexpensive. Therefore, it should be considered as the basic tool of investigation to distinguish primary from secondary Raynaud phenomenon. The capillaroscopic patterns that are found in patients with Raynaud phenomenon are widely variable, according to the various clinical subsets of the disease: normal capillaroscopic pattern, a specific capillaroscopic finding, and scleroderma-type capillaroscopic abnormalities. Several studies have demonstrated that patients who have primary Raynaud phenomenon do not exhibit capillary nailfold changes. On the contrary, patients who have mixed connective tissue disease (MCTD) (14), systemic sclerosis, and dermatomyositis demonstrate characteristic capillary nailfold abnormalities. In some rheumatic diseases, such as systemic sclerosis, the RP is a significant characteristic and is fundamentally different than the primary form of this disorder. Because of the underlying vasculopathy that is present in scleroderma, capillary nailfold is used to show the vascular changes that are ubiquitous in the small and medium arterial vessels in patients who have systemic sclerosis and are characterized by intimal proliferation with fibrosis and evidence of endothelial cell perturbation and smooth muscle cell activation (13).

Diagnostic Criteria

In particular, proposed clinical and laboratory criteria for the identification of RP include episodic attacks of acral pallor or cyanosis; no evidence of digital pitting, ulcerations, or gangrene; normal nailfold capillarioscopy results; negative antinuclear antibody testing results; and a normal erythrocyte sedimentation rate, rheumatoid factor, thyroid hormone levels, and protein levels to exclude associated rheumatic diseases and thyroid disorder. These criteria are effective in excluding the majority of patients with underlying connective tissue diseases (8). Epidemiologically, most patients with PRP tend to be women and the clinical course is usually mild, with only rare instances of tissue loss or necrosis. Clinical and laboratory criteria proposed for the identification of SRP include abnormal nailfold capillarioscopy results; positive antinuclear antibody testing results; presence of digital pitting, ulcerations, or gangrene; and evidence of other organ system involvement, including gastrointestinal, cardiopulmonary, or renal abnormalities. Patients with SRP usually have a much more complicated clinical course, with multiorgan system complications occurring frequently (11) (See also Table 10.2).

Differential Diagnosis

The main differential diagnoses are summarized in Table 10.3.

Prognosis

PR shows a rate of progression that varies widely among patients; 13% of Raynaud phenomenon patients developed a secondary disorder, many of which were connective tissue diseases (15). In some cases of PRP, attacks may last from several minutes to a few hours. In cases of SRP, affected patients develop the hallmarks of underlying disease; therefore, if an underlying disease is strongly

TABLE 10.2. Laboratory and histological findings.

- Primary Raynaud
Antinuclear antibody – negative
Erythrocyte sedimentation rate – normal
Nailfold capillaroscopy – normal
- Secondary Raynaud
Tests for underlying secondary causes (complete blood chemistry, ESR)
Positive autoantibody has low positive predictive value for an associated connective tissue disease (30%)
Antibodies to specific autoantigens more suggestive of secondary disease (e.g., scleroderma with anticentromere or antitopoisomerase antibodies)
Nailfold capillaroscopy – abnormal

TABLE 10.3. Differential diagnosis.

- Thromboangiitis obliterans
- Rheumatic arthritis
- Progressive systemic sclerosis (scleroderma)
- Systemic lupus erythematosus
- Carpal tunnel syndrome
- Thoracic outlet syndrome
- Hypothyroidism
- CREST syndrome
- Cryoglobulinemias
- Acrocyanosis
- Polycythemia
- Occupational (e.g., especially from vibrating tools)
- Drugs (e.g., chemotherapeutic agents, ergotamine, amphetamines, bromocriptine)

suspected it is important to consider specialist consultation for evaluation and treatment.

Therapeutic Management

The goals of treatment are to reduce the severity of attacks and to prevent tissue damage and loss in the fingers and toes. Prevention measures are important in primary and secondary RP regardless of the severity. Management of RP involves protecting the fingers and the toes from cold, trauma, and infection (8). Any wounds or infections should be treated early to prevent more serious infections. Avoiding emotional stresses and tools that vibrate the hand may reduce the frequency of attacks. Learning relaxation techniques and taking time to relax will further help to end an attack. Medications that can aggravate blood vessel spasm should be avoided by patients with RP such as ergotamine derivates, beta-blockers, amphetamines, and sumatriptan also is important the cessation of vasoconstrictor agents such as nicotine (8, 11). Diet is also very important and some trials have showed that fish oils containing omega-3-fatty acids may be beneficial to some patients with primary Raynaud. In addition, aspirin or clopidogrel is prescribed to decrease the risk of thrombotic complications in all cases of RP. In addition, patients should be treated for any underlying disease or condition that causes secondary Raynaud phenomenon (13). Vasodilator drugs may be of some benefit in patients whose symptoms are not adequately controlled with simpler measures which were described earlier. Patients with secondary Raynaud phenomenon are more likely than those with the primary form to be treated with medications (11). The most effective and safest drugs are calcium-channel blockers, which relax smooth muscle and dilate the small blood vessels. Low-dose nifedipine (10–30 mg PO t.i.d. or 30–120 mg sustained-release formula PO once daily) or diltiazem (30–120 mg PO t.i.d. or 120–300 mg

sustained-release formula PO once daily) has superseded topical or oral nitroglycerin for treatment of vasospasm (16). These drugs decrease the frequency and severity of attacks in about two-thirds of patients who have primary and secondary Raynaud phenomena. If adverse effects occur, decrease dosage or use another agent such as nicardipine, amlodipine, or diltiazem. These drugs also can help heal skin ulcers of the fingers or toes. On the other hand, some patients found relief with postsynaptic α_1-adrenergic antagonist which has been used with favorable response (Prazosin, 1–5 mg PO bid) because they counteract the actions of norepinephrine, a hormone that constricts blood vessels (17). Likewise angiotensin-converting enzyme inhibitors and intravenous prostaglandins have been advocated, and clinical trials have indicated some benefit. The angiotensin-receptor antagonist losartan at 25–100 mg/day has been found effective in patients with PRP and SRP in scleroderma (18). The selective serotonin uptake inhibitor fluoxetine has also been shown effective if the range dose is from 20 to 40 mg daily (19). Intravenous prostaglandins have also been used with success, such as iloprost, which when given as a 5-day infusion was beneficial in severe cases of Raynaud phenomenon; alprostadil (prostaglandin E_1 [PGE_1]) and epoprostenol (PGI_2) are considered as alternatives (20), whereas prazosin has been used with some success against primary and secondary Raynaud phenomenon (11). Recent studies have shown a role for bosentan in the treatment of severe Raynaud phenomenon associated with systemic sclerosis in which the use of intravenous prostaglandin analogues was not considered as a first-line option, because bosentan has several advantages such as rapid clinical response and oral administration absence of severe side effects. According to Ramos et al. (21), bosentan is recommended: start treatment with 125 mg daily for the first 4 weeks followed by 125 mg twice daily. This dose has shown an improvement in the ischemic lesions with healing of digital ulcer patients during the first month of therapy. Pharmological treatment of RP is summarized in Table 10.4.

In some cases, surgery should be considered; sympathectomy is indicated for pure vasospastic disease refractory to medical management (22). Digital sympathectomy has been gaining support for patients with severe or tissue-threatening disease. This may be used in patients with either primary or secondary disease, but is more commonly necessary with the secondary form. In the lower extremity, sympathectomy may produce complete and permanent relief of symptoms; however, for unclear reasons, the beneficial effects are often transient in the upper extremity. Limited improvement is seen in advanced ischemia, particularly if significant digital artery obstructive disease is present.

Table 10.4. Pharmacological treatment of Raynaud phenomenon.

Agent	Dose	Side effects
Nifedipine	10–30 mg 3 times daily (PO)	Tachycardia,
Amlodipine	5–20 mg daily (PO)	hypotension,
Diltiazem	30–120 mg 3 times daily (PO)	palpitations, constipation, anxiety
Losartan	25–100 mg daily (PO)	Dizziness, headache, fatigue, diarrhea
Prazosin	1–5 mg 2 times daily (PO)	Orthostatic hypotension, nausea, headache
Fluoxetine	20–40 mg daily (PO)	Insomnia, nauseas, diarrhea, tremors
Pentoxifylline	400 mg 3 times daily (PO)	Dyspepsia, nausea, vomiting
Epoprostenol	0.5–6 ng/kg of body weight/ min intravenously for 6–24 hr, for 2–5 days	Diarrhea, headache, rash, hypotension

References

1. Wigley FM. (2002) Clinical practice: Raynaud's phenomenon. *N Engl J Med*; 347: 1001–8.
2. Block JA, et al. (2001) Raynaud's phenomenon. *Lancet*; 357(9273): 2042–8.
3. Spencer-Green G. (1998) Outcomes in primary Raynaud phenomenon: A meta-analysis of the frequency, rates, and predictors of transition to secondary disease. *Arch Intern Med*; 158: 595–600.
4. Maricq HR, Carpentier PH, Weinrich MC, et al. (1997) Geographic variation in the prevalence of Raynaud's phenomenon: A 5 region comparison. *J Rheumatol*; 24: 879–89.
5. Raynaud M. On local asphyxia and symmetrical gangrene of the extremities (1862). New researches on the nature and treatment of local asphyxia of the extremities (1874). In: Barlow T, trans. *Selected Monographs*. London, New Sydenham Society; 1988.
6. Sangeeta DS and Wigley FM. (2007) Raynaud Phenomenon. In: John BI, David BH, John HS (eds.), *Current Rheumatology Diagnosis and Treatment*, Second Edition. McGraw-Hill.
7. Garcia-Carrasco M, Siso A, Ramos-Casals M, Rosas J, de la Red G, Gil V, Lasterra S, Cervera R, Font J, Ingelmo M. (2002) Raynaud's phenomenon in primary Sjogren's syndrome. Prevalence and clinical characteristics in a series of 320 patients. *J Rheumatol* April; 29(4): 726–30.
8. Pope JE. (2007) The diagnosis and treatment of Raynaud's phenomenon: A practical approach. *Drugs*; 67(4): 517–25.
9. Dyanne P, Westerberg DO, John RL. (2005) Approach to the patient with Raynaud's phenomenon. *Clinics in Family Practice*; 7(2): 321–34.
10. Herrick AL. (2005) Pathogenesis of Raynaud's phenomenon. *Rheumatology*; 44: 587–96.
11. Francesco B, Fredrick MW. (2005) Understanding, assessing and treating Raynaud's phenomenon. *Curr Opin Rheumatol*; 17: 752–60.
12. Cookea J, Marshallb J. (2005) Mechanisms of Raynaud's disease. *Vasc Med*; 10: 293–307.
13. Hummers LK, Wigley FM. (2003) Management of Raynaud's phenomenon and digital ischemic lesions in scleroderma. *Rheum Dis Clin North Am*; 29: 293–313.
14. Grader-Beck T, et al. (2005) Raynaud's phenomenon in mixed connective tissue disease. *Rheum Dis Clin North Am*; 31: 465.
15. Pope J. (2005) Raynaud's phenomenon (primary). *Clin Evid*; 13: 1–2.
16. Thompson AE, Pope J. (2005) Calcium channel blockers for primary Raynaud's phenomenon: A meta-analysis. *Rheumatology*; 44(2): 145–50.
17. Wise RA, Wigley FM, White B, et al. (2004) Efficacy and tolerability of a selective alpha (2C)-adrenergic receptor blocker in recovery from cold-induced vasospasm in scleroderma patients: a single-center, double-blind, placebo-controlled, randomized crossover study. *Arthritis Rheum*; 50(12): 3994–4001.
18. Dziadzio, et al. (2005) Losartan therapy for Raynaud's phenomenon and scleroderma: clinical and biochemical findings in a fifteen-week, randomized, parallel-group, controlled trial. *Arthritis Rheum*; 42(12): 2646–55.
19. Garcia-Porrua C, Margarinos CC, Gonzalez-Gay MA. (2004) Raynaud's phenomenon and serotonin reuptake inhibitors. *J Rheumatol*; 31: 2090.
20. Marasini, et. al. (2004) Comparison between iloprost and alprostadil in the treatment of Raynaud's phenomenon. *Scand J Rheumatol*; 33(4): 253–6.
21. Ramos-Casals M, Brito-Zeron P, Nardi N, Claver G, Risco G, Parraga FD, Fernandez S, Julia M, Font J. (2004) Successful treatment of severe Raynaud's phenomenon with bosentan in four patients with systemic sclerosis. *Rheumatology*; 43(11): 1454–6.
22. Maga P, Kuzdzal J, Nizankowski R, Szczeklik A, Sladek K. (2007) Long-term effects of thoracic sympathectomy on microcirculation in the hands of patients with primary Raynaud disease. *J Thorac Cardiovasc Surg*; 133(6): 1428–33.

11
Drug-Induced Autoimmunity

Martine Szyper-Kravitz and Yehuda Shoenfeld

Abstract Drug-induced autoimmunity encompasses a wide range of serological and clinical manifestations that develop after exposure to a drug. The classical and most studied example is drug-induced lupus (DIL). Although autoimmunity secondary to drugs has been recognized for more than 50 years, the introduction of new drugs has extended the spectrum and severity of clinical manifestations. Several drugs are associated with the induction of antinuclear and anti-DNA antibodies, but clinical lupus is rare, and a number of drugs are associated with antineutrophilic cytoplasmic antibody (ANCA)-positive vasculitis. The diagnosis of these conditions is not simple and requires careful elimination of other possible conditions. Although rare cases of life-threatening autoimmune conditions have been described, the majority of cases are mild and resolve after the offending drug is discontinued.

Keywords Drug-induced idiosyncratic reactions · drug-induced lupus

Drug-induced autoimmunity refers to the emergence of an autoimmune serological profile or an autoimmune condition after exposure to a drug. Most of the literature concerning drug-induced autoimmunity consists of case reports illustrating specific autoimmune conditions that developed on specific patients, and only few controlled studies have been published. Some of the postulated mechanisms have been prospectively investigated in experimental models. More recently, the induction of autoantibodies following the worldwide introduction of antitumor necrosis factor (TNF)-α in the treatment of several diseases has provided a wide database on the prevalence, clinical significance, and possible mechanisms for drug-induced autoimmunity. In this chapter, we review the current trends in drug-induced autoimmunity, including the postulated mechanisms, the range of autoimmune manifestations, and their clinical relevance.

Epidemiology

The possibility of drug-induced autoimmunity was first raised in 1945 with a report of possible sulfadiazine-induced lupus, which was followed in 1953 by hydralazine being implicated in the induction of lupus. Since then more than 100 drugs have been implicated in drug-induced lupus (DIL) (see Table 11.1 for a list of drugs). The estimate

TABLE 11.1. Most common drugs implicated in drug-induced lupus (DIL).

Antibiotics – minocycline, isoniazid
Antifungals – griseofulvin, voriconazole
Antiarrhythmics – procainamide, quinidine
Antihypertensives – hydralazine, methyldopa, captopril, acebutolol
Anticonvulsants – valproate, carbamazepine, phenytoin
Antiinflammatory – D-penicillamine, sulfasalazine
Antipsychotics – chlorpromazine
Cholesterol-lowering agents – lovastatin, simvastatin, gemfibrozil
Antithyroid – propylthiouracil
Biologic agents – interleukin 2, interferon-α,β,γ, TNF-α inhibitors

incidence of DIL is 15,000–20,000 cases per year in the USA, whereas others suggest that as many as 10% cases of systemic lupus erythematosus (SLE) may be DIL (1). The incidence and prevalence of other drug-induced autoimmune manifestations are not known. In an analysis of the French national database of pharmacovigilance in the years 1991–1994, only 0.2% of reports were suggestive of systemic autoimmunity (2). In contrast to SLE, where women are affected at a rate of 9:1 as compared with men, no sex predilection is apparent in DIL (3), although in the French report of systemic autoimmunity a female to male ratio of 3.6:1 was found (2). Also in contrast to SLE, DIL is more frequent in Caucasians than in blacks. Regarding age, patients with DIL tend to be older than those with SLE, with 63% patients aged >50 years (2, 3).

From: Y. Shoenfeld et al. (eds.): *Diagnostic Criteria in Autoimmune Diseases*, DOI: 10.1007/978-1-60327-285-8_11,
© 2008 Humana Press, Totowa, NJ

Pathogenesis

The induction of autoimmunity by drugs may involve several levels of immune control, leading to the breakdown of tolerance. In the normal development, central tolerance is achieved by the deletion of potential autoreactive thymocytes through apoptosis, whereas in the periphery, potential autoreactive cells are kept under tight control by several mechanisms. Several drugs have been shown to potentially disrupt these levels of tolerance.

Breakdown of Central Tolerance

Studying the mechanism of procaine-induced lupus, Kretz-Rommel and Rubin (4) elegantly demonstrated that two injections of procaine-hydroxylamine, a metabolite of procainamide, into the thymus of normal mice resulted in the appearance of chromatin-reactive T cells and IgG autoantibodies against chromatin, in the peripheral blood. Moreover, adoptive transfer of these chromatin-reactive T cells into naïve mice resulted in a similar autoantibody response, indicating that the egress of autoreactive T cells from the thymus to the periphery is sufficient to break B-cell tolerance and induce systemic autoimmunity. In further in vitro studies, these authors demonstrated that the drug does not affect negative selection, but rather prevents the induction of anergy in T cells and the establishment of unresponsiveness to self during positive selection (4). In another murine model, lethally irradiated bone marrow-reconstituted mice have been shown to develop a systemic autoimmune disease, after receiving high-dose cyclosporine A (CsA), which could be transferred into syngenic recipients by T cells (5). In this model, CsA appears to prevent thymic deletion by blocking signaling during negative selection in the thymus.

Breakdown of Peripheral Tolerance

Drugs implicated in the induction of lupus such as hydralazine and procainamide inhibit T-cell DNA methylation (similar to UV light). DNA methylation is a post-synthetic event, and during mitosis, methylation patterns are replicated by DNA methyltransferase (DMT). Procainamide is a competitive inhibitor of DMT, whereas hydralazine inhibits the extracellular signal-regulated kinase (ERK) pathway signaling, decreasing DMT expression and activity (6). In experimental models, Richardson's group demonstrated that treatment of human and murine $CD4^+$ T cells with DNA-hypomethylating drugs resulted in increased expression of lymphocyte function-associated antigen 1 (LFA-1), induced autoreactivity, and adoptive transfer of these autoreactive T cells into syngenic recipients, caused a lupus-like disease (6). In further studies, they demonstrated that LFA-1 overexpression (by transfection) was responsible for the autoreactivity, as adoptive transfer of the transfected, autoreactive cells into syngenic recipients caused anti-DNA antibodies, immune-complex glomerulonephritis, and pulmonary alveolitis (6). Interestingly, subsets of autoreactive T cells, hypomethylated T cell DNA, and overexpression of LFA-1 have all been described in patients with active SLE, highlighting the relevance of these experimental results for human disease (6).

Cross-Reactivity of T Cells

Cross-reactivity of T cells with self-antigens is an alternative mechanism for interference with peripheral tolerance. Pichler (7) reported that drug-specific T-cell clones (TCCs) can also react to alloantigens. The authors cloned autoreactive T cells from 100 donors with drug allergies and found that some reactive T cells reacted with the drug on different human leukocyte antigen (HLA) molecules, suggesting that drug-specific T cells may bear degenerate T-cell receptors, which are able to react with multiple antigens. In addition to a high incidence of alloreactivity of the drug-reactive T-cell receptors, he also demonstrated autoreactivity among the drug-specific TCCs, concluding that these TCCs were autoreactive and drug-reactive. The author suggests that drug-induced autoimmunity can result from the generation of broadly reactive T cells, which recognize the drug, but also HLA peptide alleles without the drug, leading to a break of tolerance to autoantigens and the emergence of autoimmunity (7).

Antigen Modification

According to the "hapten hypothesis," drugs or more commonly their reactive metabolites bind to proteins, changing their conformation and altering their recognition as "self" by the immune system. Perceived as "foreign," these proteins become the target of an immune response. Once a response is initiated, epitope spreading may occur, inducing autoimmunity to self-antigens. Examples for haptenization and epitope spreading are illustrated using heavy metals such as gold, mercury, and nickel, which bind to proteins, change their molecular and antigenic properties, and induce autoantibodies (8). Changes in the processing of antigens leading to the presentation of cryptic antigens may also contribute to the induction of the immune response, as in the case of gold, which in vitro has been found to alter the processing of proteins such as bovine ribonuclease, leading to the presentation of hidden epitopes and induction of an immune response (9). Several drugs associated with the induction of autoimmunity are oxidized to reactive metabolites, which are incriminated in the haptenization process. Interestingly, this reactivity can be transferred by lymphocytes to syngenic animals (9). Additional mechanisms by which drugs may facilitate the emergence of autoimmunity include molecular mimicry and superantigen stimulation.

The "danger hypothesis" is another plausible explanation for drug-induced autoimmunity. According to Matzinger, the default of the immune system is tolerance to most antigens, but the presentation of an antigen in the context of a "danger signal" triggers an immune response (10). Danger signals can be viral infections, physiological stress such as surgery, or reactive metabolites of drugs. This concept may explain the association of infections and stress with idiosyncratic drug reactions, such as the ampicillin idiosyncratic reaction (skin rash) among patients with Epstein–Barr virus (EBV) mononucleosis or the sulfonamide idiosyncratic reactions in HIV-infected patients (9).

Clinical Manifestations

Drug-induced autoimmunity may manifest in diverse clinical manifestations, ranging from organ-restricted to systemic diseases. In the most studied case of DIL, induced by procainamide and hydralazine, the disease is characterized by arthralgia, myalgia, pleurisy, rash, and fever, whereas pericardial, central nervous system (CNS), and renal involvement is rare. Oral ulcers, alopecia, and photosensitivity, which are typical in SLE, are rare in these cases of DIL, but purpura and erythema nodosum are more prevalent. In patients treated for more than a year with procainamide, 20% are at risk for developing symptoms, as compared with 5–8% among hydralazine-treated patients (11). To date, the therapeutic use of procainamide and hydralazine declined dramatically, and most cases of DIL are induced by other new drugs, changing the classical presentation of DIL (resembling more idiopathic SLE) and expanding the spectrum to new autoimmune manifestations.

In cases of the antiphospholipid syndrome (APS) induced by drugs such as chlorpromazine, a low frequency of thrombosis, <6% during 5 years of follow up, has been reported, as compared with a 56–87% prevalence of antiphospholipid antibodies (12). Additional drugs implicated in drug-induced APS include chlorothiazide, chlorpromazine, hydralazine, phenothiazine, procainamide, quinidine, and interferon-(INF)-α (12).

Four immune-mediated syndromes have been attributed to minocycline treatment: serum sickness, DIL, autoimmune hepatitis, and vasculitis (13). DIL and hepatitis were the most common, manifesting after a protracted use (~2 years). The most frequent symptoms are arthralgia, followed by arthritis, fever, and rash, whereas renal and CNS involvement is considered rare.

Propylthiouracil (PTU) administration has been associated with rare events of DIL and vasculitis. As patients with thyroid disease are more prone to suffer from other autoimmune conditions, they may be more susceptible to drug-induced autoimmunity. Aloush et al. (14) described three cases of DIL and one case of vasculitis, which developed in young women after prolonged treatment (>9 months) with PTU. After reviewing the literature, they identified another 30 cases of vasculitis and 12 cases of DIL after PTU treatment. Musculoskeletal symptoms were more prevalent in DIL, whereas renal and pulmonary involvement was more common among PTU-induced vasculitis. Fever, mucocutaneous lesions, serositis, and hematological and gastrointestinal involvement occurred at a lower frequency in both groups.

There have been 22 case reports of asthma patients developing Churg–Strauss syndrome (CSS) while receiving leukotriene inhibitors (15). As all the patients were being treated with inhaled or systemic corticosteroid for their asthma, and onset of CSS was often associated with steroid tapering, it has been suggested that these cases represent unmasking of undiagnosed CSS with tapering of the steroids, rather than a drug-induced disease (15). Even so, it is possible that some cases of CCS are an idiosyncratic response to leukotriene inhibitors.

The 3-hydroxy-3-methylglutaryl coenzyme A (HMG-CoA) reductase inhibitors have been associated with several cases of dermatomyositis and polymyositis (2), albeit overlap with statin-induced myopathy precludes a definite autoimmune mechanism.

Recombinant INF treatment has been associated with the emergence of thyroid autoimmunity and dysfunction, in different patient groups. Among patients with breast cancer and multiple sclerosis (MS), 30 and 7.7%, respectively, developed thyroid dysfunction, and among patients treated for hepatitis C, between 3 and 30% of previously euthyroid patients developed thyroid dysfunction (16). Interestingly, DIL has been only rarely demonstrated (0.15–0.7%).

Following the worldwide introduction of anti-TNF-α in the treatment of rheumatic and Crohn's diseases (CDs), a significant prevalence of autoimmunity have been reported, although few cases of overt disease have been published. In a retrospective national study in France encompassing all the centers prescribing anti-TNF agents for rheumatic diseases, and including more than 10,000 patients, 22 cases of DIL were identified (17). Whereas 10 patients had only anti-DNA antibodies and skin manifestations, 12 patients had at least four American College of Rheumatology (ACR) criteria for lupus. Selected cases of demyelinating syndromes resembling MS have been described following anti-TNF therapy, albeit only in patients with previous autoimmune disease [rheumatoid arthritis (RA) and CD] and not in patients with spondylarthropathy (SpA) (18), implying that the effect of anti-TNF may be secondary to an already established autoimmune milieu.

Serological Features

By definition, patients with DIL have antinuclear autoantibodies (ANAs), usually with a homogenous pattern (induced by procainamide, isoniazid, timolol, hydralazine, and phenytoin), whereas thiazides have been associated with speckled ANA patterns. Hydralazine and procainamide are associated with the induction of several autoantibodies including ANAs (>95%), antihistone, usually IgG anti-[H2a-H2B] DNA (>95%), antidenatured DNA (50%), anticardiolipin (5–15%) antibodies, and rheumatoid factor (RF) (20–30%) (11). In contrast to SLE, in DIL, the anti-DNA antibody is directed against ssDNA, anti-Sm antibodies are rare, and complement levels are within the normal range.

The most common serological findings in minocycline-induced autoimmunity are ANAs and perinuclear antineutrophilic cytoplasmic antibodies (p-ANCAs). Interestingly antihistone antibodies are found at a low frequency (13). In PTU-induced autoimmunity, a 90% prevalence of ANA, 42% prevalence of antihistone, 25% of anti-DNA, and 50% of p-ANCA were found among cases of PTU-induced lupus. In contrast, cytoplasmic ANCA (c-ANCA) was detected only in cases of PTU-induced vasculitis, a similar rate of p-ANCA was found in both conditions, but antimyeloperoxidase (anti-MPO) antibodies were found at a high frequency in PTU-induced vasculitis (14). Several additional cases of drug-induced vasculitis associated with ANCA with anti-MPO specificity have been described after exposure to minocycline, hydralazine, methimazole, and penicillamine (12, 14).

Among patients treated with INF-α, 4–19% developed some form of autoimmunity: 12% develop ANA and 8% dsDNA (19). But among hepatitis C patients, a wide range of seroconversion for thyroid autoantibodies has been reported during treatment (up to 40%) and even months after INF was terminated (16). In some of the patients, the autoantibodies disappeared months after termination of treatment, highlighting the possible direct effect of INF on the induction of the antibodies. Similarly, in patients with MS (treated with INF-β) and breast cancer, 19 and 50%, respectively, developed thyroid antibodies (16).

Increase in ANA and anti-dsDNA antibody titers occurs in all groups of patients treated with anti-TNF-α antibody or fusion proteins (19). Approximately 64% of RA patients and 49% of CD patients developed de novo ANA during infliximab treatment, and 13 and 21.5%, respectively, developed newly positive anti-dsDNA antibodies (20), albeit only about 0.2% of patients developed symptoms of SLE. Interestingly, induction of autoantibodies was higher among patients with SpAs. After 34 weeks of infliximab treatment, newly positive results for ANAs were 32.3% for RA as compared with 71.4% for SpAs, and 11.3% of RA developed anti-DNA antibodies compared with 17.1% among

SpA patients (especially non-IgG isotype) (18). In addition, in both groups, 10–15% of patients also developed antinucleosome and antihistone antibodies. A low prevalence of anti-ENA and anticardiolipin antibodies has also been described in patients treated with anti-TNF-α.

Diagnostic Criteria

To date, no diagnostic criteria for drug-induced autoimmunity have been formulated. The attribution of autoimmunity to a drug is complicated by several factors, such as the concomitant exposure to multiple drugs (poly-pharmacy), the latent period between drug exposure and the appearance of symptoms or signs of disease, and the similarities between a drug-induced reaction and a true illness. Nonetheless, the definition of drug-induced autoimmunity has to comply with several temporal criteria to establish that autoimmunity did not exist in the patient prior to the drug exposure; it developed after the introduction of the offending drug; resolution or improvement of autoimmunity followed discontinuation of the drug; and it recurs with repeated drug exposure (see Table 11.2).

Regarding the emergence of autoimmunity, the application of the above temporal criteria may be difficult. Patients may have subtle signs or be in the process of presenting an autoimmune condition, coincident with the exposure to a new drug, or they may already harbor autoantibodies without clinical disease, prior to the drug introduction. The development of autoantibodies or the emergence of an autoimmune condition may lag weeks or months after the introduction of a new drug, making a causal relationship difficult. Finally, the resolution of symptoms and the disappearance of autoantibodies may not follow the discontinuation of the suspected offending drug, as several immune processes may not be readily or rapidly reversed. In addition, by their very nature, autoimmune diseases may present insidiously or atypically, making their diagnosis a difficult task. In summary, the diagnosis of a drug-induced autoimmune condition is a process of elimination.

Prognosis

The prognosis of drug-induced autoimmunity is excellent once the causative medication is discontinued. In selected cases, corticosteroids and rarely cytotoxic agents are required. Recovery generally occurs within days or weeks.

TABLE 11.2. Proposed criteria for drug-induced autoimmunity.

1) Autoimmunity does not exist in the patient prior to the drug exposure.
2) Autoimmunity develops after the introduction of the offending drug.
3) Resolution or improvement of autoimmunity follows discontinuation of the drug (dechallenge).
4) Autoimmunity recurs with repeated drug exposure (rechallenge).

Prediction

Traditionally, a distinction has been recognized between the development of autoantibodies, following drug exposure, and the emergence of an autoimmune disease. The classical case of procaine-induced ANAs has demonstrated that although ANA positivity was detected in many patients, only a small minority developed a lupus-like disease. Similarly and more recently, a high frequency of ANAs has been detected among different groups of patients, following treatment with anti-TNF agents, but to date, only rare cases developed overt disease.

At the present time, it is not possible to predict who will develop DIL or any other drug-induced autoimmunity. Predisposing factors for DIL include slow acetylator phenotypes, HLA-DR4, complement C4 null allele, female gender, and Caucasian race (20).

Therapy

For the vast majority of patients with drug-induced autoimmunity, no specific treatment is required after the offending drug is terminated, although in selected patients, a short course of corticosteroids is necessary. In rare cases, especially when vasculitis develops, more aggressive therapy may be required.

References

1. Yung RL, Richardson BC. Drug-induced lupus. *Rheum Dis Clin North Am* 1994; 20: 61–86.
2. Vial T, Nicolas B, Descortes J. Drug-induced autoimmunity: Experience of the French Pharmacovigilance system. *Toxicology* 1997; 119: 23–7.
3. Price EJ, Venables PJW. Drug-induced lupus. *Drug Saf* 1995; 1: 283–90.
4. Kretz-Rommel A, Rubin RL. Disruption of positive selection of thymocytes causes autoimmunity. *Nat Med* 2000; 6: 298–305.
5. Bucy RP, Xu XY, Li J, Huang GO. Cyclosporine A-induced autoimmune disease in mice. *J Immunol* 1993; 151: 1039–50.
6. Oelke K, Lu O, Richardson D, Wu A, Deng C, Hanash S, Richardson B. Overexpression of CD70 and overstimulation of IgG synthesis by lupus T cells and T cells treated with DNA methylation inhibitors. *Arthritis Rheum* 2004; 50: 1850–60.
7. Pichler WJ. Drug-induced autoimmunity. *Curr Opin Allergy Clin Immunol* 2003; 3: 249–53.
8. Rao T, Richardson B. Environmentally induced autoimmune diseases: Potential mechanisms. *Environ Health Perspect* 1999; 107(Suppl. 5): 737–42.
9. Uetrecht JP. Idiosyncratic drug-reactions: Current understanding. *Annu Rev Pharmacol Toxicol* 2007; 47: 13–39.
10. Matzinger P. Tolerance, danger, and the extended family. *Annu Rev Immunol* 1994; 12: 991–1045.
11. Rubin RL. Drug-induced lupus. *Toxicology* 2005; 209: 135–47.
12. Yung R, Richardson B. Drug-induced rheumatic syndromes. *Bull Rheum Dis* 2002; 51. 1–6.
13. Elkayam O, Yaron M, Caspi D. Minocycline-induced autoimmune syndromes: An overview. *Semin Arthritis Rheum* 1999; 28: 392–7.
14. Aloush V, Litinsky I, Caspi D, Elkayam O. Propylthiouracil-induced autoimmune syndromes: Two distinct clinical presentations with different course and management. *Semin Arthritis Rheum* 2006; 36: 4–9.
15. Masi A, Hamilos DL. Leukotriene antagonists: Bystanders or causes of Churg-Strauss syndrome. *Semin Arthritis Rheum* 2002; 31: 211–7.
16. Oppenheim Y, Ban Y, Tomer Y. Interferon induced autoimmune thyroid disease (AITD): A model for human autoimmunity. *Autoimmun Rev* 2004; 3: 388–93.
17. De Bandt M, Sibilia J, Le Loët X, Prouzeau S, Fautrel B, Marcelli C, Boucquillard E, Siame JL, Mariette X. Systemic lupus erythematosus induced by anti-tumour necrosis factor alpha therapy: A French national survey. *Arthritis Res Ther* 2005; 7: R545–51.
18. De Rycke L, Kruithof E, Van Damme N, Hoffman IE, Van den Bossche N, Van den Bosch F, Veys EM, De Keyser F. Antinuclear antibodies following infliximab treatment in patients with rheumatoid arthritis or spondylarthropathy. *Arthritis Rheum* 2003; 48: 1015–23.
19. Ioannou Y, Isenberg DA. Review: Current evidence for the induction of autoimmune rheumatic manifestations by cytokine therapy. *Arthritis Rheum* 2000; 43: 1431–41.
20. Centocor, Inc. *Remicade (infliximab). Data on file.* Malvern, PA, USA: Centocor, Inc.

12
The Multiple Autoimmune Syndromes

Juan-Manuel Anaya, John Castiblanco and Adriana Rojas-Villarraga

Abstract   The common background evidence for autoimmune diseases has grown and allows us to infer that although their heterogeneity is due to a collection of diverse disorders based on epidemiology, pathology, or diagnostic criteria, in fact the underlying immunogenetic mechanism might be similar. The clinical evidence supporting the common origin of autoimmune diseases corresponds to the kaleidoscope of autoimmunity, which is the co-occurrence of various autoimmune diseases within an individual or co-occurrence within members of a family. The two better conditions that illustrate the kaleidoscope of autoimmunity are the multiple autoimmune syndromes (MAS) and the familial autoimmunity (FA). The MAS consists in the presence of three or more well-defined autoimmune conditions in a single patient. A review of the literature and cluster analysis of MAS disclosed systemic lupus erythematosus, Sjögren's syndrome, and autoimmune thyroid disease as the "chaperones" of autoimmune diseases. FA is defined as the presence of diverse autoimmune diseases on multiple members of a nuclear family. In this chapter, both the MAS and FA are discussed and illustrated in the context of the common genetic background of autoimmunity.

Keywords   Autoimmune diseases · familial autoimmune disease · familial autoimmunity · multiple autoimmune syndrome · sporadic disease

Introduction

Autoimmune diseases are chronic conditions initiated by the loss of immunological tolerance to self-antigens and which make up a heterogeneous group of disorders where multiple alterations in the immune system result in a spectrum of syndromes that either target specific organs or affect the body systematically (1). Moreover, their chronic nature has a significant impact in terms of the utilization of medical care, direct and indirect economic costs, and quality of life. Almost all autoimmune diseases disproportionately affect middle-aged women and are among the leading causes of death in this group of patients. The older the patient grows, the lower the male:female ratio becomes.

Most of the factors involved in autoimmunity can be categorized into four groups: genetic, immune defects, hormonal, and environmental. Autoimmune diseases may present as mild, subclinical or severe, or life-threatening conditions, and different patients may present with similar symptomatology and immunological phenomena indicating that these disorders may represent different expressions of similar pathogenetical processes and thus raising taxonomic questions. The term "kaleidoscope of autoimmunity" is used to describe the possible shift of one disease to another or the fact that more than one autoimmune disease may coexist in a single patient or in the same family (2, 3). Although their etiology remains poorly understood, the common features they share and a plausible common background for autoimmunity are emerging and becoming recognized (Figure 12.1) (3, 4). Characterization of the extent to which particular combinations of autoimmune diseases occur in excess of that expected on the basis of chance may offer new insights into their shared pathophysiological mechanisms.

There are three levels of evidence supporting a common origin for autoimmune diseases. The first level comes from the above-mentioned clinical evidence (i.e., the kaleidoscope of autoimmunity). The second is the pathophysiological mechanisms that are common to autoimmune diseases (Figure 12.1), and the third corresponds to the genetic evidence indicating that the genetic risk factors for autoimmune diseases may well consist of two forms: those common to many diseases and those specific for a given disorder (5).

From: Y. Shoenfeld et al. (eds.): *Diagnostic Criteria in Autoimmune Diseases*, DOI: 10.1007/978-1-60327-285-8_12,
© 2008 Humana Press, Totowa, NJ

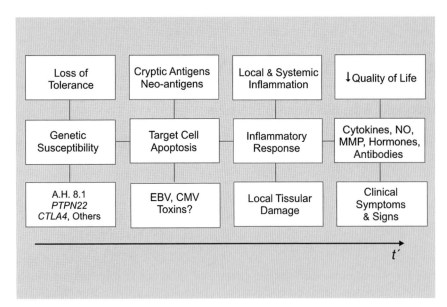

FIGURE 12.1. Fourth-stage model for the pathophysiology of autoimmune diseases. The diseases are favored by polymorphic genes (1st) that make the target cell susceptible to apoptosis (2nd), probably under an infectious or toxic insult (i.e., cigarette smoking, UV light), progressing then to organ lymphocytic infiltration (3rd) and immune system dysregulation (i.e., abnormal Treg function), and subsequent production of autoantibodies and other soluble factors (4th), all of which interfere with the organ or system function and lead to the main clinical signs and symptoms. Abbreviations – A.H. 8.1: ancestral haplotype 8.1. (*HLA-A1, cw7, B8, TNFAB*a2b3, TNFN*S, C2*C, bf*s, C4A*Q0, C4B*1, DRB1*0301, DRB3*0101, DQA1*0501, DQB1*0201*). EBV, Epstein–Barr virus; CMV, cytomegalovirus; NO, nitric oxide; MMP, metalloproteinases.

According to the first level of evidence that corresponds to the mosaic of clinical syndromes manifested in the form of co-occurrence of various autoimmune diseases within an individual or co-occurrence within members of a family, and based on the clustering of autoimmune diseases observed in various cohorts of patients (and their families) that have participated in our previous studies, we have adopted three entities found in the literature and defined a fourth.

Multiple Autoimmune Syndromes

This entity was described by Humbert and Dupond in 1988 as a syndrome(s) consisting of the presence of three or more autoimmune diseases in a single patient (6). While describing the syndrome, their observations led them to a rough classification of clusters based on the co-occurrence of autoimmune diseases, which they identified as types one through three. In multiple autoimmune syndrome (MAS)-1, the authors grouped myasthenia gravis (MG), thymoma, dermatopolymyositis (PDM), and autoimmune myocarditis together. In MAS-2, they grouped Sjögren's syndrome (SS), rheumatoid arthritis (RA), primary biliary cirrhosis (PBC), systemic sclerosis (SSc), and autoimmune thyroid disease (AITD). MAS-3 consisted of AITD, MG and/or thymoma, SS, pernicious anemia (PA), idiopathic thrombocytopenic purpura (ITP), Addison's disease (AD), type 1 diabetes (T1D), vitiligo (VIT), autoimmune hemolytic anemia (HA), and systemic lupus erythematosus (SLE) (6). The importance of this concept is the probability that having three autoimmune diseases simultaneously in one patient goes beyond epidemiological inferences or statistical chance. Thus, the previous notion argues in favor of common

pathophysiological mechanisms and genetic variants giving origin to all three diseases (Figure 12.2). Despite the great breakthrough achieved by Humbert and Dupond in providing a new taxonomy for these co-current phenotypes, on the basis of clinical evidence, the concept became subject to modifications. Initial observations that brought the concept to light were supported by neither statistical methods nor systematic approaches for clustering design. Moreover, studies assessing the risk of patients with a primary autoimmune disease developing other autoimmune diseases found an association with other autoimmune diseases not mentioned in the original report (7). In order to illustrate the magnitude of the problem concerning the risk estimate for being affected simultaneously by more than one autoimmune disease, a review of literature was carried out and a cluster analysis for MAS was performed by estimating uncorrected general distances from a categorical character matrix (Figure 12.3). Three basic, large clusters were obtained from which three main conditions stand out and might be considered the "chaperones" of the autoimmune diseases namely SLE, AITD, and SS (Figure 12.3) (3).

Polyglandular Autoimmune Syndrome, Type II

This syndrome is also universally known as *Schmidt's Syndrome* owing to a case reported by Schmidt in 1926 of two patients who presented AD and chronic lymphocytic thyroiditis. Later in 1964, in an extensive review of the literature, Carpenter included the presence of T1D in the syndrome defining the classic triad for PASII (8) (Figure 12.2). The diagnosis of PASII is based on the presence of at least two of the previously described

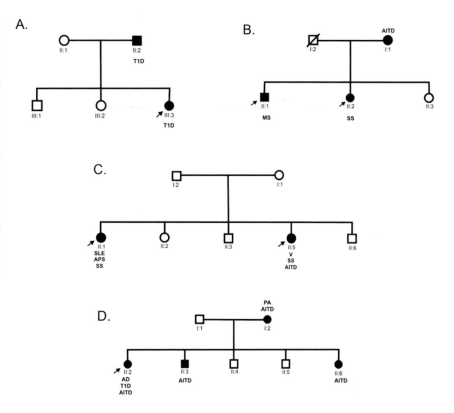

FIGURE 12.2. A. Familial autoimmune disease. In this case, a proband and a first-degree relative (i.e., her father) have type 1 diabetes (T1D). B. Familial autoimmunity. This phenomenon corresponds to the presence of different autoimmune diseases in a nuclear family. C. Multiple auto-immune syndrome. This corresponds to the presence of at least three autoimmune diseases in a single individual. In this case two siblings met criteria for MAS, although they present with different phenotypes. In addition, this family also represents a case of familial autoimmunity. D. Polyglandular autoimmune syndrome, type II. This corresponds to the presence of AD, AITD, and T1D. In this family, however, familial autoimmune disease and familial autoimmune coexist.

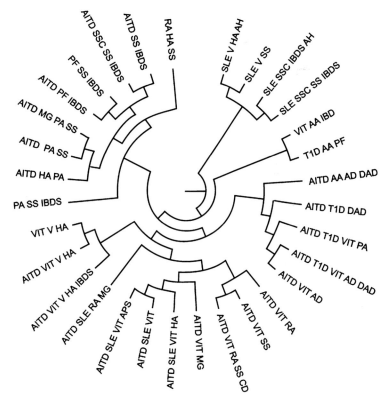

FIGURE 12.3. Multiple autoimmune syndrome clusters. The cladogram corresponds to a review of literature (3) and was obtained by unweighted pair-group method using arithmetic averages (UPGMA). Abbreviations: T1D, diabetes mellitus type 1; SLE, systemic lupus erythematosus; APS, antiphospholipid syndrome; RA, rheumatoid arthritis; SS, Sjögren's syndrome; MG, myasthenia gravis; V, vasculitis including CS, Churg–Strauss; CV, cutaneous vasculitis (diagnosed with biopsy); MP, microscopic polyangiitis; MC, mixed cryoglobulinemia; GCA, giant cell arteritis; SSc, systemic sclerosis (scleroderma); DPM, dermatopoly-myositis; IBD, inflammatory bowel disease (including Crohn's disease and ulcerative colitis); AITD, auto-immune thyroid disease; CD, celiac disease; JRA, juvenile RA; VIT, vitiligo; IBDS, inflammatory biliary diseases (including primary biliary cirrhosis and sclerosing cholangitis); AH, autoimmune hepatitis; DAD, demyelinating autoimmune diseases (including transverse myelitis and multiple sclerosis); AD, Addison's disease; AA, alopecia areata, PF, pemphigus including pemphigus vulgaris and bullous pemphigoid; HA, hemolytic anemia; PA, pernicious anemia; RP, relapsing polychondritis.

conditions in one patient. There are, nevertheless, three more types of PAS (9). PAS type I is given by the presence of oral candidiasis, hypoparathyroidism, and AD within an individual associated with mutations in the *AIRE* gene, a disorder that is inherited as an autosomal recessive disorder. PAS type III is defined as the presence of AITD, and another autoimmune disease without the presence of AD, parathyroid failure, or oral candidiasis. Finally, PAS type IV has been described as the association of two or more organ-specific autoimmune diseases. There is, nevertheless, some controversy surrounding this topic, and some authors argue that PAS types II, III, and IV are different manifestations of the same syndrome. This disagreement has strong foundations because there are several reports showing an association between T1D, AITD, CD, VIT, and AD. Moreover, these syndromes share more characteristics with each other than with PAS type I, thus making them better grouped in a common type of syndrome (9). In agreement with what previous reviewers have agreed on, we believe that MAS can include the whole grouping of PAS II. Thus the combination of the concept under a single condition that allows the association of other combinations of diseases maintains the concept of co-occurrence effectively. This is supported by studies that have found an association between organ-specific autoimmune diseases such as T1D or AITD and systemic autoimmune diseases such as SLE, SS, or RA (3) (Figure 12.3).

Familial Autoimmune Disease (FAID)

This condition is defined as the presence of one specific autoimmune disease in various members of a nuclear family (Figure 12.2). The word "familial" is used arbitrarily throughout genetic epidemiology reports on autoimmune diseases leading to a lack of consensus and hindering the interpretation of results. For instance, some reports have made the distinction between familial and sporadic based solely on the number of siblings affected. As a rule of thumb, they define familial as more than one sibling in the family being affected (10). Others use it as a term to explain the aggregation of an autoimmune disease in first-degree relatives (FDRs) of a family (11). The FAID importance is based on the fact that the presence of the same autoimmune disease in various generations of one family should require either a stronger common genetic component compared with other syndromes or a common environmental risk factor or a combination of both. There is increased evidence for an aggregation of diverse autoimmune diseases in families of patients with a single autoimmune disease (12, 13). As illustrated in Figure 12.2, a case of "sporadic" multiple sclerosis (MS) may correspond to "familial autoimmunity" once relatives are carefully investigated for the presence of other autoimmune diseases.

Thus, the family history of autoimmune diseases should be considered when performing clinical genetic analysis.

Familial Autoimmunity

As mentioned earlier, this condition is defined as the presence of diverse autoimmune diseases in multiple members of a nuclear family (Figure 12.2). Unlike the previous type of clustering, this new definition uses the term "autoimmune disease" as a trait that includes all accepted pathologies for which evidence suggests an autoimmune origin.

Prediction and Prevention

It is now clear that autoimmune diseases do not begin at the time of clinical appearance but rather many years before that. The implication of this concept lies in the possibility of predicting autoimmunity. Throughout the years, many risk factors have been found to be associated with autoimmune diseases. Of these, female gender, a family history of autoimmune diseases, and specific major histocompatibility complex (HLA) alleles were well documented (1). In addition, autoantibodies may also predict specific clinical manifestations, disease severity, and rate of progression, as well as specific clinical phenomena. The identification of these markers and the assessment of their predictive value might enable secondary prevention using specific drugs, or immunological treatment. In addition, the ability to predict the severity of the disease and its specific clinical manifestation allows tertiary prevention of disease complications. Such prevention may be accomplished by relatively simple adjustments in therapy and lifestyle. The question related to the clinical importance of the presence of antibodies in asymptomatic subjects is being resolved by prospective studies with the follow-up of autoantibody titers as well as clinical symptoms in individuals who are being evaluated.

Treatment

A diagnosis of MAS depends on the physician's accuracy and the age at onset of the first autoimmune disease (3). For example, the diagnosis of AITD (i.e., Hashimosto's thyroiditis) in a patient with a previous autoimmune disease (i.e., RA or SLE) can only be achieved when it is suspected because most of the symptoms related to hypothyroidism might be hidden by the symptoms of the underlying disease. The confirmation will be made only by appropriate tests (i.e., abnormal thyroid function tests and the presence of thyroglobulin and TPO antibodies). Each individual disease included in the MAS group should be considered and treated accordingly.

Acknowledgments. We thank Y Shoenfeld, R Cervera, RD Mantilla, and RA Levy for invaluable support. This work was supported by Colciencias (2213-04-16484) and the Fernando Chalem Rheumatology Award to J-M A.

References

1. Anaya J-M, Shoenfeld Y, Correa PA, Garcia-Carrasco M, Cervera R. *Autoimmunity and Autoimmune Disease*. Medellin, CIB; 2005.

2. Lorber M, Gershwin ME, Shoenfeld Y. The coexistence of systemic lupus erythematosus with other autoimmune diseases: The kaleidoscope of autoimmunity. *Semin Arthritis Rheum* 1994; 24: 105–13.

3. Anaya J-M, Corena R, Castiblanco J, Rojas-Villaraga A, Shoenfeld Y. The Kaleidoscope of autoimmunity: Multiple syndromes and familial autoimmunity. *Expert Rev Clin Immunol* 2007; 3: 623–35.

4. Castiblanco J, Anaya J-M. The nature and nurture of common autoimmunity. *Ann N Y Acad Sci* 2007; 1109: 1–8.

5. Anaya J-M, Gomez LM, Castiblanco J. Is there a common basis for autoimmune diseases? *Clin Dev Immunol* 2006; 13: 185–95.

6. Humbert P, Dupond JL. Multiple autoimmune syndromes. *Ann Med Interne (Paris)* 1988; 139: 159–68.

7. Sloka S. Observations on recent studies showing increased co-occurrence of autoimmune diseases. *J Autoimmun* 2002; 18: 251–7.

8. Carpenter CC, Solomon N, Silverberg SG, Bledsoe T, Northcutt RC, Klinenberg JR, Bennett IL Jr, Harvey AM. Schmidt's syndrome (thyroid and adrenal insufficiency). Review of the literature and a report of fifteen new cases including ten instances of coexistent diabetes mellitus. *Medicine* 1964; 43: 153–80.

9. Dittmar M, Kahaly GJ. Polyglandular autoimmune syndromes: Immunogenetics and long-term follow-up. *J Clin Endocrinol Metab* 2003; 88: 2983–92.

10. Radstake TRDJ, Barrera P, Albers JMC, Swinkels HL, van de Putte LBA, van Riel LBA. Familial vs sporadic rheumatoid arthritis (RA). A prospective study in an early RA inception cohort. *Rheumatology (Oxf.)* 2000; 39: 267–73.

11. Laivoranta-Nyman S, Möttönen T, Luukkainen R, Hakala M, Yli-Kerttula U, Hannonen P, Tuokko J, Toivanen A, Ilonen J. Immunogenetic differences between patients with and non-familial rheumatoid arthritis. *Ann Rheum Dis* 2000; 59: 173–7.

12. Anaya J-M, Castiblanco J, Tobon GJ, García J, Abad V, Cuervo H, Velásquez A, Angel ID, Vega P, Arango A. Familial clustering of autoimmune diseases in patients with Type 1 diabetes mellitus. *J Autoimmun* 2006; 26: 208–14.

13. Anaya J-M, Tobon GJ, Vega P, Castiblanco J. Autoimmune disease aggregation in families with primary Sjögren syndrome. *J Rheumatol* 2006; 33: 2227–34.

Part II
Systemic Vasculitis

13
Giant Cell Arteritis

Gideon Nesher

Abstract   Giantcell arteritis (GCA) involves the major branches of the aorta with predilection for the extracranial branches of the carotid artery. It occurs in individuals older than 50 years, and the incidence increases with age. The signs and symptoms of GCA can be classified into four subsets: manifestations of cranial arteritis (mainly headache, jaw claudication and visual manifestations), extracranial arteritis, systemic symptoms and polymyalgia rheumatica. Patients may develop any combination of these manifestations, which are associated with laboratory evidence of an acute-phase reaction. The only test that confirms the diagnosis is a temporal artery biopsy showing vasculitis with mononuclear cell or granulomatous inflammation usually with giant cells. However, areas of vasculitis may be missed by the biopsy and the histological examination is normal in about 15% of the cases. Some imaging modalities may aid in the diagnosis of GCA. Among these, color duplex ultrasonography of the temporal arteries is more commonly used. There are no independent validating criteria to determine whether GCA is present when a temporal artery biopsy is negative. The American College of Rheumatology (ACR) criteria for the classification of GCA may assist in the diagnosis. However, meeting classification criteria is not equivalent to making the diagnosis in individual patients, and the final diagnosis should be based on all clinical, laboratory, imaging and histological findings. Glucocorticoids are the treatment of choice for GCA. The initial dose is 40–60 mg/day for most uncomplicated cases. Addition of low-dose aspirin (100 mg/day) has been shown to significantly decrease the rate of vision loss and stroke during the course of the disease.

Keywords   Temporal arteries · headache · sedimentation rate · glucocorticoids

Description of the Disease

Giant cell arteritis (GCA) involves the major branches of the aorta with predilection for the extracranial branches of the carotid artery, including the temporal arteries. The aorta and other large arteries may also be involved.

GCA is more common among people of north European decent than among Mediterranean people and is rare among African Americans, Native Americans and Asians. GCA occurs in individuals older than 50 years, and the incidence increases with age. The age-specific incidence rates per 100,000 population increase from 2 in the age group 50–59 years to 52 in the age group 80 years and older (1). The estimated prevalence is about 1:750 persons older than 50 years (2). Women are two to three times more commonly affected.

The signs and symptoms of GCA can be classified into four subsets: manifestations of cranial arteritis, extracranial arteritis, systemic symptoms and polymyalgia rheumatica (Table 13.1). Among these, tender, prominent temporal arteries with absent pulses, jaw claudication and diplopia have the highest positive likelihood ratios for GCA diagnosis (3, 4). Patients may develop any combination of these manifestations. Patients with systemic symptoms and increased inflammatory response in laboratory testing such as very high erythrocyte sedimentation rate (ESR), anemia of inflammation and thrombocytosis tend to present less often with ischemic intracranial manifestations (5). The onset of GCA symptoms may be abrupt but in most instances symptoms develop gradually over a period of several weeks. Elevated ESR is found in more than 90% of the patients, and in 30–60% it is very high (>100 mm/h). This and other abnormalities in laboratory tests are elaborated in Table 13.2.

From: Y. Shoenfeld et al. (eds.): *Diagnostic Criteria in Autoimmune Diseases*, DOI: 10.1007/978-1-60327-285-8_13,
© 2008 Humana Press, Totowa, NJ

TABLE 13.1. Signs and symptoms of giant cell arteritis (GCA).

Clinical feature		Frequency (%)
Cranial arteritis	Headache, facial pain	70–85
	Scalp tenderness	20–40
	Prominent or tender temporal arteries	30–60
	Jaw claudication	30–40
	Vision symptoms: sudden vision loss (transient or permanent), diplopia or other ophthalmic manifestations	15–45
	Stroke, transient ischemic attacks and other neuropsychiatric manifestations	<15
	Vestibulo-auditory manifestations: hearing loss, tinnitus, vertigo	5–25
	Tongue or scalp infarction	<5
Extracranial arteritis	Aortic arch syndrome, aortic-valve insufficiency, aortic aneurysm and dissection	<15
	Clinically significant involvement of other arteries	10–20
	Peripheral neuropathies	<15
	Respiratory symptoms (cough, sore throat, hoarseness)	<15
Systemic symptoms	Fever, malaise, fatigue, anorexia, weight loss	30–60
Polymyalgia rheumatica	Bilateral aching and stiffness of the shoulder girdle, sometimes the neck and hip girdle	20–65

TABLE 13.2. Abnormalities in laboratory tests in giant cell arteritis (GCA).

Test		Frequency (%)
Acute-phase reactants	Elevated erythrocyte sedimentation rate (ESR)	90–95
	ESR ≥100 mm/h	30–60
	Elevated ESR *and/or* elevated C-reactive protein (CRP)	>95
Blood count	Anemia	35–65
	Thrombocytosis	30–60
	Leukocytosis	10–30
Liver function tests	Elevated alkaline phosphatase	30–60
	Elevated transaminases	<20
	Low albumin	10–30
Autoantibodies	Anticardiolipin	30–80

TABLE 13.3. Predictive values of temporal artery (TA) duplex ultrasonography and biopsy for giant cell arteritis (GCA) diagnosis.

	TA biopsy (%)	TA ultrasonography (%)
Positive predictive value	~100	50–90
Negative predictive value	80–90	90–95

High-resolution contrast-enhanced magnetic resonance imaging (MRI) of the temporal arteries also enables evaluation of possible inflammation of the vessel wall. Preliminary results show high sensitivity of this imaging modality (8). Angiography of the aortic arch and its branches may serve to diagnose large-vessel involvement (9). Non-invasive modalities, such as positron-emission tomography, may also be employed to detect large-vessel involvement (10), but data on their predictive values are limited.

GCA affects the vessels focally; therefore, areas of vasculitis may be missed and the histological examination is normal in about 15% of GCA patients (biopsy-negative GCA) (11). A threshold temporal artery biopsy size of 1 cm is associated with increased diagnostic yield (12). Obtaining biopsies from both temporal arteries increases the chance of a positive result by 1–14% (13, 14). It is preferable to perform the biopsy as soon as possible, but the specimen may show signs of arteritis even after 2–4 weeks of treatment (15).

There are no independent validating criteria to determine whether GCA is present when a temporal artery biopsy is negative. The American College of Rheumatology (ACR) criteria for classification of GCA (16) may assist in diagnosis.

These criteria include:

1. age at onset ≥50 years
2. a new headache
3. temporal artery abnormality such as tenderness to palpation or decreased pulsation
4. ESR ≥50 mm/h

Diagnosis and Diagnostic Criteria

The diagnosis of GCA is made primarily on clinical grounds and is bolstered by laboratory evidence of an acute-phase reaction. The only test that confirms the diagnosis of GCA is a temporal artery biopsy showing vasculitis with mononuclear cell or granulomatous inflammation usually with giant cells.

Some imaging modalities may aid in the diagnosis of GCA. Among these, color duplex ultrasonography of the temporal arteries is more commonly used. A periluminal hypo-echoic halo, probably representing vessel-wall edema, is considered highly specific for GCA (6). A recent meta-analysis concluded that when the pre-test probability of GCA is low, a negative result of ultrasonography practically excludes GCA (7). It appears that ultrasonography better serves to rule out GCA due to its high negative predictive value, whereas a positive test needs to be confirmed by a temporal artery biopsy, as the positive predictive value varies considerably among different studies (Table 13.3).

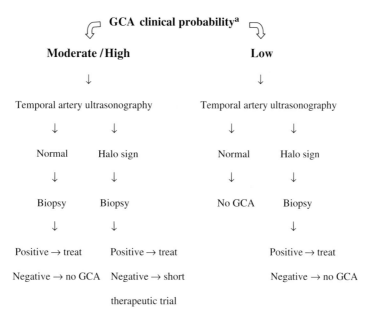

FIGURE 13.1. Suggested approach to giant cell arteritis (GCA) diagnosis.

[a] The pre-test probability is considered moderate if one of the following clinical manifestations is present *in addition* to elevated ESR and/or CRP: new headache, jaw claudication, sudden vision loss (permanent or transient), diplopia, prominent and tender temporal arteries. The probability is higher if more than one of these clinical manifestations is present, or when polymyalgia rheumatica, cerebral ischemic symptoms or systemic symptoms are present in addition to one of these manifestations.

5. abnormal artery biopsy showing vasculitis with mono-nuclear cell or granulomatous inflammation, usually with giant cells.

At least three of the criteria must be present, which yields a sensitivity of 93% and a specificity of 91%.

However, it is important to note that these are not diagnostic criteria. These classification criteria serve mainly to differentiate GCA from other types of vasculitis. They cannot effectively serve to differentiate GCA from other disease conditions. Such classification criteria work best in studying groups of patients with vasculitis and less well when used for diagnosing individual cases (17). Meeting classification criteria is not equivalent to making the diagnosis in individual patients, and the final diagnosis should be based on all clinical, laboratory, imaging and histological findings.

Based on the predictive values of tem biopsy and temporal artery duplex studies (Table 13.3), long-term experience with diagnosing and treating GCA, and data synthesis from studies, a practical approach to GCA diagnosis in suspected patients is suggested (Table 13.4).

Therapy and Course

Glucocorticoids are the treatment of choice for GCA. The initial dose is 40–60 mg/day for most cases. Starting treatment with intravenous methylprednisolone 500–1000 mg/day for 3 days may be considered in patients with vision loss (transient or permanent), diplopia, transient ischemic attacks or stroke (18).

Rapid improvement of clinical manifestations following treatment initiation is characteristic. Prompt treatment is crucial in GCA to prevent irreversible complications of acute vision loss and stroke. Thus, treatment may be started prior to confirming the diagnosis.

The average duration of treatment is 2–3 years. Relapses are experienced by 25–65% of GCA patients. Most relapses are mild, but some patients may develop vision loss or stroke while tapering glucocorticoid dosage or after discontinuation of therapy. Addition of low-dose aspirin (100 mg/day) has been shown to significantly decrease the rate of vision loss and stroke during the course of the disease, probably mediated by its anti-platelet effect (19). It is not clear whether the presence of anticardiolipin antibodies increases the rate of intracranial ischemic complications (5).

Individual cases vary greatly; therefore, the exact doses and the duration of treatment should be adjusted to the needs of the individual patient, considering both disease manifestations and glucocorticoid adverse effects. No steroid-sparing agent was proven to be widely effective thus far.

References

1. Salvarani C, Crowson CS, O'Fallon WM, Hunder GG, and Gabriel SE. Reappraisal of the epidemiology of giant cell arteritis in Olmsted County, Minnesota, over fifty-year period. *Arthritis Rheum* 2004; 51: 264–8.

2. Boesen P and Sorensen SF. Giant cell arteritis, temporal arteritis, and polymyalgia rheumatica in a Danish county. *Arthritis Rheum* 1987; 30: 294–9.

3. Smetana GW and Shmerling RH. Does this patient have temporal arteritis? *J Am Med Assoc* 2002; 287: 92–101.

4. Seo P and Stone JH. Large-vessel vasculitis. *Arthritis Rheum* 2004; 51: 128–39.

5. Nesher G, Berkun Y, Mates M, et al. Risk factors for cranial ischemic complications in giant cell arteritis. *Medicine* 2004; 83: 114–22.

6. Schmidt WA, Kraft HE, Vorpahl K, Volker L, and Gromnica-Ihle EJ. Color duplex ultrasonography in the diagnosis of temporal arteritis. *N Engl J Med* 1997; 337: 1336–42.

7. Karassa FB, Matsagas MI, Schmidt WA, and Iannidis JP. Meta-analysis: Test performance of ultrasonography for giant cell arteritis. *Ann Intern Med* 2005; 142: 359–69.

8. Bley TA, Weiben O, Uhl M, et al. Assessment of the cranial involvement pattern of giant cell arteritis with 3T magnetic resonance imaging. *Arthritis Rheum* 2005; 52: 2470–7.

9. Brack A, Martinez-Taboada V, Stanson A, Goronzy JJ, and Weyand CM. Disease pattern in cranial and large-vessel giant-cell arteritis. *Arthritis Rheum* 1999; 42: 311–17.

10. Blockmans D, Stroobants S, Maes A, and Mortelmans L. Positron emission tomography in giant cell arteritis and polymyalgia rheumatica: Evidence for inflammation of the aortic arch. *Am J Med* 2000; 108: 246–9.

11. González-Gay MA, García-Porrua C, Liorca J, et al. Biopsy-negative giant cell arteritis: Clinical spectrum and predictive factors for positive temporal artery biopsy. *Semin Arthritis Rheum* 2001; 30: 249–56.

12. Taylor-Gjevre R, Vo M, Shukla D, and Resch L. Temporal artery biopsy for giant cell arteritis. *J Rheumatol* 2005; 32: 1279–82.

13. Hall S and Hunder GG. Is temporal artery biopsy prudent? *Mayo Clin Proc* 1984; 59: 793–6.

14. Pless M, Rizzo JF III, Lamkin JC, and Lessell S. Concordance of bilateral temporal artery biopsy in giant cell arteritis. *J Neuroophthalmol* 2000; 20: 216–8.

15. Ray-Chaudhuri N, Kine DA, Tijani SO, et al. Effect of prior steroid treatment on temporal artery biopsy findings in giant cell arteritis. *Br J Ophthalmol* 2002; 86: 530–2.

16. Hunder GG, Bloch DA, Michel BA, et al. The American College of Rheumatology 1990 criteria for the classification of giant cell arteritis. *Arthritis Rheum* 1990; 33: 1122–8.

17. Hunder GG. The use and misuse of classification and diagnostic criteria for complex disease. *Ann Intern Med* 1998; 129: 417–8.

18. Dasgupta B and Hassan N. Giant cell arteritis: Recent advances and guidelines for management. *Clin Exp Rheumatol* 2007; 25(Suppl. 44): S62–5.

19. Nesher G, Berkun Y, Mates M, Baras M, Rubinow A, and Sonnenblick M. Low-dose aspirin and prevention of cranial ischemic complications in giant cell arteritis. *Arthritis Rheum* 2004; 50: 1332–7.

14
Polymyalgia Rheumatica

Gideon Nesher

Abstract Polymyalgia rheumatica is the most common inflammatory rheumatic disease of the elderly, and shares many pathogenetic and epidemiological features with giant cell arteritis. The typical symptoms are bilateral aching of the shoulder girdle, associated with morning stiffness. The neck and hip girdle may also be involved. The diagnosis of polymyalgia rheumatica is made primarily on clinical grounds. There is no single diagnostic test, but sets of diagnostic criteria have been suggested by several groups of investigators, based on the typical clinical presentation and laboratory evidence of acute-phase reaction. Other conditions that may mimic polymyalgia rheumatica must be excluded by appropriate testing and close monitoring of the disease course. Glucocorticoids at low doses (15–20 mg/day initially) are the mainstay of treatment.

Keywords Giant cell arteritis · morning stiffness · sedimentation rate · glucocorticoids

Description of the Disease

Polymyalgia rheumatica (PMR) is the most common inflammatory rheumatic disease of the elderly. PMR patients share many pathogenetic features with giant cell arteritis (GCA) (1). There is evidence for vascular inflammation with increased expression of inflammatory cytokines in the temporal arteries of PMR patients, without overt histological evidence of arteritis. Using fluorodeoxyglucose positron emission tomography, increased uptake was documented in thoracic blood vessels in PMR patients, suggestive of inflammation in these vessels (2).

Similar to GCA, the highest annual incidence rates were observed in northern Europe: 50–100 per 100,000 individuals older than 50 years. The estimated prevalence was 1:200 persons older than 50 years (3).

The typical symptom of polymyalgia rheumatica (PMR) is bilateral aching of the shoulder girdle (1). The neck and hip girdle may also be involved. Morning stiffness is also a prominent feature (Table 14.1). These symptoms are probably related to inflammation of the subacromial, subdeltoid and trochanteric bursae, and the glenohumeral or hip joints (4, 5). Onset may be acute or gradual. One-third of PMR patients without evidence of GCA have systemic manifestations such as low-grade fever, malaise and anorexia, but these are often milder than systemic symptoms in GCA patients. PMR may be associated with other GCA clinical manifestations, but may be an "isolated" phenomenon. Like GCA, PMR develops in patients older than 50 years, and is more common in women.

Diagnosis and Diagnostic Criteria

The diagnosis of PMR is made primarily on clinical grounds and is bolstered by laboratory evidence of an acute-phase reaction (Table 14.2). There is no single diagnostic test for PMR, but sets of diagnostic criteria have been suggested by several groups of investigators (Table 14.3) (3, 6, 7, 8, 9). Other conditions that may mimic PMR (such as inflammatory myopathies, elderly-onset rheumatoid arthritis (EORA), fibromyalgia, osteoarthritis, subacute infections, thyroid diseases, and occult malignancies) must be excluded by appropriate testing (10).

These sets of criteria used for diagnostic purposes are empirical. They have been defined by clinical experts who had studied the disease extensively. Each set of criteria has its own advantages and disadvantages. Recently, an international PMR Consortium has convened and initiated a multinational effort. The initial goal of the

From: Y. Shoenfeld et al. (eds.): *Diagnostic Criteria in Autoimmune Diseases*, DOI: 10.1007/978-1-60327-285-8_14,
© 2008 Humana Press, Totowa, NJ

TABLE 14.1. Clinical features of polymyalgia rheumatica (PMR).

Clinical feature	Frequency (%)
Pain in shoulder girdle	90–100
Morning stiffness	90–100
Bilateral upper arm tenderness	50–75
Neck pain	30–50
Pain in hip girdle	30–70
Distal musculo-skeletal manifestations[a]	20–50
Fever, malaise, anorexia	20–40

[a] Arthritis/arthralgia of the hands, pitting edema of the hands (RS₃PE syndrome), carpal tunnel syndrome.

TABLE 14.2. Abnormalities in laboratory tests in polymyalgia rheumatica (PMR).

Test	Frequency (%)
Elevated erythrocyte sedimentation rate (ESR)	80–95
Anemia (normocytic)	20–50
Thrombocytosis	<20
Elevated alkaline phosphatase	<20

Consortium is to standardize classification criteria and outcome measures in patients with PMR.

The finding of bilateral shoulder or hip bursitis/synovitis by ultrasonography or magnetic resonance imaging (MRI) has been reported to be present in most PMR patients, and may support a diagnosis of PMR (4, 5); however, these changes may also occur in about 20% of EORA (11).

There is a wide range (4–31%) of reported frequency of GCA in patients presenting with PMR (1). The two conditions may present together, but may sometimes be separated by long intervals and either one may present first. The approach for detecting GCA in PMR patients is a matter of controversy. One diagnostic option is to biopsy the TA routinely in all PMR patients. In this approach, the chance of missing GCA is small, as it may detect arteritis in persons with 'isolated' PMR, but the frequency of positive biopsies is very low (12, 13). Another strategy is to biopsy only those patients who have symptoms suggestive of GCA. With this approach, the results are likely to vary according to the expertise of the examining physician (14).

Severe degrees of anemia and thrombocytosis are suggestive of GCA in patients presenting with PMR symptoms. Also, poor clinical response to low-dose prednisone (15–20 mg/day) with persistent abnormalities in laboratory parameters of inflammation is also suggestive of GCA in patients presenting with "isolated" PMR (10). In such cases, ultrasonography and biopsy of the temporal arteries should be performed to rule out GCA.

It is difficult at times to distinguish between PMR patients and those with EORA and PMR-like presentation at the early stages. In 25% of EORA patients, PMR symptoms are the principal initial manifestation, and about 10% of patients with PMR presentation will eventually develop the characteristic features of RA (15, 16, 17). The lack of anti-cyclic citrullinated peptide (anti-CCP) antibodies in PMR patients may help to differentiate them in early stages from patients with EORA (18). A follow-up of several months may be required to make a definite distinction between PMR and EORA.

Therapy and Course

Glucocorticoids are the mainstay of treatment for PMR. The starting dose is 15–20 mg/day. Symptoms typically begin to abate within 1–3 days of commencing therapy.

TABLE 14.3. Criteria for diagnosis of polymyalgia rheumatica suggested by various authors.

	Healey 1984	Chuang et al. 1982	Jones and Hazleman 1981	Bird et al. 1979	Hamrin 1972
Age	>50 years	>50		>65 years	>50 years
Onset				<2 weeks	
Duration		>1 month	>2 months		>2 months
Area of pain	Neck, shoulder, or pelvic girdle	1. neck or torso, 2. shoulders or arms, 3. hips or thighs (at least 2 of 3)	shoulder and pelvic girdle	bilateral shoulder pain and stiffness	neck, shoulder or pelvic girdle (at least 2 of 3)
Morning stiffness	>1 h	>30 min	present	>1 h	
Tenderness				upper arms	
Systemic symptoms				depression, weight loss	present
Erythrocyte sedimentation rate (ESR)	Elevated	>40 mm/h*	>30 mm/h, or C-reactive protein >6 mg/l	>40 mm/h	>50 mm/h
Response to glucocorticoids	rapid, to 20 mg or less		prompt and dramatic		
Requirements for diagnosis	age must be >50, plus 3 of the other criteria	all criteria	all criteria	if any 3 criteria present – sensitivity 92% specificity 80%	criteria of age, pain, and ESR are obligatory

[a] If ESR is borderline, look instead for other evidence to support the diagnosis: change in ESR compared to pre-illness period, rapid response to low-dose steroids, history of GCA, fever, weight loss or anemia.

Prompt response to low-dose glucocorticoid therapy is typical and sometimes used to confirm the diagnosis (8, 9). After 2–4 weeks, following improvement of the clinical features of the disease together with normalization of the acute-phase reactants, the dose of glucocorticoids can be tapered while monitoring for possible recurrence of symptoms. Relapse occurs in about one-half of the patients, with response to increasing the dose to the previous level. Symptoms of GCA may develop while the glucocorticoid dose is tapered. These patients, initially diagnosed as PMR, will require a diagnostic and therapeutic approach appropriate for GCA. The duration of treatment for PMR varies from one year to several years.

References

1. Nesher G. Giant cell arteritis and polymyalgia rheumatica. In: Ball GV and Bridges SL Jr. (Eds.) *Vasculitis*. 2002, Oxford University Press, Oxford, UK.
2. Moosig F, Czech N, Mehl C, et al. Correlation between 18-fluorodeoxyglucose accumulation in large vessels and serological markers of inflammation in polymyalgia rheumatica: A quantitative PET study. *Ann Rheum Dis*, 2004;63:870–3.
3. Chuang, T.Y., Hunder, G.G., Ilstrup, D.M. and Kurland, L.T. Polymyalgia rheumatica: A 10-year epidemiologic and clinical study. *Ann Intern Med*, 1982;97:672–80.
4. Salvarani, C., Cantini, F., Olivieri, I. et al. Proximal bursitis in active polymyalgia rheumatica. *Ann Intern Med*, 1997;39:1199–207.
5. Cantini F, Nicoli L, Mannini C, et al. Inflammatory changes of the hip synovial structures in polymyalgia rheumatica. *Clin Exp Rheumatol 2005*;23:462–8.
6. Hamrin, B. Polymyalgia arteritica. *Acta Med Scand 1972*;533 (Suppl.), 1–131.
7. Bird, H.A., Esselinckx, W., Dison, A.S.J., Mowat, A.G. and Wood, P.H.N. An evaluation of criteria for polymyalgia rheumatica. *Ann Rheum Dis*, 1979;38:434–9.
8. Jones, J.G. and Hazleman, B.L. Prognosis and management of polymyalgia rheumatica. *Ann Rheum Dis*, 1981;40:1–5.
9. Healey, L.A. Long-term follow-up of polymyalgia rheumatica: Evidence for synovitis. *Semin Arthritis Rheum*, 1984;13:322–8.
10. González-Gay, M.A., García-Porrua, C., Salvarani C, Olivieri I, and Hunder GG. Polymyalgia manifestations in different conditions mimicking polymyalgia rheumatica. *Clin Exp Rheumatol*, 2000;18:755–9.
11. Lange, U., Teichmann, J., Stracke, H., Bretzel, R.G. and Neeck, G. Elderly onset rheumatoid arthritis and polymyalgia rheumatica: Ultrasonographic study of the glenohumeral joints. *Rheumatol Int*, 1998;17:229–32.
12. Healey, L.A. Relation of giant cell arteritis to polymyalgia rheumatica. *Bailliere's Clin Rheumatol*, 1991;5:371–8.
13. Schmidt, W.A and Gromnica-Ihle, E.J. Incidence of temporal arteritis in patients with polymyalgia rheumatica: A prospective study using color Doppler ultrasonography of the temporal arteries. *Rheumatology*, 2002;20:309–18.
14. Hunder, G.G. Giant cell arteritis in polymyalgia rheumatica. *Am J Med*, 1997;102:514–16.
15. Caporali R, Montecucco C, Epis O, Bobbio-Pallavicini F, Maio T, and Cimmino MA. Presenting features of polymyalgia (PMR) and rheumatoid arthritis with PMR-like onset: A prospective study. *Ann Rheum Dis*, 2001;60:1021–4.
16. Gran, J.T. and Myklebust, G. The Incidence and clinical characteristics of peripheral arthritis in polymyalgia rheumatica and temporal arteritis: A prospective study of 231 cases. *Rheumatology*, 2000;39:283–7.
17. Pease CT, Haugeberg G, Morgan AW, Montague B, Hensor EM, and Bhakta BB. Diagnosing late-onset rheumatoid arthritis, polymyalgia rheumatica, and temporal arteritis in patients presenting with polymyalgic symptoms. A prospective longterm study. *J Rheumatol*, 2005;32:1043–6.
18. Lopez-Hoyos M, Ruis de Alegria C, Blanco R, et al. Clinical utility of anti-CCP antibodies in the differential diagnosis of elderly-onset rheumatoid arthritis and polymyalgia rheumatica. *Rheumatology*, 2004;43:655–7.

15
Takayasu Arteritis

Rosa Maria Rodrigues Pereira, Jozélio Freire de Carvalho,
Maurício Levy-Neto and Eloísa Bonfá

Abstract   Takayasu arteritis (TA) is an inflammatory disease of the aorta and its primary branches that affects mainly young women. The arterial involvement may cause ischemic manifestations such as limb or abdominal claudication, visual or cerebrovascular symptoms or renovascular hypertention. Anuloaortic regurgitation secondary to aortic root dilatation may also occur. The most important parameters for diagnosis are the young age of onset and the clinical or laboratory evidence of inflammation [fever, carotidynia, elevated erythrocyte sedimentation rate (ESR)] and aortography abnormalities. Carotid and other arteries ultrasound studies showing thickened artery walls may help in the diagnosis, but the main tool for diagnosis has long been the aspect of the digital subtraction arteriography. Nowadays, the arteriography has been replaced by other contrasted enhanced arterial image studies, especially angiotomography or angioresonance. The following criteria are suggestive of the disease: (a) the concomitant presence of stenosis and aneurysm in aorta, (b) presence of stenosis of at least one aortic branch such as subclavian, common carotid, inonimate, vertebral, renal or mesenteric, especially if a few centimeters away from the arterial ostium and (c) association of thickening of the aortic wall with branch stenosis. Two diagnostic criteria sets are commonly used to classify patients as TA: the American College of Rheumatology and the Sharma modified Ishikawa's set.

Keywords   Takayasu arteritis · vasculitis · diagnosis criteria · aorta stenosis · aneurysm · aortitis

Takayasu arteritis (TA) is a chronic and progressive inflammatory disease, preferentially occlusive, that involves the aorta and its branches and may also affect the coronary and pulmonary arteries (1). This disease affects young women with a female:male ratio of 9:1. The average age of diagnosis is between 15 and 25 years of age although it has been reported as early as 3 years of age and later in life (2, 3). It has a worldwide distribution, with the greatest prevalence in Asia. In Japan, it has been estimated that 150 new cases occur each year; in contrast, the incidence is 1 to 3 new cases per million people in the United States and Europe. South America countries have been recognized as areas of relatively high incidence (4, 5).

The inflammatory process that occurs in this vasculitis may be localized to a portion of thoracic or abdominal aorta and branches, or may involve the entire extension of these vessels. Although there is considerable variability in disease expression (6), the initial vascular lesion frequently occurs in the left middle or proximal subclavian artery. As the disease progresses, the left common carotid, vertebral, brachiocephalic, right middle or proximal subclavian artery, right carotid and vertebral arteries, and aorta may also be affected.

Pathogenesis

The cause of TA remains unknown. The geographic clustering suggests that genetic and environmental factors may play an important role. Cellular and humoral immune mechanisms have been implicated in the pathogenesis of TA. The histologic findings are particularly supportive of a cell-mediated process. In this regard, natural killer cells, cytotoxic T cells and $\gamma\delta$ T lymphocytes have been demonstrated in aortic tissue from TA patients. These cells may cause vascular injury by releasing large amounts of cytolytic compound named perforin. Moreover, expression of heat shock protein-65 might facilitate recognition and

From: Y. Shoenfeld et al. (eds.): *Diagnostic Criteria in Autoimmune Diseases*, DOI: 10.1007/978-1-60327-285-8_15,
© 2008 Humana Press, Totowa, NJ

adhesion of the infiltrating cells (7). Increased expression of intracellular adhesion molecule 1 (ICAM-1) and human leukocyte antigen (HLA) class I and II antigen in the vessel wall also supports the concept of cell-mediated process.

A role for humoral immune mechanisms is suggested by the presence of hypergammaglobulinemia, rheumatoid factor and antiendothelial antibodies.

Clinical Features

Patients with TA present the following symptoms on physical examination: bruits, diminished or absent pulses and asymmetric blood pressure measurements between extremities. Because the subclavian arteries are a frequent site of vessel stenosis, blood pressure measurement in one or both arms may not be representative of aortic root pressure.

Hypertension has been reported to occur in 35–77% of TA patients (8, 9, 10, 11, 12, 13, 14). It is an important cause of morbidity in TA patients and contributes to renal, cardiac and cerebral injuries. In India, TA is the most common cause of renovascular hypertension, accounting for over 60% of all cases.

At the time of diagnosis, approximately 20% of patients with TA are clinically asymptomatic, with the disease being detected solely by abnormal vascular findings on examination. The remaining 80% of patients with TA present a variety of signs and symptoms that can be subdivided into two groups: those caused by vascular injury and those caused by systemic inflammation. The constitutional or musculoskeletal symptoms are observed in 20–40% of the patients and may dominate the presentation in approximately one-third of all cases. They are characterized by fatigue, malaise, weight loss, night sweats, fever, artralgias or myalgias.

Vascular symptoms are a direct result of current or previous arteritis. Active inflammation may cause tenderness over vessels and carotidynia, which is observed in 2–32% of patients. Vessel inflammation typically results in either stenosis or aneurysm formation. Arterial stenosis may present with signs or symptoms of diminished blood flow to regions supplied by the affected vessel, and aneurysms can rupture or cause valvular incompetence when involving the aortic root. The frequencies of common symptoms and signs are listed in Table 15.1 (8, 9, 10, 11, 12, 13, 14).

Stenosis or occlusion of vessels that supply central nervous system (vertebral and carotid arteries) may diminish perfusion and cause injury to the brain manifested by transient ischemic attacks, stroke, dizziness, syncope, headache or visual changes.

Visual symptoms chiefly result from retinal ischemia produced by narrowing/occlusion of the internal carotid circulation or as a direct complication of hypertension.

Cardiac manifestations are frequently related to aortic valvular regurgitation from dilation of the aortic root. Up to 25% of patients may also develop coronary vessel stenosis. The patients with cardiac involvement may present with dyspnea, palpitations, angina, myocardial infarction, heart failure or sudden death.

The pulmonary arteries are involved in up to 50% of cases; however, symptoms related to pulmonary arteritis are less common. Pulmonary manifestations due to pulmonary vasculitis are less common and include chest pain, dyspnea and hemoptysis. Anatomopathological studies have reported a frequency as high as 50% of pulmonary arteries involvement.

TABLE 15.1. Common symptoms and signs in Takayasu arteritis.

	Brazil (n = 73)	China (n = 530)	India (n = 106)	Japan (n = 52)	Korea (n = 129)	Mexico (n = 107)	USA (n = 60)
Fatigue (%)	–	–	–	27	34	78	43
Weight loss (%)	27.5	–	9	–	11	22	20
Musculoskeletal (%)	26	–	5	6	–	53	53
Claudication (%)	57	25	–	13	21	29	90
Headache (%)	45	–	44	31	60	57	42
Visual changes (%)	–	10	12	6	20	8	30
Syncope dizziness (%)	29	14	26	40	36	13	35
Palpitations (%)	–	–	19	23	23	43	10
Dyspnea (%)	–	11	26	21	42	72	–
Carotidynia (%)	–	–	–	21	2	–	32
Hypertension (%)	35.5	60	77	33	40	72	35
Bruit (%)	64.5	58	35	–	37	94	80
Decreased pulses (%)	85	37	–	62	55	96	60
Asymmetric blood pressure (%)	–	–	–	–	–	–	47

The most common skin lesions observed includes erythema nodosum or pyoderma gangrenosum over the legs. The lesions frequently show vasculitis of small vessels on biopsy.

Laboratorial Findings

There is no laboratory study that is diagnostic for TA, but the disease is usually associated with nonspecific findings of inflammation. In fact, acute-phase reactants such as an elevated erythrocyte sedimentation rate (ESR), increased serum C-reactive protein and alpha-2 globulin concentrations, and hypoalbuminemia are a reflection of underlying inflammatory process. These tests are not always precise or invariably reliable indicators, but usually reflect the disease activity.

Imaging Findings

Imaging of the aorta and major arteries is usually necessary to confirm the diagnosis of TA.

Arteriography: The most frequent arteriographic finding is stenosis, which occurs in 85% of patients. Vessel occlusion or irregularity is also commonly seen (Figures 15.1 and 15.2). Aneurysms may be saccular or fusiform and typically affect the aorta rather than its branches. Varying patterns of vessel involvement have been observed in different populations with lesions of the ascending aorta and aortic arch being more common in Japanese patients, whereas involvement of the abdominal aorta and renal arteries is more typical in patients from India and Brazil (8, 15, 16). Arteriography may define the localization and appearance of the arterial lesion and may also allow a therapeutic intervention (balloon dilatation and/or stent) to follow the same puncture.

Although arteriography frequently provides clear outlines of the lumen of involved arteries, it does not allow arterial wall thickening to be assessed and is an invasive test associated some risks such as an important exposure to contrast and radiation. Therefore, if a therapeutic intervention is not anticipated, a less invasive imaging technique may be preferred.

Computed tomography (CT) or magnetic resonance imaging (MRI) scans allow visualization of both vascular lumen and arterial wall thickness, improving the accuracy of TA diagnostic. It has been demonstrated that T2-weighted MRI, sensitive to liquid content, can detect arterial wall edema. Moreover, T1-weighted MRI after gadolinium injection permits visualization of the aortic wall enhancement, which could reflect inflammatory and/or fibrosis vascular lesions in TA patients. MRI improves the mapping of arterial lumen, as well as detecting aortic wall thickness disease. The degree of wall thickness and the presence of edema and/or delayed enhancement in the aortic wall could provide data regarding the diagnosis, control and follow-up of TA patients (17, 18, 19).

Diagnostic Criteria

(a) American College of Rheumatology 1990 criteria for the classification of TA (5).

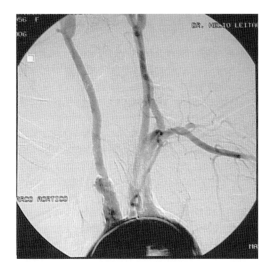 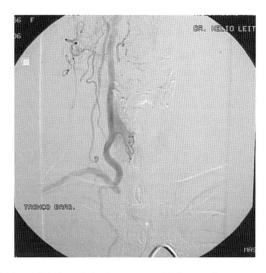

FIGURE 15.1. Arteriography. Left panel: arterial phase shows occlusion of right subclavian artery. Right panel: venosus phase shows retrograde blood flow by vertebral artery characterizing subclavian steal syndrome.

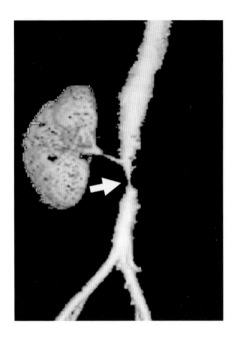

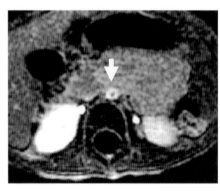

FIGURE 15.2. Left panel: magnetic resonance imaging (MRI) shaded-surface reconstruction showed aortic stenosis at the renal level (arrow) and occlusion of the left renal artery. Right panel: axial delayed enhancement in the abdominal aorta wall at the infra renal level associated with stenosis (arrow).

Criterion	Definition
Age at disease onset ≤40 years	Development of symptoms or findings related to TA at age ≤40 years
Claudication of extremities	Development and worsening of fatigue and discomfort in muscles of one or more extremities, while in use, especially the upper extremities
Decreased brachial artery pressure	Decrease pulsation of one or both brachial arteries
Blood pressure difference >10 mmHg	Difference of >10 mmHg in systolic blood pressure between arms
Bruit over subclavian arteries or aorta	Bruit audible on auscultation over one or both subclavian arteries or abdominal aorta
Arteriogram abnormality	Arteriografic narrowing or occlusion of the entire aorta, its primary branches or larger arteries in the proximal upper or lower extremities, not due to arteriosclerosis, fibromuscular dysplasia or similar causes; changes usually foci or segmental

For purposes of classification, a patient shall be said to have TA if at least three of these six criteria are present. The presence of any three or more criteria yields a sensitivity of 90.5% and a specificity of 97.8%.

(b) Sharma's criteria for TA (Ishikawa's criteria modified according to Sharma et al.) (20, 21).

Three major criteria:

1. Left mid-subclavian artery lesion: the most severe stenosis or occlusion present in the mid portion from the point 1 cm proximal to the vertebral artery orifice up to that 3 cm distal to the orifice determined by angiography.

2. Right mid-subclavian artery lesion: the most severe stenosis or occlusion present in the mid portion from the right vertebral artery orifice to the point 3 cm distal to orifice determined by angiography.

3. Characteristic signs and symptoms of at least 1 month duration: These include limb claudication, pulselessness or pulse differences in limbs, an unobtainable or significant blood pressure difference (>10 mmHg systolic blood pressure difference in limb), fever, neck pain, transient amaurosis, blurred vision, syncope, dyspnea or palpitations.

Ten minor criteria:

1. High ESR: unexplained persistent high ESR >20 mm/h (Westergren) at diagnosis or presence of the evidence in patients history.

2. Carotid artery tenderness: unilateral or bilateral tenderness of common arteries on palpation. Neck muscle tenderness is unacceptable.

3. Hypertension: persistent blood pressure >140/90 mmHg brachial or >160/90 mmHg popliteal.

4. Aortic regurgitation or Anuloaortic ectasia: aortic regurgitation by auscultation or Doppler echocardiography or angiography; or Anuloaortic ectasia by angiography or two-dimensional echocardiography.

5. Pulmonary artery lesion: lobar or segmental arterial occlusion or equivalent determined by angiography or perfusion scintigraphy, or presence of stenosis, aneurysm, luminal irregularity or any combination in pulmonary trunk or in unilateral or bilateral pulmonary arteries determined by angiography.

6. Left mid common carotid lesion: presence of the most severe stenosis or occlusion in the mid portion of 5 cm in length from the point 2 cm distal to its orifice determined by angiography.
7. Distal brachiocephalic trunk lesion: presence of the most stenosis or occlusion in the distal third determined by angiography.
8. Descending thoracic aorta lesion: narrowing, dilatation or aneurysm, luminal irregularity or any combination determined by angiography: tortuosity alone is unacceptable.
9. Abdominal aorta lesion: narrowing, dilatation or aneurysm, luminal irregularity or aneurysm combination.
10. Coronary artery lesion: documented on angiography below the age of 30 years in the absence of risk factors like hyperlipidemia or diabetes mellitus.

Presence of two major or one major and two minor criteria or four minor criteria suggests a high probability of TA.

Criticism on the Diagnosis Criteria

1. The diagnostic imaging criteria of TA are based on vascular lesions detected by conventional angiographer (CA), which represents a lumen analysis method. CA does not characterize the thickness in aortic wall; it is a limitation of this method. Alterations of aortic wall are frequently observed in TA patients, mainly in earliest period of this disease. Conversely, MRI or CT imaging scan allows visualization of both vascular lumen and arterial wall thickness, improving the accuracy of TA diagnostic.
2. In case of patients with exclusive involvement of abdominal aorta or its branches, it is not possible to fulfill Sharma's criteria. These criteria consider subclavian arteritis as the main involvement in TA diagnosis. On the contrary, the incidence of lesions in aortic branches varies depending on the geographical region analyzed, and the involvement of abdominal aorta and its branches is more frequently observed in countries as Brazil and India. Consequently, sensitivity will be decreased in these populations.

Treatment

Therapeutic approach are often guided by individual patient variables that include disease activity, the location and severity of lesions, availability of collateral circulation, nature and intensity of symptoms, and the risk of drug toxicity.

The basis of therapy for TA is glucocorticoids (GCs). The GC dose can be gradually reduced when the symptoms and laboratory inflammatory markers have improved. For patients with disease refractory to GCs, immunosuppressive agents are recommended such as methotrexate, azathioprine, mycophenolate mofetil and cyclophosphamide. Anti-tumor necrosis factor agents are also other therapeutic options in severe and unresponsive cases.

References

1. Kerr GS. Takayasu's arteritis. *Rheum Dis Clin North Am* 1995; 21: 1041–58.
2. Numano F. Differences in clinical presentation and outcome in different countries for Takayasu's arteritis. *Curr Opin Rheumatol* 1997; 9: 12–5.
3. Keystone EC. Takayasu's arteritis. In: Klippel JH and Dieppe PA, *Rheumatology*, 3rd edition. Mosby International, UK 1998; 25: 1–4.
4. Koide K. Takayasu's arteritis in Japan. *Heart Vessels* 1992; 7: 48–54.
5. Arend WP, Michel BA, Block DA, et al. The American College of Rheumatology 1990 criteria for the classification of Takayasu's arteritis. *Arthritis Rheum* 1990; 33: 1129–34.
6. Cid MC, Font C, Coll-Vinent B, Grau JM. Large vessel vasculitides. *Curr Opin Rheumatol* 1998; 10: 18–28.
7. Seko Y, Minota S, Kawasaki A, et al. Perforin-secreting killer cell infiltration and expression of a 65-kD heat-shock protein in aortic tissue of patients with Takayasu's arteritis. *J Clin Invest* 1994; 93: 750–58.
8. Sato EI, Hatta FS, Levy-Neto M, Fernandes S. Demographic, clinical, and angiographic data of patients with Takayasu's arteritis in Brazil. *Int J Cardiol* 1998; 66(Suppl. 1): S67–70.
9. Zheng D, Fan D, Liu L. Takayasu's arteritis in china: a report of 530 cases. *Heart Vessels* 1992; 7(Suppl.): S32–6.
10. Jain S, Kumari S, Ganguly NK, et al. Current status of Takayasu's arteritis in India. *Int J Cardiol* 1996; 54 (Suppl.): S111–6.
11. Ueda H, Morooka S, Ito J, et al. Clinical observations of 52 cases of aortitis syndrome. *Jpn Heart J* 1969; 10: 227–88.
12. Park YB, Hong SK, Choi KJ, et al. Takayasu's arteritis in Korea: clinical and angiographic features. *Heart Vessels* 1992; 7(Suppl.): S55–9.
13. Lupi-Herrera E, Sanchez-Torres G, Marcushamer J, et al. Takayasu's arteritis. Clinical study of 107 cases. *Am Heart J* 1977; 93: 94–103.
14. Kerr GS, Hallahan CW, Giordano J, et al. Takayasu's arteritis. *Ann Intern Med* 1994; 120: 919–29.
15. Sharma BK, Sagar AP, Singh AP, Suri S. Takayasu's arteritis in India. *Heart Vessel* 1992; 7(Suppl.): 37–43.
16. Ishikawa K, Maetani S. Long-term outcome for 120 Japanese patients with Takayasu's disease. Clinical and statistical

analyses of related prognostic factors. *Circulation* 1994; 90: 1855–60.

17. Tso E, Flamm SD, White RD, Schvartzman PR, Marcha E, Hoffman GS. Takayasu's arteritis: utility and limitations of magnetic resonance imaging in diagnosis and treatment. *Arthritis Rheum* 2002; 46: 1634–42.

18. Choe YH, Han BK, Koh EM, Kim DK, Do YS, Lee WR. Takayasu's arteritis: Assessment of disease activity with contrast-enhanced MR imaging. *Am J Roentgenol* 2000; 175: 505–11.

19. Desai MY, Stone JH, Foo TK, Hellmann DB, Lima JA, Bluemke DA. Delayed contrast-enhanced MRI of the aortic wall in Takayasu's arteritis: Initial experience. *Am J Roentgenol* 2005; 184: 1427–31.

20. Sharma BK, Jain S, Suri S, Numano F. Diagnostic criteria for Takayasu's arteritis. *Int J Cardiol* 1996; 54(Suppl.): S141–47.

21. Ishikawa K. Diagnostic approach and proposed criteria for the clinical diagnosis of Takayasu's arteriopathy. *J Am Coll Cardiol* 1988; 12: 964–72.

16
Polyarteritis Nodosa

José Hernández-Rodríguez and Maria C. Cid

Abstract Polyarteritis nodosa (PAN) is a primary systemic necrotizing vasculitis that preferentially involves medium-sized arteries. The etiology of PAN is unknown. Several viral infections, such as hepatitis B virus infection, may be associated with blood vessel inflammation, clinically and histologically indistinguishable from PAN. Clinical manifestations of PAN are heterogeneous and multisystemic. Peripheral nerve and skin are frequently involved. Other organs including gastrointestinal tract, kidney, heart, and central nervous system can be targeted, conveying a poorer prognosis. Laboratory markers reflecting a prominent acute-phase response are common but not specific. When histologic confirmation cannot be obtained, angiography of involved territories, preferentially abdominal, may disclose multiple aneurysm formation supporting the diagnosis of PAN. Current treatment policy includes high-dose corticosteroids, which are combined with immunosuppressive agents when critical organ involvement or life-threatening complications occur. IV pulse cyclophosphamide in the remission induction phase, later switched to a safer immunosuppressant for remission maintenance, is a frequently used therapeutic scheme. A recent consensus algorithm for the classification of PAN has attempted to address some of the shortenings of previous classification criteria and has also confirmed the low prevalence of PAN compared with other necrotizing systemic vasculitides.

Keywords Polyarteritis nodosa · vasculitis · classification · treatment

Polyarteritis nodosa (PAN) is a primary systemic necrotizing vasculitis characteristically involving medium-sized arteries. PAN usually targets muscular arteries ranging from 300 μm to 1 cm in diameter (1, 2). Small vessels, including arterioles, capillaries, and postcapillary venules, are not affected (1).

Epidemiology

PAN can be considered a rare disease, with an annual incidence that ranges from 0 to 1.6 cases per million inhabitants in European countries (3, 4, 5). Two different studies from Sweden and France [the latter including 7/23 patients with a concomitant hepatitis B virus (HBV) infection] have recently found a prevalence of up to 31 cases per million (6, 7). PAN affects patients with no clear sex or race predilection and can occur at all ages. The peak incidence appears to be in the fifth to sixth decades (3, 4, 5, 6, 7). Before vaccination against HBV was available, more than one-third of vasculitis patients with features suggestive of PAN were infected by HBV. Currently, less than 10% of patients with PAN lesions are HBV-infected in developed countries (8).

Pathogenesis

PAN-like lesions have been reported in chronic viral infections, particularly in association with HBV. Infection by other pathogens, including HCV, HIV, cytomegalovirus, parvovirus B19, and human T-lymphotropic virus type I, has also been found in association with similar vasculitic lesions. Vascular inflammation associated with viral infections has been thought to be triggered by immune complexes (8). However, classic PAN is not usually associated with immune-complex deposition (1). The presence of dendritic cells and the abundance of $CD4^+$ lymphocytes in vascular inflammatory infiltrates suggests that antigen-specific T-cell-mediated immune responses may also play a role in the pathogenesis of vascular inflammation in PAN (9).

Clinical Manifestations

PAN has a wide spectrum of clinical presentations and may run an indolent, subclinical course. Consequently, the diagnosis of PAN is often delayed. In other instances,

From: Y. Shoenfeld et al. (eds.): *Diagnostic Criteria in Autoimmune Diseases*, DOI: 10.1007/978-1-60327-285-8_16,
© 2008 Humana Press, Totowa, NJ

PAN may present as an acute, life-threatening disease. The occlusion or rupture of the inflamed vessels in PAN can damage any organ or territory throughout the body by producing tissue ischemia or hemorrhage. This leads to a high variety of clinical manifestations that are listed in Table 16.1. Clinical features in PAN include nonspecific constitutional manifestations such as malaise, weight loss, fever, arthralgia, and myalgia, present in a high percentage of patients (2, 8), and symptoms derived from dysfunction or damage of the targeted organs.

The most frequent focal manifestations are derived from the involvement of vessels supplying peripheral nerves and the skin (8). Peripheral nervous system involvement usually presents as mononeuritis multiplex although symmetrical peripheral neuropathy can also be observed. Cutaneous features include purpura, livedo reticularis, subcutaneous nodules, Raynaud phenomenon, and distal digital ischemia (8). Gastrointestinal tract and kidneys are also frequently affected (8). Gastrointestinal manifestations of PAN are frequently associated with a remarkable morbidity and mortality (10). Contrarily to microscopic polyangiitis (MPA), kidney involvement in PAN does not include necrotizing glomerulonephritis. Renal involvement in PAN consists of tissue infarction or hematomas (8). The latter are usually produced by rupture of renal microaneurysms. In some patients, multiple renal infarcts may lead to an acute renal failure, whereas, in others, kidney infarcts may be clinically silent from months to years (4, 8). Hypertension secondary to intrarenal artery involvement is common (4, 8).

Laboratory Features

There are no laboratory abnormalities specific for PAN. Erythrocyte sedimentation rate and C-reactive protein are commonly elevated. Chronic anemia and leukocytosis are frequently present (2, 8). Hypereosinophilia may be occasionally seen but, when present, clinical features of Churg–Strauss syndrome must be investigated and ruled out. Serologies for HBV, HCV, and other chronic viral infections are useful to diagnose viral-associated vasculitis (8). Given the unusual association of PAN with antineutrophil cytoplasmic antibodies (ANCAs), a positive ANCA test strongly supports the diagnosis of other systemic necrotizing vasculitis usually associated with the presence of ANCA, such as MPA, Wegener's granulomatosis, or Churg–Strauss syndrome (5, 11).

Histologic Diagnosis

Biopsies should be performed on symptomatic or clinically abnormal sites (e.g., muscle, sural nerve, skin, bowel, or testicle). In carefully selected individuals in whom PAN is strongly suspected, muscular biopsies from clinically affected muscles and nerves may reveal vasculitis in about 70% of patients (12). In cases in which biopsies of muscle and nerve are blindly performed, vasculitis can be seen in up to one-third of patients (2, 8, 12). Testicular biopsy was advised in the past based on that testicles are frequently involved in necropsy studies of individuals with PAN. However, testicular biopsies do not have a suitable diagnostic yield (2) and should be performed only when testicles are clinically involved and biopsies from other symptomatic territories have been negative (12). During the workup of PAN, blind renal and liver biopsies should be avoided because of the potential presence of microaneurysms and their consequent hemorrhagic complications (2, 12). PAN or other necrotizing vasculitis can also be unexpectedly diagnosed in temporal biopsies from patients with clinical suspicion of giant-cell arteritis (13). Although the main temporal arteries may be affected, involvement of the surrounding branches is more commonly seen. Necrotizing vasculitis must be always ruled out when inflammation of the temporal artery branches with a spared temporal artery is observed in a temporal artery biopsy (13).

Vascular lesions are characteristically patchy and segmental (2). PAN inflammatory infiltrates are composed

TABLE 16.1. Principal manifestations in patients with polyarteritis nodosa (PAN) (8, 10).

Clinical manifestations	Prevalence (%)
Systemic features	
Fever	31–69
Weight loss	16–66
Myalgia	30–54
Arthralgia	44–58
Cutaneous	28–58
Neurological	40–75
Mononeuritis multiplex	38–72
Central nervous system	2–28
Cranial nerve palsy	<2
Gastrointestinal tract	14–44
Abdominal pain[a]	37/38 (97)
Nausea/vomiting[a]	12/38 (32)
Diarrhea[a]	6/38 (16)
Hematochezia/melena[a]	2/38 (5)
Hematemesis[a]	3/38 (8)
Esophageal ulcerations[a]	5/38 (13)
Gastroduodenal ulcerations[a]	12/38 (32)
Colorectal ulcerations[a]	2/38 (5)
Surgical abdomen/peritonitis[a]	12/38 (32)
Renal	8–66
Cardiac	4–30
Hypertension	10–63
Eye – retinal vasculitis, retinal detachment, cotton-wool spots	3–44
Respiratory – pleural effusion	5
Testicles – orchitis/epididymitis	2–18

[a] Abdominal manifestations from a series of 38 patients with PAN (10).

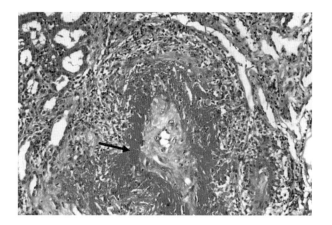

FIGURE 16.1. Typical histopathologic findings in polyarteritis nodosa: muscular artery with mixed inflammatory infiltrates and fibrinoid necrosis (arrow).

of lymphocytes, macrophages, and variable numbers of neutrophils and eosinophils (2, 9). Granulomas and giant cells are usually absent. Fibrinoid necrosis is frequently seen in active lesions (2, 9), and neutrophils are more frequently present in vessels with fibrinoid necrosis (9) (Figure 16.1). At later stages, lymphocyte and macrophage infiltration usually predominates and neoangiogenesis becomes apparent (9). In advanced lesions, vascular remodeling and healing lead to the development of intimal hyperplasia and diffuse fibrotic changes within the vessel wall (2). Severe vessel wall injury may result in the typical formation of microaneurysms (2). In PAN, vessels or vessel fragments with acute necrotizing lesions typically coexist with others with fibrotic or healing changes, representing different stages of the same inflammatory process (2, 9).

Imaging Findings

Visceral angiography may be performed in situations in which PAN is highly suspected and: (a) histologic diagnosis of vasculitis cannot be achieved, or (b) in patients predominantly experiencing symptoms suggestive of abdominal, renal, or cardiac involvement. In these patients, visceral angiography may have higher diagnostic yield than blinded muscle or peripheral nerve biopsies (12). Typical arteriographic lesions in PAN are arterial saccular or fusiform microaneurysms (1–5 mm in diameter), which can occur concomitantly with stenotic lesions, predominantly in the renal, mesenteric and hepatic artery branches. When characteristic angiographic changes are detected by an experienced radiologist, in the appropriate clinical context, the diagnosis of PAN can be established, even in absence of histologic confirmation (5, 8, 12). It must be kept in mind that conditions other than PAN may lead to multiple aneurysm formation (14).

Definition and Classification Criteria

In 1990, the American College of Rheumatology (ACR) classification criteria for PAN were established incorporating clinical, laboratory (including detection of HBV), angiographic, and histologic features (15). It is important to remark that the ACR criteria did not consider MPA as a clinicopathologic entity different from PAN. In 1994, in the Chapel Hill Consensus Conference, classical PAN was defined as a noninfectious vasculitis with distinct histopathologic features (1). PAN was also differentiated from MPA, which was considered as a systemic small- to medium-sized vessel vasculitis typically presenting with necrotizing glomerulonephritis and pulmonary capillaritis (1). The absence of pulmonary and glomerular capillary involvement in PAN has been useful in distinguishing this entity from other necrotizing vasculitides, involving small-sized vessels and frequently associated with the presence of ANCA. Both classification and nomenclature criteria are listed in Table 16.2.

TABLE 16.2. ACR criteria (15) and Chapel Hill definition (1) of polyarteritis nodosa.

1990 Criteria for the Classification of Polyarteritis Nodosa

1. Weight loss >4 kg
   Loss of 4 kg or more of body weight since illness began, not due to dieting or other factors
2. Livedo reticularis
   Mottled reticular pattern over the skin or portions of the extremities or torso
3. Testicular pain or tenderness
   Pain or tenderness of the testicles, not due to infection, trauma, or other causes
4. Myalgias, weakness, or leg tenderness
   Diffuse myalgias (excluding shoulder and hip girdle) or weakness of muscles or tenderness of leg muscles
5. Mononeuropathy or polyneuropathy
   Development of mononeuropathy, multiple mononeuropathies, or polyneuropathy
6. Diastolic blood pressure >90 mmHg
   Development of hypertension with diastolic blood pressure higher than 90 mmHg
7. Elevated blood urea nitrogen or creatinine
   Elevation of blood urea nitrogen >40 mg/dl or creatinine >1.5 mg/dl, not due to dehydration or obstruction
8. Hepatitis B virus
   Presence of hepatitis B surface antigen or antibody in serum
9. Arteriographic abnormality
   Arteriogram showing aneurysms or occlusions of the visceral arteries, not due to arteriosclerosis, fibromuscular dysplasia, or other noninflammatory causes
10. Biopsy of small- or medium-sized artery containing polymorphonuclear neutrophils
    Histologic changes showing the presence of granulocytes or granulocytes and mononuclear leukocytes in the artery wall

Patients were classified as PAN if at least 3 of the 10 criteria were present. The presence of any 3 or more criteria yielded a sensitivity of 82.2% and a specificity of 86.6%.

Definition of Polyarteritis nodosa (PAN) adopted by the Chapel Hill Consensus Conference on the nomenclature of systemic vasculitis

Necrotizing inflammation of medium-sized or small arteries without glomerulonephritis or vasculitis in arterioles, capillaries, or venules.

After these categorization systems were established, several studies have demonstrated that most patients, who met ACR classification criteria for PAN, after being reevaluated, did not meet the definition of PAN according to the Chapel Hill Consensus Conference (3, 4, 5). Therefore, the incidence of PAN has been overestimated in studies performed before the establishment of the Chapel Hill definition. Reasons for re-definition have been subsequent histologic demonstration of glomerulonephritis or small vessel involvement, ANCA positivity, or detection of HBV, HCV, or other infectious agents known to be associated with vasculitis. Consequently, many patients previously diagnosed with PAN were later re-categorized as having MPA or infection-related vasculitis.

Recently, a consensus algorithm for the classification of PAN and other necrotizing vasculitides has been proposed by combining ACR and Chapel Hill criteria, and ANCA testing and surrogate markers of vascular inflammation, including clinical, laboratory, neurophysiologic, and imaging tests (Figure 16.2) (5). This classificatory scheme has

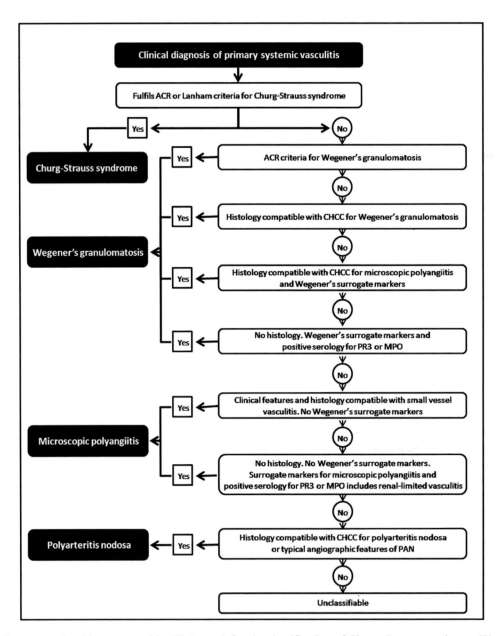

FIGURE 16.2. Consensus algorithm proposed by Watts et al. for the classification of Churg–Strauss syndrome, Wegener's granulomatosis, microscopic polyangiitis, and polyarteritis nodosa (reproduced with permission from ref 5.). ACR, American College of Rheumatology; CHCC, Chapel Hill Consensus Conference; MPO, myeloperoxidase; PR3, proteinase 3.
Note: The Lanham criteria for Churg-Strauss and the surrogate markers for Wegener's granulomatosis and microscopic polyangiitis are explained in detail in reference 5.

been already used in a large epidemiologic study analyzing different vasculitides and has definitively confirmed the low prevalence of PAN (7).

Necrotizing Arteritis Confined to Single-Organs or Systems

Patients with necrotizing vasculitis localized within a specific organ or territory with no apparent systemic involvement have been repeatedly reported (16). Although the term *PAN* defines a systemic disease (1, 15), *isolated PAN* is the term most profusely used to define these cases of localized vasculitis. Several systems can be diffusely involved by necrotizing vasculitis; these include the central nervous system, peripheral nerves, and skin. Such entities, although isolated, cannot be treated by excision, and systemic therapy is required. Necrotizing vasculitis involving single organs has been reported in the appendix, intestines, gallbladder, pancreas, breast, male and female genital organs, and urinary structures. These forms of isolated vasculitis are usually found incidentally in organs excised because of focal symptoms or local abnormalities, and can be cured by resection of the involved tissues, and systemic treatment is not usually required (16). Clinical and laboratory markers of systemic inflammatory response are weaker in patients with single-organ vasculitis than in patients with widespread systemic involvement (16). Patients with single-organ vasculitis may be carefully evaluated to exclude systemic extent at diagnosis and subjected to a tight surveillance with regard to the appearance of systemic features during follow-up because patients with apparently isolated vasculitis at presentation and later evolving to a systemic disease have been reported (16).

Disease Course and Prognosis

Contrarily to MPA and Wegener's granulomatosis, which are typically multi-relapsing diseases, PAN has been classically considered a monophasic disease with a relapse rate lesser than 10%. Nevertheless, a recent study of 10 PAN patients defined according to the Chapel Hill nomenclature criteria has shown a relapse rate higher than previously reported and similar to that seen in patients with MPA (4).

The prognosis of PAN depends on the organs involved. The French Vasculitis Study Group (FVSG) proposed the Five Factor Score (FFS), a prognosis index considering the following items: presence of severe gastrointestinal tract disease (defined as bleeding, perforation, infarction, or pancreatitis), renal involvement consisting of serum creatinine $\geq$1.58 mg/dl or proteinuria ($\geq$1 g/day), cardiac disease (infarction or heart failure), and central nervous

system involvement. When present, each of those is given a score of 1 (17). The FVSG has reported a 5-year mortality of 12% for PAN patients with FFS = 0, 26% for those with FFS = 1, and 46% when FFS is $\geq$2. The overall 7-year survival for PAN is 79% (17).

Treatment

It is important to keep in mind that the level of evidence supporting therapeutic decisions in PAN is low. As mentioned, grounds on which patients with necrotizing vasculitis have been classified as PAN patients have evolved over the years. The existing randomized clinical trials have been performed on mixed cohorts of patients with PAN and Churg–Strauss syndrome or MPA (17). The distribution of the involved organs and disease progression are the two principal determinants for treating patients with PAN. Current therapeutic approaches consider treating mild forms of primary PAN (with FFS = 0) with corticosteroids only: typically prednisone or prednisolone at doses of 1 mg/kg/day with subsequent tapering when remission is achieved (17). When prednisone cannot be tapered below 15–20 mg/day without recurrence, the addition of a second immunosuppressive agent is considered. In life-threatening situations or rapidly progressive disease, experts advise initiation of therapy with IV methylprednisolone pulses (1000 mg/day for 3 days). In the presence of critical organ involvement indicated by an FFS $\geq$1, immunosuppressants are given in addition to prednisone. Cyclophosphamide is used at doses of 2 mg/kg/day orally or as monthly intravenous doses of 0.6 g/m^2 for 6–12 months (18). According to the FVSG, monthly pulse intravenous administration is preferred to daily oral cyclophosphamide. Currently, as an extrapolation from the evidence obtained from trials performed with patients with MPA and Wegener's granulomatosis, cyclophosphamide is recommended to induce remission and a safer immunosuppressive agent such as azathioprine or methotrexate is advised to maintain remission (18). Cyclophosphamide treatment beyond 12 months is not recommended. Angiographic abnormalities can regress after treatment (10). Surgery may be required for some disease complications, such as perforation/rupture, ischemia, or hemorrhage of the gastrointestinal organs or kidneys (10).

Although biologic therapies have been used in other vasculitides with variable results (18), experience in treating patients with PAN, refractory to conventional therapies, with TNF-blocking agents remains anecdotal (19).

In patients with HBV-associated vasculitis, combination of short corticosteroid treatment with plasma exchanges and antiviral therapy (vidarabine, interferon-α2a, or lamivudine) may be effective in controlling disease activity and in facilitating viral seroconversion. The control of the viremia also helps in preventing the development of long-term hepatic complications of HBV infection (18). Relapses are rare in HBV vasculitis and never occur when viral replication has ceased and seroconversion has been achieved (10). In single-organ necrotizing vasculitis, a complete excision of the involved tissue may be curative in most cases (16).

Acknowledgment. The authors were supported by Ministerio de Educación y Ciencia (SAF 05-06250), Marató TV3 (05/0710), and Generalitat de Catalunya (SGR 0300/2005). José Hernández-Rodríguez was a research award recipient from Hospital Clínic (Barcelona, Spain) and from the RJ Fasenmyer Center for Clinical Immunology at the Cleveland Clinic Foundation (Cleveland, OH, USA).

References

1. Jennette JC, Falk RJ, Andrassy K, Bacon PA, Churg J, Gross WL et al. Nomenclature of systemic vasculitides. Proposal of an international consensus conference. *Arthritis Rheum* 1994; 37(2): 187–92.
2. Lie JT. Systemic and isolated vasculitis. A rational approach to classification and pathologic diagnosis. *Pathol Annu* 1989; 24(Pt 1): 25–114.
3. González-Gay MA, García-Porrúa C, Guerrero J, Rodríguez-Ledo P, Llorca J. The epidemiology of the primary systemic vasculitides in northwest Spain: implications of the Chapel Hill Consensus Conference definitions. *Arthritis Rheum* 2003; 49(3): 388–93.
4. Selga D, Mohammad A, Sturfelt G, Segelmark M. Polyarteritis nodosa when applying the chapel hill nomenclature – a descriptive study on ten patients. *Rheumatology (Oxford)* 2006; 45(10): 1276–81.
5. Watts R, Lane S, Hanslik T, Hauser T, Hellmich B, Koldingsnes W, et al. Development and validation of a consensus methodology for the classification of the ANCA-associated vasculitides and polyarteritis nodosa for epidemiological studies. *Ann Rheum Dis* 2007; 66(2): 222–7.
6. Mahr A, Guillevin L, Poissonnet M, Ayme S. Prevalences of polyarteritis nodosa, microscopic polyangiitis, Wegener's granulomatosis, and Churg-Strauss syndrome in a french urban multiethnic population in. *Arthritis Rheum* 2004; 2000(1): 92–9.
7. Mohammad AJ, Jacobsson LT, Mahr AD, Sturfelt G, Segelmark M. Prevalence of Wegener's granulomatosis, microscopic polyangiitis, polyarteritis nodosa and Churg

8. Lhote F, Cohen P, Guillevin L. Polyarteritis nodosa, microscopic polyangiitis and Churg-Strauss syndrome. *Lupus* 1998; 7(4): 238–58.
9. Cid MC, Grau JM, Casademont J, Campo E, Coll-Vinent B, López-Soto A et al. Immunohistochemical characterization of inflammatory cells and immunologic activation markers in muscle and nerve biopsy specimens from patients with systemic polyarteritis nodosa. *Arthritis Rheum* 1994; 37(7): 1055–61.
10. Pagnoux C, Mahr A, Cohen P, Guillevin L. Presentation and outcome of gastrointestinal involvement in systemic necrotizing vasculitides: analysis of 62 patients with polyarteritis nodosa, microscopic polyangiitis, Wegener granulomatosis, Churg-Strauss syndrome, or rheumatoid arthritis-associated vasculitis. *Medicine (Baltimore)* 2005; 84(2): 115–28.
11. Guillevin L, Lhote F, Amouroux J, Gherardi R, Callard P, Casassus P. Antineutrophil cytoplasmic antibodies, abnormal angiograms and pathological findings in polyarteritis nodosa and Churg-Strauss syndrome: indications for the classification of vasculitides of the polyarteritis nodosa group. *Br J Rheumatol* 1996; 35(10): 958–64.
12. Albert DA, Rimon D, Silverstein MD. The diagnosis of polyarteritis nodosa. I. A literature-based decision analysis approach. *Arthritis Rheum* 1988; 31(9): 1117–27.
13. Esteban MJ, Font C, Hernández-Rodríguez J, Valls-Solé J, Sanmartí R, Cardellach F, et al. Small-vessel vasculitis surrounding a spared temporal artery: clinical and pathological findings in a series of twenty-eight patients. *Arthritis Rheum* 2001; 44(6): 1387–95.
14. Molloy ES, Langford CA. Vasculitis mimics. *Curr Opin Rheumatol* 2008; 20(1): 29–34.
15. Lightfoot RW Jr, Michel BA, et al. The American College of Rheumatology 1990 criteria for the classification of polyarteritis nodosa. *Arthritis Rheum* 1990; 33(8): 1088–93.
16. Hernández-Rodríguez J, Molloy ES, Hoffman GS. Single-organ vasculitis. *Curr Opin Rheumatol* 2008; 20(1): 40–46.
17. Bourgarit A, Le Toumelin P, Pagnoux C, Cohen P, Mahr A, Le Guern V, et al. Deaths occurring during the first year after treatment onset for polyarteritis nodosa, microscopic polyangiitis, and Churg-Strauss syndrome: A retrospective analysis of causes and factors predictive of mortality based on 595 patients. *Medicine (Baltimore)* 2005; 84(5): 323–30.
18. Guillevin L, Pagnoux C. Therapeutic strategies for systemic necrotizing vasculitides. *Allergol Int* 2007; 56(2): 105–11.
19. Al-Bishri J, le Riche N, Pope JE. Refractory polyarteritis nodosa successfully treated with infliximab. *J Rheumatol* 2005; 32(7): 1371–3.

17
Microscopic Polyangiitis

Cees G.M. Kallenberg

Abstract   Microscopic polyangiitis (MPA) belongs to the antineutrophil cytoplasmic autoantibody (ANCA)-associated vasculitides (AAVs). MPA is clinically characterized by small-vessel vasculitis primarily affecting the kidneys and the lungs, but other organs may be involved as well. Renal involvement, which can be the only manifestation, is clinically apparent as rapidly progressive glomerulonephritis and histopathologically as pauci-immune necrotizing and crescentic glomerulonephritis. ANCAs in MPA are mainly directed to myeloperoxidase (MPO-ANCA). Induction treatment consists of cyclophosphamide and steroids followed by azathioprine as maintenance therapy. Other, less toxic therapeutic regimens are being tested.

Keywords   Microscopic polyangiitis · ANCA-associated vasculitis · antineutrophil cytoplasmic autoantibodies · antimyeloperoxidase antibodies · myeloperoxidase · necrotizing and crescentic glomerulonephritis

Definition

Microscopic polyangiitis (MPA) was defined by the Chapel Hill Consensus Conference (1) as "a small-vessel necrotizing vasculitis in which glomerular and pulmonary capillaries are frequently involved. Larger arteries may be involved as well."

Antineutrophil cytoplasmic autoantibodies (ANCAs) are present in most of the cases and are, in the majority of patients, directed against myeloperoxidase (MPO-ANCA). The disease belongs to the ANCA-associated vasculitides (AAVs). MPA has to be distinguished from (classic) polyarteritis nodosa (PAN), in which, according to the Chapel Hill Consensus Conference, only medium-sized and larger arteries are involved.

Epidemiology

The incidence and prevalence of MPA are not exactly known. The AAVs, mainly comprising of Wegener's granulomatosis (WG) and MPA, have been estimated to have an overall incidence of 20 per million (2). Whereas in the Northern European Caucasian population WG predominates within the group of patients with AAVs, MPA is more frequent than WG in Southern Europe and Japan. Men are slightly more affected than women. The age at presentation peaks around 60–65 years of age. There seems to be an increase in the incidence of MPA during the last two decades, which can be explained, in part, by the availability of ANCA testing.

History

Whereas PAN was described already in 1866 by Kussmaul and Maier, microscopic polyarteritis was suggested in 1985 as a disease entity by Savage et al. (3). It was recognized as a disease in which rapidly progressive glomerulonephritis, not infrequently in conjunction with pulmonary capillaritis, was a prominent finding. As this was not the case in classical PAN, MPA was considered a distinct entity. The discovery of ANCA supported the concept of MPA being a distinct disease entity because the vast majority of patients with MPA were positive for ANCA, whereas patients with classical PAN were generally ANCA negative (4). The Chapel Hill Consensus Conference (1) defined MPA as a separate condition within the group of primary vasculitides.

Pathogenesis

The etiology of MPA is largely unknown. Although (weak) associations with certain genes, including MHC genes, have been described, no strong genetic factors are involved

From: Y. Shoenfeld et al. (eds.): *Diagnostic Criteria in Autoimmune Diseases*, DOI: 10.1007/978-1-60327-285-8_17,
© 2008 Humana Press, Totowa, NJ

in MPA. Environmental factors, such as silica exposure, have been suggested (5), but their precise role in etiopathogenesis is unclear. There is, however, increased evidence that MPA is an autoimmune disease in which ANCAs, particularly those reacting with MPO, are pathogenic. First, the vast majority of patients with MPA (95%) are positive for ANCA, directed to MPO in 70% of cases and directed to proteinase 3 (PR3) in the remaining patients (4). Titers of ANCA frequently rise preceding disease activity although this is less clear for MPO-ANCA than for PR3-ANCA (6). Secondly, both MPO-ANCA and PR3-ANCA are able, in vitro, to activate

(primed) neutrophils to the production of reactive oxygen species and the release of lytic enzymes. In the presence of endothelial cells, this leads to endothelial detachment and lysis (7). The most convincing argument for a pathogenic role of MPO-ANCA comes from studies in experimental animals. Xiao et al. (8) immunized MPO-deficient mice with mouse MPO resulting in their production of anti-mouse MPO antibodies. Splenocytes from these mice were injected into immunodeficient and normal mice, which resulted in the development of severe necrotizing and crescentic glomerulonephritis, granulomatous inflammation, and systemic necrotizing vasculitis including pulmonary

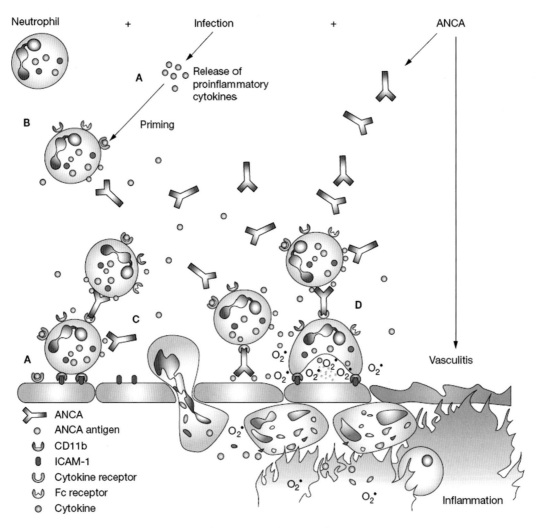

FIGURE 17.1. Schematic representation of antineutrophil cytoplasmic autoantibody (ANCA)-mediated neutrophil responses that are putatively involved in the pathogenesis of ANCA-associated small-vessel vasculitis. (A) Proinflammatory cytokines and chemokines (e.g., tumor necrosis factor α) released as a result of local or systemic infection cause upregulation of endothelial adhesion molecules (e.g., selectins, ICAM-1, and VCAM) and prime the neutrophil. (B) Neutrophil priming causes upregulation of neutrophil adhesion molecules (CD11b) and translocation of the ANCA antigens from their lysosomal compartments to the cell surface. (C) Engagement of the F(ab')₂ portion of ANCA with ANCA antigens on the cell surface and interaction of the Fc part of the antibody with Fc receptors activate the neutrophil, causing increased neutrophil-vessel wall adherence and transmigration. (D) ANCA-mediated neutrophil activation also triggers reactive oxygen radical production and possibly causes neutrophil degranulation, with consequent release of proteolytic enzymes, leading to vasculitis. (From ref. 4, with permission).

capillaritis. Immune deposits were hardly present, consistent with a so-called pauci-immune vasculitis and glomerulonephritis, which are seen also in patients with MPA (discussed below). Transfer of anti-MPO-IgG alone into recipient mice resulted in focal pauci-immune glomerulonephritis, which was strongly augmented by the simultaneous injection of lipopolysaccharide (LPS) (9). Taken together, strong evidence now exists that MPO-ANCAs are directly involved in the pathogenesis of MPA (Figure 17.1).

Clinical Manifestations

MPA belongs to the systemic vasculitides indicating that multiple organs can be affected. Major organs involved in MPA are the kidneys and the lungs. Renal involvement is manifested by microscopic hematuria with cellular casts in combination with proteinuria, which is, generally, not massive. In addition, deterioration of renal function frequently occurs clinically apparent as rapidly progressive glomerulonephritis. In 90% of patients the kidneys are involved, 30% are oliguric at the time of diagnosis, 10% end up with renal replacement therapy, and 30% of patients die (10).

MPA can be restricted to the kidneys. This ANCA-associated condition, in the majority of cases MPO-ANCA associated, is designated as idiopathic necrotizing and crescentic glomerulonephritis. Renal limited vasculitis is considered as a variant of MPA and is treated according to the guidelines for the treatment of MPA.

Lung involvement occurs somewhat less frequently and is clinically apparent as dyspnea, cough, and hemoptysis (not in all cases). The chest X-ray may show an alveolar filling pattern. Pulmonary hemorrhage is a very serious condition with a bad prognosis particularly in those patients who also have rapidly progressive glomerulonephritis (so-called renal–pulmonary syndrome) (11). As mentioned, many organs may be affected. Besides general malaise, weight loss, and fever, arthralgia/myalgia, skin involvement such as purpura, and, particularly, involvement of peripheral nerves (mononeuritis multiplex occurring in around 50% of patients) are frequent findings.

In contrast to WG, granulomatous inflammation with local tissue destruction is generally absent in MPA, and ENT abnormalities such as recurrent sinusitis, bloody nasal discharge, and cartilage destruction leading to saddle nose deformity are not characteristic for MPA.

Pathological Features

MPA is part of the AAVs that are characterized by necrotizing vasculitis of small vessels (arterioles, capillaries, venules) and lack or paucity of immune deposits within the vessel wall. In the skin, this is apparent as leukocytoclastic vasculitis. Capillaritis with fibrinoid necrosis is the typical finding in the lungs in MPA. Granulomatous inflammation is a characteristic finding in (PR3-ANCA-associated) WG but not in (MPO-ANCA-associated) MPA (12). The renal lesions are designated as necrotizing crescentic glomerulonephritis (Figure 17.2). Focal thrombosis of glomerular capillaries with fibrinoid necrosis is an early lesion that is followed by rupture of the glomerular basement membrane and extracapillary proliferation. This results in crescent formation, initially cellular crescents and later on more fibrous crescents. Periglomerular accumulation of mononuclear cells follows the glomerular inflammatory process. Deposition of immunoglobulins and complement is hardly seen (pauci-immune glomerulonephritis).

Serological Features

As MPA belongs to the AAVs, ANCAs are the diagnostic hallmark for MPA. 90–95% of patients with MPA are positive for ANCAs, the majority of whom (70%) being

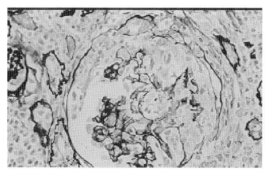 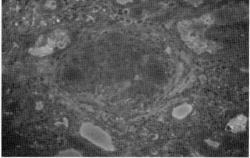

FIGURE 17.2. Necrotizing crescentic glomerulonephritis (left, silver staining) with paucity of immune deposits (right, direct immunofluorescence for IgG).

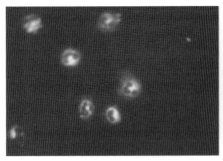

C-ANCA pattern

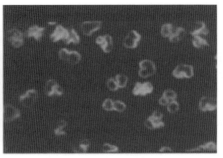

P-ANCA pattern

FIGURE 17.3. Staining of cytoplasmic components of ethanol-fixed neutrophils by indirect immunofluorescence using a serum sample from a patient with active Wegener's granulomatosis and antibodies to proteinase 3 (PR3). A characteristic cytoplasmic pattern of fluorescence (c-ANCA) is seen (left). This fluorescence pattern is different from the perinuclear pattern that can be produced by serum samples from patients with anti-MPO antibodies (p-ANCA) (right).

positive for MPO-ANCAs (13). ANCAs are routinely assessed by indirect immunofluorescence on ethanol-fixed neutrophils. A classic cytoplasmic staining pattern with accentuation of the fluorescence within the nuclear lobes is characteristic for PR3-ANCAs, whereas MPO-ANCAs produce a perinuclear staining pattern (Figure 17.3). Such a perinuclear pattern is, however, far from specific for MPO-ANCA and may be produced as well by ANCA directed to other neutrophil antigens such as lactoferrin which are not specific for the AAVs (13). Therefore, a positive test for ANCA should always be followed by an antigen-specific test, usually ELISA with specificity for PR3-ANCA and MPO-ANCA (13).

Besides ANCAs, rheumatoid factor and antiendothelial cell antibodies are frequently present in MPA. They lack, however, specificity for this disease.

Diagnostic Criteria

MPA was not included in the group of idiopathic vasculitides for which classification criteria were proposed by the American College of Rheumatology (ACR). The disease was, however, defined by the Chapel Hill Consensus Conference (1). This definition describes MPA as "necrotizing vasculitis, with few or no immune deposits, affecting small vessels (i.e., capillaries, venules, or arterioles). Necrotizing arteritis involving small- and medium-sized arteries may be present. Necrotizing glomerulonephritis is very common. Pulmonary capillaritis often occurs." In the literature, most authors use this definition to classify patients as having MPA. It is clear from the definition that histopathological evidence of pauci-immune necrotizing small-vessel vasculitis is necessary to make a diagnosis of MPA. However, no classification criteria for MPA have been formally validated with respect to sensitivity and specificity. However, an algorithm was recently proposed by Watts et al. (14) to classify patients with ANCA-associated vasculitis and PAN within a single category, that is WG, MPA, Churg–Strauss syndrome, and PAN.

Prognosis

Although no formal data are available, prognosis of idiopathic systemic vasculitides such as MPA and WG is bad without treatment (mortality of 90% after one year). The introduction of aggressive immunosuppressive treatment, in particular cyclophosphamide in combination with prednisone, has substantially improved prognosis, with cumulative patient survival at 1 and 5 years of 82 and 76%, respectively, for patients with renal involvement. End-stage renal failure occurs in 28% of patients with a mortality of around 50% (15). Death occurring during the first year of treatment was related to insufficient treatment response and infection as the most important factors. Clinically, pulmonary hemorrhage at presentation conferred a relative risk of 8.65 for patient death. Predictors for end-stage renal failure are serum creatinine at presentation, African American race, and arterial sclerosis on renal biopsy (17). Relapses occur in around 35% of patients.

Therapy

Induction treatment classically consists of cyclophosphamide with corticosteroids (prednisone, 1 mg/kg daily). Although still controversial, intravenous pulse cyclophosphamide appears as effective as oral cyclophosphamide (2 mg/kg daily) but seems less toxic, particularly in relation to infections associated with neutropenia which occur more frequently during oral cyclophosphamide. In patients presenting with a serum creatinine value of >500 μmol/l, the additional use of plasma exchange increases the rate of renal recovery when compared with intravenous methylprednisolone (18). Once remission has been obtained, maintenance treatment is advocated for another 18 months. Azathioprine is preferred for maintenance treatment as it is as effective as cyclophosphamide but less toxic (19). In view of the significant toxicity of these regimens, other drugs have been tried but data from randomized controlled trials are lacking. Both mycophenolate mofetil and rituximab are promising agents in the treatment of MPA.

References

1. Jennette JC, Falk RJ, Andrassy K, et al. Nomenclature of systemic vasculitides. Proposal of an international consensus conference. *Arthritis Rheum* 1994; 37: 187–92.
2. Watts RA, Scott DG. Epidemiology of the vasculitides. *Semin Respir Crit Care Med* 2004; 25: 455–64.
3. Savage C, Winearts C, Evans D, Rees A, Lockwood C. Microscopic polyarteritis: Presentation, pathology and prognosis. *Q J Med* 1985; 56: 467–83.
4. Kallenberg CGM, Heeringa P, Stegeman CA. Mechanisms of disease: pathogenesis and treatment of ANCA-associated vasculitides. *Nat Clin Pract Rheumatol* 2006; 2: 661–70.
5. Hogan SL, Satterly KK, Dooley MA, et al. Silica exposure in antineutrophil cytoplasmic autoantibody-associated glomerulonephritis and lupus nephritis. *J AM Soc Nephrol* 2001; 12: 134–42.
6. Kallenberg CGM, Stegeman CA, Bootsma H, Bijl M, Limburg PC. Quantitation of autoantibodies in systemic autoimmune diseases: Clinically useful? *Lupus* 2006; 15: 397–402.
7. Harper L, Savage CO. Leukocyte-endothelial interactions in antineutrophil cytoplasmic antibody-associated systemic vasculitis. *Rheum Dis Clin North Am* 2001; 27: 887–903.
8. Xiao H, Heeringa P, Hu P, et al. Antineutrophil cytoplasmic autoantibodies specific for myeloperoxidase cause glomerulonephritis and vasculitis in mice. *J Clin Invest* 2002; 110: 955–63.
9. Huugen D, Xiao H, van Esch A, et al. Aggravation of anti-myeloperoxidase antibody-induced glomerulonephritis by bacterial lipopolysaccharide: Role of tumor necrosis factor-alpha. *Am J Pathol* 2005; 167: 47–58.
10. Guillevin L, Durand-Gasselin B, Cevallos R, et al. Microscopic polyangiitis: clinical and laboratory findings in eighty-five patients. *Arthritis Rheum* 1999; 42: 421–30.
11. Niles JL, Bottinger EP, Saurina GR, et al. The syndrome of lung hemorrhage and nephritis is usually an ANCA-associated condition. *Arch Intern Med* 1996; 156: 440–5.
12. Franssen CFM, Stegeman CA, Kallenberg CGM, Gans ROB, de Jong PE, Hoorntje SJ, Cohen Tervaert JW. Antiproteinase 3- and antimyeloperoxidase-associated vasculitis. *Kidney Int* 2000; 57: 2195–206.
13. Bosch X, Guilabert A, Font J. Antineutrophil cytoplasmic antibodies. *Lancet* 2006; 368: 404–18.
14. Watts R, Lane S, Hanslik T, et al. Development and validation of a consensus methodology for the classification of the ANCA-associated vasculitides and polyarteritis nodosa for epidemiological studies. *Ann Rheum Dis* 2007; 66: 222–7.
15. Booth AD, Almond MK, Burns A, et al. Pan-Thames Renal Research Group. Outcome of ANCA-associated renal vasculitis: A 5-year retrospective study. *Am J Kidney Dis* 2003; 41: 776–84.
16. Bourgarit A, Le Toumelin PH, Pagnoux C, et al. Deaths occurring during the first year after treatment onset for polyarteritis nodosa, microscopic polyangiitis, and Churg-Strauss Syndrome. *Medicine* 2005; 84: 323–30.
17. Hogan SL, Nachman PH, Falk RJ, et al. Prognostic markers in patients with antineutrophil cytoplasmic autoantibody-associated microscopic polyangiitis and glomerulonephritis. *J Am Soc Nephrol* 1996; 7: 23–32.
18. Jayne DR, Gaskin G, Rasmussen N, et al. European Vasculitis Study Group. Randomized trial of plasma exchange or high-dosage methylprednisolone as adjunctive therapy for severe renal vasculitis. *J Am Soc Nephrol* 2007; 18: 2180–8.
19. Jayne D, Rasmussen N, Andrassy K, et al. A randomized trial of maintenance therapy for vasculitis associated with antineutrophil cytoplasmic autoantibodies. *N Engl J Med* 2003; 349: 36–44.
20. Jayne D. Part 3: Newer therapies for ANCA-associated vasculitis. *Clin Exp Rheumatol* 2007; 25(Suppl. 44): S77–9.

18
Wegener Granulomatosis

Julia U. Holle, Elena Csernok and Wolfgang L. Gross

Abstract   Wegener granulomatosis (WG) is an autoimmune disease of unknown etiology which is characterized by granulomatous lesions and small vessel vasculitis. WG is associated with antineutrophil cytoplasmic antibodies (ANCAs) directed against proteinase 3 (PR3). The disease may affect virtually any organ: however, predominant features are the involvement of the ENT tract with granulomatous disease and small vessel vasculitis affecting lung and kidneys. Immunosuppressive therapy is adapted according to stage and activity of the disease. The mainstay of therapy in life-threatening disease is cyclophosphamide (plus glucocorticoids), which is switched to less potent immunosuppressants such as azathioprine after successful induction of remission. Therapy might be needed lifelong.

Keywords   ANCA-associated vasculitis · granulomatous disease · proteinase 3

Definition

Wegener granulomatosis (WG) is an autoimmune disease of yet unknown etiology which is characterized by granulomatous lesions and small vessel vasculitis. The disease usually starts as granulomatous inflammation of the ENT tract and proceeds to a systemic phase with necrotizing small vessel vasculitis after various time. Small vessel vasculitis predominantly affects lung and kidneys and is associated with antineutrophil cytoplasmic antibodies (ANCAs) directed against proteinase 3 (PR3), a neutrophil serine protease.

Epidemiology, Classification, and Disease Stages

The incidence of WG varies between 8 per 1,000,000 and 12 per 1,000,000 per year (in Germany) (1). WG can be classified according to the nomenclature of the Chapel Hill Consensus (CHC) Conference for primary systemic vasculitides (2) and according to the classification criteria defined by the American College of Rheumatology (ACR) (3, see Table 18.1). The latter has been developed to distinguish patients with WG from other vasculitides on the basis of criteria with high sensitivity and specificity. The presence of two or more ACR criteria yields a sensitivity of 88.2% and a specificity of 92%.

The European Vasculitis Study Group (EUVAS) has developed a definition of disease stages including localized disease, which is defined as WG restricted to the upper and lower airways, an early systemic phase including any organ involvement except for renal or imminent organ failure, and generalized WG referring to full-blown disease with renal and/or imminent organ failure (4, see Table 18.2).

TABLE 18.1. Definition and classification criteria of Wegener granulomatosis (WG) according to the Chapel Hill Consensus (CHC) Conference.

CHC definition

Granulomatous inflammation involving the respiratory tract and
Necrotizing vasculitis affecting small- to medium-sized vessels
  (i.e., capillaries, venules, arterioles, and arteries)
Necrotizing glomerulonephritis is common
Cytoplasmic pattern ANCAs (C-ANCA) with antigen specificity for
  proteinase 3 (PR3) are a very sensitive marker for WG

American College of Rheumatology (ACR) classification criteria

Nasal or oral inflammation
Abnormal chest radiograph
Nephritic urinary sediment
Granulomatous inflammation on biopsy

From: Y. Shoenfeld et al. (eds.): *Diagnostic Criteria in Autoimmune Diseases*, DOI: 10.1007/978-1-60327-285-8_18,
© 2008 Humana Press, Totowa, NJ

TABLE 18.2. Disease stages according to the European Vasculitis Study Group (EUVAS) (4).

Disease stages	Organ involvement	Detection of ANCA
"Initial phase" (localized)	Upper and lower airways	−/+
Early systemic disease	Any, but no imminent organ failure, creatinine <150 μmol/l	+
Generalized disease	Any, creatinine <500 μmol/l	+
Rapid progressive GN	Creatinine >500 μmol/l	+
Refractory disease	Progress in spite of therapy	+

ANCA, antineutrophil cytoplasmic antibody.

Formerly, the term "limited disease" was used to characterize patients with predominant lung involvement and no renal manifestation.

Pathology

Genetic Background

An association with several HLA loci and alleles has been described for WG and other ANCA-associated vasculitides (5). A loss of function mutant of a tyrosine-phosphatase in T cells downregulating T-cell activity (PTPN22*W620) (6) may confer susceptibility to WG as well as to other autoimmune diseases.

Environmental Influences

Carriership of *Staphylococcus aureus* represents a risk factor for WG relapse (7), and antibiotic therapy (cotrimoxazole) may be able to control localized WG (granulomatous disease).

Pathogenetic Mechanisms

In vitro evidence suggests that PR3 (Wegener autoantigen) interacts with dendritic cells and induces their maturation into antigen-presenting cells, which are able to prime T cells for a Th1-phenotype (8). Th1-type cytokines are needed for granuloma formation. This finding points to an autoantigen-driven process ultimately leading to granuloma formation and ANCA production (Figure 18.1). In WG, granuloma formation is also supported by a certain subset of T cells (CD28⁻ T cells) that are expanded in blood, are enriched in granuloma, and represent a major source of the Th1-type cytokines (9). B cells are found in granulomatous lesions of WG, and although plasma cells producing PR3-ANCA have not yet been detected in WG granuloma, there is evidence that ANCA may be generated by affinity maturation by contact to PR3 or cross-reacting microbial antigens in granuloma (10). Today, it is widely accepted that ANCA plays a major role in inducing vasculitis. In vitro, ANCA interact with membrane PR3 (mPR3) of cytokine primed neutrophils, which results in PMN (Polymorph mono nuclear cells) activation, respiratory burst, adherence, and migration to/through endothelium (11) (ANCA cytokine-sequence theory). However, a satisfactory animal model of PR3-ANCA-induced vasculitis is still missing.

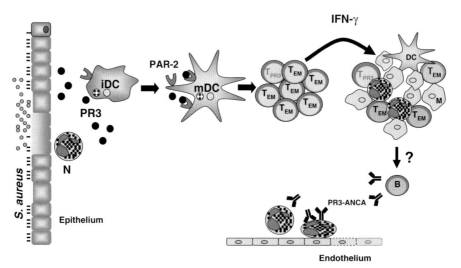

FIGURE 18.1. Hypothesis of initiation of an adaptive immune response in Wegener granulomatosis (WG): activated PMNs release PR3, which interacts with dendritic cells (DCs) (via the PAR-2-Receptor) to induce a mature, antigen-presenting DC. PR3-matured DCs prime T cells for a Th1-phenotype necessary for granuloma formation. Granuloma may be the place of ANCA production. ANCAs that are released into the circulation are a major factor in inducing small vessel vasculitis. Abbreviations: PR3, proteinase 3; iDC, immature dendritic cell; mDC, mature dendritic cell; PAR-2, protease-activated receptor-2; T$_{EM}$, effector memory T cell; T$_{PR3}$, PR3-specific T cell; B, B cell; M, macrophage; N, neutrophil.

Risk Factors for Disease and Relapse

Elevated levels of mPR3 expression are found in WG patients compared with controls and are associated with disease relapse (12). Moreover, PR3-ANCA correlate with disease activity, and persistent high titers of ANCA during remission correspond to a high risk of relapse (13).

Clinical Manifestations

Initially, patients seek medical attention for upper and/or lower airway symptoms such as nasal crusting, bleeding, and granulomatous sinusitis. Typical complications of ENT involvement in WG are saddle nose deformity and subglottic stenosis. Upon generalization of the disease, malaise, fever, weight loss, and arthralgias are common and accompany clinical signs of vasculitis. Full-blown disease is usually characterized by the involvement of the ENT tract, the lungs, and the kidneys, although virtually any other organ can be involved (see Table 18.3). Lung involvement shows nodules or diffuse infiltrates on X-ray corresponding to granulomatous disease or alveolitis and alveolar hemorrhage, respectively. WG might be complicated by intraorbital granuloma or by contiguous invasion of the cerebrum by granulomatous masses originating from the sinuses. Cerebral manifestations include pachymeningitis, cranial neuropathy, pituitary gland involvement, and cerebral vasculitis. Peripheral neuropathy, however, is more common than CNS involvement. Disease activity and damage can be scored according to disease assessment scores such as BVAS and BVAS 2003 (Birmingham Vasculitis Activity Score) and VDI (Vasculitis Damage Index) (14).

Serological Markers and ANCA Detection

ANCA Detection

Consensus guidelines currently recommend to perform an IFT (immuno-fluorescence test) together with an enzyme-linked immunosorbent assay (ELISA) to detect the ANCA pattern and the target antigen (15).

By indirect immunofluorescence, one can usually distinguish a cytoplasmic (C-ANCA) from a perinuclear pattern (P-ANCA). ANCAs detected by IFT are not specific for vasculitis, for example, ANCAs (with various target antigens) are also found in other inflammatory diseases, such as ulcerative colitis and even in infective endocarditis. Target antigens are detected by ELISA. In WG, there is usually a C-ANCA pattern found, which is due to a PR3-ANCA. ANCA is negative in about 50% of patients with localized disease, whereas PR3-ANCA can be detected in 95% of patients with generalized WG (16).

Therapy

Therapy is adapted according to disease stage and activity. For the induction of remission in severe organ- and life-threatening disease, cyclophosphamide (at 2 mg/kg body weight/day) is used in combination with steroids (FAUCI scheme). Cyclophosphamide may be administered intravenously as bolus treatment (15 mg/kg according to the CYCLOPS study protocol) with equal efficacy for induction of remission. Furthermore, methotrexate (MTX) can be used for the induction of remission in non-life threatening "early systemic" disease (17, NORAM study). For maintenance of remission, there is good evidence for the use of azathioprine (18, CYCAZAREM study). Smaller studies suggest that MTX or leflunomide may also be useful for maintenance therapy. Innovative therapies such as anti-TNF treatment and the use of rituximab

TABLE 18.3. Clinical manifestations adapted from Reinhold-Keller, E (15).

Organ site	Frequency at presentation (%)	Frequency over disease course %
E (ENT)	93	99
K (kidney)	54	70
L (lung)	55	66
Ey (eye)	40	61
H (heart	13	25
P (peripheral nerves)	21	40
C (central nervous system)	6	11
Gi (gastrointestinal)	3	6
S (skin)	21	33
A (arthralgia)	61	77
C-ANCA positive	84	

TABLE 18.4. Biochemical and serological markers of Wegener granulomatosis (WG).

Marker	Change
ESR/CRP	↑
Hemoglobin	↓ Anemia due to systemic inflammation
Ferritin	↑
sIL-2R (soluble Interleukin-2 Receptor)	↑ Shedded by activated T lymphocytes
IL-6	↑ Secreted by activated monocytes
C-ANCA/PR3	+ Titer correlates with disease activity

(anti-CD20 antibody) are currently under investigation. Infliximab has been used successfully in combination with cyclophosphamide for the induction of remission in active or refractory WG in two open prospective studies (19). However, for the maintenance of remission, anti-TNF therapy with etanercept in combination with cyclophosphamide or MTX was not efficient in increasing the rate of remission and in reducing the risk of relapse (WGET trial). Rituximab may be efficient in refractory ANCA-associated vasculitis (AAV) (20, open study). Currently, two randomized controlled trials are undertaken to investigate the effect of rituximab in AAV (RAVE, RITUXVAS).

References

1. Reinhold-Keller E, Herlyn K, Wagner-Bastmeyer R, Gross WL. Stable incidence of primary systemic vasculitides over five years: Results from de german vasculitis register. *Arthritis Rheum* 2005; 53: 93–99.

2. Jennette JC, Falk RJ, Andrassy K, Bacon PA, Churg J, Gross WL, Hagen EC, Hoffman GS, Hunder GG, Kallenberg CG. Nomenclature of systemic vasculitides. Proposal of an international consensus conference. *Arthritis Rheum* 1994; 37: 187–92.

3. Leavitt RY, Fauci AS, Bloch DA, Michel BA, Hunder GG, Arend WP, Calabrese LH, Fries JF, Lie JT, Lightfoot RW Jr. The American College of Rheumatology 1990 criteria for the classification of Wegener's granulomatosis. *Arthritis Rheum* 1990; 33: 1101–7.

4. Jayne D for the European Vasculitis Study Group (EUVAS). Update on the European Vasculitis Study Group trials. *Curr Opin Rheumatol* 2001; 13: 541–9.

5. Szyld P, Jagiello P, Csernok E, Gross WL, Epplen JT. On the Wegener granulomatosis associated region on chromosome 6p21.3. *BMC Med Genet* 2006; 7: 21.

6. Jagiello P, Aries P, Arning L, Wagenleiter SE, Csernok E, Hellmich B, Gross WL, Epplen JT. The PTPN22 620 W allele is a risk factor for Wegener's granulomatosis. *Arthritis Rheum* 2005; 52(12): 4039–43.

7. Stegemann CA, Tervaert JW, Sluiter WJ, Manson WL, de Jong PE, Kallenberg CG. Association of nasal carriage of *S. aureus* and higher relapse rates in Wegener's Granulomatosis. *Ann Intern Med* 1994; 120: 12–17.

8. Csernok E, Ai M, Gross WL, Wicklein D, Petersen A, Lindner B, Lamprecht P, Holle JU, Hellmich B. Wegener's autoantigen induces maturation of dendritic cells and licenses them for Th1 priming via the protease-activated receptor-2 pathway. *Blood* 2006; 107(11): 4440–8.

9. Komocsi A, Lamprecht P, Csernok E, Mueller A, Holl-Ulrich K, Seitzer U, Moosig F, Schnabel A, Gross WL. Peripheral blood and granuloma CD4$^+$ CD28$^-$ T cells are a major source of interferon-γ and tumor necrosis factor-α in Wegener's granulomatosis. *Am J Pathol* 2002; 160(5): 1717–24.

10. Voswinkel J, Mueller A, Kraemer JA, Lamprecht P, Herlyn K, Holl-Ulrich K, Feller A, Pitann S, Gause A, Gross WL. B lymphocyte maturation in Wegener's granulomatosis: A comparative analysis of VH genes from endonasal lesions. *Ann Rheum Dis* 2006; 65(7): 850–64.

11. Csernok E. Antineutrophil cytoplasmatic antibodies and pathogenesis of small vessel vasculitides. *Autoimmun Rev* 2003; 2(3): 158–64.

12. Rarok AA, Stegeman CA, Limburg PC, Kallenberg CG. Neutrophil membrane expression of proteinase 3 (PR3) is related to relapse in PR3-ANCA-associated vasculitis. *J Am Soc Nephrol* 2002; 13(9): 2232–8.

13. Sanders JS, Huitma MG, Kallenberg CG, Stegeman CA. Prediction of relapses in PR3-ANCA-associated vasculitis by assessing responses of ANCA titres to treatment. *Rheumatology* (2006); 45(6): 724–9.

14. Flossmann O, Bacon P, de Groot K, Jayne D, Rasmussen N, Seo P, Westman K, Luqmani R. Development of comprehensive disease assessment in systemic vasculitis. *Ann Rheum Dis* 2006; 66: 283–92.

15. Savige J, Dimech W, Fritzler M, Goeken J, Hagen EC, Jennette JC, McEvoy R, Pusey C, Pollock W, Trevisin M, Wiik A, Wong R. Addendum to the International Consensus Statement on testing and reporting of antineutrophil cytoplasmic antibodies. Quality control guidelines, comments and recommendations for testing in other autoimmune diseases. *Am J Pathol* 2003; 120: 312–8.

16. Reinhold-Keller E, Beuge N, Latza U, de Groot K, Rudert H, Nölle B, Heller M, Gross WL. An interdisciplinary approach to the care of patients with Wegener's granulomatosis: Long-term outcome in 155 patients. *Arthritis Rheum* 2000; 43(5): 1021–32.

17. de Groot K, Rasmussen N, Bacon PA, Tervaert JW, Feighery C, Gregorini G, Gross WL, Luqmani R, Jayne DR. Randomized controlled trial of cyclophosphamide versus methotrexate for induction or remission in early systemic antineutrophil cytoplasmatic antibody-associated vasculitis. *Arthritis Rheum* 2005; 52: 2461–9.

18. Jayne D, Rasmussen N, Andrassy K, Bacon P, Tervaert JW, Dadoniene J, Ekstrand A, Gaskin G, Gregorini G, de Grott K, Gross WL, Hagen EC, Mirapeix E, Petterson E, Siegert C, Sinico A, Tesar V, Westman K, Pusey C. A randomized trial of maintenance therapy for vasculitis associated with antineutrophil cytoplasmatic antibodies. *NEJM* 2003; 349: 36–44.

19. Booth A, Harper L, Hammad T, Bacon P, Griffith M, Levy J, Savage C, Pusey C, Jayne D. Prospective study of TNFalpha blockade with infliximab in anti-neutrophil cytoplasmic antibody-associated vasculitis. *J Am Soc Nephrol* 2004; 15: 717–21.

20. Keogh KA, Ytterberg SR, Fervenza FC, Carlson KA, Schroeder DR, Specks U. Rituximab for refractory Wegener's granulomatosis: Report of a prospective, open-label pilot trial. *Am J Respir Crit Care Med* 2005; 13: 13.

19
Churg-Strauss Syndrome

Philippe Guilpain and Loic Guillevin

Abstract Churg and Strauss syndrome is a primary small-vessel necrotizing vasculitis characterized by asthma, lung infiltrates, extravascular necrotizing granulomas and hypereosinophilia. Churg and Strauss syndrome is serologically associated with antineutrophil cytoplasm autoantibodies (ANCA) in about 40% of patients. ANCA status may determine two phenotypes. Churg and Strauss syndrome may be highly severe and potentially lethal. Churg and Strauss syndrome should be treated with corticosteroids, associated with immunosuppressants when poor prognosis factors are present. Treatment dramatically improved the prognosis of Churg and Strauss syndrome, and the survival rate is now about 90% at 5 years.

Keywords Churg–Strauss syndrome · vasculitis · eosinophils · ANCA · immunosuppressants

Churg and Strauss syndrome (CSS) is a primary small-vessel necrotizing vasculitis typically characterized by asthma, lung infiltrates, extravascular necrotizing granulomas and hypereosinophilia (1). CSS belongs to the group of antineutrophil cytoplasm autoantibodies (ANCA)-associated vasculitides (AAV) that also comprises microscopic polyangiitis and Wegener's granulomatosis. In CSS, ANCA may determine two phenotypes, according to their presence or their absence.

Epidemiology

In patients in the general population, CSS frequency is estimated at 2.4–6.8 per 1,000,000 patient-years. In asthma patients, the incidence is higher than in the general population (35–67 per 1,000,000 patient-years). CSS may affect patients at any age, but the maximal frequency is between 30 and 50 years. The sex ratio is approximately 1:1.

History

In 1951, Jacob Churg and Lotte Strauss pathologically individualized a subgroup of patients with necrotizing vasculitis, asthma and eosinophilia from periarteritis nodosa (1).

Pathogenesis

Some triggering factors have been suspected in CSS, including vaccinations, desensitization. Drugs (such as macrolides, carbamazepine, quinine, corticosteroid-sparing agents for asthma and more recently leukotriene modifiers) were suspected but were not proven to cause CSS. Whatever, several pathogenic factors have been identified. First, eosinophil polymorphonuclears are probably effector cells, as suggested by the increased numbers of activated eosinophils (both in blood and in tissue lesions) during the flares. Upon activation, eosinophils release their cationic cytotoxic enzymes leading to tissue damage (2). Secondly, patients with anti-myeloperoxidase (MPO) antibodies (Abs) may suffer from the deleterious effect of those Abs, which are proven both in vitro and in vivo in microscopic polyangiitis (3, 4, 5). Anti-MPO antibodies can trigger oxidative burst by the neutrophils (4) and also activate MPO to produce highly cytotoxic oxidants such as hypochlorous acid (5).

Clinical Manifestations

According to Lanham (6), CSS follows three successive phases: the prodromic phase, consisting of asthma and allergic manifestations; the second phase resulting from eosinophil infiltration of tissues and the necrotizing vasculitis phase, possibly several years (mean: 3–4 years) after

From: Y. Shoenfeld et al. (eds.): *Diagnostic Criteria in Autoimmune Diseases*, DOI: 10.1007/978-1-60327-285-8_19,
© 2008 Humana Press, Totowa, NJ

TABLE 19.1. Main clinical manifestations of CSS.

Clinical manifestations	Frequency
Asthma	~100%
Patchy pulmonary infiltrates	70%
ENT manifestations	70%
Neurological involvement, including:	50–78%
Mononeuritis multiplex	~70% of patients with nerve involvement
Symmetrical polyneuropathy	Up to 30% of patients with nerve involvement
Central nervous system involvement	Rarely noted
Heart involvement	Up to 60%
Skin lesions	40–75%
Gastrointestinal (GI) tract, including:	~40–60%
abdominal pain	30–60% of patients with GI tract involvement
diarrhoea	10–33% of patients with GI tract involvement
Kidney disease	15–50%

asthma (7, 8). Target organs are involved at various frequencies (see Table 19.1). Asthma (usually severe late onset asthma) is a cardinal feature of CSS, present in almost all CSS patients. Lung infiltrates, allergic rhinitis or sinus polyposis, mononeuritis multiplex are classically noted. Skin lesions, myalgias, gastrointestinal (GI) tract symptoms, pauci-immune glomerulonephritis and cardiac disease may be also observed. CSS can involve the myocardium, pericardium and at a lesser degree endocardium, leading to severe sequellar lesions. Thus, heart disease is a severe involvement and represents the major cause of morbidity and mortality, accounting for approximately 48% of deaths in literature series (9, 10). New methods (such as cardiac magnetic resonance imaging and gated-SPECT imaging) are under development and could improve the detection of heart involvement (11, 12). Notably, CSS patients without ANCA have more frequent cardiac disease (see below) (13, 14).

Pathological Features

Diagnosis of CSS (1) is pathologically based on the presence of eosinophilic infiltrates, extravascular necrotizing granulomas and small-vessel (granulomatous or not) angiitis. Histological demonstration of CSS may be difficult because the typical lesions rarely coexist temporally or spatially. Whereas skin biopsy often lacks diagnostic specificity, neuromuscular biopsy may be very informative when clinical and electromyographic signs are frequent.

Biochemical Features

The main laboratory abnormalities are summarized in Table 19.2.

TABLE 19.2. The main laboratory abnormalities.

Laboratory abnormalities	Frequency
Increased erythrocyte sedimentation rate	~100% during flares
Increased C-reactive protein levels	~100% during flares
Anaemia (inflammatory of blood loss)	Frequent
Blood eosinophilia (7200 ± 6700 eosinophils/mm^3)	~100% during flares
Increased serum eosinophil cationic proteins levels	~100% during flares
Increased IgE levels	75%
Rhumatoid factors	20–60%
Anti-nuclear factor	10%
Anti-neutrophil cytoplasm antibodies (ANCA)	38–50%

Serological Features

Serum ANCA can be detected in 38–50% of patients, with a perinuclear immunofluorescent-labelling pattern (p-ANCA) in 75–81% of the ANCA positive patients. P-ANCA are mostly directed against MPO as assessed by using ELISA (92–100% of the P-ANCA positive sera). ANCA titres are not clearly correlated to CSS clinical activity and not predictive of outcome. However, ANCA have a clinical signification because the presence or the absence of ANCA may determine two distinct phenotypes in CSS patients (Table 19.3) (13, 14).

Diagnosis Criteria

Diagnosis criteria are controversial in CSS. The diagnosis of CSS could not be based on the pathological criteria defined by Churg and Strauss (1), because the three distinct histological lesions are rarely observed on the same sample (6). In 1984, Lanham et al. developed Hammersmith Hospital criteria based on clinical manifestations and applicable even in the absence of pathological confirmation (6). More recently, classification criteria by the American College of Rheumatology (ACR) (15) and the Chapel Hill conference (16) have been developed but

TABLE 19.3. Relationship between anti-neutrophil cytoplasm antibodies (ANCA) status and clinical phenotype (13, 14).

Patients with ANCA	Patients without ANCA
Necrotizing crescentic glomerulonephritis	Heart involvement +++
Purpura	Pleural effusion
Alveolar hemorrhage	Pulmonary infiltrates
Mononeuritis multiplex	Fever
Sinusitis	Livedo
	Vasculitis rarely detected

TABLE 19.4. Diagnosis and classification criteria for CSS.

Criteria	Comments
Churg and Strauss (1951) (1) • Asthma • Necrotizing vasculitis involving small- to medium-sized vessels • Tissue eosinophilia • Extravascular granulomas	Diagnosis criteria Low sensibility for CSS diagnosis because the three pathological lesions are rarely present on the same sample
Hammersmith Hospital (1984) (6) • Asthma • Blood eosinophilia >1500/mm^3 • Systemic vasculitis involving at less two extrapulmonary organs	Diagnosis criteria Sensibility: 95%, specificity: 95% Criteria based on clinical findings and not on pathological findings
American College of Rheumatology (1990) (16) (4 criteria) • Asthma • Blood eosinophilia >10% • Mononeuritis simplex or multiplex • Labile lung infiltrates • Paranasal sinus abnormality • Extravascular eosinophil infiltration on biopsy findings	These classification criteria have not been developed for CSS clinical diagnosis (When ≥4 criteria are present: sensibility: 85%; specificity: 99.7%) The pathological demonstration of vasculitis is required
Chapel Hill (conference) (1994) (17) • Asthma • Blood eosinophilia • Necrotizing vasculitis involving small- to medium-sized vessels • Eosinophil-rich and granulomatous inflammation involving the respiratory tract	These classification criteria have not been developed for CSS clinical diagnosis The pathological demonstration of vasculitis is required The demonstration of granulomas is rare in the respiratory tract

they are not for diagnosis. Notably, those criteria require the presence of a necrotizing vasculitis. To date, neither the ACR (15) nor the Chapel Hill Consensus Conference (16) classification criteria distinguish patients with ANCA from those without ANCA (Table 19.4).

Prognosis

The spontaneous outcome is poor but dramatically improved with corticosteroids. Complete remission may now be obtained in about 90% of patients. Relapses may occur in about 25% of cases, often preceded by the reappearance of peripheral eosinophilia. At 10 years, survival rate is about 80%. Heart disease, treatment toxicity and infections are the main causes of death in CSS.

Prediction

Disease activity may be assessed with Birmingham Vasculitis Activity Score (BVAS) (17). CSS severity can be determined with Five Factor Score (FFS) (18) that comprises five poor prognosis factors associated with a higher death rate: proteinuria >1 g/day, renal insufficiency, creatininemia >140 μmol/l or 1.58 mg/dl, specific

cardiomyopathy, GI tract involvement and central nervous system involvement.

Therapy

Therapeutic measures depend on disease severity. In the absence of poor prognostic factor (as indicated by the FFS), CSS usually responds quickly to corticosteroids. In all cases, high doses of corticosteroids (1 mg/kg/day of prednisone or its equivalent of methylprednisolone) should be given. The most severe cases should also be treated with intravenous methylprednisolone pulses (usually 15 mg/kg for 1–3 days) at the initiation of therapy. Corticosteroids can be tapered to low doses (i.e. >10 mg/d) in several months, but their discontinuation is often impossible because of residual asthma (8). Immunosuppressant should be added to corticosteroids for patients with one or more poor prognosis factor(s) (i.e. FFS ≥1) and/or for patients with refractory or relapsing disease. In these cases, cyclophosphamide (CYC) is the gold standard, administered intravenously (600–750 mg/m^2 given at 2-week intervals for the first month, then monthly) or orally. In our experience, we prefer intravenous CYC because of less toxicity. Those patients should be treated for ≥18 months (19). When patients have achieved remission usually after 3–6 months of CYC, a less-toxic maintenance immunosuppressant (such as azathioprine) should be given (20).

Patients with refractory CSS might be managed with alternative therapies such as intravenous immunoglobulins, plasma exchanges, rituximab that have been useful in some cases, but further studies are required to demonstrate clearly the beneficial effect of these drugs in CSS.

References

1. Churg J and Strauss L. Allergic granulomatosis, allergic angiitis, and periarteritis nodosa. *Am J Pathol* 1951; 27: 277–301.

2. Guilpain P, Auclair JF, Tamby MC, et al. Serum eosinophil cationic protein: a marker of disease activity in Churg-Strauss syndrome. *Ann N Y Acad Sci* 2007; 1107: 392–9.

3. Xiao H, Heeringa P, Hu P, et al. Antineutrophil cytoplasmic autoantibodies specific for myeloperoxidase cause glomerulonephritis and vasculitis in mice. *J Clin Invest* 2002; 110: 955–63.

4. Falk RJ, Terrell RS, Charles LA, and Jennette JC. Antineutrophil cytoplasmic autoantibodies induce neutrophils to degranulate and produce oxygen radicals in vitro. *Proc Natl Acad Sci U S A* 1990; 87: 4115–9.

5. Guilpain P, Servettaz A, Goulvestre C, et al. Pathogenic effects of antimyeloperoxidase antibodies in patients with microscopic polyangiitis. *Arthritis Rheum* 2007; 56: 2455–63.

6. Lanham JG, Elkon KB, Pusey CD, and Hughes GR. Systemic vasculitis with asthma and eosinophilia: A clinical approach to the Churg-Strauss syndrome. *Medicine (Baltimore)* 1984; 63: 65–81.

7. Keogh KA and Specks U. Churg-Strauss syndrome: Clinical presentation, antineutrophil cytoplasmic antibodies, and leukotriene receptor antagonists. *Am J Med* 2003; 115: 284–90.

8. Guillevin L, Cohen P, Gayraud M, Lhote F, Jarrousse B, Casassus P. Churg-Strauss syndrome. Clinical study and long-term follow-up of 96 patients. *Medicine (Baltimore)* 1999; 78: 26–37.

9. Hellemans S, Dens J, and Knockaert D. Coronary involvement in the Churg-Strauss syndrome. *Heart* 1997; 77: 576–8.

10. Lanham JG, Cooke S, Davies J, and Hughes GR. Endomyocardial complications of the Churg-Strauss syndrome. *Postgrad Med J* 1985; 61: 341–4.

11. Petersen SE, Kardos A, and Neubauer S. Subendocardial and papillary muscle involvement in a patient with Churg-Strauss syndrome, detected by contrast enhanced cardiovascular magnetic resonance. *Heart* 2005; 91: e9.

12. Pela G, Tirabassi G, Pattoneri P, Pavone L, Garini G, and Bruschi G. Cardiac involvement in the Churg-Strauss syndrome. *Am J Cardiol* 2006; 97: 1519–24.

13. Sable-Fourtassou R, Cohen P, Mahr A, et al. Antineutrophil cytoplasmic antibodies and the Churg-Strauss syndrome. *Ann Intern Med* 2005; 143: 632–8.

14. Sinico RA, Di Toma L, Maggiore U, et al. Prevalence and clinical significance of antineutrophil cytoplasmic antibodies in Churg-Strauss syndrome. *Arthritis Rheum* 2005; 52: 2926–35.

15. Masi AT, Hunder GG, Lie JT, et al. The American College of Rheumatology 1990 criteria for the classification of Churg-Strauss syndrome (allergic granulomatosis and angiitis). *Arthritis Rheum* 1990; 33:1094–100.

16. Jennette JC, Falk RJ, Andrassy K, et al. Nomenclature of systemic vasculitides. Proposal of an international consensus conference. *Arthritis Rheum* 1994; 37: 187–92.

17. Luqmani RA, Bacon PA, Moots RJ, et al. Birmingham vasculitis activity score (BVAS) in systemic necrotizing vasculitis. *QJM* 1994; 87: 671–8.

18. Guillevin L, Lhote F, Gayraud M, et al. Prognostic factors in polyarteritis nodosa and Churg-Strauss syndrome. A prospective study in 342 patients. *Medicine (Baltimore)* 1996; 75: 17–28.

19. Cohen P, Pagnoux C, Mahr A, et al. Churg-Strauss syndrome with poor-prognosis factors: A prospective multicenter trial comparing glucocorticoids and six or twelve cyclophosphamide pulses in forty-eight patients. *Arthritis Rheum* 2007; 57: 686–93.

20. Jayne D, Rasmussen N, Andrassy K, Bacon P, Tervaert JW, Dadoniené J, Ekstrand A, Gaskin G, Gregorini G, de Groot K, Gross W, Hagen EC, Mirapeix E, Pettersson E, Siegert C, Sinico A, Tesar V, Westman K, Pusey C; European Vasculitis Study Group. A randomized trial of maintenance therapy for vasculitis associated with antineutrophil cytoplasmic autoantibodies. N Engl J Med. 2003 Jul 3;349(1):36–44.

20
Buerger Disease

Michael Ehrenfeld and Raphael Adar

Abstract Buerger disease (thromboangiitis obliterans or TAO) is a rare non-atherosclerotic vascular disease, characterized by a combination of segmental inflammation and thrombosis of medium and small size arteries and veins both in the arms and the legs. The inflammatory process leads to severe ischemic rest pain, non-healing sores, ulceration and gangrene of fingers and toes. The disease is more common in young males, though its incidence seems to be increasing among women. Buerger disease is strongly associated with tobacco abuse in any form, which most probably triggers an autoimmune response. TAO does not fulfill, however, the criteria for a classical autoimmune disease, because no autoantigen has been clearly identified to date in the disease. Various sets of diagnostic criteria have been suggested over the years and the diagnosis requires the elimination of many other diseases. Absolute discontinuation of smoking remains the essential mode of therapy. New therapeutic modalities have been recently studied in small series, all requiring further evaluation in randomized controlled trials.

Keywords Buerger disease · thromboangiitis obliterans · endarteritis · tobacco

Buerger disease, known also as thromboangiitis obliterans (TAO), is an inflammatory segmental obliterative non-atherosclerotic disease of medium to small arteries, superficial veins and, less frequently, nerves. The pathological changes are distinct and typical for vasculitis (1), involving all layers of the vessel wall, with a highly cellular inflammatory infiltrate with microabscesses and multinucleated giant cells, involving the vessel walls and vasa vasorum. This intense inflammatory infiltrate leads to the occlusive thrombus. The disease occurs predominantly in young males (77%) and cigarette smokers, and the lower extremities are the main target of vascular occlusions. The typical presenting symptoms are of distal extremity ischemia, ischemic ulcers or gangrene (2). Smoking, which is generally accepted as a risk factor for this occlusive arterial disease, may alter the immune response and increase the susceptibility to autoimmune diseases (3); thus, complete cessation of smoking remains the cornerstone of therapy. The prevalence of the disease seems to have declined in North America over the last 30 years, probably attributed to the decline in smoking. The disease is more prevalent in the Mediterranean, in the Middle East and in Asia.

Signs and Symptoms

Ischemic rest pain and ulceration of the forefoot are the typical presenting signs of the disease, and in contrast to atherosclerosis, upper extremity involvement is quite frequent (2). Patients may present with foot and arch claudication, often misdiagnosed as an orthopedic problem, leading to a delay in the diagnosis. Multiple limbs are frequently involved; thus, it has been suggested to perform an arteriogram of both upper and lower limbs, even if the patient presents with only a single-limb involvement. Table 20.1 summarizes the typical presenting signs and symptoms of TAO. The disease usually begins with involvement of the distal small arteries and veins and with time progresses to involve more proximal arteries. Large artery involvement is rare as a sole vascular involvement, and if existent, it usually occurs in association with small vessel disease. Multiple organ involvement in TAO is extremely rare, having been described in only single case reports. TAO patients may also present with Raynaud phenomenon, as well as with superficial migratory thrombophlebitis, in as much as half of the cases. Arthralgias and arthritis have also been described, even as the initial presenting manifestation (4).

From: Y. Shoenfeld et al. (eds.): *Diagnostic Criteria in Autoimmune Diseases*, DOI: 10.1007/978-1-60327-285-8_20,
© 2008 Humana Press, Totowa, NJ

TABLE 20.1. Typical presenting signs and symptoms of thromboangiitis obliterans (TAO).

Rest pain	81%
Ischemic ulcers	76%
Sensory findings	69%
Intermittent claudication	63%
Abnormal Allen test (see text)	63%
Lower extremity	50–80%
Raynaud's phenomenon	40–45%
Thrombophlebitis	40–60%
Upper extremity	10–50%
Upper and lower extremity	30–40%
Joint manifestations	12.5%

Adapted from References 2, 5, 6.

Laboratory Findings and Serological Markers

There are no specific laboratory or radiological investigations helping in the diagnosis of Buerger disease. The diagnosis is therefore established on the basis of investigations and tests aiming to eliminate other diseases that may mimic or simulate TAO.

The initial diagnostic workup includes various studies in order to exclude these conditions. Arteriosclerosis as well as a proximal embolic source should be ruled out as the main differential diagnostic diseases using both an arteriogram and an echocardiography. Although the arteriogram may be suggestive of TAO, there are no pathognomonic angiographic features in Buerger disease. Generally, the proximal arteries should be normal, both in the lower and upper limbs, with no signs of atherosclerosis, aneurysmal disease or other source of proximal emboli. The pathology, if present, is usually segmental and limited to the distal circulation (infrapopliteal and distal to the brachial artery). Typically, medium and small size vessels demonstrate tapering occlusion with collaterals with a "corkscrew" and "tree root like" configuration. These changes might be seen on the digital arteries of the fingers and toes, the tibial, peroneal, radial and ulnar arteries; thus, segmental arterial Doppler pressures might be of some help. Basic laboratory studies include a complete blood count, liver and renal function tests, fasting blood sugar and a lipid profile.

Patients should be screened for necrotizing arteritis with erythrocyte sedimentation rate (ESR), C-reactive protein (CRP), rheumatoid factor (RF), antinuclear antibody (ANA), complement measurements, antineutrophil cytoplasm antibody (ANCA), cryoglobulins, and scleroderma-specific antibodies, which would also help in ruling out other rheumatic diseases such as systemic lupus erythematosus, rheumatoid arthritis with vasculitis, and scleroderma. Hand radiographs might be of some help in excluding scleroderma calcinosis and a toxicological screen for cannabis and cocaine should be also included in the diagnostic workup. Thrombophilia including hyperhomocysteinemia and antiphospholipid antibody syndrome should also be looked for in these patients.

The putative role of autoimmune- and immune-mediated mechanisms in the pathogenesis of TAO was reviewed by us, several years ago (7). No autoantigen has been clearly identified to date in TAO. As previously stated, the disease carries an extremely strong association with tobacco use, suggesting that tobacco might be one of the environmental factors implicated in its pathogenesis. Initial studies, performed many years ago, investigated both the humoral and cellular immunity, as well as HLA associations in a group of TAO patients. B and T cells were found to be within the normal limits. ANA, RF, and smooth muscle antibodies were all not found in their patients. The authors did, however, detect circulating antibodies to heat-denatured human collagen (ACA) in 35% of the patients, and in none of the controls. All but one of the patients with these antibodies were smokers. None of the patients with arteriosclerosis were positive for these antibodies. These studies were taken a further step by another group who demonstrated significantly higher levels of all serum immunoglobulins, as compared with a control group, as well as the presence of specific antihuman arterial antibodies, which were found in all TAO patients, compared with only 5 of the 15 controls. The authors thus suggested that the angiitis or vascular damage seen in Buerger disease may be due to an autoimmune process. The Tel-Hashomer group later confirmed the initial results demonstrated by others, when significant titers of anticollagen antibodies were shown to be present in 17 of 39 patients with TAO compared with none in the controls (3). These findings were further pursued by a group of investigators who were able to demonstrate anticollagen antibodies against type I, IV, and V collagen, mainly in the subgroup of an active or severe form of the disease, as compared with healthy controls. Other investigators were able to confirm the presence of circulating immune complexes (CICs) by various techniques and even to distinguish TAO from atherosclerotic patients and normal controls by the mean values of the CICs. A search for autoantibodies in Buerger disease found 55–60% of the patients to be positive for ANCA. Antimyeloperoxidase, antilactoferin and antielastase autoantibodies were only found in the severe TAO group. Other studies were unable to confirm these findings. High titers of antiendothelial cell antibodies (AECA) were found in a small group of active TAO, compared with controls and patients in remission (8). These AECAs have been recently found to be of great importance in other vasculitides such as Kawasaki disease, in which immune-mediated vascular injury and endothelial damage are present.

Preliminary studies have looked at antiphospholipid antibodies, which are also closely related to arterial and venous thrombosis.

The role of cell-mediated immunity against tobacco antigen in TAO patients was also investigated. In this study, the authors suggested that the relation between smoking and angiitis in TAO has to do with the modulation of the immune homeostasis via the tobacco.

The Tel-Hashomer group was also able to demonstrate the presence of cellular sensitivity to human type I and/or type III collagen in the peripheral blood lymphocytes of 77% of TAO patients, compared with much lower values in healthy male controls and in patients with atherosclerosis (3, 9).

A recent study examined histological specimens of TAO patients as well as immunophenotyping of these arteries (10). Histology of the arteries clearly demonstrated a cellular infiltrate in the intima with thrombi, with an intact elastic lamina, as opposed to giant cell arteritis. The authors thus concluded that TAO is a vasculitis induced by an antigen in the intimal layer. Most of the infiltrating cells in the intima were CD3[+] T cells.

HLA associations were also studied in Buerger disease. The studies are mostly small and thus inconclusive, though it seems that genetic factors do play a role in the pathogenesis of TAO. The differences observed in the HLA antigens may be based on the genetic variability of the studied populations, as well as due to methodological differences used in the different studies.

Based on the available data in the literature, one may conclude that TAO does not fulfill the criteria for an autoimmune disease. Immune mechanisms do seem to be involved, although they might only be of a secondary importance. These mechanisms might represent an epiphenomenon consistent with the inflammatory response. Alternatively, the possibility remains that they may represent an autoimmune reaction that has yet to be elucidated.

Diagnostic Criteria

There are no universally accepted diagnostic criteria for Buerger disease. Table 20.2 describes the various sets of diagnostic criteria which have been proposed over the years for the diagnosis of TAO. The traditional diagnostic criteria of Shionoya from Japan (11, 12) are based on the following five criteria: smoking history, onset before the age of 50 years, infrapopliteal arterial occlusive disease, either upper limb involvement or phlebitis migrans, and the absence of atherosclerotic risk factors other than smoking. A definite diagnosis of Buerger disease can be made if all five criteria are present. Mills and Porter (13, 14) proposed a set of more rigid major, which are essential, and minor diagnostic criteria based on a cohort of patients evaluated in Oregon (see Table 20.2), whereas Papa and Adar (15) suggested a set of more flexible criteria of various clinical, angiographic, histopathologic and exclusionary criteria for the diagnosis of the disease. They later

TABLE 20.2. Diagnostic criteria for Buerger disease (TAO) – proposed over the years.

Criteria	Shionoya (years)	Olin (years)	Papa (years)	Mills (Oregon) (years)
Age at onset of distal extremity	<50	<45	<30–40	<45[a]
Ischemia				
Tobacco abuse	+	+	+	+[a]
Infrapopliteal distal/no prox. dis.	+	+	+	+
Upper limb disease	+		+	+[b]
Migratory SVT	+		+	+[b]
Raynaud's phenomenon			+	+[b]
Intermittent claudication (foot)			+	+[b]
Exclusion of				
• proximal embolic source		+		+
• autoimmune diseases		+		+
• trauma and local lesions				+
• hypercoagulable states		+	+	+
• atherosclerosis:				
DM/HTN	+	+	+	+
Hyperlipidemia				
Renal failure				
Confirmed distal disease via				
• Segmental Doppler and 4 limb plethysmography		+		+
• Arteriography or		+	+	+
• Histopathology		+	+	(+)
Single limb involvement (negative criterion)			+	+
Female gender (negative criterion)			+	+

[a] Major criteria.
[b] Minor criteria.
DM, diabetes mellitus; HTN, hypertension; SVT, superficial vein thrombophlebitis.

further suggested a point scoring system to help in establishing the diagnosis of Buerger disease (16). Olin had also proposed a set of diagnostic criteria, which are quite similar to those of Mills and Porter, though he did not differentiate between major and minor criteria (17).

The scoring system of Papa and Adar is described in Table 20.3a (16). This scoring system replaces the exclusionary criteria with negatively scored criteria. The objective classification of patients is an obvious advantage of this scoring system over the other sets of criteria, thus using this system, points are awarded for young age at onset, foot claudication, upper extremity involvement, superficial vein thrombosis and vasospastic phenomena. Atypical features detract points and the resultant score classifies the diagnosis of Buerger disease (TAO) as being of low,

TABLE 20.3A. Point scoring system for the diagnosis of Buerger's disease (TAO) (Papa et al.).

		Points
I. Positive points		
Age of onset	<30/30–40 years	+2/+1
Foot claudication	present/by history	+2/+1
Upper extremity	symptomatic/asymptomatic	+2/+1
Phlebitis migrans	present/by history only	+2/+1
Raynaud syndrome	present/by history only	+2/+1
Angiography; biopsy	If typical, both/either	+2/+1
II. Negative points		
Age at onset	45–50/>50 years	–1/–2
Sex/smoking	Female/nonsmoker	–1/–2
Location	Single limb/no leg involvement	–1/–2
Absent pulses	Brachial/femoral	–1/–2
AS, DM, HTN, HL	Discovered after diagnosis 5–10 years/2–5 years	–1/–2

AS, arteriosclerosis; DM, diabetes mellitus; HL, hyperlipidemia; HTN, hypertension.

TABLE 20.3B. Probability of diagnosis of Buerger disease (TAO) (Papa et al.).

Number of points	Probability of diagnosis
0–1	Diagnosis excluded
2–3	Suspected, low probability
4–5	Probable, medium probability
6 or more	Definite, high probability

medium or high probability. None of the diagnostic sets of criteria for Buerger disease have been validated; however, of the 107 patients diagnosed by Papa et al. (16) by their old criteria, the diagnosis of TAO was rejected by the point scoring system in 20 patients. Of the remaining 87 patients, the degree of certainty in the diagnosis (point scoring system versus old criteria) was lower in 31, equal in 47 and higher only in 9. The authors suggested that their point scoring system has a better ability to discriminate patients than their old previous set of criteria, thus definitely improving the specificity of the diagnosis.

Treatment of Buerger Disease (TAO)

Discontinuation of tobacco use is the only effective therapy for TAO. Patients can be reassured that if they are able to refrain from tobacco use in any form, the disease will remit and amputation will not occur as long as critical limb ischemia in the form of tissue loss or gangrene has not occurred already (18). Though many medical and surgical therapeutic options for TAO have been proposed, none have been uniformly successful. With an ischemic or necrotic lesion, local care is the other cornerstone of therapy, aiming at obtaining cleansing of the wound with creation of conditions conducive to healing. Non-steroidal anti-inflammatory agents are used as the treatment of choice for

superficial thrombophlebitis. Chronic anticoagulation has been suggested even though no clear thrombophillia has been found in TAO. Other questionable therapies that have been recommended with limited evidence for their efficacy include calcium-channel blockers, plasma expanders, cyclophosphamide and epidural spinal cord stimulation.

Intravenous administration of a prostacyclin analogue (Iloprost) was more effective than oral aspirin in a randomized trial. Healing rate of ischemic lesions as well as pain relief were significantly higher in the prostacyclin group; however, this effect was not reached with oral Iloprost (19, 20).

Recent attempts to treat TAO patients with a therapeutic angiogenesis modality using vascular endothelial growth factor (VEGF) gene therapy showed great promise with a healing effect of ischemic ulcerations and relieving the rest pain these patients suffer from. An alternative way to stimulate angiogenesis has been suggested using a Kirschner wire placed in the medullary canal of the tibia, a method that has also initially showed some promising results in reducing rest pain as well as promoting healing of existing ulcers. Other preliminary experimental therapies of TAO include implantation of bone marrow mononuclear cells including endothelial progenitor cells into ischemic limbs, autologous bone marrow transplantation, stem cell therapy using umbilical cord-blood derived multipotent stem cells, the use of an endothelin antagonist, and the use of intermittent pneumatic compressions of the foot and calf. All these modalities require further evaluation in randomized controlled trials to confirm their beneficial effects.

Finally, surgical revascularization is rarely possible due to the nature and size of the involved vessels. Occasionally bypass surgery is considered, the results of which are generally disappointing. Sympathectomy, which used to be one of the main modes of therapy in TAO, is still used today mainly for pain control and promotion of healing, in cases which are unresponsive to best available medical therapy. If all else fails, amputation should be as distal as possible, consistent with a reasonable chance of healing.

References

1. Lie JT. The rise and fall and resurgence of thromboangiitis obliterans (Buerger disease). *Acta Pathol Jpn* 1989; 39: 153–8.
2. Mills JL Sr. Buerger disease in the 21st century: diagnosis, clinical features, and therapy. *Semin Vasc Surg* 2003; 16: 179–89.
3. Adar R, Papa MZ, Halpern Z, et al. Cellular sensitivity to collagen in thromboangiitis obliterans. *N Engl J Med* 1983; 308: 1113–16.
4. Puéchal X, Fiessinger JN, Kahan A, et al. Rheumatic manifestations in patients with thromboangiitis obliterans (Buerger disease). *J Rheumatol* 1999; 26: 1764–8.

5. Olin JW, Young JR, Graor RA, et al. The changing clinical spectrum of thromboangiitis obliterans (Buerger disease). *Circulation* 1990; 82(Suppl. IV): IV3–8.

6. Puéchal X, Fiessinger JN. Thromboangiitis obliterans or Buerger disease: challenges for the rheumatologist. *Rheumatology* 2007; 46: 192–9.

7. Ehrenfeld M, Papa M, Adar R. Autoimmune mechanisms in Buerger disease. *Crit Ischemia* 2001; 11: 7–13.

8. Eichhorn J, Sima D, Lindschau C, et al. Antiendothelial cell antibodies in thromboangiitis obliterans. *Am J Med Sci* 1998; 315: 17–23.

9. Papa M, Bass A, Adar R, et al. Autoimmune mechanisms in thromboangiitis obliterans (Buerger disease): The role of tobacco antigen and the major histocompatibility complex. *Surgery* 1992; 111: 527–31.

10. Kobayashi M, Ito M, Nakagawa A, et al. Immunohistochemical analysis of arterial wall cellular infiltration in Buerger disease (endarteritis obliterans). *J Vasc Surg* 1999; 29: 451–8.

11. Shionoya S. What is Buerger's disease? *World J Surg* 1983; 7: 544–51.

12. Shionoya S. Diagnostic criteria of Buerger disease. *Int J Cardiol* 1998; 66 (Suppl. I): s243–5.

13. Mills JL, Porter JM. Buerger disease: A review and update. *Semin Vasc Surg* 1993; 6: 14–23.

14. Mills JL. Buerger disease in the 21st century: diagnosis, clinical features, and therapy. *Semin Vasc Surg* 2003; 3: 179–89.

15. Papa MZ, Adar R. A critical look at thromboangiitis obliterans (Buerger disease). *Vasc Surg* 1992; 5: 1–21.

16. Papa MZ, Rabi I, Adar R. A point scoring system for the clinical diagnosis of Buerger disease. *Eur J Vasc Endovasc Surg* 1996; 11: 335–9.

17. Olin JW. Thromboangiitis obliterans (Buerger disease). In: Rutherford RB, (ed.) *Rutherford's Vascular Surgery*. 6th ed. Philadelphia: Elsevier-Saunders, 2005: 404–19.

18. Ballman KV. Long term survival and amputation risk in thromboangiitis obliterans (Buerger's disease). *JACC* 2004; 44: 2410–1.

19. Fiessinger JN, Schafer M. Trial of iloprost versus aspirin treatment for critical limb ischemia of thromboangiitis obliterans. The TAO study. *Lancet* 1990; 335: 555–7.

20. The European TAO Study Group. Oral Iloprost in the treatment of thromboangiitis obliterans (Buerger disease): a double blind, randomized, placebo-controlled trial. *Eur J Vasc Endovasc Surg* 1998; 15: 300–7.

21
Behçet Disease

Gerard Espinosa

Abstract   Behçet disease (BD) is a systemic vasculitis characterized by recurrent oral and genital ulcers, and ocular inflammation, but it may also involve the joints, skin, central nervous system and gastrointestinal tract. Although it has a world-wide distribution, it is more prevalent in the countries along the Silk Road. The aetiology of the disease remains unknown.

The diagnosis is based on clinical grounds, and classification criteria proposed by the International Study Group perform well in a clinical context. To date, the treatment of BD remains largely empirical and considerable differences exist in practical approaches to treatment. The primary goals of management are symptom control, early suppression of inflammation and prevention of end-organ damage. Regarding prognosis, the main associates of mortality in BD are major vessel pathology and neurologic involvement.

Keywords   Behçet disease · recurrent oral ulcers · vasculitis

Behçet disease (BD) is characterized by recurrent oral and genital ulcers and uveitis, but cutaneous, articular, neurologic, or vascular manifestations have also been observed (1).

Epidemiology

The geographical distribution of BD is distinctive. Although it has a world-wide distribution, it is more prevalent in the countries along the Silk Road, an ancient trading route between the Mediterranean and East Asia (2). In Turkey, the prevalence is estimated to be between 110 and 420 per 100,000, whereas that in Japan is 13–20 per 100,000, and the prevalence in the UK and the USA is estimated at 1–2 per 100,000 (1). It has only occasionally been reported in individuals of African origin.

History

One of the earliest descriptions of an illness that bears similarities to BD is found in Hippocrates' writings from ancient Greece in 450 BC (3). It was not until 1871 that individual features such as recurrent relapsing hypopyon uveitis, oral aphthae, and combined orogenital ulcerations were described. These features were usually attributed to tuberculosis or syphilis and in 1937 Hulusi Behçet proposed that this triple-symptom complex might be a separate disease entity (4). Behçet saw his first patient with recurrent aphthous stomatitis, genital ulcers, erythema nodosum, and visual disturbances in 1924. In 1930, he documented his second patient and in 1936 his third, and proposed that these signs constituted a specific disease entity. Finally, BD was formally recognized at the International Congress of Dermatology in 1947.

Pathogenesis

The etiology of BD remains unknown, but the most widely held hypothesis of disease pathogenesis is that a profound inflammatory response is triggered by an infectious agent in a genetically susceptible host (5). A combination of genetics, infectious agents, immune dysregulation and inflammatory mediators, heat shock proteins, oxidative stress, lipid peroxidation, coagulation abnormalities (6), and environmental factors have also been implicated (7).

The most plausible environmental trigger is an infectious agent, and evidence of ongoing or previous infection with a variety of viral and bacterial agents has been sought. These include *herpes simplex virus 1*, the hepatitis viruses,

From: Y. Shoenfeld et al. (eds.): *Diagnostic Criteria in Autoimmune Diseases*, DOI: 10.1007/978-1-60327-285-8_21,
© 2008 Humana Press, Totowa, NJ

and *parvovirus B19*. Potential bacterial triggers include mycobacteria, *Borrelia burgdorferi*, *Helicobacter pylori* and a variety of streptococcal antigens (5). Most recently, antibodies to *Saccharomyces cerevisiae* have been proposed as a serological marker of disease, but the clinical relevance of this finding is uncertain.

In every population studied, the most closely associated risk factor for disease, and in some countries for disease severity, is HLA-B51 (2). However, the biological mechanism whereby specific HLA-B alleles confer disease susceptibility remains unknown. In addition, the relative risk of disease associated with HLA-B51 varies widely in different ethnic populations, and the disease-associated alleles are present at high frequency in some populations in whom the disease is virtually unknown.

Clinical Manifestations

BD is multisystemic in nature, and any organ or system in the body may be affected. Signs and symptoms are illustrated in Table 21.1, but there is a considerable variation in the pattern of system involvement of BD worldwide (8). Recurrent aphthous ulceration is the sine qua non of BD; they are painful and appear in the gingiva, tongue, and buccal and labial mucosal membranes. Genital ulcers are morphologically similar to oral ulcers but frequently heal by scarring. They usually occur on the scrotum and penis in men and on the vulva in women.

Ocular lesions occur in the uvea and retina resulting in various symptoms, including blurred vision, eye pain, photophobia, lacrimation, floaters, and periglobal hyperemia. Skin disease in the form of erythema nodosum is common, particularly in females. It usually occurs on the front of the legs and may resolve but remain in hyperpigmented areas. Other cutaneous lesions described in patients with BD are pseudofolliculitis and acneiform nodules. Synovitis, arthritis, and/or arthralgia may occur, and the joints most frequently affected are the knees, followed by the wrists, ankles, and elbows. Destructive changes rarely occur in the joints.

TABLE 21.1. Symptoms and signs of Behçet disease (BD).

	Prevalence (%)
Mouth ulcers	100
Genital ulcers	94
Cutaneous involvement	70–80
Erythema nodosum	40–60
Articular involvement	40
Eye involvement	30–70
Vascular involvement	7–50
Gastrointestinal involvement	5–20
Central nervous system involvement	5–10

The concept of vasculo-Behçet has been adopted for cases in which vascular complications are present and often dominate the clinical features. Venous involvement is more common and may result in both superficial thrombophlebitis and deep venous thrombosis. Arterial complications are less common than venous involvement (9). Like occlusive lesions, arterial aneurysms are caused by vasculitis that begins in the vasa vasorum (10).

Gastrointestinal manifestations, including dysphagia, epigastric pain, colicky abdominal pain, bleeding, and diarrhea, are primarily caused by mucosal ulcerations and/or perforations (11).

The neurological involvement in BD primarily affects the central nervous system and includes parenchymal (with pyramidal signs, hemiplegia/paresis, behavioural changes; movement disorders, such as hemichorea, hemiballismus, and hemidystonia; hypersomnia, cranial nerve palsies, and aseptic meningitis) and nonparenchymal involvement (intracranial hypertension, because of dural sinus thrombosis). Peripheral neuropathy and myopathy are rare (12).

Pathological Features

BD is characterized by the presence of vasculitis, involving particularly venules. Lesions are characterized by perivascular lymphocytic and monocytic cellular infiltration, with or without fibrin deposition in the vessel wall. Significant neutrophil infiltration in the absence of infection is also seen, particularly in early lesions.

Biochemical and Serological Features

Laboratory findings are non-specific in BD. Moderate anemia and peripheral neutrophil leukocytosis are observed in some patients. Autoantibodies such as rheumatoid factor, antinuclear antibody, antineutrophil cytoplasmic antibody, and antiphospholipid antibody are usually negative. Importantly, non-specific markers of inflammation such as C-reactive protein level and erythrocyte sedimentation rate can be normal despite active disease. HLA typing is generally not useful in a diagnostic context because of the lack of sensitivity of the association with HLA-B51.

Diagnostic Criteria

There is no specific test or histologic finding in BD. Several sets of diagnostic criteria have been suggested for BD over the years. Classification criteria have been published by the International Study Group in 1990 (13) (Table 21.2). They were a consequence of the consensus among investigators

TABLE 21.2. International study group criteria for the diagnosis of Behçet disease.

Recurrent oral ulceration	Minor aphthous, major aphthous, or herpetiform ulceration observed by physician or patient, which have recurred at least three times in a 12-month period
And two of the following:	
Recurrent genital ulceration	Aphthous ulceration or scarring, observed by physician or patient
Eye lesions	Anterior uveitis, posterior uveitis, or cells in vitreous on slit lamp examination; or retinal vasculitis observed by ophthalmologist
Skin lesions	Erythema nodosum observed by physician or patient, pseudofolliculitis or papulopustular lesions; or acneiform nodules observed by the physician in post-adolescent patients not on corticosteroid treatment
Positive pathergy test	Read by physician at 24–48 h

The findings are applicable only in the absence of other clinical explanations.

and have been widely adopted to ensure that groups of patients entering into studies would be comparable.

The pathergy test is performed by introducing a 20-gauge or smaller sterile needle 5 mm obliquely into the patient's flexor aspect of the avascular forearm skin without injection of saline under sterile conditions. At 24–48 h after the pricking, the puncture site becomes inflamed and the test is considered positive if there is an indurated erythematous small papule or pustule formation of more than 2 mm in diameter, which usually resolves within 3 or 4 days. Although the test is positive in more than 60% of Middle Eastern patients with BD, it occurs in about 15% of Korean patients and 5% of Caucasians, reducing its diagnostic value in these groups.

The differential diagnosis of BD should include Reiter's syndrome, sarcoidosis, Stevens–Johnson syndrome, and inflammatory bowel disease (Crohn's disease and ulcerative colitis with extragastrointestinal involvement). Other causes of periodic fevers, such as familial Mediterranean fever (14) or hyper IgD syndrome, aphthous stomatitis, pharyngitis and cervical adenitis (PFAPA) syndrome, should be considered in children. Patients with significant neurological involvement may occasionally be misdiagnosed as having multiple sclerosis. Other chronic systemic diseases associated with recurrent aphthous ulceration include systemic lupus erythematosus and mixed connective tissue disease.

Prognosis

The mortality of patients with BD ranges from 0.9% during the course of a single year's follow-up to 3.9% at 10 years (15). Recently, Kural-Seyahi et al. (16) reported the mortality and overall morbidity in a cohort of 387 patients with BD followed during 20 years. The main associates of mortality were major vessel pathology (especially pulmonary arterial aneurysm) and neurologic involvement. Mortality was specifically increased among young males and, interestingly, tended to decrease significantly over the time. However, central nervous system involvement and major vessel disease were exceptions, because they can have their onset late, up to 10 years, during the disease course.

Therapy

The main objectives of BD treatment are to relieve symptoms, control inflammation, minimize functional disability, and prevent recurrences and end-organ damage. The choice of treatment depends on the clinical presentation and the severity of the manifestations. Combination drug therapy is preferred and results in a better outcome.

Mucocutaneous lesions are commonly treated with topical corticosteroids (CS). Colchicine, pentoxifylline, and thalidomide also are used for mucocutaneous lesions, but the toxicity of thalidomide limits its application (17). Joint involvement responds to non-steroidal anti-inflammatory drugs, colchicine, and CS.

The management of ocular inflammation depends on its severity. Topical midryatic agents and topical CS are given in cases of anterior uveitis. Acute attacks of mild posterior uveitis, intermediate uveitis, vitritis, and cystoid macular edema, especially if unilateral, in turn, can be treated with periocular CS injections. Systemic administration of CS, azathioprine (AZA), cyclosporine-A (CSA), chlorambucil, or cyclophosphamide has been effective in suppressing eye inflammation. However, only AZA has been shown in controlled trials to be beneficial. Most clinicians currently use combination therapy, which includes CS, AZA, and CSA (18).

When the central nervous system is involved, treatment most commonly consists of combination therapy with pulse CS and pulse cyclophosphamide or chlorambucil, although serious adverse effects limit its usage as a first-line agent for an acute attack. CSA and tacrolimus are not advised for the treatment of central nervous system involvement because of their increased rate of neurotoxicities (12).

Severe vasculitis is treated with CS and immunosuppressive agents, although controlled studies have not shown benefit. However, most relapses have been associated with discontinuation of treatment. Anticoagulants agents are used for deep venous thrombosis in addition to the administration of immunosuppressive agents.

In resistant cases of severe and refractory ocular manifestations or those with mucocutaneous or articular features that require high doses of CS, interferon(IFN)-α may be used (19).

Recently, an expert panel with specific expertise in BD management formulated recommendations for optimal use of anti-TNF agents in these patients (20). In general, TNF-blocking agents should be used with caution only for selected patients with severe disease. Patients with two or more relapses of posterior uveitis per year, or active CNS disease and/or selected patients with intestinal inflammation, or arthritic and mucocutaneous manifestations that reduce significantly the quality of life would fit this category. More interestingly, a single infusion of infliximab (5 mg/kg) can be used as a first-line agent for sight-threatening, bilateral posterior eye segment inflammation, when the fast-onset of response is considered to be critical to prevent fixed retinal lesions and thus permanent visual loss.

References

1. Sakane T, Taneko M, Suzuki N, Inaba G. Behcet's disease. *N Engl J Med* 1999; 341: 1284–91.
2. Verity DH, Marr JE, Ohno S, Wallace GR, Stanford MR. Behçet's disease, the silk road and HLA-B51: historical and geographical perspectives. *Tissue Antigens* 1999; 54: 213–20.
3. Feigenbaum A. Description of Behçet's syndrome in the Hippocratic third book of endemic diseases. *Br J Ophthalmol* 1956; 40: 355–6.
4. Behçet H. Über rezidiverende, apthöse durch ein Virus verursachte Geschwüre am Mund, am Auge und an der Genitalen. *Dermatol Wochenschr* 1937; 105: 1152–7.
5. Direskeneli H. Behçet's disease: Infectious aetiology, new autoantigens, and HLA-B51. *Ann Rheum Dis* 2001; 60: 996–1002.
6. Espinosa G, Font J, Tassies D, et al. Vascular involvement in Behçet's disease: Relation with thrombophilic factors, coagulation activation, and thrombomodulin. *Am J Med* 2002; 112: 37–43.
7. Evereklioglu C. Current concepts in the etiology and treatment of Behçet Disease. *Surv Ophthalmol* 2005; 50: 297–350.
8. Yazici H, Fresko I, Yurdakul S. Behcet's syndrome: disease manifestations, management, and advances in treatment. *Nat Clin Pract Rheumatol* 2007; 3: 148–55.
9. Atzeni F, Sarzi-Puttini P, Doria A, Boiardi L, Pipitone N, Salvarani C. Behçet's disease and cardiovascular involvement. *Lupus* 2005; 14: 723–6.
10. Calamia KT, Schirmer M, Melikoglu M. Major vessel involvement in Behçet disease. *Curr Op Rheumatol* 2004; 17: 1–8.
11. Bayraktar Y, Ozaslan E, Van Thiel DH. Gastrointestinal manifestations of Behcet's disease. *J Clin Gastroenterol* 2000; 30: 144–54.
12. Diri E, Espinoza LR. Neuro-Behçet's Syndrome: Differential diagnosis and management. *Curr Rheumatol Rep* 2006; 8: 317–22.
13. International Study Group for Behcet's Disease Criteria for diagnosis of Behcet's disease. *Lancet* 1990; 335: 1078–80.
14. Espinosa G, Arostegui JI, Plaza S, et al. Behçet's disease and hereditary periodic fever syndromes: Casual association or causal relationship? *Clin Exp Rheumatol* 2005; 23(4 Suppl. 38): S64–6.
15. Yazici H, Basaran G, Hamuryudan V, et al. The ten-year mortality in Behcet's syndrome. *Br J Rheumatol* 1996; 35: 139–41.
16. Kural-Seyahi E, Fresko I, Seyahi N, et al. The long-term mortality and morbidity of Behçet syndrome. A 2-decade outcome survey of 387 patients followed at a dedicated center. *Medicine (Baltimore)* 2003; 82: 60–76.
17. Lin P, Liang G. Behçet disease: recommendation for clinical management of mucocutaneous lesions. *J Clin Rheumatol* 2006; 12: 282–6.
18. Kaklamani VG, Kaklamanis PG. Treatment of Behçet's disease: An update. *Semin Arthritis Rheum* 2001; 30: 299–312.
19. Kötter I, Günaydin I, Zierhut M, Stübiger N. The use of interferon-α in Behçet disease: review of the literature. *Semin Arthritis Rheum* 2004; 33: 320–35.
20. Sfikakis PP, Markomichelakis N, Alpsoy E, et al. Anti-TNF therapy in the management of Behçet's disease – review and basis for recommendations. *Rheumatology* 2007; 46: 736–41.

22
Susac Syndrome

Manuel Francisco Ugarte and Ricard Cervera

Abstract   Susac syndrome is a microangiopathy causing small infarcts in the brain, cochlea, and retina. It is characterized by the clinical triad of acute or subacute encephalopathy, sensorineural hearing loss, and retinal branch artery occlusions. This syndrome is probably an immune-mediated endotheliopathy that affects the microvasculature of the brain, retina, and inner ear, but it has also been postulated that Susac syndrome can be due to a thrombotic occlusion of the small vessels of these organs.

The diagnosis is made by the presence of the triad of acute or subacute encephalopathy, sensorineural hearing loss, and retinal branch artery occlusions. When this triad is not completed, the imaging techniques can help with the diagnosis.

The treatment includes immunosuppression (with high-dose steroids and cytotoxic drugs) and anticoagulation.

Keywords   Susac syndrome · microangiopathy

Susac syndrome is a microangiopathy causing small infarcts in the brain, cochlea, and retina. It is characterized by the clinical triad of acute or subacute encephalopathy, sensorineural hearing loss, and retinal branch artery occlusions.

Epidemiology

The most commonly affected demographic group is represented by young women, the female : male sex ratio is 3:1, and the age at onset is usually between 20 and 40 years. Susac syndrome has been reported in North America, Europe, and Asia. A higher incidence during Spring and Summer has been described (1).

History

The first case report was made by Susac et al. (2) in 1979. They described two women with a progressive neurologic disorder, multifocal retinal branch artery occlusion, and hearing loss.

Pathogenesis

Preliminary evidence suggests that Susac syndrome is an immune-mediated endotheliopathy that affects the microvasculature of the brain, retina, and inner ear. Anti-endothelial cell antibodies may play a role in either mediating or reflecting the endothelial cell injury (3,4).

It has also been postulated that this syndrome could be a form of presentation of the catastrophic antiphospholipid syndrome, because it is characterized by multiple organ involvement because of thrombotic occlusions of the small vessels and the presence of antiphospholipid antibodies has been reported in some patients (5).

Clinical Manifestations

The triad (encephalopathy, inner ear involvement, and retinal artery occlusions) is clinically obvious at onset in only 20% of cases (6). However, this triad is usually completed after several years of follow-up (from 0 to 3). The frequencies of organ involvement at presentation are described in Table 22.1 (1).

Brain involvement usually presents as encephalopathy, ranging from mild memory loss or personality changes to confusion (1,7, 8,9). Patients can also present headache or

From: Y. Shoenfeld et al. (eds.): *Diagnostic Criteria in Autoimmune Diseases*, DOI: 10.1007/978-1-60327-285-8_22,
© 2008 Humana Press, Totowa, NJ

TABLE 22.1. Symptoms and signs of Susac Syndrome at presentation.

Organ involvement	Prevalence (%)
Retinal involvement	46
Brain involvement	80
Cochlea involvement	52
Complete triad	20

paresthesia. At physical examination, corticospinal syndrome, Babinsky sign, ataxia, frontal lobe syndrome, and hypoesthesia are the most common findings (1). Amenorrhea, which has been related to hypothalamic or pituitary involvement, has also been described (9).

Inner ear involvement usually presents as a bilateral hearing loss, and involves low and medium frequencies. It is caused by apical cochlear damage because of occlusion of the cochlear end arterioles. Clinical findings also include tinnitus and vertigo (1).

Eye involvement usually is referred as scotoma or visual acuity loss. Visual fields are frequently abnormal. Fundoscopic examination reveals retinal ischemic whitening, cotton-wool patches, periarterial whitening, box-car segmentation, and cherry red spot (9,10). Optic disk pallor may occur in the later stages. Retinal artery wall plaques have sometimes been described (10). They are yellow and usually located away from arterial bifurcations, which helps to distinguish them from visible emboli. These plaques are known as Gass plaques and are a helpful finding in making the diagnosis: they reflect a focal disturbance of the endothelium with subsequent deposition of atheromatous material, are sometimes refractile, and their presence does not suggest an embolic disorder, but rather Susac syndrome (10). Nevertheless, fundoscopy is less sensitive than fluorescein angiography for detecting new occlusions (1).

Imaging Findings

Brain Involvement

Brain computed tomography scan is usually normal in Susac syndrome, except for atrophy, which may develop during follow-up. Brain magnetic resonance imaging (MRI) typically shows bilateral gray and white matter lesions (11,12). They are numerous and often small (3–7 mm), are predominantly supratentorial (but may also involve infratentorial compartment), and present as hypointensities in T1-weighted images and small T2 and FLAIR hyperintensities (11,12). The cerebellum, cerebellar peduncles, brainstem, deep gray basal ganglia, and thalamus are frequently involved. The *corpus callosum* is always involved. Although any part of the *corpus callosum* may be affected, the central portion is preferentially involved with microinfarcts that are typically small but may be large and have a "snowball" appearance. Occasionally, linear defects (spokes) may extend from the callosal septal surface to the superior margin of the *corpus callosum*. Central callosal holes ultimately develop and may be patognomonic (11,13,14). Gadolinium enhancement of gray and white matter lesions is found in up to 70% of patients (11). Coronal and sagittal planes are essential to avoid missing lesions of *corpus callosum*. Diffusion-weighted imaging and apparent diffusion coefficient have been proved to be sensitive to the histologic and physiologic changes associated with brain infarction. During the acute phase, infarcted cerebral tissue is hyperintense on diffusion-weighted MRI and has reduced apparent diffusion coefficient (15). In Susac syndrome, hyperintense lesions have been reported, with reduced apparent diffusion coefficient (16).

Eye Involvement

Retinal arteriolar branch occlusions and arterial wall hyperfluorescence are typical features of Susac syndrome on fluorescein angiography. Although the most frequent cause of retinal occlusions is clearly embolic (cardiac disease or carotid stenosis), arterial wall hyperfluorescence is not a usual finding in embolic occlusions. Arteriolar multifocal fluorescence is frequent in Susac syndrome (17). Retinal branch artery occlusions and arterial wall hyperfluorescence are not parallel: they are not always detected in the same site nor at the same time. Arterial wall hyperfluorescence zones may represent preocclusive lesions, and may be taken as an indicator of active disease (18).

Laboratory Findings

Despite extensive laboratory investigation, no consistent abnormalities have been found. The erythrocyte sedimentation rate and C-reactive protein may be elevated. Minor elevations of the antinuclear and antiphospholipid antibodies can be found. Elevation of factor VIII and von Willebrand factor antigen levels may occur. These elevations may be due to endothelial perturbation. The factors are stored in the Weibel-Palade bodies membrane bound to the endothelium and may be released during endothelial damage. Although their elevation may be due to acute phase reactants, their close association with the endothelium would be consistent with endotheliopathy (9,13).

Cerebrospinal fluid examination may show a lymphocytic pleocytosis and proteins are usually elevated during the encephalopathic episode. The presence of oligoclonal bands and elevated IgG index may be misinterpreted as being due to multiple sclerosis.

Pathological Features

Most of the reports that included brain biopsy results described small foci of necrosis (microinfarcts) within the cerebral cortex and white matter, with loss of neurons, axons, and myelin. Only a few reports have provided detailed information about the microvasculature. The characteristics included endothelial cell necrosis with sloughing of dead cells into vascular lumina, endothelial cell denudement of capillaries and venules, mural and intra-luminal fibrin deposition, basement membrane zone thickening due to a combination of basement membrane reduplication (lamellation) and collagen deposition, and intense deposition of C4d and C3d within the majority of capillaries. Perivascular and intramural lymphocytic infiltration has been also described (3,19).

Diagnosis

There are no established diagnostic criteria for this syndrome, but the triad of acute or subacute encephalopathy, sensorineural hearing loss, and retinal branch artery occlusions must be present. However, in cases lacking any of these three findings at presentation, brain MRI (specially if there are lesions in the *corpus callosum*), and eye examination (fundoscopy and fluorescein angiography) may be helpful for the diagnosis (Table 22.2).

Prognosis

Three major clinical courses have been described in patients with Susac syndrome: monocyclic, polycyclic and chronic continuous (19). However, independently of which of these courses the disease has, patients frequently have sequelae. Brain sequelae is reported in 66.7%, but is usually mild (behavioral or personality changes, loss of memory and concentration, slight cognitive disturbances, ataxia, and hemiparesia) (1). Eye sequelae is reported in 27.5% (mainly, mild visual loss) (1). Inner ear sequelae is reported in 89.7% (uni- or bilateral hearing loss).

TABLE 22.2. Diagnostic criteria for Susac syndrome.

Acute or subacute encephalopathy
Retinal branch artery occlusions
Sensorineural hearing loss

The diagnosis is made when the three clinical manifestations are present. In cases lacking any of the three findings at presentation, brain MRI (especially if there are lesions in the *corpus callosum*) and eye examination (fundoscopy and fluorescein angiography) may be helpful for the diagnosis.

Although Susac syndrome is thought to be self-limited, late relapses may occur, especially in the retina. No death directly related to Susac syndrome has been reported.

Treatment

No clinical trials have been performed for the treatment of Susac syndrome, but strong immunosuppressive therapy has been postulated for this condition. During the first week, it is recommended the use of high dose steroids (i.e., three pulses of intravenous methylprednisolone followed by high-dose oral prednisone). Intravenous immunoglobulins (2 g/kg) are also recommended and this dose can be repeated every month for 6 months. Cytotoxic drugs (i.e., cyclophosphamide, mycophenolate mofetil, and methotrexate) can also be used (19). Anticoagulation therapy can be helpful, especially in those cases with antiphospholipid antibodies (5).

References

1. Aubert-Cohen F, Klein I, Alexandra JF, Bodaghi B, Doan S, Fardeay CM, Lavallée P, Peitte JC, Le Hoang P, Papo T. Long-term outcome in Susac syndrome. *Medicine* 2007; 86: 93–102.
2. Susac JO, Hardman JM, Selhorst JB. Microangiopathy of the brain and retina. *Neurology* 1979; 29: 313–6.
3. Magro CM. Susac syndrome – an autoimmune endotheliopathy. 1st Susac Symposium. Ohio State University, Columbus OH, April 2005.
4. Waldman J, Knight D. Antiendothelial cell antibodies in Susac's syndrome. 1st Susac Symposium. Ohio State University, Columbus OH, April 2005.
5. Bucciarelli S, Cervera R, Martinez M, Latorre X, Font J. Susac's syndrome or catastrophic antiphospholipid syndrome. *Lupus* 2004; 13: 607–8.
6. Susac JO. Susac syndrome: The triad of microangiopathy of the brain and retina with hearing loss in young men. *Neurology* 1994; 44: 591–3.
7. O'Halloran HS, Pearson PA, Lee WB, Susac JO, Berger JR. Microangiopathy of the brain, retina, and cochlea (Susac syndrome). A report of five cases and a review of the literature. *Ophtalmology* 1998; 105: 1038–44.
8. Papo T, Biousse V, Le Hoang P, Fardeu C, N'Guyen N, Houn DL, Aumaitre O, Bousser MG, Godeau P, Piette JC. Susac syndrome. *Medicine (Baltimore)* 1998; 77: 3–11.
9. Petty GW, Engel AG, Younge BR, Duffy J, Yanagihara T, Lucchineti CF, Bartleson JD, Parisi JE, Kasperbauer JL, Rodriguez M. Retinocochleocerebral vasculopathy. *Medicine (Baltimore)* 1998; 77: 12–40.
10. Egan RA, Ha Nguyen T, Gass JD, Rizzo JF III, Tivman J, Susac JO.Retinal arterial wall plaques in Susac syndrome. *Am J Ophthalmol* 2003; 135: 483–6.
11. Susac JO, Murtagh FR, Egan RA, Berger JR, Bakshi R, Lincoff N, Gean AD, Galetta SL, Fox RJ, Costello FE,

Lee AG, Clark J, Layzer RB, Daroff RB.MRI findings in Susac's syndrome. *Neurology* 2003; 61: 1783–1787.

12. White ML, Zhang Y, Smoker WR.Evolution of lesions in Susac syndrome at serial MR imaging with diffusion-weighted imaging and apparent diffusion coefficient values. *Am J Neuroradiol* 2004; 25: 706–13.

13. Susac JO, Egan RA, Rennebohm RM, Lubow M. Susac's syndrome: 1975–2005 microangiopathy/autoimmune endotheliopathy. *J Neurol Sci* 2007; 257: 270–2.

14. Gross M, Eliashar R.Update on Susac's syndrome. *Curr Opin Neurol* 2005; 18: 311–4.

15. Lansberg MG, Thies VN, O'Brien MW, Ali JO, de Crespigny AJ, Tong DC, Moseley ME, Albers GW. Evolution of apparent diffusion coefficient, diffusion-weighted and T2-weighted signal intensity of acute stroke. *Am J Neuroradiol* 2001; 22: 537–44.

16. Xu MS, Tan CB, Umapathi T, Lim CC. Susac syndrome: Serial diffusion-weighted MR imaging. *Magn Reson Imaging* 2004; 22: 1295–8.

17. Recchia FM, Brown GC. Systemic disorders associated with retinal vascular occlusion. *Curr Opin Ophthalmol* 2000; 11: 462–7.

18. Susac JO.Susac's syndrome. *Am J Neuroradiol* 2004; 25: 351–2.

19. Rennebohm RM, Susac JO.Treatment of Susac's syndrome. *J Neurol Sci* 2007; 257: 215–20.

23
Goodpasture Disease

Thomas Hellmark and Mårten Segelmark

Abstract   Goodpasture disease is a prototype of autoimmune disease. The disease can be transferred with the antibodies and there is a strong correlation with certain HLA genes. The pathogenic epitope on the NC1 domain of the α3-chain of type IV collagen is well characterized and only antibodies against this epitope correlate with disease. The diagnosis is made on the combination of rapidly progressive renal failure and the demonstration of anti-glomerular basement membrane (GBM) antibodies. The course is sometimes complicated by severe lung hemorrhage, and untreated Goodpasture disease has a poor prognosis. Early diagnosis and treatment with immunosupressive agents and plasma exchange leads to improved prognosis. Owing to its clinical significance and high predictive value, anti-GBM antibody analysis is indicated in most cases of unknown renal failure with microhematuria, especially if progression is rapid.

Keywords   Anti-glomerular basement membrane nephritis · glomerulonephritis · basement membrane · reno-pulmonary syndrome

Goodpasture disease, also known as anti-GBM disease, is a rare autoimmune disease. Patients develop autoantibodies against the noncollagenous domain 1 of the α3-chain of type IV collagen (α3(IV)NC1) (1), leading to glomerulonephritis and lung hemorrhage. Patients experience a rapid progression to renal failure and death if the disease is not recognized and treated early. The disease has been extensively studied which has led to a better understanding of autoimmunity in general.

Epidemiology

Published patient series have come from New Zealand, Australia, United Kingdom, the United States, China, and Scandinavia and estimated frequencies vary from 0.5 to 1 cases per million inhabitants per year. There are two peaks of age-dependent incidence, in the third and in the seventh decades. The disease is uncommon before puberty and the male-to-female ratio is approximately equal (2, 3, 4).

History

For more than 50 years, Goodpasture syndrome has been used to describe patients presenting with acute or sub acute reno-pulmonary syndromes of unknown etiology in recognition of a case report by EW Goodpasture in 1919 (5, 6). When the technique for direct immunofluorescence (IF) was introduced, it was shown that such patients often had a continuous linear deposit of immunoglobulins along their glomerular basement membrane (Figure 23.1). A pathogenic role of these antibodies was demonstrated by elution from human kidneys and transfer to primates (7). The term Goodpasture syndrome was then used for the triad of lung hemorrhage, renal failure, and anti-GBM antibodies. Today, the term is preferred for glomerulonephritis caused by antibodies directed against α3(IV)NC1, with or without lung hemorrhage.

Pathogenesis

Numerous animal models have been described showing the pathogenic role of the anti-GBM antibodies. In a classic experiment, primates developed glomerulonephritis after injection of autoantibodies eluted from the kidneys of a nephrectomized patient suffering from anti-GBM disease (7). Indirect proof of the pathogenic potential of the antibodies was given by the reappearance of disease in a renal transplant given to a patient with persistent high levels of circulating anti-GBM antibodies. Temporal relationships between relapse and reoccurrence of autoantibodies have

From: Y. Shoenfeld et al. (eds.): *Diagnostic Criteria in Autoimmune Diseases*, DOI: 10.1007/978-1-60327-285-8_23,
© 2008 Humana Press, Totowa, NJ

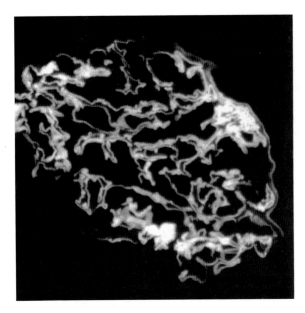

FIGURE 23.1. Direct IF of human kidney biopsy. IgG is visualized and a linear staining is found along the GBM. This picture is identical to staining using anti-α3(IV) monoclonal antibodies.

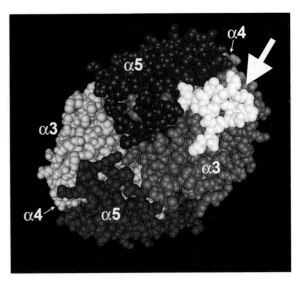

FIGURE 23.2. A model of the NC1 hexamer of type IV collagen found in the GBM. Each type IV collagen molecule is composed of one α3, one α4, and one α5 chain. The two α4 NC1 domains bind to each other, whereas the α3 binds an α5 NC1 domain. The amino acids identified as the epitope of the pathogenic antibodies is indicated on one of the α3 molecules in white and the large arrow. The proposed positions of the six α(IV) NC1 domains found in the human GBM are indicated. Note that the two α4(IV) domains are positioned on the back of the molecule. This picture of the NC1 hexamer is modeled from the NCBI MMDB entry #29412 using the Cn3D software (NCBI).

also been reported. The titer of circulating anti-GBM antibodies, as measured by ELISA, has been shown to have prognostic importance (3).

Patients of this disease have a polyclonal immune response and develop autoantibodies to different parts of the antigen (8, 9). Two major epitopes have been identified (10), but only antibodies against one reflect the toxicity of the antibodies (11). This epitope is situated near the triple helical junction (Figure 23.2). The epitope is a cryptotope and accessibility for the anti-GBM antibodies is normally limited. The cryptic properties have recently been shown to be due to cross-linking of the NC1 hexamer of type IV collagen (12). However, it has been shown that oxidants can open up the structure, as can certain subpopulations of anti-GBM antibodies (10).

There is evidence for a T-cell component in anti-GBM disease. The autoantibody IgG subclass distribution is compatible with a T-cell mediated reaction toward a protein antigen. A mononuclear interstitial cell infiltrate is invariably seen in human anti-GBM disease, consisting mainly of CD4$^+$ cells. Animal models indicate a role of autoreactive T cells. Transfer of anti-GBM antibodies alone can induce disease but always with a mild glomerulonephritis. Furthermore, immunization with a short peptide, i.e. the T-cell epitope, can induce florid glomerulonephritis without measurable levels of anti-GBM antibodies (13, 14).

Genetic studies have revealed a strong link to exist between anti-GBM disease and HLA-DRB1*1501 and DRB1*1502. Most reports stem from Caucasian populations where the DRB1-15 antigen is found in 70–80% of patients, compared with 20–30% of the controls. A

negative link is found between HLA-DR7 and DR1, thus acting protective (4).

Clinical Manifestations

The typical presentation is that of a reno-pulmonary syndrome i.e. the combination of renal and pulmonary insufficiency. However, many other types of presentations have been described. Most patients report some form of general prodromal symptoms such as fatigue and malaise but usually only confined to the preceding few weeks or months. In some series, more than 50% of the patients present with only renal involvement. Virtually all have microhematuria, many have macrohematuria, and rapidly progressive renal insufficiency is common. Sometimes the progression is explosive leading to anuria within days, while a minority of cases experience a protracted course where the renal function is preserved for several months. Proteinuria is usually modest but occasional patients present with nephrotic syndrome. The presenting symptoms for patients with lung involvement are hemoptysis, exertional dyspnoea, cough, and fatigue. The hemorrhage occurs mainly into the alveolar spaces and may result in marked iron deficiency anemia or exertional dyspnoea

TABLE 23.1. Symptoms and signs of Goodpasture disease at presentation.

Signs and symptoms	Prevalence	Comments
Rapidly progressive GN	99%	
Lung involvement	30–60%	
Malaise, fatigue, and weight loss	70–90%	Related to anemia, uremia, or degree of inflammation
Arthralgia and myalgia	Rare	May not be related to Goodpasture disease
Hypertension		Late event due to advanced renal failure with fluid retention

even in the absence of hemoptysis. There are reports that environmental factors such as cigarette smoke or other inhaled fumes may predispose for lung manifestations of the disease. In rare cases, patients have disease manifestations that are confined to the lungs. Signs and symptoms at presentation are listed in Table 23.1.

Pathological Features

Light microscopy typically reveals general widespread crescent formation. The percentage of glomeruli exhibiting crescents often exceeds 80%, and the percentage usually correlates to renal function as well as outcome after treatment. The typical finding in direct IF microscopy is a linear staining of IgG along the GBM, often accompanied by C3 deposition. Other staining patterns are sometimes seen, especially in mild cases with preserved renal function as well as in severely damaged glomeruli (Table 23.2)

TABLE 23.2. Laboratory findings.

Method	Finding	Comment
Light microscopy of renal tissue	Extensive crescent formation, diffuse proliferative glomerulonephritis with variable degree of necrosis, glomerulosclerosis, and tubular loss	
IF on renal tissue	Linear binding of IgG along the glomerular basement membrane	Can occasionally be seen in SLE, diabetes mellitus, renal transplants, and in some normal kidneys
	C3 deposition	Found in approximately 75% of cases
	IgA or IgM	Found in 10–15%
Urine analysis	Hematuria, proteinuria	
s-Creatinine	Elevated	

Serological Features

Anti-GBM antibodies are per definition present in all patients with Goodpasture disease; however, different detections methods may yield discrepant results. Circulating anti-GBM antibodies can be detected using indirect IF, western blotting, or ELISA. In indirect IF, serum from the patient is overlaid a section of normal kidney. A good substrate and a good pathologist are needed because unspecific staining can be difficult to distinguish from the true linear staining pattern. Low levels of circulating autoantibodies cannot usually be detected with indirect IF. Many labs have their in-house anti-GBM assay or western blotting method, and there are several commercially available ELISA kits on the market. The performances of these assays depend on the purity of the antigen preparation, but are generally good (15). Tissue-bound anti-GBM antibodies can be visualized by direct IF of renal biopsy specimens (Figure 23.1). This method can give false-positive results in cases of diabetes and in biopsies from renal transplants. In patients presenting as reno-pulmonary syndromes, anti-GBM antibodies can usually be found in around one-third of the cases; in patients with rapidly progressive glomerulonephritis without pulmonary symptoms, less than 5% have circulating anti-GBM.

Many patients (20–35%) with anti-GBM antibodies also have anti-neutrophil cytoplasmic antibodies (ANCAs), mostly with specificity for myeloperoxidase (MPO-ANCA). Some double-positive patients have features typical for Wegener's granulomatosis or Microscopic polyangiitis, but virtually all published cases have severe renal disease. We recommend that ANCA and anti-GBM be analyzed in parallel in patients with renal disease (Table 23.3).

Diagnostic Criteria

The diagnosis of Goodpasture disease relies on the detection of anti-GBM antibodies in conjunction with glomerulonephritis and/or lung hemorrhage. The diagnosis is problematic only when features of other diseases simultaneously present.

Prognosis

Prognosis of anti-GBM disease is highly dependent on the stage of the renal disease at time of diagnosis. When detected before s-creatinine has risen above 600 micromol/l (5 mg/dl), there is a good chance of renal recovery, if treatment with immunosupressive agents and plasma

TABLE 23.3. Serological findings.

Serological feature	Prevalence
Anti-GBM	100%
ANCA (mostly MPO-ANCA)	20–35%

exchange is rapidly instituted (3, 16). In such patients, the amounts of epitope-specific circulating antibodies seem to convey prognostic information. In some patients with low levels of circulating antibodies, who often tend to be MPO-ANCA positive, IF on kidney biopsy fails to show the typical linear pattern. This in conjunction with reports of the coincidental reappearance of symptoms with rising anti-GBM levels, suggest that low levels of anti-GBM antibodies may lack clinical significance. It is, however, prudent to wait with renal transplantation for several months after anti-GBM antibodies have fallen below the detection level.

Prediction

In the setting of moderate renal failure and microscopic hematuria, anti-GBM antibodies herald a nephrological emergency. A positive test indicates that the patient is at great risk of developing permanent renal failure as well as life-threatening lung hemorrhage unless decisive therapeutic measures are instituted. A negative test, especially in conjunction with negative tests for ANCA, conveys a message that toxic therapies safely can be withheld for a few days, for instance until biopsy reports return. In the setting of oliguric renal failure, a positive test points toward end-stage renal disease.

ELISA using purified NC1 domains of type IV collagen has become the gold standard for detecting anti-GBM antibodies for many nephrologists, making sensitivity and specificity impossible to calculate. False-positive reactions occur mainly in SLE and other diseases with polyclonal activation. Normally approximately 1% of samples sent to a laboratory contain unspecific reactivities. This can be controlled for by always checking for background reactivities in each sample. Studies comparing indirect IF with commercial ELISA kits have shown a concordance between such assays of approximately 90%. Discrepancies between assays and false-positive test typically exhibit results close to the cutoff level for positive results. The PPV and NPV are very high and have been estimated to be 95% or more (15).

Therapy

Standard therapy includes extracorporeal removal of auto-antibodies using either plasmapheresis or protein A adsorption combined with cyclophosphamide and corticosteroids to reduce antibody production. Intensive plasmapheresis can usually control the disease within two to three weeks, but additional treatment sessions are often needed to prevent rebounding titers. Cyclophosphamide therapy is usually tapered after three months and if anti-GBM antibodies no longer can be detected by ELISA, no further cytotoxic agents are necessary. Anti-GBM antibodies rarely reoccur after the first year, but ANCA-positive patients may experience clinical relapse in conjunction with rising ANCA levels.

References

1. Wieslander J, Bygren P, Heinegard D. Isolation of the specific glomerular basement membrane antigen involved in goodpasture syndrome. *Proc Natl Acad Sci USA* 1984; 81: 1544–1548.

2. Cui Z, Zhao MH, Xin G, Wang HY. Characteristics and prognosis of Chinese patients with anti-glomerular basement membrane disease. *Nephron Clin Pract* 2005; 99: c49–55.

3. Segelmark M, Hellmark T, Wicslander J. The prognostic significance in goodpasture's disease of specificity, titre and affinity of anti-glomerular-basement-membrane antibodies. *Nephron Clin Pract* 2003; 94: c59–c68.

4. Salama AD, Levy JB, Lightstone L, Pusey CD. Goodpasture's disease. *Lancet* 2001; 358: 917–920.

5. Stanton MC, Tange JD. Goodpasture's syndrome (pulmonary haemorrhage associated with glomerulonephritis. *Australas Ann Med* 1958; 7: 132–144.

6. Goodpasture EW. The significance of certain pulmonary lesions in relations in relation to the etiology of influenza. *Am J Med Sci* 1919; 158: 863–870.

7. Lerner RA, Glassock RJ, Dixon FJ. The role of anti-glomerular basement membrane antibody in the pathogenesis of human glomerulonephritis. *J Exp Med* 1967; 126: 989–1004.

8. Hellmark T, Johansson C, Wieslander J. Characterization of anti-GBM antibodies involved in goodpasture's syndrome. *Kidney Int* 1994; 46: 823–829.

9. Hellmark T, Segelmark M, Unger C, Burkhardt H, Saus J, Wieslander J. Identification of a clinically relevant immunodominant region of collagen IV in goodpasture disease. *Kidney Int* 1999; 55: 936–944.

10. Hudson BG, Tryggvason K, Sundaramoorthy M, Neilson EG. Alport's syndrome, goodpasture's syndrome, and type IV collagen. *N Engl J Med* 2003; 348: 2543–2556.

11. Hellmark T, Burkhardt H, Wieslander J, Goodpasture disease. Characterization of a single conformational epitope as the target of pathogenic autoantibodies. *J Biol Chem* 1999; 274: 25862–25868.

12. Borza DB, Bondar O, Colon S et al. Goodpasture autoantibodies unmask cryptic epitopes by selectively dissociating autoantigen complexes lacking structural reinforcement: novel mechanisms for immune privilege and autoimmune pathogenesis. *J Biol Chem* 2005; 280: 27147–27154.

13. Lou YH, Anti-GBM glomerulonephritis: a T cell-mediated autoimmune disease. *Arch Immunol Ther Exp (Warsz)* 2004; 52: 96–103.

14. Bolton WK, Chen L, Hellmark T, Wieslander J, Fox JW. Epitope spreading and autoimmune glomerulonephritis in rats induced by a T cell epitope of goodpasture's antigen. *J Am Soc Nephrol* 2005; 16: 2657–2666.

15. Sinico RA, Radice A, Corace C, Sabadini E, Bollini B. Anti-glomerular basement membrane antibodies in the diagnosis of goodpasture syndrome: a comparison of different assays. *Nephrol Dial Transplant* 2006; 21: 397–401.

16. Levy JB, Turner AN, Rees AJ, Pusey CD. Long-term outcome of anti-glomerular basement membrane antibody disease treated with plasma exchange and immunosuppression. *Ann Intern Med* 2001; 134: 1033–1042.

24
Kawasaki Disease

Jordi Anton and Rosa Bou

Abstract   Kawasaki disease is an acute systemic vasculitis of still unknown etiology. Diagnosis is based on clinical criteria that include fever, exanthema, conjunctivitis, changes in the extremities, erythema of oral mucosa and lips, and cervical lymphadenopathy. However, these criteria have low sensitivity and specificity and therefore, other clinical and laboratory features may be helpful in establishing the diagnosis, especially for cases of atypical or incomplete Kawasaki disease. Prognosis depends on the extent of cardiac involvement; coronary aneurysms develop in 20–25% of untreated patients, which may lead to myocardial infarction and sudden death. Treatment with high-dose intravenous immuno-globulin is effective in reducing the risk of coronary aneurysms in most cases, and together with aspirin, is the treatment of choice for initial Kawasaki disease.

Keywords   Child · fever · mucocutaneous lymph node syndrome · coronary aneurysm · intravenous immunoglobulins

Kawasaki disease (KD) is a systemic vasculitis that affects small and medium-sized vessels (1). It is an inflammatory process, self-limited, but potentially life threatening depending on the extent of cardiac involvement. The disease was first described by Tomisaku Kawasaki in 1967, in 50 children with a mucocutaneous lymph node syndrome, with high fever and a characteristic desquamation of fingers and toes (2).

Epidemiology

Even though KD is markedly more prevalent in Asian countries, it has a universal distribution and can be manifested in any race and ethnic group. It is a pediatric disease and in most of the series, 85% of patients are less than 5 years old; it is also more common in boys (male/female ratio 1.5–2.1/1).

Pathogenesis

The etiology of KD is still unknown, although clinical, laboratory, and epidemiological features suggest an infectious origin. However, many studies have failed to identify a unique infectious agent in KD. It has also not been proved to be related to exposure to any drug or as a response to a superantigen. On the contrary, activation of immune system is an evident characteristic of KD, and concentrations of many proinflammatory cytokines and chemokines are being studied in patients with KD, which may lead to improved anti-inflammatory therapy in the future. Finally, a reasonable open hypothesis is that KD is an inappropriate and exaggerated immune response to one or multiple environmental or infectious agents that elicits the disease in a genetically susceptible individual.

Clinical Manifestations

(Percentages of appearance enclosed in brackets) (3).

Fever (100%): The fever in KD is typically high spiking and remittent (in many cases >40°C). It is often resistant to antipyretics.

Changes in Extremities (93%): Erythema and edema of hands and feet, which is sometimes painful, is a frequent manifestation of KD at the onset of the disease, and for lasts 1–3 days. Desquamation of fingers and toes appears in the convalescence phase (2–3 weeks after onset of fever); therefore, it is useful only to confirm the diagnosis and not to decide when to start treatment. A subtle perineal desquamation may also be observed at the early stages of the disease. Approximately 1 or 2 months after the onset of fever, small transverse grooves across fingernails may appear (Beau's lines).

Exanthema (95%): The exanthema in KD is polymorphous and nonspecific. It is often an erythematous,

From: Y. Shoenfeld et al. (eds.): *Diagnostic Criteria in Autoimmune Diseases*, DOI: 10.1007/978-1-60327-285-8_24,
© 2008 Humana Press, Totowa, NJ

maculopapular rash, but occasionally other rashes such as scarlatiniform and micropustular, and erythroderma can also appear. It has not been described as bullous or vesicular eruption. It can be seen during the acute phase of illness, often during the first 5 days of fever. The exanthema is usually extensive, affecting predominantly the trunk, but it can also be limited to the perineal region.

Conjunctival Injection (90%): The conjunctivitis is bilateral, painless, and nonpurulent, affecting the bulbar conjunctiva (sparing the limbus). It usually begins shortly after the onset of fever and is transient (sometimes can only be seen on the first day during the acute phase of the illness). A mild acute iridocyclitis or anterior uveitis may also be noted by a slit lamp (4).

Changes in Lips and Oral Cavity (93%): The lips are dry and cracked, with hemorrhagic erythema; there is a characteristic strawberry tongue with prominent papilla, and a diffuse erythema of oropharyngeal mucosal surfaces. Ulcers and pharyngeal exudates are not suggestive of KD.

Lymphadenopathy (43%): It is usually unilateral and confined to the anterior cervical triangle. There has to be at least one adenopathy ≥1.5 cm in diameter (to fulfill diagnostic criteria), although multiple adjacent enlarged nodes may be detected using cervical ultrasound.

Other Clinical Findings: Clinical findings other than the classical diagnostic criteria are common in KD and may help us in diagnosis. Gastrointestinal manifestations including vomiting, diarrhea, and abdominal pain are present in approximately one-third of the patients. Gallbladder distention (hydrops) can also occur in KD (5); in some patients, liver enlargement and jaundice have also been reported.

Characteristically, patients with KD have marked irritability, to the point that only if it is not present, other diagnosis should be considered. This may reflect aseptic meningitis that is found in those KD patients who have had a lumbar puncture. Transient sensorineural hearing loss and facial paralysis are rarely present (6).

Arthritis and arthralgia may also be observed during the acute phase or convalescence, which affects both small and large joints. Induration and erythema at the site of a previous vaccination with Bacille Calmatte-Guérin has also been described (7).

Cardiac manifestations such as myocarditis and pericarditis occur during the acute phase of illness, whereas coronary aneurysms are formed in later stages.

Laboratory Findings

A specific laboratory test for the diagnosis of KD does not exist. However, some investigations can be performed to help with the diagnosis.

Conventional blood test may show leukocytosis and elevated acute-phase reactants—C reactive protein, erythrocyte sedimentation rate (frequently >100 mm/h)—

and normocytic normochromic anemia. Thrombocytosis typically develops in the second or third week of disease. Other findings include elevated liver enzymes, lipid profile alterations (decrease in cholesterol and high-density lipoprotein levels and increase in triglycerides) (8), hypoalbuminemia, hyponatremia, and more rarely hiperbilirrubinemia.

Urinalysis may reveal sterile pyuria, whereas the analysis of cerebrospinal fluid shows evidence of aseptic meningitis with pleocytosis; glucose and protein levels are normal.

Echocardiography

During the acute phase of illness, an echocardiographic evaluation may reveal signs of myocarditis with decreased ejection fraction, pericarditis, mitral regurgitation and perivascular brightness of the coronary wall. Coronary aneurysms generally appear during the convalescence phase (from second week). Ideally, echocardiography should be performed at least while diagnosis, at weeks 2 and between 6 and week 8 of illness (9).

Course of the Disease: The course of KD can be divided into three phases (10):

1. *Acute febrile phase (1st–2nd week)*: KD appears suddenly with high fever and irritability, and as the disease progresses other symptoms develop: adenitis, conjunctivitis, erythema and edema of hands and feet, and changes in oral mucosa. If untreated, these symptoms last for 12–15 days and then disappear. Common analytical findings in this stage are leucocytosis and increase in acute-phase reactants, with normal or slightly low hemoglobin and normal platelets.
2. *Subacute phase (3rd–6th week)*: Once the patient has been treated with immunoglobulin, fever disappears, symptoms return to normal and a typical periungal desquamation of finger and toes is usually seen. Laboratory tests may show marked thrombocytosis and anemia, with normalization of leukocytosis and acute-phase reactants. It is in this phase that coronary aneurysms develop.
3. *Convalescence phase*: Most patients are asymptomatic at this stage, although Beau lines may be observed in fingernails. Blood tests return to normal and coronary aneurysm could either disappear or not, and they may become symptomatic in the form of myocardial infarction.

Diagnostic Criteria

The diagnosis of KD is based on the presence of at least 5 days of fever, and ≥4 of the five principal clinical features (Table 24.1) (9).

TABLE 24.1. Diagnostic criteria for Kawasaki disease.

Fever of ≥5 days[a] and presence of ≥4 principal features[b]:
1. Changes in extremities:
    Acute phase: erythema of palms and soles, and edema of hands and feet
    Subacute phase: desquamation of fingers and toes.
2. Polymorphous exanthema
3. Bilateral bulbar conjunctival injection.
4. Changes in lips and oral mucosa: erythematous and cracked lips, strawberry tongue, and oral and pharyngeal hyperemia.
5. Cervical lymphadenopathy (>1.5 cm diameter).
Exclusion of other diseases with similar findings[c].

[a] Patients with at least 5 days of fever and <4 principal criteria can be diagnosed with KD when coronary artery abnormalities are detected.
[b] In the presence of ≥4 principal criteria, KD diagnosis can be made on day 4 of illness, or even before by experienced clinicians who have treated many KD.
[c] See Table 24.2.

Atypical/Incomplete KD

Regardless of how the diagnostic criteria are applied, they have both low sensitivity and specificity. Some patients with suspected KD do not fulfill the diagnostic criteria, and diagnosis is made based on coronary artery abnormalities. These cases would be the so-called "incomplete KD". The term "atypical KD" should be reserved for patients who have atypical symptoms that are not common in classical KD, such as renal impairment, acute surgical abdomen, and pleural effusion (9). Children under one year of age are more frequently affected with an incomplete form of KD and, therefore, it is important that a correct diagnosis be made and early treatment started in these patients, because in addition, they are at higher risk of developing coronary aneurysms than older children. In such cases, clinicians should pay attention to other clinical or laboratory findings not included in the diagnostic criteria that are useful in corroborating the diagnosis.

Differential Diagnosis

Because KD has unspecific symptoms that are similar to those of other diseases, a precise differential diagnosis is required to carry out an adequate treatment and not to underdiagnose or overdiagnose—especially in atypical and incomplete KD cases. Diseases with similar clinical features are listed in Table 24.2.

Treatment

Although the exact mechanism of action is not clear, effective therapy exists for most patients with acute KD. Treatment with aspirin and intravenous immunoglobulin (IVIG) are still current recommendations, which has

TABLE 24.2. Differential diagnosis of KD.

Infectious diseases	Adenovirus, measles, parvovirus, herpesvirus
	Scarlet fever
	Infectious mononucleosis
Immune reactions	Steven-Johnson syndrome
	Toxic shock syndrome
	Systemic onset juvenile idiopathic arthritis
Rheumatic diseases	Polyarteritis nodosa
	Systemic lupus erythematosus
	Rheumatic fever

been seen to reduce the risk of developing coronary aneurysm from 20–25% to less than 5% if administered within the first 10 days of illness (11, 12).

High-dose aspirin (80–100 mg/Kg daily divided in four doses) is used during the acute phase of illness for its anti-inflammatory and anti-pyretic effect, although more recent studies suggest that other less-toxic nonsteroidal anti-inflammatory agents or lower doses of aspirin would also be effective. Once the fever has disappeared in the 48–72 h period, aspirin is reduced to an anti-platelet dose (3–5 mg/Kg in a single daily dose) for six–eight weeks, and is then discontinued if platelet count and acute-phase reactants have returned to normal and there are no signs of coronary abnormalities in the echocardiography.

Treatment with IVIG should be administered early in the course of the disease, preferably within the first 10 days of illness (if possible between day 5 and 7). Recommended doses are 2 gr/kg in an 8–12 h infusion. In patients presenting after day 10 of illness, IVIG should only be administered in those having either persistent fever or aneurysms with signs of systemic inflammation (increased acute-phase reactants). Patients with persistent or recrudescent fever for 36 h or more after the IVIG infusion (10–20% of patients do not respond to a single dose) will require a second dose of IVIG (13).

For those still unresponsive, there are other optional therapies that have been effective in series of cases. Probably, the most accepted one would be to administer pulsed intravenous methylprednisolone (30 mg/Kg for 1–3 days). Other optional treatments include infliximab, cyclophosphamide, ulinastatin, and pentoxifiline (14).

References

1. Ozen S, Ruperto N, Dillon MJ, Bagga A, Barron K, Davin JC, et al. EULAR/PReS endorsed consensus criteria for the classification of childhood vasculitides. *Ann Rheum Dis* 2006; 65(7):936–941.
2. Kawasaki T. Acute febrile mucocutaneous syndrome with lymphoid involvement with specific desquamation of the fingers and toes in children [in Japanese]. *Arerugi.* 1967; 16:178.
3. Royle JA, Williams K, Elliott E, Sholler G, Nolan T, Allen R, et al. Kawasaki disease in Australia, 1993–95. *Arch Dis Child* 1998; 78(1):33–39.

4. Smith LB, Newburger JW, Burns JC. Kawasaki syndrome and the eye. *Pediatr Infect Dis J* 1989; 8(2):116–118.

5. Suddleson EA, Reid B, Woolley MM, Takahashi M. Hydrops of the gallbladder associated with Kawasaki syndrome. *J Pediatr Surg* 1987; 22(10):956–959.

6. Amano S, Hazama F. Neural involvement in Kawasaki disease. *Acta Pathol Jpn* 1980; 30(3):365–373.

7. Garcia PS, Staines BT, Hernandez B, V, Yamazaki Nakashimada MA. [Reactivation of the scar of BCG vaccination in Kawasaki's disease: clinical case and literature review]. *Rev Alerg Mex* 2006; 53(2):76–78.

8. Chiang AN, Hwang B, Shaw GC, Lee BC, Lu JH, Meng CC et al. Changes in plasma levels of lipids and lipoprotein composition in patients with Kawasaki disease. *Clin Chim Acta* 1997; 260(1):15–26.

9. Newburger JW, Takahashi M, Gerber MA, Gewitz MH, Tani LY, Burns JC, et al. Diagnosis, treatment, and long-term management of Kawasaki disease: a statement for health professionals from the Committee on Rheumatic Fever, Endocarditis, and Kawasaki Disease, Council on Cardiovascular Disease in the Young, American Heart Association. *Pediatrics* 2004; 114(6):1708–1733.

10. Saundel R, Petty R. Kawasaki disease. In: J Cassidy, R Petty, R Laxer, C Lindsley. *Textbook of Pediatric Rheumatology*. Elsevier Saunders; 2005, pp. 521–538.

11. Durongpisitkul K, Gururaj VJ, Park JM, Martin CF. The prevention of coronary artery aneurysm in Kawasaki disease: a meta-analysis on the efficacy of aspirin and immunoglobulin treatment. *Pediatrics* 1995; 96(6): 1057–1061.

12. Nagashima M, Matsushima M, Matsuoka H, Ogawa A, Okumura N. High-dose gammaglobulin therapy for Kawasaki disease. *J Pediatr* 1987; 110(5):710–712.

13. Wallace CA, French JW, Kahn SJ, Sherry DD. Initial intravenous gammaglobulin treatment failure in Kawasaki disease. *Pediatrics* 2000; 105(6):E78.

14. Newburger JW, Fulton DR. Kawasaki disease. *Curr Treat Options Cardiovasc Med* 2007; 9(2):148–158.

25
Cogan Syndrome

Aharon Kessel and Elias Toubi

Abstract   Typical Cogan syndrome (CS) includes ocular involvement that is primarily interstitial keratitis (IK) with audiovestibular involvement such as sudden onset of nausea, vomiting, tinnitus, vertigo along with progressive hearing loss. The time interval between ocular and audiovestibular involvement may be as long as 2 years. A typical CS type includes patients with classic relapsing pattern of autoimmune-type vestibuloauditory symptoms in addition to the presentation of other types of inflammatory eye disease, with or without IK. Another group includes patients with more than 2 years between the onset of the ophthalmogic symptoms and the audiovestibular manifestations. A third group includes patients with typical ocular manifestations associated, within 2 years, with audiovestibular symptoms different from Meniere-like episodes.

Keywords   Autoimmunity · progressive hearing loss · interstitial keratitis

Introduction

The earliest description of nonsyphilitic keratitis coexisting with vestibuloauditory disturbances was published by Morgan and Baumgarther in 1934 (1). In 1945, the ophthalmologist David G. Cogan described four patients with the same symptoms and classified this entity as "Cogan syndrome" (CS) (2). Fifteen years later, Cody and Williams called attention to the systemic manifestations of this syndrome (3). Some authors divide CS into typical and atypical varieties based on the type of ocular inflammation present (3, 4): typical CS manifests primarily with IK, whereas atypical CS may exhibit other inflammatory ocular involvement such as iritis, episcleritis in addition to or in place of IK. Atypical CS is usually associated with systemic inflammatory vascular disease and carries a less-favorable prognosis than typical CS (4).

Epidemiology

CS is a rare disease occurring primarily in young adults and with no apparent sexual predilection (4, 5). A recent review of 60 patients from the Mayo Clinic (Rochester, MN), who were followed from 1940 to 2002, indicated that the average age at onset of disease (defined as the point when both eye and ear findings were noted) was 38 years (range 9–70 years) (6).

Pathogenesis

Although the pathogenesis of CS remains obscure, autoimmune-mediated cellular or humoral processes have been postulated by many investigators. This opinion has been supported by the findings of antibodies against inner ear and corneal tissues along with the presence of a lymphocytic and plasma cell infiltrates in the cornea and the inner ear (7). In an elegant study, Lunardi et al. found that DEP-1/CD148 is a pathogenetically relevant autoantigen target in CS. It is a widespread cell-surface antigen that is expressed in endothelial cells and supporting cells within the sensorineural epithelia in the inner ear as well as in nerve and glial cells. In this regard, the injection of purified antibodies to DEP-1/CD148 into Balb/c mice resulted in hearing loss (8). Histological analysis of the inner ear showed degeneration of the sensory receptors and supporting structures of the cochlea and vestibular apparatus and demyelination and atrophy of the vestibular and cochlear branches of the eight cranial nerves (9). Several authors have noted an upper respiratory tract infection immediately preceding in 50% of cases of CS, suggesting an infectious origin. However, surveying for

From: Y. Shoenfeld et al. (eds.): *Diagnostic Criteria in Autoimmune Diseases*, DOI: 10.1007/978-1-60327-285-8_25,
© 2008 Humana Press, Totowa, NJ

infections is usually negative. The possible suspected infections include Chlamydia, *Mycoplasma pneumoniae*, Epstein–Barr virus, Herpes Simplex virus, Varicella-Zoster virus, Cytomegalovirus and influenza A and B. Thus, it has been suggested that CS can be triggered by vaccination and infection, which may lead in some cases to a hypersensitivity response with possible cross immunity to similar proteins in the tissues of the audiovestibular system, eye or other organs, as well as those associated with vasculitis (10). The connection of CS with vasculitis and the response to corticosteroids and immunosuppressive drugs also support an immune-mediated condition.

Clinical Findings

In the review by Gluth et al., the most common presenting symptoms present when first evaluated by a physician were sudden hearing loss in 50% of patients, balance disturbance in 40%, ocular irritation in 32%, photophobia in 23%, tinnitus in 13% and blurred vision in 10%. Interestingly, only 5% of the patients were initially presented with both vestibuloauditory and ophthalmologic symptoms. In this series, 47% of patients presented initially with only vestibuloauditory signs and 33% had only ophthalmologic symptoms. Seven percent of patients were initially presented with constitutional symptoms including myalgia, arthralgia, headache, rash and fever. In most patients (85%), both vestibuloauditory and ophthalmologic symptoms developed in less than 2 years (6).

Ophthalmic Manifestations

The typical presentation of CS is, in most cases, the occurrence of bilateral IK (6, 11). IK tend to appear in close proximity to episodes of audiovestibular dysfunction. IK is rarely asymptomatic, and most of the patients are clinically manifested by intense photophobia, lacrimation, eye pain and disturbances in visual acuity. On examination of patients with IK, early typical findings include subepithelial peripheral corneal stromal infiltrate. Consequently, secondary neovasclarization may frequently ensue. In most cases, both eyes are affected during the disease course, with great variability in symptoms from one eye to the other, and from day to day. The ocular manifestations may have a relapsing course with periodic attacks occurring during the years. Patients were designated as having atypical CS if another significant inflammatory eye lesion in addition to, or rather than, IK was present (Table 25.1). In the atypical CS group, the ocular manifestation also tends to appear in both eyes (11).

A moderate and usually transient decrease in visual acuity is not infrequent in CS, but amaurosis or blindness may also occur.

TABLE 25.1. Ocular manifestations of Cogan syndrome.

Typical	Atypical
Interstitial keratitis	Scleritis/episcleritis
Subepithelial peripheral corneal stromal infiltrates	Retinal artery occlusion
	Choroiditis
	Retinal hemorrhage/vasculitis
	Papillitis
	Isolated conjuctivitis[a]
	Isolated subconjunctival haemorrhage[a]
	Isolated iritis[a]
	Uveitis

[a] Only if it is associated with Meniere-like episodes within an interval of 2 years.

Audiovestibular Manifestations

In both typical and atypical CS, the classical audiovestibular presentation is sudden onset of nausea, vomiting, tinnitus, vertigo and hearing loss, which is usually bilateral (4). Hearing loss may initially fluctuate with repeated attacks but generally develops progresses to irreversible bilateral deafness in 52–85% of patients (6, 12). In their review, Gluth et al. (6) reported that the most common otolaryngologic symptoms that appeared in their patients during the disease course included hearing loss (100%), vertigo (90%), tinnitus (80%), ataxia (53%) and oscillopsia (25%). Vestibular function tests such as bilateral absence vestibular responses to caloric testing and bilateral weak vestibular responses to caloric testing were abnormal in most patients. Additionally, physical examination revealed spontaneous and/or gaze-induced nystagmus at some point of their disease in 20% of the patients. Usually the hearing loss in CS is classified as sensorineural, preferentially affecting medium to high frequencies, although a mechanical component has also been reported (13). These manifestations, along with the visual symptoms, usually occur either concurrently or sequentially within a few weeks to months. Rarely, years may separate the appearance of visual and audiovestibular manifestations (12).

Systemic Manifestations

General constitutional symptoms such as, headache, arthralgia, fever, weight loss, fatigue, arthritis and myalgia are common among the patients (5, 6). Systemic manifestations occur in 50–75% of patients. Respiratory symptoms include dyspnea, hemoptysis and pleuritic chest pain. Gastrointestinal manifestations include nausea, vomiting and diarrhea (6). Neurologic symptoms of CS are present in approximately 50% of cases and include headaches, psychosis, coma, convulsion, neuropathy and stroke (14). The two most serious systemic complications are vasculitis and cardiovascular involvement. The prevalence of vasculitis in CS patients is reported to be 12–15% (5, 6, 15). Vasculitis can involve all layers of different sized vessels. Clinically, vasculitis has been documented in the skin, kidneys, subcutaneous nodules, coronary and cerebral arteries and muscles (15). Cardiovascular involvement is present in 10% of CS patients (4, 5). The most characteristic cardiovascular manifestation of CS is aortitis with aortic insufficiency. Other manifestations include, aortic dilatation, aortic valvular insufficiency, congestive heart failure, pericarditis, arrhythmias and silent coronary artery disease (16). The comparison of the distribution of clinical features between cases of typical CS and atypical CS shows that patients having atypical CS present significantly more frequent musculoskeletal and neurological manifestations and lymphadenopathy (11). Additionally, atypical CS has also been reported to be associated with other systemic diseases such as sarcoidosis, rheumatoid arthritis, juvenile idiopathic arthritis, Sjogren syndrome, Crohn disease, ulcerative colitis and Wagener's granulomatosis (11).

Laboratory and Radiological Data

Laboratory abnormalities have been found in CS patients but none are diagnostic. They include an elevated erythrocyte sedimentation rate (ESR), leukocytosis with neutrophilia, anemia and thrombocytosis (6). Non-specific markers of inflammation such as C-reactive protein and high levels of gamma globulin have also been found. Low titers of rheumatoid factor, antinuclear antibodies and cryoglobulins were detected in a few patients (5). By definition, serological tests for syphilis are negative. Antibodies against the inner ear and cornea may support the clinical suspicion but are not consistently detected in CS or correlate with disease activity. Results of computed tomography (CT) and magnetic resonance imaging (MRI) have been reported in CS patient evaluation. Some authors reported that in CT and MRI there was evidence of narrowing or obliteration of parts of the vestibular labyrinth that are related to the risk of permanent hearing loss (13, 17). However, in the review by Gluth et al., CT (14 patients) and MRI (20 patients) of the head were normal or nondiagnostic in all cases (6).

Treatment

Glucocorticosteroids are the primary treatment for CS. Ocular manifestations in CS typically respond well to topical corticosteroids and cycloplegics, such as atropine eye drops. Recently, topical cyclosporin A was used successfully in the treatment of severe anterior segment inflammation (18). Systemic treatment is indicated for severe or resistant eye involvement. At the onset of audiovestibular dysfunction, rapid initiation of high-dose corticosteroids (1–1.5 mg/kg

of prednisone daily) is recommended. If there is no response after 2 weeks, the steroids are rapidly tapered (5). Many reports have documented resolution of the hearing loss with a similar regimen but no controlled studies have been performed (4, 5). If hearing improves, steroids are tapered slowly and continued for 2–6 months. In a 5-year follow-up, 95% of the untreated patients had permanent hearing loss. About 55% of the patients treated with systemic steroids within 2 weeks of initial hearing loss experienced hearing improvement, compared with only 8% of patients who were treated after 2 weeks (4). Vasculitis and other prominent systemic complications of CS usually respond well to systemic corticosteroids. For severe unresponsive vasculitis, immunosuppressive drugs such as cyclosporin A (0.5–2 mg/kg/day) or cyclophosphamide (1.5–2.0 mg/kg/day) in conjunction with prednisone have been used successfully (19). Good response to treatment with methotrexate has also been reported in a few cases (11). Recent reports suggested that, in cases of relapse despite therapy with corticosteroids and immunosuppressive agents, treatment with anti-TNF-α should be started (20). Patients with profound hearing loss after unsuccessful treatment with anti-inflammatory drugs are candidates for cochlear implantation.

Diagnostic Criteria

The diagnosis of CS is mainly based on clinical issues. Unlike other systemic collagen or autoimmune diseases, it is not associated with a specific autoantibody. The laboratory profile (elevated ESR and leukocytosis) of the disease is a reflection of the extent of the inflammation and cytokine cascade and therefore no laboratory or radiographic test is diagnostic of CS. Hence, the diagnosis of CS is based on clinical findings of both ocular and audiovestibular abnormalities in the setting of a negative laboratory work-up for syphilis or other immune-mediated disease. When a patient presents without IK or the audiovestibular symptoms are not present concomitantly, the diagnosis of CS becomes highly questionable. The differential diagnosis of CS should include diseases causing an IK, audiovestibular diseases associated with eye findings and systemic diseases that include ocular and ear manifestations (Table 25.2). The other difficulty in gathering diagnostic criteria arises from the low incidence of reported cases of the disease. Until now, approximately 250 cases have been reported in the English literature. It can be assumed that the true frequency is higher. In summary, typical CS-type criteria should include ocular involvement that is primarily IK with audiovestibular involvement which is similar to Meniere disease (sudden onset of nausea, vomiting, tinnitus and vertigo) along with progressive hearing loss. The time interval between ocular and audiovestibular involvement may be as long as 2 years.

TABLE 25.2 Differential diagnosis of Cogan syndrome.

Infectious
    Congenital and acquired syphilis
    Chlamydial infections
    Mumps
    Herpes Zoster
    Rubeola
Immune-mediated diseases
    Polyarthritis nodosa
    Wegener granulomatosis
    Rheumatoid arthritis
    Relapsing polychondritis
    Temporal arteritis
    Sjogren's syndrome
    Behçet's syndrome
    Sacroidosis
    Systemic lupus erythematosis
Others
    Vogt-Koyanagi-Harada syndrome
    Susac syndrome

Atypical CS type can be diagnosed in three groups of patients. The first group includes patients with classic relapsing pattern of autoimmune-type vestibuloauditory symptoms in addition to the presentation of other types of inflammatory eye disease, with or without IK (Table 25.1). The second group includes patients with more than 2 years between the onset of the ophthalmogic symptoms and the audiovestibular manifestations. The third group includes patients with typical ocular manifestations associated, within 2 years, with audiovestibular symptoms different from Meniere-like episodes.

It seems important that primary physicians should suspect, as early as possible, the diagnosis of CS. These patients could benefit from early referral to specialized centers, where early initiation of immunosuppressive drugs could prevent permanent hearing loss and the need for cochlear implants.

References

1. Morgan RF, Baumgartner CJ. Menier's disease complicated by recurrent interstitial keratitis: Excellent result following cervical ganglionectomy. *West J Surg* 1934; 42: 628.
2. Cogan DS. Syndrome of nonsyphilitic interstitial keratitis and vestibuloauditory Symptoms. *Arch Ophthalmol* 1945; 33: 144–9.
3. Cody DTR, Williams HL. Cogan's syndrome. *Laryngoscope* 1960; 70: 477.
4. Haynes BF, Kaiser-Kupfer MI, Mason P, Fauci AS. Cogan syndrome: studies in Thirteen patients, long-term follow-up, and a review of the literature. *Medicine* 1980; 59: 426–41.
5. Vollertsen RS, Mcdonald TJ, Younge BR, Banks PM, Stanson AW, Ilstrup DM. Cogan's syndrome: 18 cases and a review of the literature. *Mayo Clin Proc* 1986; 61: 344–61.
6. Gluth MB, Baratz KH, Matteson EL, Driscoll CLW. Cogan syndrome: a retrospective review of 60 patients throughout a half century. *Mayo Clin Proc* 2006; 81(4): 483–8.
7. Arnold W, Gebbers JO. Serum antibodies against corneal and internal ear tissues in Cogan's syndrome. *Laryngol Rhinol Otol* 1984; 63: 428–32.
8. Lunardi C, Bason C, Leandri M et al. Autoantibodies to innear ear and endothelial antigens in cogan's syndrome. *Lancet* 2002; 360: 915–21.
9. Clair EWS, McCallum RM. Cogan's syndrome. *Curr Opin Rheumatol* 1999; 60: 69–71.
10. Berrocal GJR, Vargas JA, Vaquero M, Ramony Cajal S, Ramirez-Camacho RA. Cogan's syndrome: An oculo-audiovestibular disease. *Postgrad Med J* 1999; 75: 262–4.
11. Grasland A, Pouchot J, Hachulla E, et al. Typical and atypical cogan's syndrome: 32 cases and review of the literature. *Rheumatology* 2004; 43: 1007–15.
12. McDonald TJ, Vollertsen RS, Younger BR. Cogan's syndrome: audiovestibular Involvement and prognosis in 18 patients. *Laryngoscope* 1985; 95: 650–4.
13. Majoor MHJM, Albers FWJ. Casselman JW. Clinical relevance of magnetic resonance imaging and computed tomography in cogan's syndrome. *Acta Otolaryngol* 1993; 113: 625–31.
14. Bicknell JM, Holland JV. Neurologic manifestations of Cogan syndrome. *Neurology* 1978; 28: 278–81.
15. Vollertsen RS. Vasculitis and Cogan's syndrome. *Rheum Dis Clin North Am* 1990; 16: 433–8.
16. Livingston JZ, Casale AS, Hutchins GM, Shapiro EP. Coronary involvement in cogan's syndrome. *Am Heart J* 1992; 123(2): 528–30.
17. Casselman JW, Majoor MHJM, Albers FW. MR of the inner ear in patients with cogan syndrome. *Am J Neuroradiol* 1994; 15: 131–8.
18. Shimura M, Yasuda K, Fuse N, Nakazawa M, Tamai M. Effective treatment with topical cyclosporin A of a patient with cogan syndrome. *Ophthalmologica* 2000; 214: 429–32.
19. Allen NB, Cox C, Cobo M, et al. Use of immunosuppressive agents in the treatment of severe ocular and vascular manifestations of cogan's syndrome. *Am J Med* 1990; 88: 296–301.
20. Fricker M, Baumann A, Wermelinger F, Villiger PM, Helbling A. A novel therapeutic option in cogan disease? TNF-α blockers. *Rheumatol Int* 2007; 27: 493–5.

26
Henoch-Shoenlein Purpura

Margalit Lorber

Abstract   Henoch-Shoenlein Purpura (HSP) is a multisystem disorder of unknown etiology affecting predominantly the skin, joints, gastrointestinal tract, and the kidneys but other organs can be affected as well. It is one of the most common causes of vasculitic disorders in children. No specific autoantibodies have been detected in HSP, but the presence of IgA depositions in both skin and kidney biopsies and the presence of IgA-containing circulating immune complexes support the immunological pathogenesis. The natural history of the disease is cure in most cases, although recurrence and end-stage kidney disease are described. The treatment consists of corticosteroids and immunosuppressive drugs.

Keywords   IgA · vasculitis · kidney

Henoch-Shoenlein Purpura (HSP) is a multisystem disorder affecting predominantly the skin, joints, gastrointestinal tract and the kidneys but other organs can be affected as well. It is one of the most common causes of vasculitic disorders in children (1, 2).

This is a variant of acute leukocytoclastic vasculitis of the immunoglobulin A (IgA)–mediated type. This disorder is characterized by a purpuric rash occurring on the lower region of the legs. The rash varies from macular-papular to vesiculobullous with ulceration. Systemic symptoms are arthritis, abdominal pain, gastrointestinal bleeding, hematuria, and cardiac and neurological changes.

Epidemiology

The annual incidence is 13.5–18/100,000 children (3, 4). Although this condition can affect any person from 6 months to adulthood, 50% of cases occur in children under 5 years of age and 75% in children under 10 years. Boys are affected more than girls in a 1.5–2:1 ratio. In the northern countries HSP occurs mainly between November and January (5). In one-half to two-thirds of children, an upper respiratory tract infection precedes the clinical onset of HSP by 1–3 weeks. Caucasians are more affected than non-Caucasians.

History

William and Heberden were the first to note Henoch-Schoenlein (or Henoch-Schonlein) purpura (HSP) in the early 1800s. However, Schonlein first described the combination of acute purpura and arthritis in children in 1837, and Henoch reported the manifestations of abdominal pain and nephritis in 1874.

Pathogenesis

The etiology of HSP remains unknown. However, IgA clearly plays a critical role in the immunopathogenesis of HSP, as evidenced by increased serum IgA concentrations, IgA-containing circulating immune complexes, and IgA deposition in vessel walls and renal mesangium. HSP is almost exclusively associated with abnormalities involving IgA1, rather than IgA2. The predominance of IgA1 in HSP may be the consequence of abnormal glycosylation of O-linked oligosaccharides unique to the hinge region of IgA1 molecules (6, 7). IgA aggregates or complexes with complement deposited in target organs, resulting in elaboration of inflammatory mediators, including vascular prostaglandins such as prostacyclin, which may play a central role in the pathogenesis of HSP vasculitis.

From: Y. Shoenfeld et al. (eds.): *Diagnostic Criteria in Autoimmune Diseases*, DOI: 10.1007/978-1-60327-285-8_26,
© 2008 Humana Press, Totowa, NJ

A subpopulation of human lymphocytes bears surface Fc and/or C3 receptors (complement receptor lymphocytes), which can bind circulating immune complexes or C3 generated by activation of the alternative complement pathway. Such immune complexes appear in HSP and may be part of the pathogenetic mechanism. Some have speculated that an antigen stimulates the production of IgA, which, in turn, causes the vasculitis. Allergens, such as foods, horse serum, insect bites, exposure to cold, and drugs such as ampicillin, erythromycin, penicillin, quinidine, and quinine may precipitate HSP. Infectious causes include bacteria such as Haemophilus, Parainfluenzae, Mycoplasma, Legionella, Yersinia, Shigella, or Salmonella and viruses such as adenoviruses, Epstein-Barr virus, parvovirus B19, and varicella which may precipitate HSP as well.

Vaccines such as those against cholera, measles, paratyphoid A and B, typhoid, and yellow fever have also been implicated (8).

Clinical Manifestations

The signs and symptoms are listed in Table 26.1.

Palpable purpura usually occurs first on the lower limbs and then spreads to the buttocks. Purpura is usually most prominent over the buttocks, the posterior aspects of the lower legs, and the elbows. Scalp edema can occur. Hemorrhagic vesicles and bullae are rare. In most patients, skin lesions are the first sign of HSP. Hives, angioedema, and target lesions can also occur. Vesicular eruptions and swelling and tenderness of an entire limb have been noted. Erythema multiforme–like lesions can be present.

The most serious complication of HSP is **renal involvement**, which occurs in 50% of older children but is serious in only approximately 10% of patients. In 80% of patients, renal involvement becomes apparent within the first 4 weeks of illness. The main kidney histopathological abnormalities of HSP-renal disease and IgA nephropathy are summarized in Table 26.2. The common and different clinical aspects of HSP-renal disease and IgA nephropathy are listed in Table 26.3.

Abdominal pain and bloody diarrhea may precede the typical purpuric rash of HSP in 14–36% of patients, complicating the initial diagnosis and even resulting in unnecessary laparotomy. Gastrointestinal (GI) manifestations occur in approximately 50% of cases and usually consist of

TABLE 26.1. Symptoms and signs of HSP at presentation.

	Prevalence
Purpura	90%
Hematuria, proteinuria	50%
Abdominal pain	75%
Arthralgia/arthritis	60–85%

TABLE 26.2. Renal Histopathology in HSP and IgA nephropathy

	HSP	IgA nephropathy
Sclerosis	3%	35%
Mesangial sclerosis	6%	42%
Endothelial proliferation	65%	30%
Thin basement-membrane nephropathy	6%	0%
Electronically dense deposits	Sparse, loose, widely spread in glomerular mesangium subendothelial area, intrabasement membranes	Dense, lumpy limited in mesangium, paramesangium
IgG glomerular deposits	72%	20%
Linear IgG deposits in the glomerular capillary wall	6%	0%
IgA and immunoglobulin M (IgM) and/or C3 deposit		
Capillary wall staining for IgA	70%	43%

TABLE 26.3. HSP and IgA nephropathy.

	HSP	IgA nephropathy
Extrarenal manifestation	Common	Rare
IgA nephropathy	+	+
Both occur in the same family	+	+
Same prevalence in certain geographical areas	+	+
Changes in IgA (9)	+	+
Age at onset >12y (10,11)	10%	26%
Abdominal pain	60%	3%
Purpura	90%	0
Arthralgia	50%	0
Renal pathology (Table 3)	+	+
Long-term remission	73%	20%
Urinary podocytes excretion (12)	+	+

colicky abdominal pain, melena, or bloody diarrhea. Hematemesis occurs less frequently. Intussusception should be suspected in HSP patients with abdominal pain and/or melena. Barium enema is frequently therapeutic.

Arthralgias occur in 60–85% of patients with HSP. The pain most commonly affects the knees and ankles and less frequently the wrists and fingers. Arthritis is very rare. HSP leaves no permanent joint deformities. Less frequent manifestations occur in other organs, mostly by vasculitis. Cardiac manifestations: vasculitis involving the myocardium, pulmonary manifestations: pulmonary hemorrhage or severe bilateral pulmonary hemorrhage, urinary manifestations: stenosing uteritis, priapism, penile edema, or orchitis. Central nerve system (CNS) involvement: vasculitis involving the CNS and intracranial hemorrhage.

Eye manifestations: Bilateral subperiosteal orbital hematomas have been noted. Adrenal hematomas have occurred. In rare patients, acute pancreatitis is the sole presenting feature of HSP (13).

Serological Features

There is no immunoserological marker in HSP. Elevated levels of serum IgA and IgA-containing circulating immune complexes are frequently detected in HSP. IgA1 in the circulation and glomerular deposits of patients with IgA nephropathy (IgAN) and children with HSP is aberrantly glycosylated; the hinge-region O-linked glycans are galactose deficient (6). The neoepitopes on IgA1 responsible for the formation of pathogenic immune complexes were recently identified. These studies may lead to the development of non-invasive diagnostic assays and future disease-specific therapy (7). Serum levels of IgA anticardiolipin antibody (aCL) are elevated in the initial active stage of adult HSP, suggesting that the IgA aCL may play some role in the onset of adult HSP (14).

Diagnostic Criteria

The former criteria for the diagnosis of HSP are the American College of Rheumatology 1990 criteria (15). The four criteria, of which two are necessary to make the diagnosis, were: age <20 years at onset, palpable purpura, "bowel angina"—diffuse abdominal pain or bowel ischemia usually with bloody diarrhea, and biopsy evidence of granulocytes in the walls of the arterioles or venules. The new (revised) criteria, from 2006 are listed in Table 26.4.

Prognosis

HSP is fatal only in the rarest of cases. Initial attacks of HSP can last several months, and relapses are possible. Kidney damage related to HSP is the primary cause of morbidity and mortality. Patients with no renal symptoms at onset have a good outcome at adulthood. Overall, an estimated 2% of cases of HSP progress to renal failure; as many as 20% of children who have HSPN and are treated in specialized centers require hemodialysis. The renal prognosis appears to be worse in adults than in children. Women during pregnancy have a high rate of complications, such as hypertension, proteinuria, or both (17).

Therapy

Several modes of treatment have been used. Currently, no widely accepted treatment protocols exist for patients with significant renal involvement. Corticosteroids (CS) are still the drug of choice, either as intravenous pulse methylprednisolone or oral prednisone.

Cyclosporin A has been described as an optional therapy in combination with CS. The results show effectiveness in both reducing proteinuria and improving the histological grade. The histological grade of the International Study of Kidney Disease in Children (ISKDC) was improved in all patients who received a follow-up kidney biopsy (18). Azathioprine with CS is an effective combination which shows reduction in proteinuria and serum creatinine and improvement in creatinine clearance in a high percentage of the treated children in a long-term follow-up (19). Tonsillectomy combined with steroid therapy was described by few groups as a therapeutic modality for children with HSP, in combination with CS. Tonsillectomy was performed after 1–4 cycles of methylpredisolone during oral CS. In all patients, proteinuria disappeared without any case of recurrence of both HSP and HSP nephritis. Early tonsillectomy was correlated with better outcome.

Treatment of children with HSP nephritis associated with nephritic-range proteinuria and significant histopathological changes on biopsy, including crescentic nephritis with high-dose corticosteroids plus oral cyclophosphamide is effective, safe, and significantly reduces proteinuria.

TABLE 26.4. Diagnostic criteria for Henoch-Schoenlein purpura (16).

The diagnosis is made when palpable purpura is present (mandatory criteria) in addition to at least one of the following four criteria
1. Diffuse abdominal pain
2. Any biopsy showing predominant IgA deposition
3. Arthritis[a] or arthralgia
4. Renal involvement (any hematuria and/or proteinuria)

[a]Acute, any joint

References

1. Cassidy JT, Petty RE. Vasculitis. In: Text book of Pediatric Rheumatology, 3rd ed. Philadelphia, Wb Saunders Company 1995; pp. 365–422.
2. Allen DM, Diamond LK, Howell DA. Anaphylactoid purpura in children (Schoenlein-Henoch syndrome): review with follow-up of renal complications. *Am J Dis Child* 1960; 99: 833–54.
3. Stewart M, Savage JM, Bell B, McCord B. Long term renal prognosis of Henoch-Shoenleine purpura in an unselected childhood population. *Eur J Pediatr* 1988; 147: 113–15.
4. Neilsen HE. Epidemiology of Henoch-Schoenlein purpura. *Acta Paediatr Scand* 1988; 77: 125–31.
5. Robson WLM, Leung AKC. Henoch-Schoenlein purpura. *Adv Pediatr* 1994; 41: 163–94.

6. Lau KK, Wyatt RJ, Moldovenau Z, Tomana M, Julian BA, Hogg RJ, Lee JY, Huang WQ, Mestecky J, Novak J. Serum levels of galactose-deficient IgA in children with IgA nephropathy and Henoch-Schonlein purpura. *Pediatr Nephrol* 2007; 22(12): 2067–72.

7. Novak J, Moldoveanau Z, Renfrow MB, Yanagihara T, Suzuki H, Raska M, Hall S, Brown R, Huang WQ, Goepfert A, Kilian M, Poulsen K, Tomana M, Wyatt RJ, Julian BA, Mestecky J. IgA nephropathy and Henoch-Schoenlein purpura nephritis: aberrant glycosylation of IaA1, formation of IgA1-containing immune complexes, and activation of mesangial cells. *Contrib Nephrol* 2007; 157: 134–8.

8. Lane SE, Watts R, Scott DG. Epidemiology of systemic vasculitis. *Curr Rheumatol Rep* 2005; 7(4): 270–5.

9. Coppo R, Basolo B, Piccoli G, Mazzucco G, Bulzomi MR, Roccatello D, De Marchi M, Carbonara AO, Barbiano di Belgiojoso G. IgA1 and IgA2 immune complexes in primary IgA nephropathy and Henoch-Schonlein nephritis. *Clin Exp Immunol* 1984, Sep; 57(3): 583–90.

10. Li YT, Lv JC, Li GT, Jiang L, Song YH, Zhang H. Comparative analysis of clinicopathological findings and outcome of Henoch-Schonlein nephritis and IgA nephropathy in adults. *Beijing Da Xue Xue Bao* 2007; 39(5): 458–61.

11. Zhou JH, Huang AX, Liu TL, Kuang YJ. A clinico-pathological study comparing Henoch-Schonlein purpura nephritis with IgA nephropathy in children. *Zhonghua Er Ke Za Zhi* 2003, Nov; 41(11): 808–12.

12. Hara M, Yanagihara T, Kihara I. Cumulative excretion of urinary podocytes reflects disease progression in IgA nephropathy and Schonlein-Henoch purpura nephritis. Biochemical features: *Clin J Am Soc Nephrol* 2007; 2(2): 231–8.

13. Carlson JA, Chen KR. Cutaneous vasculitis update: small vessel neutrophilic vasculitis syndromes. *Am J Dermatopathol* 2006; 28(6): 486–506.

14. Kawakami T. Vasculitis from the dermatological point of view. *Nihon Rinsho Meneki Gakkai Kaishi* 2007; 30(3): 156–64.

15. Mills JA, Michel BA, Bloch DA, Calabrse LH, Hunder GG, Arend WP, et al. The American College of Rheumatology 1990 criteria for the classification of Henoch-Schonlein purpura. *Arthritis Rheum* 1990; 33: 1114–21.

16. Ozen S, Ruperto N, Dillon MJ, Bagga A, Barron K, Davin JC, Kawasaki T, Lindsley C, Petty RE, Prieur A, Ravelli A, Woo P. EULAR/PReS endorsed consensus criteria* for the classification of childhood vasculitides. *Ann Rheum Dis* 2006; 65: 936–41.

17. Ronkainen J, Nuutinen M, Koskimies O. The adult kidney 24 years after childhood Henoch-Schonlein purpura: a retrospective cohort study. *Lancet* 2002; 360(9334): 666–70.

18. Shin JI, Park JM, Shin YH, Kim JH, Lee JS, Jeong HJ. Henoch-Schonlein purpura nephritis with nephritic-range poteinuria: histological regression possibly associated with cyclosporine A and steroid treatment. *Scand J Rheumatol* 2005; 34(5): 392–5.

19. Shin JI, Park JM, Shin YH, Kim JH, Lee JS, Kim PK, Jeong HJ. Can azathioprine and steroids alter the progression of severe Henoch-Schonlein nephritis in children? *Pediatr Nephrol* 2005; 20(8): 1087–92.

27
Cryoglobulinemic Syndrome

Suk Seo and Natalie Julia Török

Abstract   Cryoglobulinemia (CG) is a systemic inflammatory syndrome that generally involves small to medium vessel vasculitis because of cryoglobulin-containing immune complexes. It is now recognized that the majority of clinically significant CG have concurrent chronic hepatitis C virus (HCV) infection. Ineffective immune response to HCV has been hypothesized as a culprit. Clinical course of CG, however, is protean, and successful treatment of HCV does not guarantee resolution of CG. The role of HCV in the pathogenesis of CG and basis for its current treatment practice are discussed here.

Keywords   Cryoglobulinemia · cryoglobulin · chronic hepatitis C

Background/Historical Note

Cryoglobulins are a mixture of immunoglobulins and complement components that precipitate at temperature lower than 37C°. Cryoglobulinemia (CG) literally means the presence of cryoglobulins in a patient's serum, but it is a term often used to refer to a clinically apparent systemic inflammatory syndrome that generally involves small to medium vessel vasculitis secondary to cryoglobulin-containing immune complexes.

Before the identification of the hepatitis C virus (HCV) in 1989, CG was largely termed "essential" in patients who did not have associated lymphoproliferative or autoimmune diseases. It is now recognized that up to 90% of patients with clinically evident CG have chronic HCV infection. Therefore, anti-HCV treatment options offer a chance for causal therapy of the majority of patients with CG. In this chapter, we describe the current diagnostic approaches based on the classification of CG and a brief summary of the treatment options.

Diagnostic Criteria

Classification and Pathomechanism

Although the phenomenon of cryoprecipitation and associated hyperviscosity was described in the 1930s, the association of CG with so-called Meltzer's triad (palpable purpura, arthralgia, and myalgia) was not described until the 1960 s (1, 2).

In 1974, Brouet et al. devised the current system of classification of the three types of CG based upon its immunochemical composition and reported frequency of each type (Table 27.1) (3). Because of the biochemical basis for Brouet's classification, it is not surprising that the pathogenicity and clinical findings generally correlate with its corresponding types.

Type I GC is caused by hypersecretion of monoclonal antibodies (IgG or IgM, and much less likely IgA and free light chains) because of underlying lymphoproliferative disorders such as multiple myeloma, Waldenstrom's macroblobulinemia, or chronic lymphocytic leukemia. The hypersecretion leads to clinical symptoms and signs related to hyperviscosity, by aggregating to form immune complexes and precipitating in vivo depending upon antibody-specific conditions of temperature, pH, CG concentration, and weak noncovalent factors.

Unlike the type I GC, the type II and III (mixed) CG have rheumatoid factor-binding activity differentiated by its clonality (the type II with the monoclonal Ig with RF activity and the type III with the polyclonal Ig with RF

TABLE 27.1. Brouet classification for cryoglobulinemia (1).

Type	Prevalence (%)	Immunoglobulins
I	25	Monoclonal IgM, Monoclonal IgG
II	25	Monoclonal IgM
III	50	Polyclonal IgM

From: Y. Shoenfeld et al. (eds.): *Diagnostic Criteria in Autoimmune Diseases*, DOI: 10.1007/978-1-60327-285-8_27,

activity). Most cases of type II CG are associated with chronic HCV infection. Although the type III CG is sometimes seen in chronic autoimmune disorders as well as hematological malignancies, the majority of the type III CG patients also have chronic HCV infection.

In CG patients with HCV, anti-HCV antibody and HCV RNA are found in high concentrations in the cryoprecipitate, as well as the vessel walls of affected organ. It is now known that HCV proteins are important in the different steps of the pathogenesis. HCV core protein is a ligand for IgM/IgG complex and serves as a binding site for the vascular endothelium through the globular domain of the C1q receptor. This interaction, in turn, activates the complement cascade, with complement fragments (C3a, C5a) acting as chemotactic mediators (4). Furthermore, the HCV core protein has also shown to inhibit suppressor T-cell proliferative responses (5). Therefore, the potential mechanism for CG development could be that the HCV core in the cryoglobulin complex may inhibit the suppression of B-cell clones that produce RF autoantibodies, which causes further progression of CG production.

Rarely, CG is also seen in some patients with Epstein–Barr virus and human immunodeficiency virus (HIV) and human T-cell lymphotropic virus-1 (HTLV-1), as well as chronic systemic infections secondary to bacteria or fungi. In such cases, how cryoglobulins are produced and which antigen triggers this process is still largely speculative. Increased prevalence of the mixed-type CG is also reported in patients with chronic liver diseases of non-HCV-related etiologies (6). The association of CG with chronic hepatitis B virus (HBV) infection in particular has been disputed as the prevalence of cryoglobulins in HBV-infected patients is similar to that in other chronic liver diseases (6).

At the present time, there is no clear consensus on the diagnostic criteria of the CG syndrome. Correct diagnosis and management requires a careful consideration of combined clinical, laboratory, and pathological data.

Clinical Presentation

Majority of patients with detectable type I GC are asymptomatic with only rare history suggestive of Raynaud's phenomenon, digital ischemia, livedo reticularis, and palpable purpura that usually occur on the lower extremities. However, the classic description of type I GC is related to the hyperviscosity resulting in focal thrombotic events, such as gangrene and catastrophic cardiovascular, pulmonary, renal, or neurological events.

Although most CG patients have HCV (therefore would have type II or III CG), HCV-infected patients develop CG in 30–50% of cases (7). Among these, only 2–15% of cryoglobulin-positive patients develop symptoms attributed to it, with cutaneous manifestation seen in nearly all patients with GC syndromes (7). Indeed, as in type 1, the cutaneous

TABLE 27.2. Frequency of clinical and serologic features of essential mixed cryoglobulinemia associated with hepatitis C virus infection (8).

Fatigue	100%	Peripheral neuropathy	50%
Monoclonal rheumatoid factor	99%	Splenomegaly	40%
Reduced complement level (C4)	95%	Raynaud's phenomenon	25%
Cutaneous vasculitis	95%	Sjögren's syndrome	25%
Palpable purpura	90%	Neurocognitive impairment	25%
Hepatitis	85%	Lymphadenopathy	15%
Arthralgias	75%	Skin ulcers	15%
Female gender	70%	Thyroiditis	5%
Glomerulonephritis	55%	Low-grade non-Hodgkin lymphoma	5%

finding is one of the earliest systemic signs seen in the mixed-type CG. Dore et al. reported the frequency of specific symptoms, signs, and associated disease states seen in the patients with mixed CG and HCV at the initial presentation (Table 27.2) (8). However, it is important to note that the clinical manifestations of CG are protean, and significant overlap exists among different types of CG, contrary to the historical descriptions of CG. Symptoms often wax and wane over time, each episodes lasting weeks to months, with spontaneous remissions and exacerbations.

Clinically apparent major end-organ damage is rare in the mixed CG, with an exception of renal dysfunction, which is present in approximately 20% of patients at the time of diagnosis (9). Histological examination is very characteristic of GC-induced renal disease, and most CG patients with renal complications have hematuria, proteinuria, and hypocomplementemia, although the plasma creatinine concentration itself is initially normal or only mildly elevated (10, 11, 12). However, acute renal failure and/or the nephrotic syndrome may be seen in some patients.

In more recent studies, other clinical features were added, including an evolution to low-grade non-Hodgkin lymphoma, observed in some patients with CG. Indeed, HCV is also a lymphotropic virus and it is worth noting that 6–28% of patients with type II cryoglobulinaemia develop symptomatic lymphoma after 4–10 years of follow-up (13).

Laboratory Data

Persistently elevated cryocrit (>1% for 3–6 months) is often used for confirmation of diagnosis. In real practice, however, the diagnosis is often delayed because of improper handling of the blood collection, although the patient may have clinical history otherwise suggestive of CG. Because it requires coordinated effort by the patient and the laboratory personnel for accurate measurement of cryoglobulins, false-negative results are often reported. If clinically the suspicion is high, revisiting the steps for special handling of the blood sample and communication with the laboratory may be necessary.

Flamm et al. (14) and Peng et al. (15) summarized key steps in correctly measuring cryoglobulin. First, the blood is collected at fasting state because lipids may interfere with the test. When drawing blood, it is also important to know that the routine laboratory testing for cryoglobulin is performed only on serum because plasma treated with anticoagulants can cause false-positive result by formation of cryofibrin and heparin-precipitable complexes. For correct detection, blood samples must be constantly kept at 37°C on the way to the laboratory (use pre-warmed tube). After it is spun in temperature-controlled centrifuge, the serum is cooled to 4°C then observed for precipitation over a 48- to 72-h period. It is important to remember that the cryoprecipitate for type 1 CG is usually observed within hours, whereas it may take up to 1 week for cryoprecipitate formation of the mixed CG. The tube is then centrifuged in the cold. A cryocrit is then determined by measuring the packed (centrifuged) volume of the precipitate as a percentage of the original serum volume at 4°C.

Approximately 40% of normal individuals possess CG, but their quantity is usually too small for detection by cryocrit (measurable level by cryocrit is generally 1% or 1 mg/dL). Highest cryocrit (approaching 50%) is generally seen in type I CG **whereas 2–7% in type II, and 1–3% in type III. Although the cryocrit itself can suggest the type of CG, there is no correlation between the cryocrit and the severity of organ involvement. The type of abnormal protein (IgM or IgG), hence a specific type of CG, can be determined by immunoelectrophoresis and immunofixation, but the more sensitive methods for detection of oligoclonal components of type III cryoglobulins are immunoblotting and two-dimensional electrophoresis.

The presence of cryoglobulin in the serum can affect other blood tests, which may hinder prompt diagnosis of CG in some cases. High cryoprecipitates can interfere with automated analyzers in measurement of complete blood count, resulting in pseudothrombocytosis and/or pseudoleukocytosis, which can be mistaken for primary bone marrow dysfunction as seen in type I CG. Cryoprecipitates may also deplete HCV antibody and HCV antigens from the serum, leading to a false-negative hepatitis serology, which can delay the correct diagnosis. When suspicion for underlying chronic hepatitis C is high, but the initial serologic test is negative for HCV, dual measurement of serum and cryoprecipitate for HCV antibody and HCV antigen could avoid this problem. In addition, HCV RNA should be tested by using PCR.

Complements may be important adjuncts in the diagnosis and monitoring treatment response because diminished serum complement components may reflect ongoing consumption by CG. Type I CG typically produces few serological complement abnormalities, but mixed CG sera often demonstrate reduced levels of all complements, except the levels of C3 that are generally unaffected, or only mildly diminished. It is important to remember that such changes in complement levels are not specific or sensitive to CG, and are seen in other active connective tissue diseases, which may or may not be associated with the type III CG.

Histological Data

In rare cases where a definitive diagnosis cannot be made based on clinical presentation and laboratory data, direct immunohistochemistry on involved tissues can often confirm that cryoglobulins are responsible for the patient's signs and symptoms. Biopsy of purpuric skin lesion is most commonly performed, and more invasive procedures such as nerve or renal biopsy is reserved for those patients whose diagnosis is otherwise in doubt. In the skin, typical pathological finding would be leukocytoclastic vasculitis. Direct immunofluorescence microscopy of acute lesions often reveals deposits of IgM, IgG, and/or C3 complements. Peripheral nerve biopsy will show pauci-inflammatory occlusive small vessels in type I GC and necroinflammatory epineural vasculitis in the mixed GC. All three main types of cryoglobulinaemic vasculitis can lead to kidney disease, most typically causing type I membranoproliferative glomerulonephritis, and rarely, mesangioproliferative glomerulonephritis. Renal biopsy may show striking influx of macrophages that is not seen in any other types of proliferative glomerulonephritis. Patients suspected of having type I CG should have bone marrow biopsy to rule out underlying hematological conditions such as multiple myeloma.

Prognosis

Mortality and morbidity in a patient with CG often depend on concomitant diseases, but patients with renal involvement and lymphoproliferative disorder have worse prognosis overall. A meta-analysis of 19 studies published between 1994 and 2001, CG was associated with increased risk of cirrhosis and higher overall mortality with chronic hepatitis C (16).

Cryoglobulin levels also may decrease and clinical symptoms of CG often improve as underlying conditions (i.e., HCV or primary malignancies) are successfully treated. However, as mentioned earlier, there is no correlation between the cryocrit and the severity of end-organ involvement or treatment response.

Treatment

Because HCV has a clear biological role in the pathogenesis of CG in most patients, one must consider eradicating HCV with antiviral therapy. Interferon-based treatment reduces viral replication rate (even without complete or permanent elimination), inhibits lymphocyte proliferation and immunoglobulin synthesis, and improves immune complex clearance by enhancing macrophage activity. Current standard treatment for HCV is PEG-interferon α plus ribavirin. The rate of sustained viral response to PEG-interferon plus ribavirin is comparable in hepatitis C patients with or without CG. In a recent randomized control study with 18 patients affected by mixed CG, the efficacy and safety of PEG-interferon α-2b in combination with ribavirin was confirmed for the initial treatment of HCV-associated CG (17).

When considering antiviral therapy on CG patients with HCV, physicians should pay particular attention to the patient's renal function. Using ribavirin (and to a lesser degree, PEG-interferon) is contraindicated in patients with significant renal insufficiency (Cr Clearance <50 mg/dL), which may be more common in HCV with CG versus HCV without CG. Although there are anecdotal reports of successful treatment of patients with moderate renal insufficiency with a proportionate reduction in ribavirin dose, this approach has not been well studied (18).

Moreover, interferon-based therapy should be considered with a caveat in that its direct immunomodulating effect can induce de novo autoimmune diseases that may aggravate clinical manifestations of CG. In active CG, some advocate first using immunosuppression with steroids and cyclophosphamide. In the most severe cases, additional use of plasma exchange may be beneficial, particularly in active cryoglobulinemic nephropathy. Because immunosuppressive medications increase HCV RNA level and serum cryoglobulin, they should be administered in low doses and reduced as soon as possible, and one may consider initiating antiviral therapy once the disease activity is stabilized in few months.

The latest attempt against the abnormal B-cell clones driven by HCV is the anti-CD 20 monoclonal antibody rituximab. This agent has previously shown activity in B-cell lymphomas and autoimmune disorders. Recent studies showed rituximab resulted in a significant and rapid improvement of clinical signs and end-organ function, and a decline of RF activity and cryocrit in most patients with CG, including patients who were resistant to PEG-interferon. However, because rituximab decreases anti-HCV antibody titers and increases viremia, the long-term effect of rituximab on the progression of liver disease is not known (19).

It is also important to note that CG is also seen in HCV-negative patients or patients who have achieved complete HCV clearance. Furthermore, clinical recovery from CG is observed in patients with persistent viral replication. Such cases demand more complete understanding of CG and its pathophysiology.

References

1. Meltzer, M, Franklin, EC. Cryoglobulinemia–a study of twenty-nine patients. I. IgG and IgM cryoglobulins and factors affecting cryoprecipitability. *Am J Med* 1966; 40: 828.

2. Meltzer, M, Franklin, EC, Elias, K, et al. Cryoglobulinemia – a clinical and laboratory study. II. Cryoglobulins with rheumatoid factor activity. *Am J Med* 1966; 40: 837.

3. Brouet J, Clauvel J, Danon F. Biologic and clinical significance of cryoglobulins. A report of 86 cases. *Am J Med* 1974; 57(5): 775–88.

4. Sansonno D, Dammacco F. Hepatitis C virus, cryoglobulinemia, and vasculitis: immune complex relations. *Lancet Infect Dis* 2005; 5: 227–36.

5. Yao Z, Nguyen D, Hiotellis A, Hahn Y. Hepatitis C virus core protein inhibits human T lymphocyte responses by a complement-dependent regulatory pathway. *J Immunol* 2001; 167: 5264–72.

6. Lunel F, Musset L, Cacoub P, et al. Cryoglobulinemia in chronic liver diseases: role of hepatitis C virus and liver damage. *Gastroenterology* 1994; 106: 1291–300.

7. Cacoub P, Costedoat-Chalumeau N, Lidove O, et al. Cryoglobulinemia vasculitis. *Curr Opin Rheumatol* 2002; 14: 29–35.

8. Dore MP, Fattovich G, Sepulveda AR, Realdi G. Cryoglobulinemia Related to Hepatitis C Virus Infection Cryoglobulinemia related to hepatitis C virus infection. *Dig Dis Sci* 2007 April; 52(4): 897–907. Epub 2007 February 16.

9. Monti, G, Galli, M, Invernizzi, F, et al. Cryoglobulinaemias: a multi-centre study of the early clinical and laboratory manifestations of primary and secondary disease. GISC. Italian Group for the Study of Cryoglobulinaemias. *QJM* 1995; 88: 115.

10. Gorevic, PD, Kassab, HJ, Levo, Y, et al. Mixed cryoglobulinemia: Clinical aspects and long-term follow-up of 40 patients. *Am J Med* 1980; 69: 287.

11. D'Amico, G, Colasanti, G, Ferrario, F, Sinico, RA. Renal involvement in essential mixed cryoglobulinemia. *Kidney Int* 1989; 35: 1004.

12. Misiani, R, Bellavita, P, Fenili, D, et al. Hepatitis C virus infection in patients with essential mixed cryoglobulinemia. *Ann Intern Med* 1992; 117: 573.

13. Vallat L, Benhamou Y, Gutierrez M, et al. Clonal B cell populations in the blood and liver of patients with chronic hepatitis C virus infection. *Arthritis Rheum* 2004; 50: 3668–78.

14. Steven Flamm, Sanjiv Chopra, Burton Rose. Clinical manifestations and diagnosis of essential mixed cryoglobulinemia, UpToDate version 15.1, August 21, 2006.

15. Stanford Peng, Peter Schur. Overview of cryoglobulins and cryoglobulinemia, UpToDate version 15.1, August 21, 2006.

16. Kayali Z, Buckwold V, Zimmerman B, Schidt W. Cryoglobulinemia, and cirrhosis: A meta-analysis. *Hepatology* 2002; 36: 9978–85.

17. Mazzaro C, Zorat F, Caizzi M. Treatment with peg-interferon alfa-2b and ribavirin of hepatitis C virus-associated mixed cryoglobulinemia: A pilot study. *J Hepatol* 2005; 42: 632–8.

18. Zuckerman, E, Keren, D, Slobodin, G, et al. Treatment of refractory, symptomatic, hepatitis C virus related mixed cryoglobulinemia with ribavirin and interferon-alpha. *J Rheumatol* 2000; 27: 2172.

19. Sansonno D, De Re V, Lauletta G. Monoclonal antibody treatment of mixed cryoglobulinemia resistant to interferon a with an anti-CD20. *Blood* 2003: 101: 3818–26.

28
Hypersensitivity Angiitis

Shimon Pollack

Abstract Hypersensitivity vasculitis (HSV) or angiitis is also termed allergic vasculitis and has been defined to describe vasculitis of small blood vessels which is believed to be secondary to hypersensitivity mechanisms. This is a relatively common condition characterized clinically by the development of palpable purpuric rash over the lower limbs, buttocks, and forearms. With the exception of the skin, other organs and tissues such as joints and kidneys may also be involved. The main symptoms and signs are palpable purpura, fever, arthralgia, proteinuria, and microscopic hematuria. HSV is typically associated with chronic bacterial and viral infections and also with the use of various drugs. Histological examination of purpuric lesions reveals prominent vasculitis with endothelial swelling, intense polymorph or lymphocyte infiltration, and disintegration of polymorphs (leucocytoclasis), resulting in "nuclear dust". The small blood vessels may also be thrombosed with fibrinoid changes and epidermal necrosis. The course of HSV is variable; it may last for 2–3 weeks or even several years.

Keywords Leukocytoclasis · palpable purpura · immune complexes

Hypersensitivity vasculitis (HSV) or angiitis is a small blood vessel vasculitis which is believed to be secondary to hypersensitivity mechanisms (1, 2, 3, 4). It is characterized by the development of palpable purpuric rash, mostly over the lower limbs (Figure 28.1). Histological examination shows intense polymorph or lymphocyte infiltration and disintegration of polymorphs (leucocytoclasis), resulting in "nuclear dust" (Figure 28.2). The course of HSV is short in general and does not last for more than 3 weeks. However, in rare cases, repeated bouts of vasculitis may last for years.

History and Classification

A broad and heterogenous group of syndromes may result from the inflammation and damage to small blood vessels. The heterogeneity and overlap between syndromes have been major impediments to the development of a coherent classification for the various vasculitides.

The concept that inflammatory vascular disease secondary to hypersensitivity or allergic mechanism should exist as a distinct nosologic entity was first proposed in 1948 by Zeek et al. (5). Certain features, such as the prominent involvement of the skin and the observation that these vasculitic syndromes appeared to be precipitated by use of serum or drugs, suggested a difference between HSV and other forms of small-vessel vasculitis that were recognized at that time (6).

Thus, in accordance with the old and classical classification of Fauci et al. in 1978 (2), hypersensitivity angiitis is being related to either endogenous antigens (connective tissue diseases or malignancies) or exogenous antigens (infections, drug reactions, or serum sickness) and is grouped together with other small-vessel vasculitides such as Henoch-Schönlein purpura, cryoglobulinemia, or microscopic polyangiitis (Table 28.1). It may be the primary manifestation of a disease (like in cutaneous leukocytoclastic angiitis) or, alternatively, a secondary component of another primary disease (like in autoimmune diseases or malignancies).

Despite these distinguishing features, difficulties have arisen in defining HSV as a distinct illness. In many patients, no inciting antigen could be found (7). In spite of that, the American College of Rheumatology (ACR) has developed some 18 years ago distinct criteria for the classification of HSV as a separate definable clinical syndrome Ref. (4) and (Table 28.2).

From: Y. Shoenfeld et al. (eds.): *Diagnostic Criteria in Autoimmune Diseases*, DOI: 10.1007/978-1-60327-285-8_28,
© 2008 Humana Press, Totowa, NJ

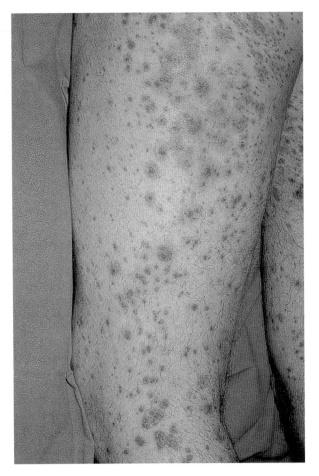

FIGURE 28.1. Purpuric rash and palpable purpura.

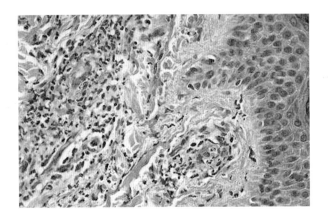

FIGURE 28.2. Leukocytoklastic vasculitis.

In this chapter, we will refer mainly to HSV-defined clinical entities, namely HSV related to infection, drugs, and malignancies and also to related clinical entities such as serum sickness, urticarial vasculitis, and cutaneous vasculitis.

TABLE 28.1. Small vessel vasculitis[a].

Wegener's granulomatosis
Churg-Strauss syndrome
Microscopic polyangiitis (polyarteritis)
Henoch-Schönlein purpura
Essential cryoglobulinemic vasculitis
Cutaneous leukocytoclastic angiitis
Hypersensitivity angiitis

[a] Modified from Jennette JC et al Nomenclature of systemic vasculitides. Proposal of an International Consensus Conference *Arth Rheum* 1994; 37:189.

TABLE 28.2. 1990 Criteria for the classification of hypersensitivity vasculitis[a].

Criterion	Definition
Age at disease onset >16 years	Development of symptoms after age 16
Medication at disease onset	Medication was taken at the onset of symptoms that may have been a precipitating factor
Palpable purpura	Slightly elevated purpuric rash over one or more areas of the skin; does not blanch with pressure and is not related to thrombocytopenia
Maculopapular rash	Flat and raised lesions of various sizes over one or more areas of the skin
Biopsy including arteriole and venule	Histological changes showing granulocytes in a perivascular extravascular location

[a] hypersensitivity vasculitis is defined if at least 3 of these 5 criteria are present. The presence of any 3 or more criteria yield a sensitivity of 71% and specificity of 83.9%.

Modified from Calabrese et al. The American College of Rheumatology 1990 criteria for the classification of hypersensitivity vasculitis. *Arthritis Rheum* 1990; 33: 1110.

Immunopathogenesis

Zeek, in his first classification scheme for vasculitides, coined the term "hypersensitivity" for allergic vasculitis in relation to animal models of vasculitis induced by the administration of exogenous antigens (allergens) such as horse serum and sulfonamides (8). In this animal vasculitic model, a prominent cutaneous involvement has been observed together with involvement of small blood vessels, i.e. arterioles, venules, and capillaries. All lesions were approximately the same age and the vasculitis reaction was self-limited. The identification of an inciting antigen in this model raised the possibility of an immune-complex mechanism. However, in many patients who fit the clinical and pathological picture of the disease, no inciting antigen can be identified (7). Thus, the 1994 Chapel Hill Consensus Conference on nomenclature of the vasculitides (9) proposed an alternative term for hypersensitivity vasculitis—cutaneous leucocytoclastic angiitis. However, these two histopathological patterns appear to represent two distinct processes. In addition, although most lesional skin biopsies of HSV demonstrate a neutrophil predominance, others show primarily lymphocytic infiltration (7).

Diagnosis

The diagnosis of hypersensitivity vasculitis should be considered in any patient with palpable purpura associated with an unexplained systemic illness. Sometimes there are also certain clinical abnormalities, such as polyarthralgia/polyarthritis and microscopic hematuria, which suggest a diagnosis of a multisystem disease (see Table 28.3). A number of nonvasculitic diseases may also produce some or all of these abnormalities. Thus, the clinical approach should especially exclude certain infectious diseases such as Rocky Mountain spotted fever, Lyme disease, syphilis, disseminated gonococcal infection, and some cases of bacterial endocarditis (most cases of bacterial endocarditis produce small-vessel vasculitic disease). Also, atrial myxoma and cocaine abuse should be considered and excluded. Once these diseases and others have been excluded, it is important to establish in a short course the diagnosis of HSV. Whereas most HSV syndromes resolve spontaneously or require mild treatment only, certain types may require a more aggressive therapy. The definitive diagnosis is usually made upon biopsy of involved skin with the typical pathological finding of leucocytoclastic vasculitis: perivascular polymorphonuclear leukocytes with fragmentation and extravasation of erythrocytes with fibrinoid necrosis of vessel wall (Figure 28.2). Immunofluorescence staining shows variable quantities of immunoglobulin (mostly IgG) and complement deposition. Laboratory tests may add some support to the diagnosis, and additional imaging measures may help,

TABLE 28.3. Clinical and laboratory features of 93 patients with HSV[a].

Criterion	% positive
Palpable purpura	63
Neutrophils around arterioles or venules	54
Medications at onset	53
Transient arthralgias	46
ESR > 50 mm (Westergren)	40
Hematuria (gross or micro)	37
Low C4	36
Cutaneous ulcers or pitted scars	33
Monoarthritis or oligoarthritis	30

[a] Modified from Michel BA, Hunder GG, Bloch DA, Calabrese LH. Hypersensitivity vasculitis and Henoch-Schönlein purpura: a comparison between the 2 disorders. *J Rheumatol* 1992; 19:723.

TABLE 28.4. Work-up for patients with possible HSV[a].

Skin biopsy with immunofluorescence
Complete blood count
Serum creatinine
Liver transaminases
Serum and urine electrolytes
Urinalysis with microscopy
Chest radiograph
Antinuclear antibody assay (ANA)
Serum complement levels
Antineutrophil cytoplasmic antibodies (ANCA)
Cryoglobulins
Hepatitis C antibody
ESR

[a] Modified from ref. 20 Rich RR, Fleisher TA, Shearer WT, Kotzin BL, Schroeder Jr HW (Ed): *Clinical Immunology – principles and practice.* 2nd Edition, Mosby 2001, p. 67.14.

sometimes, to establish a more defined diagnosis (see Table 28.4). If an offending antigen, such as a drug, is recognized, it should be removed if possible. If an underlying disease such as an infection or a neoplasm is recognized, it should be treated appropriately. If there is no recognizable underlying disease, treatment should be initiated according to the clinical manifestations that are present.

Differential Diagnosis

The single most difficult disorder to differentiate from HSV is Henoch-Schönlein purpura (HSP). Some have suggested in the past that because of the very similar clinical picture, it may represent HSV with a different allergic reaction to some other exogenous antigens (10). However, the results of established immunopathological studies, with the demonstration of circulating IgA immune complexes and IgA deposits in vascular lesions of HSP, support the distinction of HSP from HSV (11). Thus, HSP will be discussed separately in detail in another chapter of this book.

Drugs act probably as haptens to stimulate an immune response. Also, certain infections such as chronic bacteremia (e.g. bacterial endocarditis), hepatitis, and HIV may chronically stimulate immune response and be associated with immune-complex formation and the generation of HSV. Chronic bacterial infections that may be complicated by HSV should be treated efficiently and carefully because HSV in these cases may progress to a more systemic disease, such as adult Henoch-Schönlein purpura, and have the potential to display a severe prognosis (12).

Leukocytoclastic vasculitis predominantly involving the skin with occasional involvement of other organ systems may be the presenting sign of some neoplasms (1). In most cases, surgical removal of tumor and/or appropriate therapy is associated with the disappearance of vasculitic lesions. Several immunopathological mechanisms underlying the malignancy-associated vasculitis have been proposed. Cytokine production by malignant cells may be one of the precipitating factors that lead to vasculitis (13).

Patients with leukocytoclastic angiitis which is confined exclusively to the skin are diagnosed as localized cutaneous vasculitis. The pattern of disease associations with localized cutaneous vasculitis includes underlying systemic illness like infection or malignancy and also connective tissue disease (14, 15, 16). Some patients also have drug etiology—up to 10–20% (16). The annual incidence of localized cutaneous angiitis is at 15.4/million (14), which is higher than the annual incidence of both Wegener's granulomatosis (8.5/million) and microscopic polyangiitis (3.6/million). Some patients may initially be diagnosed as having cutaneous leukocytoclastic angiitis but will subsequently be found to have systemic form of small-vessel vasculitis.

Hypersensitivity reactions commonly cause rash also, which may be presented as urticarial lesions. If urticarial lesions persist for at least 24 hours and sometimes leave traces of hyperpigmentation, urticarial vasculitis should be considered. Three subtypes are known (17): (a) normocomplementemic form, which is generally idiopathic and benign; (b) hypocomplementemic form, which is often associated with a systemic inflammatory disease; and (c) hypocomplementemic urticarial vasculitis syndrome (HUVS), which is a potentially severe condition associated with autoantibodies to C1q. The lesions of urticarial vasculitis are often accompanied by stinging or burning and not by pruritus as in common urticaria. The classic histological picture is of leukocytoclastic vasculitis. Most patients with urticarial vasculitis have the hypocomplementemic subtypes (17) and are likely to manifest signs of an underlying systemic autoimmune disease.

Vasculitis may be the result of an ongoing reaction to an unidentified antigenic stimulus (18) as in essential mixed cryoglobulinemia (EMC). Although rheumatoid factor is present in most patients, the inciting antigen is still undefined. In the broad sense, EMC may represent a chronic form of HSV. Indeed, small amounts of cryoglobulins are frequently found in HSV, probably as part of an immune-complex reaction. Thus, the differentiation of EMC from HSV may pose theoretical and also practical problems. EMC is also characterized by palpable purpura and vasculitis of small vessels with leukocytoclasia. However, in contrast to HSV, ECM is not self-limited and generally runs a chronic course (19).

Treatment

Once the diagnosis of HSV has been established, a decision regarding treatment must be made. Management strategy is largely empiric. The type, intensity, and duration of therapy are based on the degree of disease severity in an individual patient. When there is an involvement of organs and tissues except skin or synovial membranes, glucocorticoids should be instituted immediately. Cytotoxic/immunosuppressive

therapy should be added only if an adequate response does not result or if remission can only be achieved or maintained with high doses of steroids. Many of the side-effects of glucocorticoid therapy are marked by decrease in frequency and severity in patients on alternate-day regimens compared to daily regimens.

On the contrary, many of the HSV syndromes resolve with only symptomatic treatment (nonsteroidal anti-inflammatory drugs and/or H_1 antihistamines) or after the removal of the offending agent, as in infection or malignancy. Colchicine, hydroxychloroquine, or dapsone may also be tried for persistent disease.

As in every other disease, it should be remembered that each patient requires individual decision-making and should be practiced in order to provide maximal therapeutic efficacy with minimal toxic side-effects.

References

1. Fauci, AS, Haynes BF, Katz P: The spectrum of vasculitis: clinical, pathologic, immunologic and therapeutic considerations. *Ann Intern Med* 1978; 89:660–76.
2. Calabrese LH, Clough ID: Hypersensitivity vasculitis group (HVG): a case-oriented review of a continuing clinical spectrum. *Cleve Clin Q* 1982; 49:17–42.
3. Michel BA, Hunder GG, Bloch DA, Calabrese LH: Hypersensitivity vasculitis and Henoch-Schönlein purpura: a comparison between the 2 disorders. *J Rheumatol* 1992; 19:721–8.
4. Calabrese LH, Michel BA, Bloch DA et al. The American College of Rheumatology 1990 criteria for the classification of hypersensitivity vasculitis. *Arthritis Rheum* 1990; 33:1108 113.
5. Zeek PM, Smith CC, Weeter JC: Studies on periarteritis modosa. III. The differentiation between the vascular lesions of periarteritis modosa and hypersensitivity. *Am J Pathol* 1948; 24:889–917.
6. Zeek PM: Periarteritis modosa and other forms of necrotizing angiitis. *N Engl J Med* 1953; 248:764–71.
7. Ekenstam EA, Callen JP: Cutaneous leukocytoclastic vasculitis: clinical and laboratory features of 82 patients seen in private practice. *Arch Dermatol* 1984; 120:848–489.
8. Zeek PM: Periarteritis modosa: a critical review. *Am J Clin Pathol* 1952; 221:777–91.
9. Jennette JC, Falk RJ, Andrassy K et al. Nomenclature of systemic vasculitides. Proposal of an International Consensus Conference. *Arthritis Rheum* 1994; 37:187–92.
10. Heng MCY: Henoch-Schönlein purpura. *Br J Dermatol* 1985; 112:235–40.
11. Kauffman RH, Herman WA, Meyer WL, Daha MR, van Es LA: Circulating IgA immune complex in Henoch-Schönlein purpura: a longitudinal study of their relationship to disease activity and vascular deposition of IgA. *Am J Med* 1980; 69:859–66.
12. Saulsbury FT. Clinical update: Henoch-Schönlein purpura. *Lancet* 2007; 369:976–8.
13. Motzer RJ, Bander HN, Nanus DM: Renal cell carcinoma. *N Engl J Med* 1996; 335:865–75.

14. Watts RA, Joliffe VA, Grattan CEH, Elliott J, Lockwood M, Scott DGI: Cutaneous vasculitis in a defined population-clinical and epidemiological association. *J Rheumatol* 1998; 25:920–4.

15. Jessop SJ. Cutaneous leucocytoclastic vasculitis: a clinical and aetiological study. *Br J Rheumatol* 1995; 34:942–5.

16. Sanchez NP, Van Hale HM, Su WPD. Clinical and histo-pathologic spectrum of necrotising vasculitis. *Arch Dermatol* 1985; 121:325–40.

17. Wisnieski J: Urticarial vasculitis. *Curr Opin Rheumatol* 2000; 12:24–32.

18. Leonard H. Calabrese, BA. et al. The American College of Rheumatology 1990 criteria for the classification of hyper-sensitivity vasculitis. *Arthritis Rheum* 1990; 33:1108–13.

19. Gorevic PD, Kassab HJ, Levo Y, Kohn R, Maltzer M, Prose P, Franklin EC: Mixed cryoglobulinemia: clinical aspects and long-term follow-up of 40 patients. *Am J Med* 1980; 69:287–308.

20. Rich RR, Fleisher TA, Shearer WT, Kotzin BL, Schroeder Jr. HW. (Eds): *Clinical Immunology – Principles and Practice.* 2nd Edition, Mosby 2001, pp 67.13–15.

Part III
Idiopathic Inflammatory Myopathies

29
Polymyositis

Georgina Espígol and Josep M. Grau

Abstract Polymyositis (PM) represents one of the three major forms of idiopathic inflammatory myopathies. Its prevalence is not known because of overdiagnosed cases [muscular dystrophies, inclusion body myositis (IBM)]. PM usually presents in middle age, particularly in women. Pathogenic mechanisms include the abnormal expression of major histocompatibility complex (MHC)-class I antigens and the activation of CD8 cells. The clinical pattern consists in a subacute or chronic proximal muscle weakness, with a marked increment of serum CK values. The diagnosis of muscle pathology requires an experienced team because some muscular dystrophies and IBM may resemble PM. In contrast to dermatomyositis, neoplastic-associated cases do exist but in a lesser proportion. PM may be associated with other autoimmune diseases or with some infectious diseases. In most cases, a satisfactory clinical response can be obtained with corticosteroids and immunosuppressive agents, but a fatal evolution may occur in a small percentage of cases.

Keywords Inflammation · myositis · MCH class I · dystrophy

Polymyositis (PM) is one of the three major forms of inflammatory myopathies. It is defined as a subacute myopathy that basically affects adults and presents with weakness of the proximal muscles.

Epidemiology

Inflammatory myopathies are uncommon diseases. They can be differentiated into three major subsets: dermatomyositis (DM), PM and inclusion body myositis (IBM) (1, 2). PM is rare in childhood and is mainly seen after the second decade of life, being more common in females. The prevalence of PM is unknown. The incidence of the different forms of inflammatory myopathies has been estimated using outdated criteria and in addition a few studies not distinguished between PM and IBM (1,3).

Pathogenesis

The association with other autoimmune disorders and the response to immunotherapies supported the autoimmune origin of PM, although target antigens have not been identified. Recent studies of the molecular immunology of autoantibodies, the MHC and other genetic factors have emphasized their role in the pathogenesis of this disease (4). In PM, CD8-T cells invade MHC antigens, expressing muscle fibers (5). Expression of cytokines has been demonstrated in mononuclear cells in affected muscles and may contribute to local inflammatory response and to perpetuation of the autoimmune response. Therefore, better knowledge of the immune mechanisms will allow identification of new potential therapeutic targets (6).

Clinical Manifestations

PM presents with muscle weakness that evolves over several weeks or months. The pattern of muscular weakness is nonselective.

Patients report difficulty with everyday tasks such as climbing steps, rising from a seat, or lifting objects. Distal muscles are affected late, and facial muscles remain normal. Patients with myalgias but normal strength do not have PM (1,7).

Weakness of the respiratory muscles develops in some cases of severe PM and may lead to the need for assisted ventilation (8).

Extramuscular findings are more common in DM but may also occur in PM. Cardiac manifestations include myocarditis, arrhythmias or congestive cardiac failure.

From: Y. Shoenfeld et al. (eds.): *Diagnostic Criteria in Autoimmune Diseases*, DOI: 10.1007/978-1-60327-285-8_29,

TABLE 29.1. Features the patient *does not* have (7).

Rash (characteristic of dermatomyositis)
Family history of neuromuscular diseases
Exposure to myotoxic drugs, especially penicillamine, zidovudine, and
　(rarely) statins
Endocrine disease (hypothyroidism, hyperthyroidism,
　hypoparathyroidism, hypercortisolism)
Neurogenic disease (exclude by electromyography and neurological
　examination)
Dystrophies[a] and metabolic myopathies (excluded by history and muscle
　biopsy)
Inclusion body myositis (excluded by clinical examination and muscle
　biopsy)

[a] Dysferlin deficiency and facioscapulohumeral muscular dystrophies in
particular because severe inflammation can be found in muscle biopsies.

These manifestations may sometimes occur in hypertensive patients because of long-term steroid treatment. Arthralgias may occur even without an association with connective tissue diseases. Other symptoms such as fever, weight loss or Raynaud's phenomenon appear in association with other connective tissue diseases. Interstitial lung disease is more common in patients with anti-Jo-1 or other antisynthetase antibodies (9).

PM may be associated with many autoimmune diseases and viral infections such as systemic lupus, rheumatoid arthritis, vasculitis, HIV and HTLV-1 infection. Although significantly less frequent than in adult DM patients, there is an association with malignant disorders, the most common being the ovaries and breast in females and the lung and gastrointestinal tracts in males. The highest risk in PM is during the 1- to 5-year period after diagnosis of the myopathy and in patients over 50 years of age (10), making surveillance for early diagnosis highly recommended. Screening with a complete physical examination and complementary tests (according to age and personal history) should be made yearly (6,11).

PM should be considered as a syndrome that occurs alone or in association with other disorders such as autoimmune diseases or viral infections. All myopathies have a lot of manifestations in common and could be difficult to separate them. PM remains a diagnosis of exclusion. PM as a stand-alone entity is uncommon (Table 29.1) (7).

Diagnosis

The diagnosis of PM requires clinical manifestations and three laboratory tests: serum muscle enzyme concentrations, electromyography and muscle biopsy.

The main serum muscle enzyme is creatine kinase (CK) (up to 50-fold normal). Other enzymes, aspartate and alanine aminotransferases, lactate dehydrogenase and aldolase may also be elevated but CK is always increased in patients with active disease (7,12).

Electromyography shows a myopathic process with increased spontaneous activity with fibrillations, complex repetitive discharges and positive sharp waves (7).

Pathology

Muscle biopsy is the definitive examination for the diagnosis. Whenever possible it should be performed before initiating treatment. An open biopsy provides a larger tissue sample that allows not only conventional microscopic examination but also immunohistochemical studies and electron microscopy. In some cases, the biopsy is normal or shows minimal changes. Some studies have suggested that magnetic resonance imaging (MRI) may be helpful to diagnose a myopathy and to also select a biopsy site (13).

The positive biopsy shows multifocal lymphocytic infiltrates surrounding and invading healthy muscle fibers (Figure 29.1). The muscle cells express MHC-class I antigens (Figure 29.2) and the lymphocytes are CD8$^+$ cells (5). Dalakas et al. refer to this lesion as the CD8/MHC-I complex (7).

Serological Features Autoantibodies

The most common autoantibodies in PM are the antisynthetases directed against aminoacyl tRNA synthetases. The antibody against histidyl-tRNA synthetase, anti-Jo-1, is the best known and has a high specificity for the 'antisynthetase syndrome' (myositis, arthritis and Raynaud's phenomenon). The pathogenic importance of these autoantibodies remains unclear (6,14). In rare cases of PM with associated signal recognition particle (SRP) antibodies the prognosis is poor.

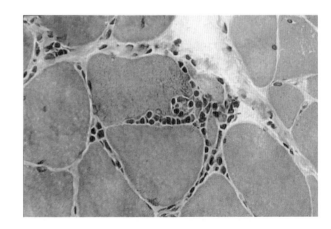

FIGURE 29.1. Lymphocytic infiltrate surrounding and invading an otherwise normal cell. Gomori's trichrome on frozen tissue.

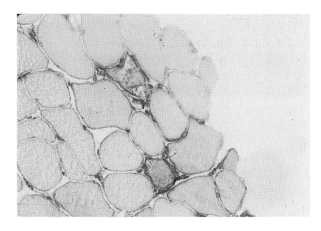

FIGURE 29.2. Abnormal MHC class I expression in the sarcolemma of muscle cells. Immunohistochemistry on frozen tissue.

Diagnostic Criteria

Several criteria proposed have not been successful. For instance, the criteria proposed by Bohan and Peter do not distinguish between PM and IBM. Because histopathology and immunopathology are mandatory to achieve a diagnosis of PM, Dalakas proposed the term definite PM if a patient has an acquired, subacute myopathy fulfilling the inclusion and exclusion criteria, raised concentrations of serum CK and primary inflammation in the muscle biopsy (7) (Table 29.2).

Treatment

Few controlled trials have been published and most of the experience with the use of drugs has arisen from case reports. Corticosteroids are the main initial treatment for inflammatory myositis, although their efficacy has not been established in randomized studies. Not all patients respond to the use of these drugs and many have iatrogenic

complications. Second line agents such as immunosuppressives or intravenous immunoglobulin should be considered when the disease is not controlled with corticosteroids (relapses, ineffectiveness of 3 months of high-dose prednisone and rapidly progressive disease). The medical approach must be individualized. New therapies directed to cytokine modulation and the use of monoclonal antibodies are promising (6,7,15).

References

1. Dalakas MC. (1991) Polymyositis, dermatomyositis and inclusion-body myositis. *N Engl J Med* 325: 1487–98.
2. Dalakas MC. (2001) Polymyositis, dermatomyositis and inclusion-body myositis. In: Braunwald E, Fauci AS, Kasper DL, Hauser SL, Longo DL, Jameson JL, (eds.), Harrison's Principles of Internal Medicine, 15th edn. New york, McGraw-Hill, 2524–29.
3. Mastaglia FL, Philips BA. (2002) Idiopathic inflammatory myopathies: epidemiology, classification and diagnostic criteria. *Rheum Dis Clin North Am* 28: 723–41.
4. Hohlfeld R, Engel AG, Goebels N, Behrens L. (1997) Cellular immune mechanisms in inflammatory myopathies. *Curr Opin Rheumatol* 9: 520–6.
5. Dalakas MC. (2002) Muscle biopsy findings in inflammatory myopathies. *Rheum Dis Clin North Am* 28: 779–98.
6. Mastaglia FL, Garlepp MJ, Phillips BA, Zilko PJ. (2003) Inflammatory myopathies: clinical, diagnostic and therapeutic aspects. *Muscle Nerve* 27(4): 407–25.
7. Dalakas MC, Hohlfeld R. (2003) Polymyositis and dermatomyositis. *Lancet* 362: 971–82.
8. Selva-O'Callaghan A, Sanchez-Sitjes L, Muñoz-Gall X, et al. (2000) Respiratory failure due to muscle weakness in inflammatory myopathies: maintenance therapy with home mechanical ventilation. *Rheumatology* 39: 914–6.
9. Grau JM, Miro O, Pedrol E, Casademont J, Masanés F, Herrero C, Haussmann G, Urbano-Marquez A. (1996) Interstitial lung disease related to dermatomyositis. Comparative study with patients without lung involvement. *J Rheumatol* 23: 1921–6.
10. Zantos D, Zhang Y, Felson D. (1994) The overall and temporal association of cancer with polymyositis and dermatomyositis. *J Rheumatol* 21: 1855–9.
11. Sparsa A, Liozon E, Herrman F, et al. (2002) Routine vs extensive malignancy search for adult dermatomyositis and polymyositis. *Arch Dermatol* 138: 969–71.
12. Targoff IN. (2002) Laboratory testing in the diagnosis and management of idiopathic inflammatory myopathies. *Rheum Dis Clin North Am* 28: 859–90.
13. Park JH, Olsen NJ. (2001) Utility of magnetic resonance imaging in the evaluation of patients with inflammatory myopathies. *Curr Rheumatol Rep* 3: 334–5.
14. Miller FW. (1993) Myositis-specific autoantibodies: touchstones for understanding the inflammatory myopathies. *JAMA* 270: 1846–9.
15. Cordeiro AC, Isenberg DA. (2006) Treatment of inflammatory myopathies. *Postgrad Med J* 82; 417–24.

TABLE 29.2. Diagnostic criteria for PM (7).

Criterium	Definite	Probable
Myopathic muscle weakness	Yes	Yes
Electromyographic findings	Myopathic	Myopathic
Muscle enzymes	High (up to 50-fold normal)	High (up to 50-fold normal)
Muscle-biopsy findings	Primary inflammation, with the CD8/MHC-1 complex and no vacuoles	Ubiquitous MHC-1, but no CD8+ infiltrates or vacuoles
Rash or calcinosis	Absent	Absent

30
Dermatomyositis

Andrea Doria, Chiara Briani, Anna Ghirardello, Sandra Zampieri, Piercarlo Sarzi-Puttini and Riccardo Rondinone

Abstract   Dermatomyositis (DM) is an acquired disease, characterized by complement-mediated microangiopathy which results in an inflammatory infiltrate primarily affecting skin and muscle. The major clinical manifestations are proximal muscle weakness and skin rash. However, articular, esophageal, and pulmonary manifestations may coexist. The increase of muscle enzymes, particularly creatine kinase (CK), and characteristic electromyographic and histopathologic findings are the prominent laboratory features. Bohan and Peter's diagnostic criteria, proposed in 1975, have been widely accepted and used until now. However, muscle immunopathology, myositis-specific autoantibodies testing, and the use of muscle ultrasound (US) or Magnetic Resonance Imaging (MRI) have been recently introduced in the diagnostic work-up of patients with myositis. Although the role of these new investigations in diagnosing DM is still to be fully elucidated, they may assist clinicians in the management of difficult cases increasing the diagnostic accuracy of the old criteria.

Keywords   Dermatomyositis · idiopathic inflammatory myopathies · cancer · connective tissue disease

Dermatomyositis (DM) is an idiopathic inflammatory myopathy (IIM) characterized by an inflammatory infiltrate primarily affecting the skeletal muscle and skin.

Polymyositis (PM) and inclusion body myositis (IBM) are the other two major categories of IIM. Although IIM might share some similarities, they have distinct clinical, histopathological, immunological, and pathogenetic features and it is crucial to distinguish the three disorders because they differ in prognosis and response to treatment.

Classification

According to Bohan and Peter (1, 2), DM can be subdivided into 4 groups: idiopathic DM, juvenile DM, DM associated with cancer, and DM associated with other connective tissue diseases. Other DM subsets have been subsequently identified (3, 4, 5), including amyopathic DM (ADM), in which the disease affects only the skin; hypomyopathic DM, in which cutaneous manifestations of DM are associated with subclinical evidence of myositis; post-myopathic DM, in which patients with previous classic DM present a recovery of the myositis, but skin rashes remain active; DM sine dermatitis, in which no rash is detected but the biopsy sample is typical for DM; and the last subset in which DM is drug induced (Table 30.1.).

TABLE 30.1. Classification of dermatomyositis.

1. Idiopathic DM
2. Juvenile DM
3. DM associated with cancer
4. DM associated with other connective tissue diseases
5. Amyopathic DM
6. Hypomyopathic DM
7. DM sine dermatitis
8. Drug-induced DM

DM: dermatomyositis.

Epidemiology

DM is the most common IIM in all age group; however, it is a rare disease. The reported incidence of DM and PM ranges between 2 and 8 new cases per 1,000,000 inhabitants per year with a prevalence between 5 and 11 cases per 100,000 individuals (4, 5). Hengstman GJ et al. suggested a latitude gradient with an increasing relative prevalence of DM along with geographical latitude in Europe (6). The cause of the gradient is unknown and both genetic and environmental factors may be involved. DM affects both children and adults with an overall female/male ratio of about 2:1. However, inside each subgroup of DM there are

From: Y. Shoenfeld et al. (eds.): *Diagnostic Criteria in Autoimmune Diseases*, DOI: 10.1007/978-1-60327-285-8_30,

sex-related differences: the female/male ratio is 1:1 in juvenile DM, 1:2 in cancer-associated DM, and 9:1 in the forms associated with other connective tissue diseases.

Pathogenesis

DM is a microangiopathy that affects skin and muscle, where early activation and deposition of complement causes lysis of endomysial capillaries and muscle ischemia (7). DM is commonly regarded as an autoimmune rheumatic disease; however, the causative autoantigen is yet to be identified. A recent study on a large population showed that African-American and European-American patients with DM shared the risk factor HLA-DRB1*0301, whereas these two ethnic groups differed regarding HLA risk for anti-Mi-2 antibodies which was DRB1*0302 in the former and DRB1*0701 in the latter group (8).

Clinical Manifestations

DM is primarily characterized by muscular and cutaneous manifestations (3, 4, 5). The main symptoms are weakness, affecting mainly the proximal muscles, and myalgias. The onset of DM may be acute (days) or insidious (several months), with patients complaining of increasing fatigue while rising from a chair, lifting their arms, climbing steps, combing their hair or hanging clothes. Distal muscles are involved late in DM. The extensor muscles of the neck may be involved, causing difficulty in holding up the head (head drop). In severe cases, the respiratory and oropharyngeal muscles are involved causing dysphagia and respiratory difficulties. In some cases, a lack of coordination of the swallowing muscles occurs which may lead to *ab ingestis* pneumonia. Myalgias are less frequent than muscular weakness, and, when present, accompany the weakness. The most common clinical signs are reduction of the muscular strength in the proximal muscles, contractures and, late in the course of the disease, muscular atrophy (40% of cases).

Skin manifestations sometimes accompany, but more often precede by several months or years the signs of muscle involvement (1, 3, 4, 5). A classification of skin manifestations observed in DM is reported in Table 30.2 (9). The most common and peculiar skin manifestations are (a) violaceous erythematous papules which may be observed on the extensor surface of metacarpophalangeal, proximal and distal interphalangeal joints (Gottron's sign), and, less frequently, on the elbows, knees, malleoli, and other bony prominences (Gottron's papules); (b) heliotrope rash, i.e. a purplish erythema of the eyelids, often associated with periorbital edema; (c) symmetrical macular violaceous erythema (photosensitive rash) overlying the face, neck, upper chest, and the extensor surface of the arms. Other cutaneous manifestations may also be observed, including

TABLE 30.2. Cutaneous manifestations of dermatomyositis.

Skin lesions pathognomonic of DM
1. Gottron's papules
2. Gottron's sign

Skin lesions highly characteristic of DM
1. Periorbital violaceous (heliotrope) erythema with or without associated edema of the eyelids and periorbital tissue.
2. Grossly visible periungual telangiectasia with or without dystrophic cuticles.
3. Symmetrical macular violaceous erythema overlying the dorsal aspect of the hands and fingers (where it can track the extensor tendon sheaths), extensor aspects of the arms and forearms, deltoids, posterior shoulders and neck (the shawl sign), V-area of anterior neck and upper chest, central aspect of the face and forehead.

Skin lesions compatible with DM
1. Poikiloderma atrophicans vasculare (poikilodermatomyositis)
2. Calcinosis cutis

DM: dermatomyositis.

periungual teleangiectasia with or without dystrophic cuticles, vasculitic skin manifestations consisting of subcutaneous nodules, erythema, periungual infarctions, and digital ulcers, calcifications in the subcutaneous tissues leading to subcutaneous painful hard nodules which can ulcerate the overlying skin with leakage of calcareous material, and Raynaud's phenomenon which is more common in patients with idiopathic DM and in DM associated with connective tissue diseases.

Arthralgias, interstitial lung disease, cardiac abnormalities, and renal involvement as a result of a persistent myoglobinuria or glomerulonephritis are other manifestations of DM (3, 4, 5).

In children, DM resembles the adult disease, except for more frequent subcutaneous calcifications, vasculitic skin changes, and extramuscular manifestations.

Patients with inflammatory myopathies have a higher risk of malignancy than the normal population. Cancer seems to be more common in patients with DM than in those with PM (3, 4, 5). In DM, it has been reported to occur in approximately 30% of cases with a higher occurrence in men and in old age (3, 4, 5).

Finally, DM can overlap with other connective tissue diseases, particularly systemic sclerosis.

Pathological Features

Histopathologically, in DM the inflammation is perivascular or in the interfascicular septae and around fascicles; the inflammatory infiltrate consists primarily of B cells, macrophages, and CD4+ cells (5, 7). Early in the inflammatory process, there is activation of the complement that leads to the formation and deposition of the C5b-C9 complement membrane attack complex (MAC) on or around the endomysial blood vessels, with consequent capillary necrosis, microinfarcts, inflammation, endofascicular hypoperfusion, and eventually perifascicular atrophy, which is the characteristic histological feature of DM. The skin lesions show perivascular inflammation with CD4-positive cells in the dermis; in chronic stages there is dilatation of superficial capillaries.

Laboratory Abnormalities

High serum levels of muscular enzymes are characteristic of the disease (5). The most sensitive muscle enzyme is serum creatine kinase (CK), which increases in the acute phase. Elevation in serum aldolase, lactate dehydrogenase (LDH), and aspartate and alanine aminotransferase (AST and ALT) may also occur. Myoglobin is a protein present in skeletal and cardiac muscle, but not in other tissues, whose blood concentration can rise during muscular diseases, and can also be present in the urine. During the active phases of the disease, serum inflammation indexes (erythrocyte sedimentation rate (ESR), C-reactive protein) may also be increased.

Serological Features

Anti-nuclear antibodies are detected in 50% of cases by indirect immunofluorescence and in 80% by ELISA. Traditionally, autoantibodies associated with IIM have been divided into myositis-specific autoantibodies (MSA) and myositis-associated autoantibodies (MAA), the latter occurring also in autoimmune diseases without myositis (10, 11, 12). MSA are present in 30–40% of patients with DM. Anti-Mi-2 antibodies are directed against a nuclear protein of 7 subunits, which is part of a protein complex involved in gene transcription (11). Anti-Mi-2 antibodies are present in 25% of patients with DM and seem to be associated with acute onset of disease, good prognosis, and good response to the therapy (10).

Autoantibodies directed against cytoplasmic aminoacyl tRNA synthetases, especially anti-hystidil-tRNA synthetase (anti-Jo-1) antibodies, are reported in 10–25% of patients with DM in association with pulmonary fibrosis (10, 12). Anti-SRP antibodies are occasionally observed in DM patients (10). A new antibody to a 155-kd antigen or Se antigen, which appears to be a marker of ADM, has been recently described (3). Finally, the most common MAA in DM is anti-Ro/SSA (10). When other MAA are detected, an overlap syndrome is suggested (10).

Electromyography

Like in other IIM, needle electromyography (EMG) shows increased spontaneous and insertional activity with fibrillation potential, complex repetitive discharges, positive sharp waves, small polyphasic motor units potentials (MUPs), and early recruitment. The amount of spontaneous activity reflects an ongoing disease activity. Late in the course of the disease, insertional activity may be decreased as a consequence of fibrosis. These abnormalities may be observed in 70–90% of patients; however, they are not specific because they can be detected in other muscular diseases.

Muscle Biopsy

Muscle biopsy is the gold standard in the diagnosis of IIM and is indicated before the beginning of treatment. Generally, the biopsy is performed in the proximal muscles of the legs, choosing areas with active muscle involvement. The characteristic histological findings were reported earlier under the section Pathological Features.

Muscle Magnetic Resonance Imaging (MRI)

MRI represents the gold standard of the imaging study of muscle diseases, providing a detailed anatomic view of the extent of muscle damage. In DM, T2-weighted images and short-tau inversion recovery (STIR) show symmetric alterations with edematous aspects, particularly in the musculature close to the limbs which correlate very well with the disease activity (4).

Muscular Ultrasound

Muscular Ultrasound (US), although still not widely used, is a promising noninvasive method which seems to have a high sensitivity in the diagnosis of myositis (4). In DM, the acute inflammatory aspects, revealed by US hypoechogenicity, prevail on muscular hypotrophy/atrophy characteristic of chronic forms and are shown by US hyperechogenicity.

Diagnostic Criteria

The diagnosis of DM is based on the presence of characteristic skin manifestations associated with inflammatory myopathy. Skin manifestations are recognized by physical examination and they do not usually require histological confirmation. Inflammatory myopathy is suspected on the basis of clinical features and confirmed by laboratory tests, including high serum muscle enzyme concentration, electromyography and muscle biopsy abnormalities. More recently, autoantibodies (MSA and MAA), muscle MRI, and US have been introduced in the diagnostic work-up of patients with IIM. However, the role of these new investigations in the diagnosis of DM has not yet been clarified.

Several diagnostic criteria for IIM have been proposed; however, none of them has been properly validated. Bohan and Peter criteria (1, 2) have been widely accepted and used till now. They include four muscular criteria (symmetric proximal muscle weakness, serum elevation of skeletal-muscle enzymes, the classic EMG and muscle-biopsy abnormalities of inflammatory myopathy) and one cutaneous criterion, i.e. the typical skin rashes of DM (Table 30.3.). According to these criteria, the diagnosis of PM is considered definite, probable, and possible in presence of 4, 3, or 2 muscular criteria, respectively, whereas the diagnosis of DM is considered definite, probable, and possible when skin rash is associated with 3, 2, or 1 muscular criteria, respectively. It is worthy to note that these criteria incorporate exclusion of other diagnosis. The Bohan and Peter criteria showed high sensitivity when tested in patients with PM and DM, and high specificity when tested against patients with other connective tissue diseases. However, their specificity has never been evaluated in patients with neuromuscular conditions which may mimic IIM. One of the major criticisms addressed to Bohan and Peter criteria was that they cannot distinguish PM from IBM or other myopathies, particularly dystrophies (5), leading to misdiagnosis and inappropriate therapy. Therefore, in order to increase the specificity of Bohan and Peter criteria, it has been suggested to add MSA and muscle RMN findings (13). Because the advances in muscle immunopathology now let us to discriminate among the different inflammatory myopathies, Dalakas and Hohfeld have recently proposed muscle biopsy–based diagnostic criteria (4). One of the most interesting aspects of these new criteria is to have emphasized the role of the MHC-1/CD8 complex as a specific marker in differentiating PM and IBM from other muscular diseases,

TABLE 30.3. Bohan and Peter diagnostic criteria for dermatomyositis (Ref. 1, 2).

1) Symmetric proximal muscle weakness determined by physical examination
2) Elevation of serum skeletal muscle enzymes, including CK, aldolase, serum glutamate oxaloacetate and pyruvate transaminases, and lactate dehydrogenase
3) The electromyographic triad of short, small, polyphasic motor unit potentials; fibrillations, positive sharp waves, and insertional irritability; and bizarre, high-frequency repetitive discharges
4) Muscle biopsy abnormalities of degeneration, regeneration, necrosis, phagocytosis, and an interstitial mononuclear infiltrate
5) Typical skin rash of DM. Including a heliotrope rash and Gottron's sign/papules

The diagnosis of DM is considered definite, probable, and possible when skin rash is associated with 3, 2, or 1 muscular criteria, respectively.
Exclusion criteria: central or peripheral neurologic diseases, muscular dystrophies, granulomatous and infectious myositis, metabolic and endocrine myopathies, and myastenia gravis.

TABLE 30.4. Dalakas and Hohlfeld diagnostic criteria for dermatomyositis (Ref. 5).

Criterion	Myopathic DM		Amyopathic DM
	Definite	Probable	Definite
Myopathic muscle weakness	Yes	Yes	.No
Serum skeletal muscle enzymes	High or normal	High	High or normal
Electromyographic findings	Myopathic	Myopathic	Myopathic or non-specific
Muscle biopsy abnormalities	Perifascicular, perimysial or perivascular infiltrates; perifascicular atrophy		Non-specific or diagnostic for DM
Rash or calcinosis	Present	Not detected	Present

DM: dermatomyositis.

particularly dystrophies. According to these criteria (Table 30.4), the diagnosis of DM is definite if myopathy is accompanied by characteristic rash and histopathology. If no rash is detected but the biopsy sample is typical for DM, the diagnosis is probable. Finally, if the typical DM rash is present but muscle weakness is not apparent, the clinical diagnosis is ADM. This classification was also criticized because of a low sensitivity of some items leading to non-diagnostic muscle biopsy in some patients with myositis. The major concerns were: the pathogenesis of myositis is patchy, the reading of the biopsies is subjective, and the specialized immunopathology testing for CD8 and MHC-1 is not widely available (14). It has also been argued that biopsy abnormalities characteristic of PM and DM are nonspecific (except for perifascicular atrophy) and do not clearly distinguish PM from DM or any myopathy with necrosis, including IBM and muscular dystrophies (15, 16). Even the MHC-1/CD8 complex is not pathognomonic of PM because it was occasionally seen in patients with IBM and dystrophies (15, 16). However, a muscle biopsy–based diagnostic criteria SEEM to be less useful for the diagnosis of DM than for PM or IBM. In fact, in DM skin manifestations, including Gottron's papules and sign and heliotrope rash are very specific features, making the histological diagnosis not always necessary.

A new classification of IIM based on overlap syndrome features and autoantibodies (MSA and MAA) has been proposed. This classification was tested in patients affected with IIM according to Bohan and Peter criteria and seems to be more accurate in dividing patients into IIM subcategories, particularly in distinguishing patients with PM or DM from those with myositis associated with overlap syndrome (17).

The International Myositis Assessement and Clinical Study Group (IMACS)—a multidisciplinary coalition of more than 100 experts in adult and juvenile IIM—has recently tried to develop a consensus on these issues (18). Both adult and pediatric specialists agreed that probable

TABLE 30.5. Proposed minimal set of hallmark cutaneous manifestations of DM for the purpose of defining amyopathic DM for future clinical studies.

Major cutaneous criteria:
- "Heliotrope rash"
- Gottron's papules
- Gottron's sign of DM

Minor cutaneous criteria
- Macular violaceous erythema (with or without associated scale/hyperkeratosis, pigmentary change, and/or telangiectasia) involving:
  - Scalp and/or anterior hairline
  - Malar eminences of face and/or forehead and/or chin
  - V-area of neck and/or upper chest (open collar area; V-sign)
  - Nape of the neck and/or posterior aspects of shoulders (shawl sign)
  - Extensor surfaces of the arms and/or forearms
  - Linear streaking overlying extensor tendons of the dorsal aspects of the hands
  - Periungual areas
  - Lateral surface of thighs and/or hips
  - Medial malleoli

  (Involvement of each of the above anatomical region qualifies as a single minor criterion)
- Periungual nailfold telangiectasia and/or cuticular hemorrhage/infarct and/or dystrophic cuticles
- Poikiloderma (concurrence of hyperpigmentation, hypopigmentation, telangiectasia, and superficial atrophy)
- Mechanic's hand lesions
- Cutaneous calcinosis
- Cutaneous ulcers
- Pruritus and/or cutaneous burning sensation

The hallmark cutaneous manifestations of DM will be presumed to be present if the following conditions are met: presence of two major criteria or one major criterion and two minor criteria (biopsy of at least one skin lesion should show changes consistent with cutaneous DM).

or definite PM and DM as defined by Bohan and Peter criteria are appropriate for enrolling patients into clinical trials. However, in order to rule out other forms of myopathies and to distinguish PM from IBM, abnormal biopsy results consistent with PM have been considered mandatory. Conversely, although experts concurred that Gottron's sign/papules or heliotrope rash alone would be sufficient to distinguish DM from PM or IBM, adult specialists were unable to reach a consensus on whether muscle biopsy has to be considered mandatory, and left this decision to the investigators of the individual clinical trials (for children, muscle biopsy criteria are not required when pathognomonic skin rashes are present).

Finally, the diagnosis of ADM has to be made when hallmark manifestations of classical DM persist for 6 months or longer with no clinical evidence of proximal muscle weakness and no serum muscle enzyme abnormalities, provided that they do not fulfill exclusion criteria, i.e. either the treatment with systemic immunosuppressive agents for two consecutive months or longer within the first six months after the skin disease onset, or the previous use of any drug capable of inducing isolated DM-like skin changes. This raised the question of the definition of "hallmark cutaneous manifestations of classical DM," and therefore a set of classification criteria has been proposed (Table 30.5) (19).

Prognosis

As DM is responsive to immunotherapy in most cases, the prognosis of the disease significantly improved after the introduction of steroids, immunosuppressants, and/or Intravenous Immunoglobulin (IV Ig). Early diagnosis and treatment are crucial for avoiding atrophic changes of the muscle with consequent loss of function. Mortality is mostly related to cardiopulmonary disease, malignancies, and infections.

Prediction

No disease predictive factors have been identified to date. Factors predictive of a bad prognosis are old age at onset, myositis severity, dysphagia, cardiac and pulmonary involvement, poor response to therapy, and the presence of malignancy (3). CK levels and the extent of muscular involvement at onset do not seem to be determinants for the prognosis.

Therapy

Corticosteroids remain the elective drugs for the treatment of DM (3, 4, 5). Starting therapy consists of prednisone 1–2 mg/Kg orally for 2–4 weeks, and then it should be gradually tapered to the lowest effective dosage. In some cases, IV methylprednisolone may be considered.

Among the immunosuppressants, methotrexate (7.5–20 mg/week), azathioprine (1.5–2.5 mg/kg/day), and cyclophosphamide (1–2 mg/kg/day orally or 0.75–1 g/m^2 intravenously per month for 5–6 months) are currently used (3, 4, 5, 20). In some cases, cyclosporine A (3–4 mg/kg/day) has also been reported to be efficacious alone or in association with other immunosuppressants. Emerging evidence points to the efficacy of different immunosuppressive agents (mycophenolate mofetil and tacrolimus), biological agents (tumor necrosis factor-TNF inhibitor and anti-CD20), and IV Ig (2 g/kg/month) (20).

The cutaneous manifestations of DM may be triggered or worsened by exposure to ultraviolet light and therefore the avoidance of excessive sun exposure and the use of sunscreens are required. Moreover, cutaneous manifestations may be controlled by the application of topical corticosteroids or the more recent class of calcineurin inhibitors, such as tacrolimus and pimecrolimus (3). Antimalarials, such as hydroxychloroquine sulfate or choroquine phosphate, may be used in patients with ADM and in resistant cases may be associated with quinacrine (3).

References

1. Bohan, A., and Peter, J.B. (1975) Polymyositis and dermatomyositis (first part). *N Engl J Med* **292**, 344–7.
2. Bohan, A., and Peter, J.B. (1975) Polymyositis and dermatomyositis (second part). *N Engl J Med* **292**, 403–7.
3. Callen, J.P., and Wortmann, R.L. (2006) Dermatomyositis. *Clin Dermatol* **24**, 363–73.
4. Briani, C., Doria, A., Sarzi-Puttini, P., and Dalakas, M.C. (2006) Update on idiopathic inflammatory myopathies. *Autoimmunity* **39**, 161–70.
5. Dalakas, M.C., and Hohlfeld. R. (2003) Polymyositis and dermatomyositis. *Lancet* **362**, 971–82.
6. Hengstman, G.J.D., van Venrooij, W.J., Vencovsky, J., Moutsopoulos, H.M., and van Engelen, B.G.M. (2000) The relative prevalence of dermatomyositis and polymyositis in Europe exhibits a latitudinal gradient. *Ann Rheum Dis* **59**, 141–2.
7. Dalakas, M.C. (1998) Molecular immunology and genetics of inflammatory muscle diseases. *Arch Neurol* **55**, 1509–12.
8. O'Hanlon, T.P., Rider, L.G., Mamyrova, G., et al. (2006) HLA Polymorphisms in African Americans with idiopathic inflammatory myopathy. Allelic profiles distinguish patients with different clinical phenotypes and myositis autoantibodies. *Arthritis Rheum* **3670**, 3681.
9. Euwer, R.L. and Sontheimer, R.D. (1994) Dermatologic aspects of myositis. *Curr Opin Rheumatol* **6**, 583–589.
10. Ghirardello, A., Zampieri, S., Tarricone, E., et al. (2006) Clinical implications of autoantibody screening in patients with autoimmune myositis. *Autoimmunity* **39**, 217–21.
11. Ghirardello, A., Zampieri, S., Iaccarino, L., Tarricone, E., Gambari, P.F., and Doria, A. (2005) Anti-MI-2 antibodies. *Autoimmunity* **38**, 79–83.
12. Zampieri, S., Ghirardello, A., Iaccarino, L., Tarricone, E., Gambari, P.F., and Doria, A. (2005) Anti-JO-1 antibodies. *Autoimmunity* **38**, 73–78.
13. Targoff, I.N., Miller, F.W., Medsger, T.A., and Oddis, C.V. (1997) Classification criteria for idiopathic inflammatory myopathies. *Curr Opin Rheumatol* **9**, 527–35.
14. Miller, F.W., Rider, L.G., Plotz, P.H., Isenberg, D.A., and Oddis, C.V. (2003) Diagnostic criteria for polymyositis and dermatomyositis. *Lancet* **362**, 1762–3.
15. Amato, A.A., and Griggs, R.C. (2003) Unicorns, dragons, polymyositis, and other mythological beasts. *Neurology* **61**, 288–90.
16. Nirmalananthan, N., Holton, J.L., and Hanna, M.G. (2004) Is it really myositis? A consideration of the differential diagnosis. *Curr Opin Rheum* **16**, 684–91.
17. Troyanov, Y., Targoff, I.N., Tremblay, J.L., Goulet, J.R., Raymond, Y., and Senecal, J.L. (2005) Novel classification of idiopathic inflammatory myopathies based on overlap syndrome features and autoantibodies: analysis of 100 French Canadian patients. *Medicine* **84**, 231–49.
18. Oddis, C.V., Rider, L.G., Reed, A.M., Ruperto, N., Brunner, H.I., Koneru, B., Feldman, B.M., Giannini, E.H., and Miller, F.W., International Myositis Assessment and clinical Studies Group. (2005) International consensus guidelines for trials of therapies in Idiopathic Inflammatory myopathies. *Arthritis Rheum* **52**, 2607–15.
19. Sontheimer, R.D. (2002) Dermatomyositis. An overview of recent progress with emphasis on dermatological aspects. *Dermatol Clin* **20**, 387–408.
20. Choy, E., Hoogendijk, J., Lecky, B., and Winer, J. (2005) Immunosuppressant and immunomodulatory treatment for dermatomyositis and polymyositis. *Cochrane Database Syst Rev* **20** CD003643.

31
Clinically Amyopathic Dermatomyositis

Richard D. Sontheimer, Pedram Gerami and Hobart W. Walling

Abstract   There has been increased interest recently in the concept of dermatomyositis (DM) skin disease occurring for unusually long periods (<6 months) without the development of muscle weakness (i.e., amyopathic DM [syn. DM sine myositis]). This interest has been heightened by the realization that adult-onset clinically amyopathic DM (CADM) and classic DM patients might have similar levels of risk for systemic complications such as interstitial lung disease and internal malignancy. Contrastingly, in juvenile-onset CADM, patients might have a significantly lower risk of the complications of severe calcinosis and cutaneous vasculitis compared with those with juvenile-onset classical DM. This chapter will provide an overview of the diagnostic criteria for CADM, a comparison of the clinical and laboratory features of CADM and classical DM, and a discussion of management issues of DM skin disease including topical and systemic therapy.

Keywords   Dermatomyositis · amyopathic · hypomyopathic · sine myositis

Description of the Disease

Over the past 15 years, there has been a widening interest within the dermatology community in the concept of DM skin disease occurring for unusually long periods of time without the development of muscle weakness (i.e., DM sine myositis). This interest was sparked in part by the renaming of DM sine myositis as "amyopathic DM"[1] in order to direct attention to the need for more work in this area (1). The concept of "amyopathic DM" then evolved into one of "clinically- amyopathic DM" (CADM) (see Table 31.1 for definitions) (2). Our recent work in this area has demonstrated that there are important similarities and differences in CADM patients relative to classic DM patients. Importantly, adult-onset CADM and classic DM patients might have a similar risk for systemic complications such as interstitial lung disease and internal malignancy. Contrastingly, in juvenile-onset CADM, patients might have a signifi-

cantly lower risk of the complications of severe calcinosis and cutaneous vasculitis compared with patients with juvenile-onset classical DM (3, 4).

Further interest in CADM has developed as a result of the realization that it is not as rare as previously thought. Before 1990, DM sine myositis was thought to be an extremely rare entity as reflected by the fact that there was virtually no written record of it in the medical literature. In the early 1990s, amyopathic DM was estimated to account for 10–20% of the DM patients seen in Dermatology clinics at USA academic healthcare centers. Today, CADM patients are recognized to account for even higher percentages of the DM patients.

The authors of this chapter have recently presented systematic reviews of the published literature on adult-onset CADM (5) and juvenile onset CADM (3). This chapter will summarize these and related efforts to better understand the clinical and prognostic significance of CADM.

Diagnostic Criteria

The definitions of amyopathic DM and CADM, as presented in Table 31.1, hinge upon the presence of the hallmark inflammatory cutaneous manifestations of DM.

---

[1] A designation originally coined by the rheumatologist, Carl M. Pearson, M.D. who was a highly visible leader in the field of DM/PM research in the United States during the second half of the 20th century.

From: Y. Shoenfeld et al. (eds.): *Diagnostic Criteria in Autoimmune Diseases*, DOI: 10.1007/978-1-60327-285-8_31,
© 2008 Humana Press, Totowa, NJ

TABLE 31.1. Definitions of terms relating to cutaneous DM.[a]

Terms(abbreviation)	Definitions
Amyopathic DM (ADM)[b]	A subset of DM patients characterized by biopsy-confirmed hallmark cutaneous manifestations of classical DM occurring for 6 months or longer with no clinical evidence of proximal muscle weakness and no serum muscle enzyme abnormalities. If more extensive muscle testing is carried out, the results should be within normal limits (if such results are positive/abnormal, the patient can be classified as having "hypomyopathic dermatomyositis" [see below]). Exclusion criteria for amyopathic DM include: 1. Treatment with systemic immunosuppressive therapy for two consecutive months or longer within the first six months after skin disease onset (such therapy could prevent the development of clinically significant myositis). 2. Use of drugs known to be capable of producing isolated DM-like skin changes (e.g., hydroxyurea) at the onset of cutaneous changes.
Classical DM (CDM)[b]	Patients having the hallmark cutaneous manifestations of DM, proximal muscle weakness, and objective evidence of muscle inflammation characteristic of DM.
Clinically-amyopathic DM (CADM)[b]	An umbrella designation used to refer to amyopathic DM and/or hypomyopathic DM patients as defined here (i.e., clinically amyopathic DM = amyopathic DM + hypomyopathic DM). This designation was coined to emphasize the fact that the predominant _clinical_ problem is skin disease in patients so affected.
Clinically amyopathic DM evolving into classical DM (CADM → CDM)[b]	A working designation for those individuals in whom the onset of clinically significant muscle disease (i.e., weakness) appears _greater than_ 6 months after an initial disease presentation as CADM.
Cutaneous DM	A clinicopathological pattern of skin change seen only in DM (syn. hallmark cutaneous lesions of DM).
DM siné myositis[b]	A term of primarily historical significance that is synonymous with amyopathic DM.
Hallmark cutaneous lesions of DM	Skin lesions that alone or in combination are seen only in patients with some form of DM (syn. cutaneous DM)
Hypomyopathic DM[b]	Patients with cutaneous DM and no clinical evidence of muscle disease (i.e., weakness) that are found to have subclinical evidence of myositis upon laboratory, electrophysiological, and/or radiological evaluation.
Idiopathic inflammatory dermato-myopathies (IIDM)	A more inclusive umbrella designation proposed by one of the authors (RDS) for the spectrum of illness that is currently referred to conventionally as the "idiopathic inflammatory myopathies"
Idiopathic inflammatory myopathies (IIM)	The traditional umbrella designation for the spectrum of illness that results from characteristic clinicopathological patterns of autoimmune inflammatory injury of skin and skeletal muscles.
Premyopathic DM (PRPDM)[b]	A holding designation for patients having hallmark DM skin lesions without muscle weakness for _less than_ 6 months.

[a] Adapted from prior publication (2) with publisher's permission.
[b] Each of the indicated DM clinical subgroups can be subcategorized according to age of onset, i.e., adult-onset clinically amyopathic DM and juvenile-onset clinically amyopathic DM.

Experienced dermatologists and rheumatologists have little difficulty in recognizing these hallmark skin changes of DM and distinguishing them from cutaneous manifestations of related disorders such as lupus erythematosus (LE). However, it is curious that the minimal set of individual DM skin changes that must be present in order to justify a diagnosis of cutaneous DM (syn. DM-specific skin disease) has never been agreed upon. One of the authors of this chapter (RDS) previously proposed an approach to identifying a minimal set of hallmark cutaneous manifestations of DM for defining amyopathic DM for research studies (4) (Table 31.2). However, to date there has been no formal effort to test and validate this approach.

Some clinicians, including the authors of this chapter, feel that some of the individual hallmark skin changes of DM are pathognomonic of this illness (e.g. the concurrent presence of Göttron papules and periungual/nail fold telangectasia) while others are highly characteristic (eg,

periorbital heliotrope erythema, Göttron's sign). It is this diagnostic certainty of the hallmark skin lesions of DM with characteristic histologic changes that has led to the concept of DM skin disease existing in some individuals for long periods of time as isolated clinical entities (i.e. amyopathic DM and hypomyopathic DM).

The early definition of amyopathic DM was the presence of biopsy-confirmed hallmark skin changes of DM for 6 months or longer without clinical evidence of proximal muscle weakness or muscle enzyme abnormalities (6). This definition was subsequently criticized by others on the basis that had more extensive muscle testing been carried out in such patients not exhibiting weakness (e.g., electromyography [EMG], muscle biopsy, magnetic resonance imaging, muscle spectroscopy, muscle ultrasonography), subclinical evidence of myositis might be identified. And in fact that is the case in some patients. This resulted in the addition of the term "hypomyopathic DM" to the DM lexicon and the coining of the umbrella designation

TABLE 31.2. A proposed minimal set of hallmark cutaneous manifestations of DM needed for defining amyopathic DM for future clinical studies.[a]

For this purpose, the hallmark cutaneous manifestations of DM will be presumed to be present if the following conditions are met: Presence of two major criteria or one major criterion and two minor criteria. (A biopsy of at least one skin lesion should show changes consistent with cutaneous DM.)

➤**Major cutaneous criteria:**

■ Heliotrope erythema

Macular violaceous erythema with or without associated scale of the eyelids and/or periorbital skin. Secondary or associated cutaneous findings such as scale, pigmentary change, telangiectasia and/or edema can also be present.

■ Gottron's papules

Violaceous papules or small plaques overlying the dorsal or dorsal-lateral aspects of interphalangeal and/or metacarpophalangeal joints. When fully formed, these papules become slightly depressed at the center which can assume a white, lacy appearance. Associated scale/hyperkeratosis, pigmentary change, and/or telangiectasia may be present.

■ Gottron's sign

Macular violaceous erythema with or without associated scale/hyperkeratosis, pigmentary change, and/or telangiectasia involving extensor aspects of the knuckles and/or elbows and/or knees and/or medial malleoli.

➤**Minor cutaneous criteria:**

■ Macular violaceous erythema (with or without associated scale/hyperkeratosis, pigmentary change, and/or telangiectasia) involving:
  • Scalp and/or anterior hairline
  • Malar eminences of face and/or forehead and/or chin
  • V-area of neck and/or upper chest (open collar area; V-sign)
  • Nape of the neck and/or posterior aspect of shoulders (shawl sign)
  • Extensor surfaces of the arms and/or forearms
  • Linear streaking overlying extensor tendons on the dorsal aspects of the hands
  • Periungual areas
  • Lateral surface of thighs and/or hips (holster sign)
  • Medial malleoli

(involvement of each above-mentioned anatomical region qualifies as a single minor criterion)

■ Periungual nailfold telangiectasia and/or cuticular hemorrhage/infarct and/or dystrophic cuticles

■ Poikiloderma (concurrence of hyperpigmentation, hypopigmentation, telangiectasia, and superficial atrophy)

■ Mechanic's hand lesions

■ Cutaneous calcinosis

■ Cutaneous ulcers

■ Pruritus

[a] This criteria set was originally presented and discussed at the Third Annual Meeting of the Medical Dermatology Society in San Francisco on March 20th, 1997.
Table reprinted here from prior publication (4) with the publisher's permission.

"CADM" to emphasize the fact that while hypomyopathic DM patients might have abnormalities on muscle testing their only clinically manifest problem is DM-specific skin disease for extended periods of time. It might be presumed that patients with hypomyopathic DM would be at high risk for subsequently developing frank muscle weakness due to myositis. However, to date this has not been found to be the case (5, 3). In fact in our extensive review of the literature, patients with HDM often continued to be asymptomatic after prolonged periods of follow-up.

Tools for Assessing Cutaneous Disease Activity and Injury

Progress in better understanding the clinical significance and optimal management of DM skin disease has been hindered by the absence of validated tools for assessing changes in skin disease activity and injury. Werth and coworkers have recently begun to address this issue by developing the Cutaneous Dermatomyositis Disease Area and Severity Index (CDASI) (7).

This instrument was patterned after the Cutaneous Lupus Activity and Severity Index (CLASI), which has been shown to be a valid and reproducible measure of cutaneous LE disease activity and injury (8). The CDASI was recently compared with two other preliminary indices relating to dermatomyositis skin disease activity, the DM Skin Severity Index (DSSI), and the DM Cutaneous Assessment Tool (CAT). In a systemic comparison of these three instruments by 10 dermatologists in 16 DM patients, the CDASI was found to be the optimal outcome measure for studies of cutaneous DM (7). Validated instruments such as these that reproducibly measure changes in DM skin disease activity and injury over time provide a new outcome measure for future clinical trials of DM.

Comparison of Features in CADM and Classical DM

Table 31.3 presents a comparison of the signs and symptoms of CADM patients to those with classical DM. A comparison of laboratory findings of CADM patient to those of classical DM patients is presented in Table 31.4.

Can the Course of the Disease be Predicted?

CADM is currently a clinical diagnosis supported by cutaneous histopathological findings (the clinical and histopathological manifestations of CADM are indistinguishable from those of classical DM). As such, there is currently no way to predict the initial appearance of CADM. Preliminary studies have suggested that individuals who develop CADM might have an immunogenetic predisposition that is different from that of patients with classical DM. However, the predictive value of several autoantibody specificities that have been suggested in preliminary studies to be associated with CADM (eg, 155 kDa, 140 kDa, Se) (9, 10) has yet to be determined.

TABLE 31.3. Comparison of signs and symptoms (numerals represent %).

	CADM[a]		Classical DM[b]	
	Adult-onset	Juvenile-onset	Adult-onset	Juvenile-onset
Hallmark skin lesions	100[c]	100[c]	100[c]	100[c]
Clinically evident muscle weakness	0[c]	0[c]	100[c,d]	100[c,d]
Male/female ratio	27/73	8/9	1/2	1/2
Interstitial lung disease	13	0	10–40	rare
Risk of internal malignancy	14	NS[e]	20	NS
Calcinosis cutis	Rare	4	20[f]	50[f]
Pruritus	Frequent	Frequent	Frequent	Frequent
Photosensitivity	NR	NR	30–50	NR
Late onset weakness (>6 mos)	13	26	NA[g]	NA
Cutaneous vasculopathy	0	0	10[f]	20[f]

[a] Data from references (5, 3).
[b] Consensus values from general rheumatology and dermatology literature.
[c] By definition.
[d] The Bohan and Peter classification of DM requires the presence of the hallmark DM rash plus one or more of the following criteria: (a) symmetric muscle weakness, (b) muscle biopsy evidence of myositis, (c) elevation of muscle enzymes, and (d) electromyographic evidence of myositis. (Definite DM—three of the four criteria plus rash; probable DM—two of the criteria plus rash; possible DM—one criterion plus rash.) Thus, it is theoretically possible to make a diagnosis of classical DM without the presence of muscle weakness. However, it has been the authors' experience that many modern rheumatologists would probably question the diagnosis of DM in the absence of a typical pattern of symmetrical muscle weakness. Therefore, CADM patients have traditionally been excluded from modern epidemiological studies of DM performed outside of Dermatology.
[e] Not significantly elevated.
[f] Rates dependent upon length of period of observation.
[g] Not applicable.

Therapy and Prevention

When possible, the hallmark inflammation skin changes of cutaneous DM should be managed with sun avoidance and sun protection including the use of broad-spectrum, photostable sunscreen having a sun protection factor of 30 or more. Local therapy should begin with topical corticosteroids and topical antipruritics. Typically, stronger topical corticosteroid preparations (class I-II) are required. Solution, spray, or foam-based corticosteroid preparations are best for pruritic scalp involvement while creams, ointments, and gels are best for other areas of the body. Nonsteroidal topical immunomodulators such as tacrolimus ointment and pimecrolimus cream can be used in steroid-sensitive areas such as the periocular tissue, face, and intertriginous areas.

However, most patients with active cutaneous DM will require some form of systemic therapy to control the

TABLE 31.4. Laboratory findings in CADM and classical DM (numerals represent %).

	CADM		Classical DM	
	Adult-onset	Juvenile-onset	Adult-onset	Juvenile-onset
Elevated creatine kinase	38[a]	33	85	85
Elevated ESR[b]	25	22	50	50
Autoantibodies				
ANA	63	53	40–60	50–80
Jo-1	4	0	20	5
Mi-2	NR[c]	NR	15	5
140 kD	100[d]	NR	15[d]	NR
155 kD	74[e]	NR	21[d]	29[d]
Se	60[e]	NR	NR	NR

[a] By definition, all patients with amyopathic DM have normal muscle enzymes. In our systematic reviews of the CADM patients having the hypomyopathic DM subphenotype, 14 of 37 (38%) adult-onset patients and 1 of 3 (33%) juvenile-onset patients had elevated creatine kinase levels.
[b] Erythrocyte sedimentation rate.
[c] Not reported.
[d] Single unconfirmed report.
[e] Unconfirmed preliminary observation (9).

inflammation and pruritus (11). Systemic corticosteroids when indicated for systemic disease activity such as myositis or interstitial lung disease can be of benefit for the cutaneous inflammation. However, because of associated adverse effects, long-term systemic corticosteroids should not be relied upon when treating isolated DM skin disease. Other agents that can be of benefit include single-agent or combination therapy with the aminoquinoline antimalarials (hydroxychloroquine, chloroquine, quinacrine). In addition, Dapsone can provide a steroid-sparing effect for cutaneous DM activity in patients with mild to limited forms of skin disease. Oral therapy with long-acting, non-sedating antihistamines during the day (e.g. cetirizine, fexofenadine) and long-acting sedating antihistamines during the evening (doxepin) can also provide symptomatic benefit while trying to control the active inflammation with the above-mentioned immunomodulatory agents.

Some patients with widespread, highly symptomatic, refractory forms of cutaneous DM can experience psychosocial and occupational disability unless the skin disease activity is controlled. Such patients might require traditional systemic immunomodulatory therapy with agents such as high-dose intravenous immunoglobulin, methotrexate, azathioprine, and/or mycophenolate mofetil. Anecdotal evidence would suggest that different classes of recombinant biological immunomodulators might also be of benefit for refractory cutaneous DM (e.g., TNF-alpha inhibitors—etanercept, infliximab, adalimumab; memory B-cell depleters—retuximab; costimulatory pathway inhibitors—efalizumab).

There was an initial current of thought that early aggressive systemic therapy of CADM patients might prevent the subsequent delayed development of clinically significant muscle weakness. However, the preponderance of the published data to date addressing this issue would suggest that this is not the case and that both adult-onset and juvenile-onset CADM patients should be managed conservatively with symptomatic measures and carefully observed for the appearance of any systemic manifestations/associations of DM (muscle weakness, interstitial lung disease, internal malignancy) (5, 3). This is particularly important because juvenile CADM patients do not typically develop the severe degree of calcinosis or vasculitis that is characteristic of juvenile classic DM. At the outset of their illness, adult-onset CADM patients like adult-onset classical DM patients should undergo a careful surveillance examination for associated internal malignancy. Such exams should be repeated every 6–12 months for several years after the initial presentation of DM.

Acknowledgments. Dr. Sontheimer's contributions to the preparation of this work was supported by The Richard and Adeline Fleischaker Chair in Dermatology Research at the University of Oklahoma Health Sciences Center.

References

1. Euwer RL, Sontheimer RD. Amyopathic dermatomyositis (dermatomyositis siné myositis). Presentation of six new cases and review of the literature. J Am Acad Dermatol 1991; 24:959–966.
2. Sontheimer RD. Would a new name hasten the acceptance of clinically-amyopathic dermatomyositis (dermatomyositis sine myositis) as a distinctive subset within the idiopathic inflammatory dermatomyopathies spectrum of clinical illness? J Am Acad Dermatol 2002; 46:626–636.
3. Gerami P, Walling H, Lewis J, Doughty L, Sontheimer RD. A systematic review of juvenile-onset clinically-amyopathic dermatomyositis. Brit J Dermatol 2007; 157:637–44.
4. Sontheimer RD. Dermatomyositis: An overview of issues of interest to dermatologists[Review]. Dermatologic Clin 2002; 20(3):387–408.
5. Gerami P, Schope JM, McDonald L, Walling HW, Sontheimer RD. A systematic review of adult-onset clinically amyopathic dermatomyositis (dermatomyositis sine myositis): a missing link within the spectrum of the idiopathic inflammatory myopathies. J Am Acad Dermatol 2006; 54(4):597–613.
6. Euwer RL, Sontheimer RD. Amyopathic dermatomyositis: A review. J Invest Dermatol 1993; 100:124S–127S.
7. Quain RD, Bangert CC, Costner MK et al. Comparison of the reliability and validity of outcome instruments for cutaneous dermatomyositis. J Invest Dermatol 127, S59. 2007.
8. Albrecht J, Taylor L, Berlin JA et al. The CLASI (Cutaneous Lupus Erythematosus Disease Area and Severity Index): An outcome instrument for cutaneous lupus erythematosus. J Invest Dermatol 2005; 125(5):889–894.
9. Targoff IN, Trieu EP, Sontheimer RD. Autoantibodies to 155 kD and Se autoantigens in patients with clinically-amyopathic dermatomyositis. Arthritis Rheum 43[Suppl. 9], S194. 2000.
10. Sato S, Hirakata M, Kuwana M et al. Autoantibodies to a 140-kd polypeptide, CADM-140, in Japanese patients with clinically amyopathic dermatomyositis. Arthritis Rheum 2005; 52(5):1571–1576.
11. Sontheimer RD. The management of dermatomyositis: current treatment options. Expert Opin Pharmacother 2004; 5(5):1083–1099.

32
Sporadic Inclusion Body Myositis

Josep M. Grau and Albert Selva-O'Callaghan

Abstract Sporadic inclusion body myositis (sIBM) is the most common acquired muscle disease in elderly individuals, particularly men. Its prevalence varies among ethnic groups, but it is estimated at 35 per one million people over 50 years. Genetic as well as environmental factors and autoimmune processes might both have a role in its pathogenesis. Unlike other inflammatory myopathies, sIBM causes very slowly progressive muscular weakness and atrophy. It has a distinctive pattern of muscle involvement and different forms of clinical presentation. In some cases a primary autoimmune disease coexists. Diagnosis is suspected on clinical grounds and is established by a typical muscle pathology. The rule for sIBM is its refractoriness to conventional forms of immunotherapy.

Keywords Inclusion body · myositis · myopathy · inflammation

Sporadic inclusion body myositis (sIBM) is one of the three main subsets of inflammatory myopathies, the other two being polymyositis and dermatomyositis. Although in all these conditions there are inflammation in the endomysium, muscle fiber necrosis, elevation of serum muscle enzymes, and varying degrees of muscle weakness, sIBM is often misdiagnosed as polymyositis. sIBM should be distinguished from hereditary inclusion body myopathies (hIBM) in which histologic and ultrastructural findings resemble those of sIBM with one clear exception: the absence of inflammation.

Epidemiology

The prevalence of sIBM is estimated at between 4.5 and 9.5 per one million rising to 35 per million for people over 50 years old. A number of discrepancies suggest that these numbers underestimate the true prevalence of this myopathy. On the basis of clinical reports from reference centers worldwide, it seems that sIBM is the most common acquired myopathy in patients above 50 years, affecting men slightly more frequently than women (1, 2).

History

In 1971, Yunis and Samaha coined the term IBM for the definition of a myopathy that clinically resembled a chronic polymyositis but was pathologically characterized by the presence of vacuoles containing cytoplasmic degradation products with fibrillary nuclear and cytoplasmic inclusions. A few years earlier, some authors had reported clinical cases suggestive of IBM. Since then, large series of patients have been described.

Pathogenesis

Although the underlying cause of sIBM is unclear, it seems that at least two processes might occur in parallel: a primary immune process because of T-cell-mediated cytotoxicity and a non-immune process characterized by vacuolization and intracellular accumulation of amyloid-related molecules probably because of MHC-class I-induced stress (2).

Recently, Choi et al. (3) demonstrated the elevated expression of transglutaminases 1 and 2 in the vacuoles of sIBM, co-localized with amyloid-related proteins. They suggest that these enzymes participate in the formation of insoluble amyloid deposits and may thereby contribute to progressive and debilitating muscle disease. This topic has recently been explored by Selva et al. (4) with interesting results. Genetic factors are presumed to play a role in sIBM based on an association between sIBM and certain human leukocyte antigen (HLA) genes, in particular HLA-DR3. This association is present in nearly 75% of the cases, but this figure may vary in different ethnic groups (2, 5, 6).

From: Y. Shoenfeld et al. (eds.): *Diagnostic Criteria in Autoimmune Diseases*, DOI: 10.1007/978-1-60327-285-8_32,
© 2008 Humana Press, Totowa, NJ

Clinical Manifestations

sIBM causes weakness and atrophy of the distal and proximal muscles, and involvement of the quadriceps and deep
finger flexors are clues to early diagnosis. The pattern is
sometimes asymmetric resembling a motor neuron disease.
Neck flexors and extensors are frequently affected. Heat
drop and camptocormia (selective atrophy and weakness
of paraspinal muscles) may occur, even as a form of clinical
presentation. Dysphagia occurs in up to 60% of patients
with sIBM and again may be the form of presentation in rare
cases. Sensory function is normal as well are tendon reflexes,
but they become diminished or absent as the atrophy of
major muscles occur. The clinical course is always chronic
or very chronic, lasting for years after the onset of symptoms
and the diagnosis of the disease. Disease progression is slow
but steady resembling that of a muscular dystrophy.

Differential Diagnosis

sIBM is often misdiagnosed as polymyositis or other diseases and is frequently only suspected retrospectively when
a patient with presumed polymyositis does not respond to
therapy. In a patient complaining of falls because of weakness at the knees and feet with atrophic thighs and without
paresthesias or cramps the most plausible diagnosis is
sIBM. Useful data regarding differential diagnoses are
summarized in Table 32.1.

Pathological Features

The common findings in muscle biopsy are perivascular
and endomisial inflammatory infiltrates of varying degrees,
rimmed vacuoles in atrophic fibers (Figure 32.1), the presence of partial cellular invasion by CD8 cells, frequent
cytochrome oxidase (COX)-negative cellules, amyloid
deposits, and the upregulation of MHC-class I antigens in
healthy muscle cells. Nuclear and/or cytoplasmic filamentous inclusions of 16–20 nm are seen in electron microscopy
examination (7) (Figure 32.2). On some occasions, an

TABLE 32.1. Differential diagnoses (prominent data
for each condition).

Motor neuron disease:
  Hyperreflexia, cramps, fasciculations
  Typical EMG
Polymyositis:
  Subacute (weeks to months)
  Proximal and symmetrical muscle weakness
  High CK levels
Vacuolar myopathies (myofibrillar myopathies, hIBM):
  Lack of inflammation, negative MHC-HLA-class I

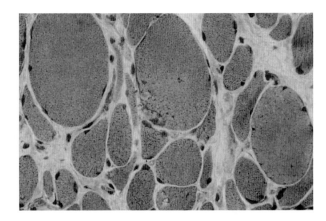

FIGURE 32.1. Rimmed vacuoles in two muscle fibers. Note also
the marked variability in fiber size and the excess of connective
tissue. Gomori's trichrome in frozen tissue.

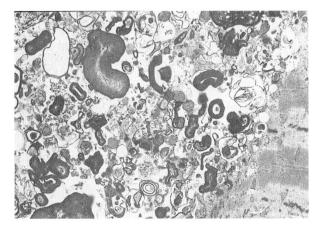

FIGURE 32.2. Cytoplasmic filamentous inclusions in a case of
sporadic inclusion body myositis (sIBM). Electron-microscopy.

additional muscle biopsy must be performed if pathological
changes are suggestive but not consistent.

Biochemical Features

Creatine kinase (CK) serum levels are moderately elevated
but can be normal. Unlike other inflammatory conditions,
acute phase reactants are normal in sIBM.

Serological Features

Different autoantibodies can be detected in a percentage of
sIBM patients. Antinuclear antibodies (20%), rheumatoid
factor (13%), anticardiolipin antibodies (10%), and anti-Ro
antibodies (10%) are the most frequently reported. In about
10% of the cases dysproteinemia can also be detected (8).

Associated Immune Disorders

Several autoimmune disorders have been reported in association with sIBM (2, 8, 9, 10), including pernicious anemia, dermatitis herpetiformis, psoriasis, Sjögren's syndrome, SLE, rheumatoid arthritis, common variable immunodeficiency, idiopathic thrombocytopenic purpura, Hashimoto's thyroiditis, dermatomyositis, and gluten sensitivity enteropathy. Unlike dermatomyositis, sIBM should not be considered as a paraneoplastic condition.

Diagnostic Criteria

The definite diagnostic procedure is a biopsy of the muscle. Although pathological features individually are all nonspecific and can also be seen in other myopathies and neurogenic disorders, their co-occurrence in the same biopsy allows the diagnosis of sIBM. Table 32.2 shows the proposed diagnostic criteria for sIBM. The criteria for diagnosis of sIBM were first proposed by Griggs et al. in 1995, with minor modifications in 2002 and were finally reviewed by Dalakas in 2007. Table 32.3 presents the diagnostic categories (definite, probable, and possible sIBM) (1, 2, 11).

Prognosis

The severity of the disease is poorly associated with the degree of inflammatory changes found in muscle biopsies, and although treatment with corticosteroids might reduce

TABLE 32.2. Proposed diagnostic criteria for sporadic inclusion body myositis.

Clinical features:
  Duration of illness >6 months
  Age at onset >30 years
  Slowly progressive muscle weakness and atrophy: selective pattern with early involvement of quadriceps femoris and finger flexors (frequently not symmetric)
  Dysphagia
Laboratory features:
  Serum CK levels might be high but can be normal
  EMG: myopathic or mixed patterns, with both short- and long-duration motor unit potentials and spontaneous activity
Muscle biopsy:
  Myofiber necrosis and regeneration
  Endomysial mononuclear cell infiltrate (in variable degree)
  mononuclear cell invasion of non-necrotic fibers (mainly CD8)
  MHC-class I expression in otherwise morphologically healthy muscle fibers
  Vacuolated muscle fibers (rimmed vacuoles)
  Ubiquitin-positive inclusions and amyloid deposits in muscle fibers
  Nuclear and/or cytoplasmic filamentous inclusions of 16–20 nm on electron microscopy
  COX-negative fibers

TABLE 32.3. Diagnostic categories.

Definite sporadic inclusion body myositis:
  Characteristic clinical features with biopsy confirmation: inflammatory myopathy with autoaggressive T cells, rimmed vacuoles, COX-negative fibers, amyloid deposits or filamentous inclusions, and upregulation of MHC-class I expression. With these pathological findings, the presence of other laboratory features are not mandatory.
  Atypical pattern of weakness and atrophy but with diagnostic biopsy features.
Probable sporadic inclusion body myositis:
  Characteristic clinical and laboratory findings but incomplete biopsy criteria (e.g., features of necrotizing inflammatory myopathy with T-cell invasion but absence of rimmed vacuoles, amyloid deposits, filamentous inclusions, and COX-negative fibers)
Possible sporadic inclusion body myositis:
  Atypical pattern of weakness and incomplete biopsy criteria

the inflammation, it does not stop the degenerative changes and has little or no effect on the degree of weakness. sIBM is a relentlessly progressive disorder: most patients requiring a walking aid after 5 years and the use of wheelchair by about 10 years. sIBM patients often die because of a complication of their debilitating progressive disease (aspirative pneumonia) or for an unrelated condition.

Therapy

Most patients do not respond to antiinflammatory, immunosuppressant, or immunomodulatory drugs currently available. Corticosteroids, cytotoxic drugs, intravenous immunoglobulins, antithymocyte globulin, and cytokine-based therapies have been used with poor results on follow-up (1, 2). A small proportion of patients do respond, at least initially, and this probably represents a subgroup in whom the disease is diagnosed early and/or is associated with a primary autoimmune condition (12). In some centers, an initial 3- to 6-month trial of prednisone and methotrexate or azathioprine is recommended.

Other empirical therapies such as coenzyme Q10, carnitine, and even statins have been used or are under investigation. Exercise therapy and orthotic appliances have confirmed their efficacy in stabilizing muscle strength and functional ability.

References

1. Needham M, Mastaglia FL. (2007) Inclusion body myositis: Current pathogenetic concepts and diagnostic and therapeutic approaches. *Lancet Neurol* 6: 620–31.
2. Dalakas MC. (2006) Sporadic inclusion body myositis. Diagnosis, pathogenesis and therapeutic strategies. *Nat Clin Pract Neurol* 2: 437–47.

3. Choi YC, Park GT, Kim TS, Sunwoo IN, Steinert PM, Kim SY. (2000) Sporadic inclusion body myositis correlates with increased expression and cross-linking by transglutaminases 1 and 2. *J Biol Chem* 275: 8703–10.

4. Selva A. Casellas F, de Torres I, Palou E, Grau JM, Vilardell M. (2007) Celiac disease and antibodies associated with celiac disease in patients with inflammatory myopathy. *Muscle Nerve* 35: 49–54.

5. Garlepp MJ, Laing B, Zilko PJ, Ollier W, Mastaglia FL. (1994) HLA associations with inclusion body myositis. *Clin Exp Immunol* 98: 40–5.

6. Jain A, Sharma MC, Sarkar C, Bhatia R, Singh S, Handa R. (2007) Major histocompatibility complex class I and II detection as a diagnostic tool in idiopathic inflammatory myopathies. *Arch Pathol Lab Med* 131(7): 1070–6.

7. Mendell JR, Sahenk Z, Gales T, Paul L. (1991) Amyloid filaments in inclusion body myositis: Novel findings provide insight into nature of filaments. *Arch Neurol* 48: 1229–34.

8. Koffman BM, Rugiero M, Dalakas MC. (1998) Immune-mediated conditions and antibodies associated with sporadic inclusion body myositis. *Muscle Nerve* 21: 115–7.

9. Bielsa S, Madroñero AB, Grau JM, Porcel JM. (2007) Inclusion-body myositis associated with systemic sclerosis. *Med Clin (Barc)* 128: 278.

10. Badrising UA, Schreuder GMT, Giphart MJ, et al. (2004) Associations with autoimmune disorders and HLA class I and II antigens in inclusion body myositis. *Neurology* 63: 2396–8.

11. Griggs RC, Askanas V, Di Mauro S, et al. (2005) Inclusion body myositis and myopathies. *Ann Neurol* 38: 705–13.

12. Quartuccio L, De Marchi G, Scott CA, Ferraciolini G, Beltrami CA, de Vita S. (2007) Treatment of inclusion body myositis with cyclosporin-A or tacrolimus: Successful long-term management in patients with earlier active disease and concomitant autoimmune features. *Clin Exp Rheumatol* 25(2): 246–51.

33
Antisynthetase Syndrome

Ira N. Targoff

Abstract   Autoantibodies to many of the aminoacyl-transfer RNA synthetases have been identified, the most common of which is directed at histidyl-tRNA synthetase (anti-Jo-1). Most individual patients have AuAbs to only one of these enzymes, but each autoantibody has been associated with a similar set of clinical manifestations including inflammatory myopathy, interstitial lung disease, arthritis, Raynaud's phenomenon, and mechanic's hands. The antisynthetases were first recognized as myositis, autoantibodies, and myositis is present in over 95% of anti-Jo-1 patients in most studies, but some patients have interstitial lung disease, or occasionally arthritis, without myositis, particularly those with certain of the non-Jo-1 antisynthetases. Clinically similar myositis and other connective tissue disease features can occur in association with other autoantibodies, but when associated with an antisynthetase autoantibody, it has been referred to as the antisynthetase syndrome. Patients often do not have all features of the syndrome. Although there are no defined criteria for this condition, patients with two major clinical features along with the autoantibody could reasonably be considered to have the syndrome. Identifying patients as having antisynthetases may be helpful in diagnosis, patient characterization, and patient management.

Keywords   Polymyositis · interstitial lung disease · autoantibodies

Introduction

The aminoacyl-tRNA synthetases (aaRS) are cellular enzymes that catalyze the binding of an amino acid to a corresponding transfer RNA. The amino acid can then be incorporated into a polypeptide chain at the ribosome. Each amino acid has a separate aaRS enzyme, which must be distinct enough to enable it to specifically recognize the amino acid and the transfer RNAs for that amino acid, in order to maintain the fidelity of the translation process. These enzymes are immunologically distinct; autoantibodies (AuAbs) to one of the enzymes generally do not cross-react with other aaRSs, and most patients with AuAbs to one of the enzymes do not have AuAbs to others, with occasional exceptions. However, the clinical pictures observed in association with each of the described anti-aaRS AuAbs have shared very significant similarities, leading to the use of the term "antisynthetase syndrome".

History

Anti-Jo-1 AuAbs, named for the prototype patient, were first described in 1980 using immunodiffusion against calf thymus extract, as the most common precipitin among patients with polymyositis (PM) (1). It was determined that anti-Jo-1 was directed against histidyl-tRNA synthetase when protein A-assisted immunoprecipitation showed the antigen to be a protein associated with a specific transfer RNA, identified as a transfer RNA for histidine, and that the AuAbs specifically inhibited the activity of the histidyl-tRNA synthetase but not other aaRSs (2). Subsequent reports confirmed the strong association of anti-Jo-1 with inflammatory myopathy in different populations, particularly clinical PM (3). In addition, early reports noted the marked increase in interstitial lung disease (ILD) in anti-Jo-1-positive compared with antibody-negative myositis, and later, an increase in other extra-muscular, connective tissue disease features was observed (Table 33.1) (4, 5). Shortly thereafter, two other AuAbs that immunoprecipitated different sets of transfer RNAs were shown by specific inhibition to be directed at threonyl-tRNA synthetase (anti-PL-7, for "precipitin line") and alanyl-tRNA synthetase (anti-PL-12) (5, 6). Three other antisynthetases have since been found by using similar methods of immunoprecipitation of proteins and transfer RNAs, and specific enzyme inhibition (autoantibodies to gly-RS, ile-RS, asn-RS (7, 8)), and later confirmed by demonstrating reaction with recombinant proteins and/or microsequencing techniques. A preliminary report identified AuAbs to

From: Y. Shoenfeld et al. (eds.): *Diagnostic Criteria in Autoimmune Diseases*, DOI: 10.1007/978-1-60327-285-8_33,
© 2008 Humana Press, Totowa, NJ

TABLE 33.1. Anti-synthetases autoantibodies.

Name	Antigen	Molecular weight (kDa)[a]	Test	Frequency (%)[b]	HLA[c]	Clinical	Comments (Ref)
Jo-1	Histidyl-tRNA synthetase -tRNA[his]	50	ID; IPP; WB; EIA	18–20 (6% for tRNA)	HLA-DR3 HLA-DQA1 *0501 or *0401	Myo(95); ILD(80); Arth(60); RP(60); MH(70); Fever	1) PM > DM 2) Adult > child 3) anti-tRNA only with anti-enzyme
PL-7	Threonyl-tRNA synthetase	80	ID; IPP; EIA	<3	HLA-DQA1 *0501 or *0401	(see Jo-1)	May have more DM than anti-Jo-1
PL-12	Alanyl-tRNA synthetase -tRNA[ala]	110	ID; IPP; EIA	<3 (<3 for tRNA)	(Similar to PL-7)	(see Jo-1; lower frequency myo, 60–80%- less in Japan)	Most anti-enzyme have anti-tRNA
OJ	Isoleucyl-tRNA synthetase Multi-enzyme complex	150 170 130 75	IPP; WB; AAI	<2 <1	(Similar to PL-7)	(see Jo-1; Lower freq myo)	Ile-RS usual main antigen; leu-RS, lys-RS can be seen with ile-RS
EJ	Glycyl-tRNA synthetase	75	IPP; WB	<2	(Similar to PL-7)	(see Jo-1)	More DM than anti-Jo-1
KS	Asparaginyl -tRNA synthesis	65	IPP	<2		(see Jo-1; less myo)	Some with only ILD
YRS	Tyrosyl-tRNA synthetase		IPP	<1		Myo + ILD	Single patient preliminary report
Zo	Phenylalanyl- tRNA synthetase		IPP	<2		Myo + ILD	Single patient report

[a] Molecular weight is that of subunits (His-tRNA synthetase is a dimer of 50 kDa subunits).

[b] Frequency is that in all myositis in most US studies. Percents are estimated from available studies and experience.

[c] In Japanese patients, anti-synthetases were associated with HLA-DQA*0102 and *0103.

Arth – arthritis; DM – dermatomyositis; EIA – enzyme immunoassay; Freq – frequency; ID – immunodiffusion; ILD – interstitial lung disease; IPP – immunoprecipitation; kDa – kilodaltons; MH – mechanic's hands; Myo – myositis; PM – polymyositis; RP – Raynaud's phenomenon; WB – Western immunoblotting. Adapted from Targoff IN. Laboratory testing in the diagnosis and management of idiopathic inflammatory myopathies. *Rheum Dis Clin North Am.* 2002; 28: 859–890.

tyrosyl tRNA synthetase using immunoprecipitation, enzyme inhibition, and mass spectrometry for microsequencing (9). Most recently, AuAbs reacting with phenylalanyl-tRNA synthetase were described, that immunoprecipitated the α and β components, which were independently identified by mass spectroscopy (10). Seven of these 8 antisynthetases were initially found in patients who had myositis, and anti-KS was later found in myositis patients (8). Each AuAb has also been seen in association with ILD (alone or with myositis).

Epidemiology

Several studies have found the frequency of anti-Jo-1 in adult inflammatory myopathy to be in the range of 20% (4, 11). Of the AuAbs considered to be relatively "myositis-specific" (MSAs), anti-Jo-1 has consistently been the most frequent overall. In most populations, the non-Jo-1 anti-synthetases are each individually, and usually collectively, much less frequent than anti-Jo-1. Each is usually present in <1%–5% of myositis patients. The relative frequency of the different non-Jo-1 anti-synthetases has varied in

different populations. Some studies suggest anti-EJ may be more common in Asian populations.

Clinical Manifestations

In most studies, myositis has been the most consistent and frequent clinical manifestation in anti-Jo-1 patients, usually present at some point in the course in the range of 95% (93–100%). Clinical PM, as defined by the Bohan and Peter criteria (see chapter on PM), is usually the most common form associated with anti-Jo-1 (3, 12), but typical dermatomyositis (DM) can occur, and in some studies can be as common (4). In some studies, groups with non-Jo-1 antisynthetases, such as anti-EJ, have had more DM than PM. Studies suggest that this also may vary with the population studied. Antisynthetases occasionally occur in juvenile myositis, but in a considerably smaller proportion than in adult myositis. There have been very rare reports in inclusion body myositis; in one reported case, the clinical course was more typical of PM (13). As compared to patients without the antibodies, the myositis of antisynthetase patients may be more likely to recur after initial suppression as treatment is withdrawn (4). No other clinical differences from antibody-negative myositis have been consistently observed.

Although the antisynthetases as a group are considered MSAs, the frequency of myositis with certain non-Jo-1 antisynthetases has been lower than with anti-Jo-1. With anti-PL-12, anti-KS, and anti-OJ, some studies have found ILD to be more frequent than myositis (7, 8). The observed relative frequency of myositis and ILD may be affected by referral patterns and by the clinical groups screened. There may also be differences between ethnic groups; the frequency of myositis with anti-PL-12 and anti-KS was lower in Japanese than in US patients (6, 8). ILD may be the most important extra-muscular feature of the syndrome because of prognostic and therapeutic implications. Some patients are asymptomatic or do not have progressive disease, but ILD may be severe, and acute respiratory distress syndrome has been observed. Almost all antisynthetase patients have myositis, ILD, or both. Arthritis is also common and can occasionally be the predominant manifestation. It is typically symmetrical, often involving fingers, wrists, and knees, and is usually non-erosive, although it can be deforming. An erosive form associated with calcinoses in the distal fingers has been observed. An increase in the frequency of Raynaud's phenomenon has been observed in some studies (4). A skin manifestation may occur, referred to as "mechanic's hands," marked by hyperkeratotic lines along the edges of the fingers (4). This is not specific for antisynthetase patients, and it can be seen with other AuAbs (anti-U1RNP and anti-PM-Scl). In general, the antisynthetases would be better considered specific for the antisynthetase syndrome than for myositis in particular.

Pathogenesis

A detailed pathologic picture has been described in patients with PM, marked by endomysial infiltration of lymphocytes with CD8$^+$-T cells that surround and invade non-necrotic muscle fibers. A different pattern was observed for DM, with perimysial inflammation, more prominent B cells, and vasculopathy with complement deposition and capillary loss. In the one study comparing the pathology of anti-Jo-1-associated myositis to that of antibody-negative PM and DM (14), neither pattern was observed. Infiltration tended to be perimysial as in DM, even in the absence of the DM rash. But the features of vasculopathy, complement deposition, and reduced capillary index, were not observed. Changes suggestive of fasciitis were observed that were not seen in most with PM or DM. These findings support considering antisynthetase patients as a separate syndrome, but further study is needed.

The role of antisynthetases in the pathogenesis of antisynthetase clinical manifestations is unknown. In a recent preliminary report, immunization of mice with Jo-1 antigen reproduced antisynthetase features. However, in another animal model, myositis was induced by expression of MHC Class I on muscle fibers, and some of the animals developed anti-Jo-1, suggesting the antibody was a secondary phenomenon not involved in pathogenesis. The relevance of either model to human disease is not yet clear. The recent observation that anti-Jo-1 levels can vary with disease activity (15), confirming previous reports, also suggests that antibody production is tied to fundamental disease mechanisms.

Relatively little information is available about the histology of the ILD of anti-Jo-1 patients. One study found nonspecific interstitial pneumonia to be the predominant pattern, but other patterns can occur, including bronchiolitis obliterans organizing pneumonia. The well-documented strong association of the anti-Jo-1 with ILD often makes lung biopsy unnecessary.

Serological Features

As noted, eight antisynthetases have been described (Table 33.1). Each antibody immunoprecipitates one or more proteins, along with a characteristic transfer RNA or set of transfer RNAs (Figure 33.1). In each case, the AuAb reacts with the synthetase enzyme, but some patients may also have AuAbs that react directly with the tRNA. This is most common with anti-PL-12 patients (6), most of whom have anti-tRNA^{ala}, while about a third of anti-Jo-1 patients have anti-tRNA^{his}. These antibodies appear to be unusual with other antisynthetases. The others presumably immunoprecipitate the transfer RNA indirectly by their reaction with the synthetase enzyme. No clinical differences have been observed between anti-Jo-1 patients with and without anti-tRNA autoantibodies. Most anti-OJ sera react with isoleucyl-tRNA synthetase, which is a component of a multienzyme complex of aaRS that contains the aaRS enzymes for 9 amino acids. Immunoprecipitation with anti-OJ shows the multiple proteins of the complex and one or two tRNAs, which appear to be tRNA^{ile} (7). Inhibition and blotting data suggest that some patients with anti-OJ react with other components of the synthetase complex; usually these are in addition to isoleucyl-RS (7). Most antisynthetase sera inhibit the activity of the enzyme antigen. It is not yet known whether autoantibodies to the other 4 aaRSs can occur (cysteine, serine, valine, tryptophan). However, antibodies that immunoprecipitate significant amounts of specific unidentified transfer RNAs are rare among myositis patients. Some studies have demonstrated areas of common epitopes, including an area in the N-terminal region for anti-Jo-1.

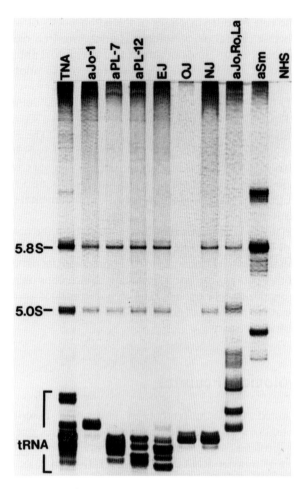

FIGURE 33.1. Immunoprecipitation for nucleic acids using anti-aminoacyl-tRNA synthetase sera. Protein A-Sepharose was coated with anti-synthetase sera, then incubated with HeLa cell extract, followed by phenol-extraction and analysis by 7 M urea, 10% polyacrylamide gel electrophoresis developed with silver stain. TNA = total nucleic acid; a = anti; NHS = normal human serum; TRNA = transfer RNA. Sera used are marked at top, including anti-Jo-1, anti-PL-7, anti-PL-12, anti-Sm, prototype sera for anti-EJ and anti-OJ along with another anti-OJ serum (NJ), a serum with anti-Jo-1 along with anti-Ro/SSA and anti-La/SSB, and NHS. Each anti-synthetase shows a recognizable set of tRNAs that can be distinguished from total tRNA and from each other. (From Targoff IN. Autoantibodies to aminoacyl-transfer RNA synthetases for isoleucine and glycine: Two additional synthetases are antigenic in myositis. *J. Immunol* 1990; 144: 1737–43.).

However, no clinical differences have yet been associated with differences in targeted epitopes.

AuAbs reacting with the 52 kDa form of Ro/SSA antigen have been observed to occur frequently in myositis, and are significantly more common in anti-Jo-1 and other antisynthetase patients than in antibody negative myositis (16). An unusual feature is that this frequently occurs in patients without anti-Ro60 or anti-La. It has been suggested that this finding can be used to aid in diagnosis of

myositis. Anti-Ro60 and anti-La do occur in some patients with anti-Jo-1, however, and may be more common than in other myositis patients. Anti-U1RNP has also been observed in association with antisynthetases, although less commonly. It is unusual for individual patients to have more than one antisynthetase, but this has been rarely observed. Similarly, most antisynthetase patients do not have other myositis autoantibodies (anti-Mi-2, anti-PM-Scl, or anti-SRP).

Diagnostic Criteria

The antisynthetase syndrome has not been formally defined, and criteria have not been developed. The term is generally used only for patients shown to have an anti-synthetase AuAb. The manifestations of the antisynthetase syndrome are not specific for this condition, nor is any combination of symptoms. Thus, a patient with myositis, ILD, arthritis, and mechanic's hands who does not have an antisynthetase is not considered to have the antisynthetase syndrome. A similar clinical picture can be seen in association with anti-U1RNP, with specific antibodies to other U-RNPs such as anti-U2RNP or anti-U5RNP, or with anti-PM-Scl, and other autoantibodies. The physician can recognize the possibility of the syndrome, but the antibody cannot be reliably predicted from the clinical picture. However, as a group, those with antisynthetases are distinctive in the prominence of myositis and significant ILD.

It is important to use a method that is as specific for detection of the antibody as possible, because the value of the antibody is in its disease specificity. ELISA is currently clinically available only for anti-Jo-1; this test is usually highly sensitive but has the potential for false positives. Confirmation of positives by a second detection method is often helpful, particularly when clinically unexpected. Immunodiffusion is also used for detection of anti-Jo-1. Although less sensitive, it is an intrinsically more specific method. Immunoprecipitation is often used to look for myositis AuAbs and can detect all of the described antisynthetases. This is most specific when tests for both the transfer RNAs and the proteins are used to demonstrate the presence of the antibody.

Patients with anti-synthetases almost always have some component of the antisynthetase syndrome, usually including either myositis or ILD. Occasional patients have had only arthritis. Because this can be the presenting feature, additional patients may go through a period of time when arthritis is the only feature evident. Sometimes treatment of one component (such as arthritis) may delay appearance of another. Limitations from ILD may delay recognition of weakness. It would be exceedingly rare for a patient with an antisynthetase to lack evidence of myositis, ILD, or arthritis.

Patients who have only one of these clinical manifestations could be considered to have the individual conditions (PM, ILD, or inflammatory arthritis). Thus, to consider the condition to instead be the antisynthetase syndrome, the patient should have at least two of the recognized manifestations that have been associated with the antibody (that occur more frequently in association with the antibody), including those in Table 33.1. If one of these features were myositis, the patient could be considered to have "overlap myositis" according to the recent clinical and antibody classification of Troyanov et al. (17).

In order to be considered to have PM, ILD, or inflammatory arthritis, the patient would be expected to satisfy criteria as discussed in this volume under the individual conditions. However, the antisynthetase AuAbs also have value in diagnosis of these conditions. The AuAbs are very rare among normal individuals and those with other myopathies, especially as detected by reliable and specific techniques. It has been suggested that the antibodies could be useful as part of a criteria set for diagnosis of myositis (18). The question often arises as to whether muscle biopsy is necessary in antisynthetase-positive patients with a clinical picture consistent with PM based on history, physical examination, muscle enzymes, electromyography and/or magnetic resonance imaging, and the exclusion of complicating issues such as use of medications with potential to cause myopathy, hypothyroidism, or others. The presence of other features of the antisynthetase syndrome would further support the diagnosis. However, such patients would not satisfy Bohan and Peter's criteria for definite PM, which were formulated before the availability of myositis autoantibody testing. Although formal studies are not available to answer this question, it might be considered that such patients would have a high likelihood of PM even if the biopsy were normal. The primary clinical value of a muscle biopsy in such a circumstance would thus be to exclude other causes of myopathy; however, as in the case noted above with anti-Jo-1 and histologic IBM, the antibody may be more relevant to patient management than the muscle biopsy results. We have previously suggested that because of their high disease specificity, addition of an MSA (including any antisynthetase) to the Bohan and Peter criteria set would be a simple way to incorporate antibodies, and thus increase the sensitivity, without significantly degrading specificity. Thus, unlike with the original Bohan and Peter criteria, patients could be considered to have definite PM without a biopsy. Criteria for the use of antisynthetases in diagnosis of ILD are not available. It may be reasonable to use the finding of an antisynthetase similarly to how one might use the knowledge of an associated connective tissue disease in approaching a patient with suspected ILD.

The antibodies may also help predict later development of extra-muscular features in patients with myositis. The presence of an antisynthetase is thought to increase the risk that a myositis patient will develop ILD, or that an ILD patient will develop myositis. Antisynthetase patients often present with manifestations other than myositis. In one study, myositis was an uncommon initial presentation; it was present in only 4 of 18 anti-Jo-1 patients at onset, but 14 over the course of disease (19). Patients may present with the ILD, with signs of myositis, such as an elevated CK, incidentally noted during initial evaluation or developing later. Since fever may also be present, the initial impression may be that of pneumonia. Arthritis can be a common presenting feature (19), often leading to an initial diagnosis of rheumatoid arthritis. This suggests that early recognition of the antibody could help with prediction of later manifestations. A clue to the possible presence of an antisynthetase would include a cytoplasmic pattern by indirect immunofluorescence testing. Testing might also be considered in patients with ILD, even if the patient carries a diagnosis of rheumatoid arthritis or another connective tissue disease.

The recent study demonstrating variation of anti-Jo-1 level with myositis activity supports a potential role in predicting or diagnosing an exacerbation of myositis (15).

Therapy

The approach to treatment of antisynthetase-associated myositis is similar to that used for treatment of other PM patients. It is usually started with high-dose corticosteroids. An immunosuppressive agent (usually methotrexate or azathioprine) is added when there is resistant disease, disease that recurs as treatment is withdrawn, or significant steroid side effects. Some start an immunosuppressive agent with the corticosteroids initially, particularly for severe disease. Because antisynthetase-associated myositis is more likely to recur, these patients might also be considered for this approach. A disadvantage of methotrexate in this group, which has frequent ILD, is the potential for methotrexate to induce hypersensitivity pneumonitis. They may have less pulmonary reserve, and there may be diagnostic confusion. However, one retrospective analysis suggested that methotrexate may be more effective than azathioprine in this group. Agents used for resistant PM and DM, such as tacrolimus, have been used in antisynthetase patients. Whether B-cell targeted therapies such as rituximab will be more effective in this group than antibody-negative myositis is not known.

Antisynthetase-associated ILD has been treated in a similar manner to ILD in other connective tissue diseases. For progressive disease not responding to corticosteroids, immunosuppressive agents including cyclophosphamide have been used. In a recent report, a series of patients with antisynthetase-associated ILD responded well to tacrolimus, suggesting a promising alternative warranting further study (20).

References

1. Nishikai M, Reichlin M. Heterogeneity of precipitating antibodies in polymyositis and dermatomyositis: Characterization of the Jo-l antibody system. *Arthritis Rheum* 1980; 23: 881–888.

2. Mathews MB, Bernstein RM. Myositis autoantibody inhibits histidyl-tRNA synthetase: A model for autoimmunity. *Nature* 1983; 304: 177–179.

3. Arnett FC, Targoff IN, Mimori T, Goldstein R, Warner NB, Reveille JD. Interrelationship of major histocompatibility complex class II alleles and autoantibodies in four ethnic groups with various forms of myositis. *Arthritis Rheum* 1996; 39: 1507–1518.

4. Love LA, Leff RL, Fraser DD, et al. A new approach to the classification of idiopathic inflammatory myopathy: Myositis-specific autoantibodies define useful homogeneous patient groups. *Medicine* 1991; 70: 360–374.

5. Marguerie C, Bunn CC, Beynon HLC et al. Polymyositis, pulmonary fibrosis and autoantibodies to aminoacyl-tRNA synthetase enzymes. *Q J Med* 1990; 77: 1019–1038.

6. Bunn CC, Bernstein RM, Mathews MB. Autoantibodies against alanyl-tRNA synthetase and tRNA^{ala} coexist and are associated with myositis. *J Exp Med* 1986; 163: 1281–1291.

7. Targoff IN, Trieu EP, Miller FW. Reaction of anti-OJ autoantibodies with components of the multi-enzyme complex of aminoacyl-tRNA synthetases in addition to isoleucyl-tRNA synthetase. *J Clin Invest* 1993; 91: 2556–2564.

8. Hirakata M, Suwa A, Takada T. Clinical and immunogenetic features of patients with autoantibodies to asparaginyl-transfer RNA synthetase. *Arthritis Rheum* 2007; 56(4): 1295–1303.

9. Hashish L, Trieu EP, Sadanandan P, Targoff IN. Identification of autoantibodies to tyrosyl-tRNA synthetase in dermatomyositis with features consistent with anti-synthetase syndrome. *Arthritis & Rheumatism* 52 (supplement): S312. 2005. Abstract.

10. Betteridge Z, Gunawardena H, North J, Slinn J, McHugh N. Anti-synthetase syndrome: a new autoantibody to phenylalanyl transfer RNA synthetase (anti-Zo) associated with polymyositis and interstitial pneumonia. *Rheumatology* 2007; 46(6): 1005–1008.

11. Targoff IN. Laboratory testing in the diagnosis and management of idiopathic inflammatory myopathies. *Rheum Dis Clin North Am* 2002; 28(4): 859–890.

12. Chinoy H, Salway F, Fertig N, et al. In adult onset myositis, the presence of interstitial lung disease and myositis specific/associated antibodies are governed by HLA class II haplotype, rather than by myositis subtype. *Arthritis Research Therapy* 2006; 8(1): R13.

13. Hengstman GJ, ter Laak HJ, van Engelen BG, van Venrooij BG. Anti-Jo-1 positive inclusion body myositis with a marked and sustained clinical improvement after oral prednisone. *Journal of Neurology, Neurosurgery Psychiatry* 2001; 70(5): 706.

14. Mozaffar T, Pestronk A. Myopathy with anti-Jo-1 antibodies: pathology in perimysium and neighbouring muscle fibres. *J Neurol Neurosurg Psychiatry* 2000; 68: 472–478.

15. Stone KB, Oddis CV, Fertig N, et al. Anti-Jo-1 antibody levels correlate with disease activity in idiopathic inflammatory myopathy. *Arthritis Rheum* 2007; 56(9): 3125–3131.

16. Rutjes SA, Vree Egberts WT, Jongen P, Van Den Hoogen F, Pruijn GJ, van Venrooij WJ. Anti-Ro52 antibodies frequently co-occur with anti-Jo-1 antibodies in sera from patients with idiopathic inflammatory myopathy. *Clin Exp Immunol* 1997; 109: 32–40.

17. Troyanov Y, Targoff IN, Tremblay JL, Goulet JR, Raymond Y, Senecal JL. Novel classification of idiopathic inflammatory myopathies based on overlap syndrome features and autoantibodies: analysis of 100 French Canadian patients. *Medicine* 2005; 84(4): 231–249.

18. Targoff IN, Miller FW, Medsger TA, Jr., Oddis CV. Classification criteria for the idiopathic inflammatory myopathies. *Curr Opin Rheumatol* 1997; 9: 527–535.

19. Schmidt WA, Wetzel W, Friedlander R et al. Clinical and serological aspects of patients with anti-Jo-1 antibodies – an evolving spectrum of disease manifestations. *Clin Rheumatol* 2000; 19(5): 371–377.

20. Wilkes MR, Sereika SM, Fertig N, Lucas MR, Oddis CV. Treatment of antisynthetase-associated interstitial lung disease with tacrolimus. *Arthritis Rheum* 2005; 52(8): 2439–2446.

34
Granulomatous Myositis

Sergio Prieto and Josep M. Grau

Abstract   Granulomatous myositis is extremely infrequent. Epitheliod granuloma on muscle biopsy is nearly always associated with sarcoidosis, but other causes have been reported, including an idiopathic form. Symmetrical proximal or distal muscle weakness is the rule in the clinical presentation and is sometimes associated with dysphagia. Although the clinical profile together with electromyography (EMG) studies may be useful, definite diagnosis requires a pathological examination. Systemic glucocorticoids are the treatment of choice, but the clinical outcome is not always satisfactory.

Keywords   Granulomatous myositis · sarcoidosis

Epidemiology

On the basis of a large series of muscular biopsies and in pathological terms, the estimated prevalence of granulomatous myositis is 0.4%, regardless of the clinical manifestations (1). There is little information on granulomatous myositis because most papers include only case reports or short series of patients.

Similar to sarcoidosis, this disease is more frequent in women, while idiopathic forms are more often seen in men. The onset of the disease occurs in the 50 s and in cases associated with sarcoidosis the average time from the diagnosis to the initial systemic clinical manifestations is 12 months (2, 3).

Etiology

Table 34.1 shows the different causes of granulomatous myositis. Sarcoidosis is the most frequent (1), followed by the idiopathic forms and those associated with infections. The remaining causes are considered anecdotical. There is controversy regarding the idiopathic forms

because some authors consider them as an exceptional form of sarcoidosis.

Clinical Manifestations

Muscle involvement in sarcoidosis is asymptomatic in 50–80% of the cases (4). In symptomatic cases, muscle weakness and dysphagia is the form of presentation of granulomatous myositis.

Muscle weakness is symmetrical and bilateral. Lower limbs are particularly affected in cases of sarcoidosis (2), while distal involvement as well as upper limbs are more frequently affected in the idiopathic forms (3).

The different forms of clinical presentation in the sarcoidosis-related cases are summarized in Table 34.2.

Dysphagia is not constant but is frequent in both sarcoidosis-related cases and in idiopathic forms (3, 5).

TABLE 34.1.   Etiology of granulomatous myositis.

- Sarcoidosis (the most frequent)
- Idiopathic
- Infectious diseases: Tuberculosis (6), Syphillis (7) *Pneumocystis jirovecci* (8).
- Neoplastic diseases: Lymphoma (9).
- Intestinal inflammatory disease (10).
- Graft-versus-host disease (11).
- Foreign-body reaction (12).
- Thymoma/Myasthenia Gravis (13).

From: Y. Shoenfeld et al. (eds.): *Diagnostic Criteria in Autoimmune Diseases*, DOI: 10.1007/978-1-60327-285-8_34,
© 2008 Humana Press, Totowa, NJ

TABLE 34.2.   Sarcoid myopathy. Clinical forms.

| 1. Chronic. The most frequent. Insidious and late evolution. |
| 2. Acute. Frequent at the onset of the disease. |
| 3. Palpable nodule. Rare cases. |

Pathological Features

The presence of granulomas in muscle biopsy is mandatory for diagnosis. Granulomata are typically located between the muscle cells. Cellular infiltrate contains giant cells (Langerhans), epithelial cells, macrophages and T cells in a lesser proportion. A mononuclear perivascular infiltrate can also be found. (Figure 34.1).

Biochemical Features

There are no specific biochemical abnormalities in granulomatous myopathy. Serum creatine kinase (CK) levels are typically normal.

Diagnosis

Typical muscle biopsy findings are mandatory for achieving a definite diagnosis. Electromyography (EMG) may show a myopathic pattern with spontaneous fibrillations and a reduction in amplitude and duration of the potentials. EMG can be useful in the selection of muscle biopsy. The same occurs with the presence of erythema nodosum, increasing the possibility of finding a typical granuloma in muscle tissue. With respect to EMG studies, there are no differences between sarcoidosis-related and idiopathic forms of granulomatous myositis. The remaining diagnostic tests such as thoracic CT scan, angiotensin-converting enzyme (ACE) serum values, ^{67}Ga scintigraphy or biopsy

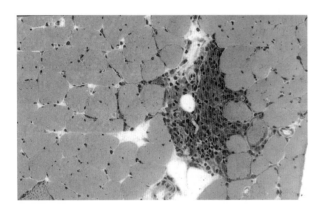

FIGURE 34.1. Sarcoid granuloma in a case of chronic sarcoidosis. H & E on frozen tissue.

TABLE 34.3.   Treatment of granulomatous myositis.

| - Systemic glucocorticoids. |
| - Methotrexate. |
| - Cyclophosphamide. |
| - Cyclosporine. |
| - Azathioprine. |
| - Infliximab. |
| - Adalimumab. |

of the other organs are used to rule out secondary forms, mainly sarcoidosis.

Therapy

The various therapies used in the treatment of granulomatous myositis are described in Table 34.3. Systemic corticosteroids are the treatment of choice at 0.5–1.0 mg/kg body weight for 4–6 weeks with a gradual dosage reduction. In refractory cases and in those requiring prolonged steroid treatment, methotrexate at 10–20 mg per week represents a valid option. No beneficial effects have been reported with the use of the remaining classical immunosuppresive agents. Experimental biological approaches with infliximab and adalimumab have been successfully used in refractory cases of sarcoidosis (3).

Prognosis

The clinical outcome in granulomatous myositis varies widely. While good response is obtained with corticosteroids in acute myopathic symptomatic cases, poor response is the rule in chronic cases (4). There are also differences among the idiopathic forms and sarcoidosis-related cases, with a better outcome observed in the latter (3).

Globally, there are no major disabilities for patients with granulomatous myositis, although complete recovery is achieved in only 10% of the cases (3).

References

1. Prayson RA. (1999) Granulomatous myositis. Clinicopathologic study of 12 cases. *Am J Clin Pathol* **112,** 63–8.
2. Mozaffar T, Lopate G, Pestronk A. (1998) Clinical correlates of granulomas in muscle. *J Neurol* **245,** 519–24.
3. Le Roux K et al. (2007) Granulomatous myositis: a clinical study of thirteen cases. *Muscle Nerve* **35,** 171–7.
4. Silverstein A, Siltzbach LE. (1969) Muscle involvement in sarcoidosis. Asymptomatic, myositis, and myopathy. *Arch Neurol* **21,** 235–41.
5. Wolfe SM, Pinals RS, Aelion JA, Goodman RE. (1987) Myopathy in sarcoidosis: clinical and pathologic study of four

cases and review of the literature. *Semin Arthritis Rheum* **16**, 300–6.

6. Wang JY et al. (2003) Tuberculous myositis: a rare but existing clinical entity. *Rheumatology* **42**, 83–84.

7. Adams RD, Victor M. Principles of Neurology. (1993) 5th ed. New York: McGraw-Hill; p. 1202.

8. Pearl GS, Sieger B. (1996) Granulomatous Pneumocystis carinii myositis presenting as an intramuscular mass. *Clin Infect Dis* **22(3),** 577–8.

9. Min HS et al. (2006) An autopsy case of aggressive CD30+ extra-nodal NK/T-cell lymphoma initially manifested with granulomatous myositis. *Leuk Lymphoma* **47(2),** 347–52.

10. Nakamura Y et al. (2002) Muscle sarcoidosis following malignant lymphoma: diagnosis by MR imaging. *Skeletal Radiol* **31**, 702–5.

11. Kaushik S et al. (2002) Granulomatous myositis: a manifestation of chronic graft-versus-host disease. *Skeletal Radiol* **31**, 226–9.

12. Vogel H. (1999) Pathologic finding in nerve and muscle biopsies from 47 women with silicone breast implants. *Neurology* **53**, 293–7.

13. Herrmann DN, Blaivas M, Wald JJ, Feldman EL. (2000) Granulomatous myositis, primary biliary cirrosis, pancytopenia and thymoma. Muscle Nerve **23**, 1133–6.

35
Eosinophilic Myositis

Albert Selva-O'Callaghan and Josep M. Grau

Abstract   Eosinophilic myositis (EM) constitutes a group of rare, clinically and pathologically heterogeneous disorders characterized by eosinophil infiltration of skeletal muscle. Parasitic infection is the commonest cause worldwide, but it can also be a feature of other conditions such as hypereosinophilic syndrome or muscle dystrophies. Most cases have no known etiological factor and are considered as idiopathic. EM should be distinguished from dermatomyositis and other systemic diseases such as Churg-Strauss granulomatosis. Idiopathic EM can be classified into three subtypes: focal EM, eosinophilic polymyositis, and eosinophilic perimyositis. Pathological studies are mandatory to differentiate and diagnose these entities.

Keywords   Eosinophilic polymyositis · perimyositis · focal eosinophilic myositis

Eosinophilic myositis (EM) constitutes a group of rare, clinically and pathologically heterogeneous disorders characterized by eosinophilic infiltration of skeletal muscles or, in the absence of eosinophil muscle infiltration, by the damage attributed to cytotoxicity caused by major basic protein (MBP) released by eosinophils (1, 2, 3, 4). Peripheral blood and/or bone marrow hypereosinophilia is common. The main causes of skeletal muscle eosinophil infiltration are parasitic infections and idiopathic inflammatory muscle disorders therefore, diagnosis of idiopathic EM may be achieved after exclusion of parasitic infections, systemic disorders with hypereosinophilia such as Churg-Strauss granulomatosis (CSG), or intake of various drugs or toxics. Occasionally, EM is the muscle expression of a hypereosinophilic syndrome (5, 6). In this case, muscle damage or dysfunction is caused by toxicity derived from eosinophils and helps to define the hypereosinophilic syndrome.

Clinical Manifestations

Idiopathic EM is classified into three subtypes: focal EM, eosinophilic polymyositis, and eosinophilic perymyositis. The clinical and laboratory data are reflected in Table 35.1 and 35.2.

Focal Eosinophilic Myositis

This is considered a benign entity, which usually affects the lower limbs mimicking deep-vein thrombosis. Pain and calf swelling are typical manifestations and the absence of systemic symptoms is characteristic. Laboratory tests demonstrate raised creatine kinase levels and electromyography and image techniques such as magnetic resonance imaging (MRI) reveal focal myositis features. Muscle biopsy shows deep eosinophilic muscle infiltration with invasion of muscle fibers and necrosis (1, 3, 7). Symptoms usually resolve spontaneously.

Eosinophilic Polymyositis

This is a systemic disease. Proximal muscle weakness is indistinguishable from idiopathic polymyositis, although pitting edema is more frequent in EM. Serum creatine kinase levels are markedly elevated indicating extensive damage and some authors have reported cardiac involvement as a frequent manifestation, at times in the context of a hypereosinophilic syndrome. Histopathology reveals a diffuse perivenular and deep muscle eosinophil infiltrate with CD8[+] and CD4[+] T cells and macrophages affecting the endomysium and muscle fibers. MRI can be useful in defining the extent of muscle involvement and directing muscle biopsy (8). Prednisone (0.5–1 mg/kg/d) is the therapy of choice.

From: Y. Shoenfeld et al. (eds.), *Diagnostic Criteria in Autoimmune Diseases*, DOI: 10.1007/978-1-60327-285-8_35,
© 2008 Humana Press, Totowa, NJ

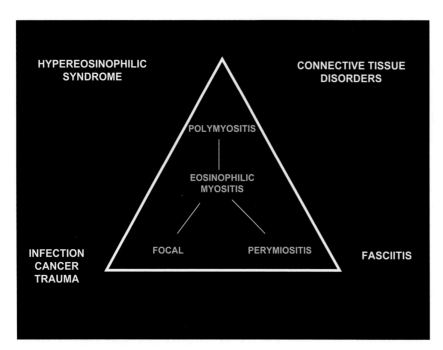

Eosinophilic Perimyositis

Myalgias and mild muscle weakness are usually seen in patients diagnosed with perimyositis, a benign condition as a rule. Histopathological studies in these patients show that muscle fibers are normal, and perimysial eosinophilic infiltrate observed at the muscle surface extends into the fascia. Perimyositis can be related to eosinophilic fasciitis. Peripheral blood eosinophilia is variable. In rare cases, corticosteroid therapy is needed to improve symptomatology.

The relationship between eosinophilic muscle disease and the pathological proposals of the different subtypes of eosinophilic myositis are shown in Figures 35.1 and 35.2 (from Hall FC, et al (1), modified).

Diagnosis

Establishing the diagnosis of EM requires rigorous evaluation to exclude an underlying infectious process (1, 2, 3, 4). Careful evaluation of patients with EM should include

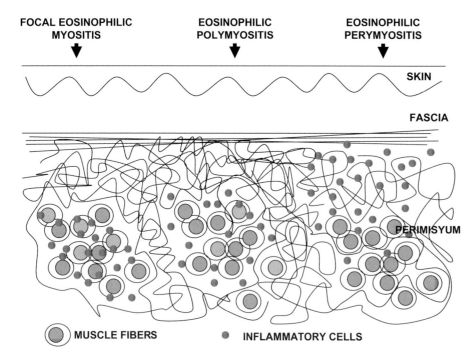

FIG 35.2 Drawing representing the different subtypes of eosinophilic myositis

investigation for parasitic infection, the commonest cause of eosinophilia worldwide, which can cause systemic disease. Blood serologies for trichinosis, echinoccocosis, toxoplasmosis, toxocarosis, schistosomiasis, distomatosis, filariosis, borreliosis, some viruses (*coxsackie* and Epstein-Barr virus), and parasite studies in stool are generally recommended. Systemic cancer, rarely, and lymphoproliferative disorders such as Ki-1 lymphoma, monoclonal T-cell expansion, and Kimura disease can be confused or accompanied by EM (9).

Systemic diseases such as CSG, polyarteritis nodosa (PAN), and dermatomyositis (DM) or polymyositis (PM) can resemble EM (10). Histology shows vasculitis in CSG and PAN, whereas eosinophilia is uncommon in inflammatory myopathies (DM, PM). Nevertheless, is important to keep in mind that PM is considered as an exclusion diagnosis; thus, eosinophilic polymyositis may occur as a part of other well-recognized diseases such as the hypereosinophilic syndrome, which may have therapeutic implications. Imatinib, an inhibitor of tyrosine kinase, and mepolizumab, a human monoclonal antibody against interleukin IL-5, seem to be effective in the treatment of different manifestations of the hypereosinophilic syndrome. A mutation of the gene encoding calpain-3, a muscle-specific protein, has recently been described in six patients with idiopathic eosinophilic myositis (11, 12), and calpainopathy should be taken into account as a possible cause of EM, at least in a subset of patients. This issue is relevant because this type of dystrophy does not benefit from glucocorticoid or immunosuppressive therapy.

In the case of perimyositis, inflammation is localized in the perimysium. This subtype of EM can resemble eosinophilic fasciitis as well as two well-known syndromes related to ingestion of toxic substances: the toxic oil syndrome, which appeared in Spain in 1981 in patients who consumed rapeseed oil, and the eosinophilia-myalgia syndrome, described in New Mexico in 1989 after consumption of contaminated L-tryptophan. Both diseases present with eosinophilia and internal organ involvement in addition to cutaneous and muscle disease (2, 10).

TABLE 35.1. Main signs and symptoms in patients diagnosed with eosinophilic myositis (3).

Muscle pain, cramping, or tenderness	68
Upper or lower extremity swelling edema	45
Muscle weakness	16
Arthralgias/arthritis	10
Myocarditis/pericarditis	10
Vasculitis	6
Inflammatory eye disease	6
Raynaud's phenomenon	6
Eosinophilic pneumonia	3
Angioedema	3

Values are expressed in percentages.

TABLE 35.2. Laboratory findings in patients diagnosed with eosinophilic myositis (3).

Eosinophilia	77
↑ ESR	77
↑ CPK	68
↑ Aldolase	44
Rheumatoid factor (+)	33
ANA (+)	6

ESR: erythrocyte sedimentation rate. CPK: creatine kinase. ANA: antinuclear antibodies. Eosinophilia: peripheral eosinophil count of $>0.5 \times 10^9/l$. Values are expressed in percentages.

TABLE 35.3. Proposed criteria for diagnosis of patients with suspected eosinophilic myositis.

(I) Focal eosinophilic myositis[a]
Major
1. Pain and calf swelling (other muscles can be affected)
2. Deep eosinophilic infiltration with muscle fiber invasion and necrosis on muscle biopsy
Minor
a) Elevated serum levels of creatine kinase and aldolase
b) MRI or electromyographic evidence of focal myositis
c) Absence of systemic illness
d) Eosinophilia $> 0.5 \times 10^9/l$
Exclusion
(i) Deep-vein thrombosis, cellulitis, parasitic infections

(II) Eosinophilic polymyositis[b]
Major
1. Proximal weakness affecting limb-girdle muscles. (may be severe)
2. Widespread deep infiltration of eosinophils into muscle, with eosinophilic cuffing, on histology study. Myonecrosis and endomysium inflammation are usually present. In the absence of eosinophil infiltration, deposition of major basic protein (MBP) should be demonstrated by specific immunostaining
Minor
a) Elevated serum levels of creatine kinase and aldolase
b) Eosinophilia $> 0.5 \times 10^9/l$
c) Systemic illness with frequent cardiac involvement
d) Corticosteroids are needed
Exclusion
(i) Hypereosinophilic syndrome, cell T clonality, dermatomyositis, vasculitis (Churg Strauss syndrome), drugs, calpainopathy, parasitic infections

(III) Eosinophilic perimyositis[c]
Major
1. Myalgias, proximal mild weakness
2. Eosinophilic infiltrate confined to fascia and superficial perimysium, absence of myofiber necrosis
Minor
a) Absence of systemic manifestations
b) Normal creatine kinase and aldolase levels
c) Eosinophilia $> 0.5 \times 10^9/l$
Exclusion
(i) Toxic oil syndrome, myalgia-eosinophilia, exposure to inorganic or organic substances

[a] The presence of two major criteria or one major and all the three minor criteria allows diagnosis.
[b] The presence of both major criteria or one major and two minor criteria allows diagnosis.
[c] The presence of either major criteria or major criteria number 2 and the two minor criteria allows diagnosis.

Pathology

Histopathological findings usually help to confirm the diagnosis of EM, and in cases caused by parasitic infection, it can be seen on microscopy as in *Trichinella spiralis*. It should be noted that on occasions eosinophils may be not apparent on muscle biopsy, with immunostaining being necessary to identify eosinophilic major basic protein (MBP), which may, nonetheless, be positive (12, 13). MBP, which is stored in the crystalloid cores of eosinophils, is responsible for muscle fiber damage owing to cytotoxicity as the result of non-enzymatic physical interactions (13).

Diagnostic criteria

Till now no specific or systematized diagnostic criteria have been defined for these different subtypes of EM. We propose a set of criteria taking into account the current knowledge of these disorders. (Table 35.3)

Treatment and prognosis

In general terms, the prognosis of EM is good (1, 2, 3, 4, 10), especially in the localized forms of focal EM. More generalized forms can benefit from glucocorticoid therapy at a dose of 0.5–1 mg/kg body weight. Occasionally, EM appears as a manifestation of a hypereosinophilic syndrome (more than 6 months with persistent hypereosinophilia of more than $1,500 \times 10^9/l$ with no known etiology and organ damage or dysfunction as a result of local release of the toxic contents of eosinophils), and may therefore be catastrophic (14). In these rare cases, the determination of the abnormal fusion *FIP1L1* and *PDGFRA* genes is mandatory to confirm the diagnosis, because treatment with imatinib mesylate could improve the clinical picture (6). Mepolizumab, a fully humanized anti-IL-5 monoclonal antibody, seems to produce sustained eosinophil reductions and may be a therapeutic option in patients with clinically poor prognosis or in those

who do not response to corticosteroids. Patients with perimyositis within a more generalized toxic disease do not always have a favorable outcome.

References

1. Hall FC, Krausz T, and Walport MJ. (1995) Idiopathic eosinophilic myositis. *QJ Med* **88**, 581–6.
2. Serratrice G, Pellisier JF, Roux H, and Quilichini P. (1990) Fasciitis, perimyositis, myositis, polymyositis and eosinophilia. *Muscle Nerve* **13**, 385–95.
3. Kaufman LD, Kephart GM, Seidman RJ, Buhmer D, Qvarfordt I, Nässberger L, et al. (1993) The spectrum of eosinophilic myositis. Clinical and immunopathogenic studies of three patients and review of the literature. *Arthritis Rheum* **36**, 1014–24.
4. Pickering MC, and Walport MJ. (1998) Eosinophilic myopathic syndromes. *Curr Opin Rheumatol* **10**, 504–10.
5. Bosch JA. (2001) Hypereosinophilic syndrome. *Med Clin (Barc)* **117**, 375–6.
6. Wilkins HJ, Crane MM, Copeland K, and Williams WV. (2005) Hypereosinophilic syndrome: an update. *Am J Haematol* **80**, 148–57.
7. Kobayashi Y, Fujimoto T, Shiiki H, Kitaoka K, Murata K, and Dohi K. (2001) Focal eosinophilic myositis. *Clin Rheumatol* **20**, 369–71.
8. Hundt W, Stäbler A, and Reiser M. (1999) MRI findings of muscle involvement in idiopathic hypereosinophilic syndrome. *Eur Radiol* **9**, 525–8.
9. Dunand M, Lobrinus JA, Spertini O, and Kuntzer T. (2005) Eosinophilic perimyositis as the presenting feature of a monoclonal T-cell expansion. *Muscle Nerve* **31**, 646–51.
10. Watts RA. (2001) Eosinophilia and musculoskeletal disease. *Curr Opin Rheumatol* **13**, 57–61.
11. Krahn M, Lopez de Munain A, Streichenberg N, Bernard R, Pécheux C, Testard H, et al. (2006) *CAPN3* Mutations in patients with idiopathic eosinophilic myositis. *Ann Neurol* **59**, 905–11.
12. Brown RH, and Amato A. (2006) Calpainopathy and eosinophilic myositis. *Ann Neurol* **59**, 875–7.
13. Murata K, Sugie K, Takamure M, Fujimoto T, and Ueno S. (2003) Eosinophilic major basic protein and interleukin-5 in eosinophilia myositis. *Eur J Neurol* **10**, 35–38.
14. Ishizawa K, Adachi D, Kuboi K, Yamaguchi T, Mitsuhashi T, Shimizu Y,. (2006) Multiple organ involvement in eosinophilic polymyositis: an autopsy report. *Hum Pathol* **37**, 231–5.

36
Eosinophilic Fasciitis

Albert Selva-O'Callaghan and Josep M. Grau

Abstract Eosinophilic fasciitis (EF) is an uncommon scleroderma-like syndrome with an unknown etiology and pathogenesis. Peripheral blood eosinophilia, hypergammaglobulinemia, and elevated erythrocyte sedimentation rate are the main laboratory findings. Full-thickness wedge biopsy of the clinically involved skin is essential for establishing an accurate diagnosis. Differential diagnosis includes systemic sclerosis and other fasciitis syndromes caused by substances such as L-tryptophan myalgia-eosinophilia and toxic oil syndrome. Diagnosis of EF can be established by clinical, laboratory, and histological findings. Nevertheless, universally accepted criteria are lacking. Corticosteroids are effective in the treatment of EF. Some patients improve spontaneously.

Keywords Eosinophilic fasciitis· scleroderma-like· eosinophilia

Eosinophilic fasciitis (EF) is a scleroderma-like disorder first described by Shulman (1) in 1974. This skin fibrosis disorder is relatively uncommon and occurs in a sporadic rather than epidemic form. It can be localized, with disease involving one extremity, or less frequently generalized, affecting the four extremities, the trunk and abdomen, causing ventilatory restriction in some cases. EF is characterized by induration of the skin, peripheral eosinophilia, and hypergammaglobulinemia. The onset of the disease is usually abrupt and, in some cases, follows excessive physical activity, and positivity for *Borrelia* serology testing had occasionally been reported (2). Associated hematological diseases and autoimmune thyroid disorders have rarely been reported in some series. Visceral and extracutaneous involvements in FE are unusual (3).

Clinical Manifestations

Painful and erythematous swellings of the affected extremities are the main cardinal clinical features. Edema is progressively replaced by thickening of the skin which is firmly bound to the underlying tissue. *Peau d'orange* appearance (Figure 36.1) and the *"groove"* sign (Figure 36.2), a longitudinal depression in the skin along the course of blood vessels, are characteristic findings in these patients. Skin induration can lead to joint contractures with limited mobility. EF can easily be differentiated from systemic sclerosis

(SSc), because of the absence of sclerodactylia. The facies is spared and the typical features of SSc are not found in EF. Physical examination does not reveal microstomia, teleangiectasias, or sclerodactylia. Raynaud's phenomenon is usually absent in patients with EF, and capillaroscopy does not reveal the distinctive nailfold microvascular findings generally seen in SSc. Main clinical and laboratory data of EF are reflected in Tables 36.1 and 36.2.

Pathological features. A full-thickness wedge biopsy of the involved skin usually reveals characteristic findings (4). Fascia *muscularis* shows accumulation of lymphocytes,

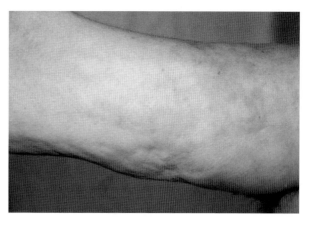

FIGURE 36.1. Thickened skin (*Peau d'orange* appearance) in a case of eosinophilic fasciitis.

From: Y. Shoenfeld et al. (eds.), *Diagnostic Criteria in Autoimmune Diseases*, DOI: 10.1007/978-1-60327-285-8_36,
© 2008 Humana Press, Totowa, NJ

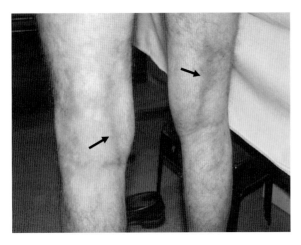

FIGURE 36.2. Longitudinal depressions in the skin (arrows). Groove sign in eosinophilic fasciitis.

macrophages, and plasma cells but not always eosinophils or their degranulation product (major basic eosinophilic protein) are found in the tissue affected, which do not contravene the diagnosis. Fascia *muscularis* is usually 2–15 times the thickness of normal fascia and is firmly adherent to the subjacent skeletal muscle. The dermis and epidermis are usually normal. The epimysium near the fascia and perimysium among muscle fibers are often inflamed given the so-called perimyositis (Figure 36.3) (5, 8).

Diagnosis. Universally accepted diagnostic criteria in patients with EF are lacking. Most articles and rheumatology textbooks state that patients can be diagnosed with EF, a scleroderma-like disorder, when characteristic skin lesions, which can affect trunk and extremities are present,

TABLE 36.1. Main signs and symptoms in patients diagnosed with eosinophilic fasciitis.

References	(2)	(7)	(8)	(9)
Skin induration	100	96	100	100
Localized[a]	–	60	30	74
Diffuse[b]	–	40	70	26
Erythema	100	–	10	–
Pitting edema	82	44	70	–
Hyperpigmentation	9	–	30	–
Facial edema	9	6	0	–
Groove sign	18	–	40	–
Peau d'orange	–	21	20	–
Contractures	27	56	40	–
Fever	–	–	20	–
Weight loss (> 15%)	–	–	40	–
Ventilatory restriction	0	7	40	–
Perymyositis	–	7	60	–
Raynaud's	0	2	10	–
Sclerodactylia	9	0	0	–
Pruritus	–	–	30	–
Arthritis	–	40	20	–

[a] Localized: either lower extremities or forearms, asymmetric.
[b] Diffuse: skin induration of trunk, abdomen, and four extremities.

TABLE 36.2. Laboratory findings in patients diagnosed with eosinophilic fasciitis.

References	(2)	(7)	(8)	(9)
Eosinophilia	64	63	100	92
Hypergammaglobulinemia	18	34	40	50
ANA	18	6	10	22
Autoantibodies	0	4	0	–
Aldolase	–	–	40	–
Cytopenias	9	2	10	–
Thyroid dysfunction	1	–	10	–
Borrelia burgdorferi serology	2	–	0	–
Elevated ESR	64	29	–	74

Eosinophilia: $> 0.5 \times 10^9$/l. ANA: antinuclear antibodies. ESR: erythrocyte sedimentation rate.

and the distal fingers, toes, and facies are clinically spared. Exclusion of SSc is mandatory and investigation of known causes of scleroderma-like syndromes such as the toxic oil syndrome, silica exposure, gadolinium administration in patients with renal failure, and L-tryptophan-induced eosinophilia myalgia-epidemic syndrome is necessary. Typically, there is no involvement of internal organs such as the lung or kidney in patients with EF, and the characteristic autoantibodies which help diagnosis of SSc (anti-topoisomerase or Scl-70 and anticentromere) are absent. The Raynaud's phenomenon, which is nearly constant in SSc patients, is rare if not exceptional in EF, as is the peripheral microvascular damage in the nailfold study with capillaroscopy. Deep cutaneous biopsy including the fascia *muscularis* is essential for diagnostic support. Biopsy findings usually show striking inflammation and thickening of the fascia. Even in the absence of tissue eosinophils, the thickened fascia and its lymphocyte infiltration allow the diagnosis. Magnetic resonance imaging (MRI) and serum aldolase concentration seem to be useful in the diagnosis and follow-up of patients diagnosed with FE (10, 11).

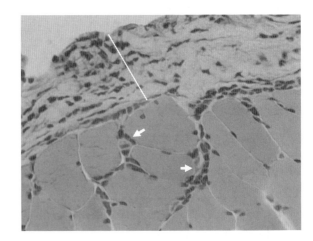

FIGURE 36.3. Thickened fascia (barr) and moderate inflammatory infiltrate in eosinophilic fasciitis.

Diagnostic criteria. Some authors have attempted to define diagnostic criteria for EF, at least to include or exclude patients published as a case report or small series in the medical literature. Three years after the initial description of Shulman (1), Bennett et al (5) suggested that cardinal manifestations of EF should include the following five items: (i) localized nature of the skin involvement, (ii) pronounced thickening of the subcutaneous fascia, (iii) absence of visceral changes and Raynaud's phenomenon, (iv) association with eosinophilia and hypergammaglobulinemia, and (v) beneficial response to corticosteroids. In a recent review of the literature, Endo et al (9) included patients with EF when: (i) the characteristic clinical findings are present (symmetric swelling, induration and/or tightness of the skin and subcutaneous tissues, mainly affecting the extremities; (ii) the characteristic histopathological findings are shown, including deep fascia, or in patients with MRI revealing inflammation and/or thickening of the deep fascia. Finally, other authors (2) have defined the following criteria in a study on patients with EF from a single center in Switzerland: (i) characteristic skin lesions such as cutaneous erythema and induration, cutaneous swelling of the upper and/or lower extremities; and (ii) fascial biopsy with histopathological findings such as thickening of the fascia with chronic inflammatory infiltrate containing eosinophils.

In our opinion, some of the previous commented issues related to EF are more important than others, and suggest that some, such as cutaneous induration, which respects the acral zones or typical fascia thickening with inflammatory infiltration, and not necessarily eosinophils, should be included as main or major diagnostic criteria, while other features such as elevated erythrocyte sedimentation rate (ESR), hypergammaglobulinemia, or even peripheral eosinophilia may help achieve diagnosis but alone does not allow correct diagnosis of EF. Exclusion of SSc by clinical as well as immunological and capillaroscopic studies is essential, as recommended to discard exogenous substances that could be responsible for this disorder. Studies are needed to determine the validity of these criteria or the positive and negative predictive value, but the rarity of EF and the small number of new cases made this topic difficult to address.

Taking into account the case reports and published series of patients with EF, it seems logical to define the following criteria, described in Table 36.3.

Therapy and prognosis. Although some patients improve spontaneously without treatment, the mainstay therapy in patients with EF includes an initial full dose of glucocorticoids (1 mg/kg/d), which usually resolve the edema and induration. This clinical improvement can take weeks or months and is heralded by resolution of peripheral blood eosinophilia. Cimetidine, a histamine 2 antagonist, may be useful in combination with prednisone (12). Antimalarials, methotrexate, cyclosporine and, recently,

TABLE 36.3. Proposed criteria for the diagnosis of patients with suspected FE.

Major criteria[a]
1. Swelling, induration and thickening of the skin and subcutaneous tissue, symmetrical or not, diffuse (extremities, trunk and abdomen) or localized (extremities)
2. Fascial thickening with accumulation of lymphocytes and macrophages with or without eosinophilic infiltration (obtained after a full-thickness wedge biopsy of clinically involved skin)

Minor criteria
(a) Eosinophilia $> 0.5 \times 10^9/l$
(b) Hypergammaglobulinemia $> 1.5\,gr/l$
(c) Muscle weakness and/or elevated levels of aldolase
(d) Groove sign and/or *Peau d'orange*
(e) Hyperintense fascia on T2-weighted images on MRI
Exclusion criteria: patients diagnosed with systemic sclerosis.

[a] Presence of both major criteria or one major criteria plus 2 minor criteria, allows the diagnosis of eosinophilic fasciitis.

mycophenolate mofetil and infliximab, chimeric monoclonal antibody with specificity to tumor necrosis factor alpha, have been reported in sporadic and refractory cases (13). Fortunately, few patients present with refractory fibrosis and generalized involvement, which includes the trunk, abdomen, and the four extremities. In these cases, aggressive therapy not only with steroids but also with other coadjuvant immunosuppressive drugs seems warranted. Physical therapy should be recommended in all cases to prevent or improve joint contractures.

References

1. Shulman LE. (1974) Diffuse fasciitis with hypergammaglobulinemia and eosinophilia: a new syndrome? *J Rheumatol* **1**, 46.
2. Antic M, Lautenschlager S, Itin PH. (2006) Eosinophilic fasciitis 30 years after- what do we really know? Report of 11 patients and review of the literature. *Dermatology* **213**, 93–101.
3. Doyla JA. (1984) Eosinophilic fasciitis: extracutaneous manifestations and associations. *Cutis* **34**, 259–61.
4. Barnes L, Rodnan GP, Medsger TA, and Short D. (1979) Eosinophilic fasciitis. A pathologic study of twenty cases. *Am J Pathol* **96**, 493–518.
5. Serratrice G, Pellisier FJ, Roux H, and Qulichini P. (1990) Fasciitis, perimyositis, myositis, polymyositis, and eosinophilia. *Muscle Nerve* **13**, 385–95.
6. Bennett RM, Herron A, and Keogh L. (1977) Eosinophilic fasciitis. Case report and review of the literature. *Ann Rheum Dis* **36**, 354–9.
7. Lakhanpal S, Ginsburg WW, Michet CJ, Doyle JA, and Moore SB. (1988) Eosinophilic fasciitis: clinical spectrum and therapeutic response in 52 cases. Semin *Arthritis Rheum* **17**, 221–31.
8. Trallero-Araguás E, Selva-O'Callaghan A, Simeón-Aznar CP, Sanjurjo-Golpe E, García-Patos V, and Vilardell-Tarrés M.

(2005) Eosinophilic fasciitis: analysis of a series of 10 patients. *Med Clin (Barc)* **125**, 145–8.

9. Endo Y, Tamura A, Matsushima Y, Iwasaki T, Hasegawa M, Nagai Y, et al. (2007) Eosinophilic fasciitis: report of two cases and a systematic review of the literature dealing with clinical variables that predict outcome. *Clin Rheumatol* **26**, 1445–51.

10. Fujimoto M, Sato S, Ihn H, Kikuchi K, Yamada N, and Takehara K. (1995) Serum aldolase level is a useful indicator of disease activity in eosinophilic fasciitis. *J Rheumatol* **22**, 563–5.

11. Nakajima H, Fujiwara S, Shinoda, and Oshawa N. (1997) Magnetic resonance imaging and serum aldolase concentration in eosinophilic fasciitis. *Internal Medicine* **36**, 654–6.

12. Naschitz JE, Boss JH, Misselevich I, Yeshurun D, and Rosner I. (1996) The fasciitis-panniculitis syndromes. Clinical and pathologic features. *Medicine (Baltimore)* **75**, 6–16.

13. Drosou A, Kirsner RS, Welsh E, Sullivan TP, and Kerdel FA. (2003) Use of infliximab, an anti-tumor necrosis alpha antibody for inflammatory dermatoses. *J Cutan Med Surg* **7**, 382–386.

Part IV
Other Immune-Mediated Systemic Diseases

37
Sarcoidosis

Juan Mañá

Abstract Sarcoidosis is a multisystemic granulomatous disease of unknown etiology. The available evidence suggests that the disease results from an exposure of genetically susceptible hosts to specific environmental agents, which trigger a Th1 immunological response in the involved organs, leading to granuloma formation. Sarcoidosis usually presents with bilateral hilar lymphadenopathy, and pulmonary, cutaneous and ocular involvement, although any organ can be affected. The diagnosis is based on a compatible clinical and radiological picture, demonstration of noncaseating granulomas with negative cultures for mycobacteria and fungus, and exclusion of other granulomatous diseases. In general, an acute onset, particularly Löfgren's syndrome, has a good prognosis, whereas an insidious presentation heralds a chronic disease. Corticosteroids should be administered when severe and progressive disease involves major organs such as lungs, eyes, <u>heart and</u> central nervous system. Several drugs may be useful as alternative therapies in cases refractory to corticosteroid treatment.

Keywords Sarcoidosis · Löfgren's syndrome · granulomatous diseases

Sarcoidosis is a multisystemic disease of unknown etiology characterized by the accumulation of T lymphocytes, mononuclear phagocytes and noncaseating granulomas in the affected organs. It frequently presents with bilateral hilar lymphadenopathy (BHL), and pulmonary, cutaneous and ocular involvement, although any organ can be affected. The diagnosis requires the exclusion of other granulomatous diseases (1, 2).

Epidemiology

Sarcoidosis occurs throughout the world. However, because of the lack of a precise definition and the fact that some cases are asymptomatic, the true incidence is unknown. The prevalence ranges from 10 to 40 per 100,000 in the USA and Europe. Most of patients are young and middle-aged adults with a slight predominance in women, more evident in Löfgren's syndrome (LS). Afro-American and Asian Indians have more severe disease, whereas asymptomatic cases are more common in Caucasian. LS is more frequent in the Northern European countries and Spain, and predominates during the spring months. Spatial clusters of illness have suggested person-to-person transmission or shared exposure to environmental agents

(1). Recent studies have demonstrated that several environmental and occupational factors may trigger the disease (3, 4).

Etiology

The cause of sarcoidosis is not known. The available evidence suggests that the disease results from an exposure of genetically susceptible hosts to specific and persistent environmental agents, which trigger a heightened cellular immune response in the involved organs. Recently, multiple studies have focused on the relationship between sarcoidosis and human leukocyte antigen phenotypes. Genetic factors are important in defining the pattern of disease presentation and prognosis (5). Although some studies have speculated on a role for Mycobacterium spp in the etiology of the disease, to date there is not evidence that sarcoidosis is caused by an infectious agent.

Immunopathogenesis

Sarcoidosis characterizes by a Th1 immunological response. Initially there is accumulation in the involved organs of activated CD4$^+$ T lymphocytes and mononuclear

From: Y. Shoenfeld et al. (eds.): *Diagnostic Criteria in Autoimmune Diseases*, DOI: 10.1007/978-1-60327-285-8_37,
© 2008 Humana Press, Totowa, NJ

phagocytes, which release interleukin (IL)-2, interferon-γ, and other cytokines, leading to the formation of noncaseating granulomas. Granulomas may resolve spontaneously or evolve to fibrosis with permanent tissue damage. Tumor necrosis factor-α plays a role in the inhibition of apoptosis in the granuloma, which contributes to the persistence of inflammation and evolution to fibrosis (6).

Clinical Presentation and Organ Involvement

Sarcoidosis is occasionally discovered by chance in an asymptomatic individual, usually as BHL on chest X-ray (CXR). The onset of sarcoidosis may be acute or insidious. Acute, or subacute, sarcoidosis develops over a period of weeks or a few months, and it usually heralds a good prognosis. It is characterized by mild constitutional symptoms such as fatigue, malaise, anorexia, weigh loss, low-grade fever, arthralgias, and respiratory symptoms. One of the most typical forms of acute sarcoidosis is LS. It consists in the association of erythema nodosum with BHL, sometimes with pulmonary involvement, on CXR. Some patients present only a periarticular ankle inflammation without erythema nodosum, which has been considered a clinical variant of LS. Polyarthralgias, low-grade fever, anterior uveitis, and transient unilateral facial paralysis may be present as well (7). On the contrary, an insidious onset for several months is usually associated with respiratory complaints without constitutional symptoms, or with symptoms referable to organs other than the lung. It rather correlates with a chronic course and permanent organ damage (8).

Intrathoracic

Intrathoracic involvement occurs in 90% of cases, so 10% of patients have isolated extrathoracic sarcoidosis (stage 0). The inflammatory process is mainly located on alveoli, small bronchi, and small blood vessels and predominates on the upper lung zones. Patients may be asymptomatic or present dry cough and dyspnea with exercise. Associated bronchial hyperreactivity may be present. Hemoptysis is rare. Rales are not frequent. Table 37.1 summarizes the classical radiological stages of sarcoidosis. Hilar bilateral and right paratracheal adenopathy and reticulonodular infiltration with upper lung zone predominance is the most typical pattern. Atypical radiological findings include large nodules, alveolar infiltrates, hilar calcification, pleural effusion, and pneumothorax. External compression by enlarged hilar adenopathies or endobronchial involvement may cause distal atelectasis. The evolution to fibrosis may cause large airway distortion with severe dysfunction (9).

TABLE 37.1 Chest X-ray stages in pulmonary sarcoidosis[a]

	% at onset	% with resolution
Stage 0: Normal chest X-ray (CXR)	<10%	
Stage I: Bilateral hilar lymphadenopathy (BHL) without pulmonary involvement	50%	65%; <10% progress to pulmonary involvement
Stage II: BHL with pulmonary involvement	30%	20–50%
Stage III[b]: Pulmonary involvement without BHL	10–15%	<20%

[a] Classification based on CXR. Although high-resolution thoracic CT and gallium-67 scan may suggest a different stage, it is not necessary to change the criteria since these tests are indicated only in a limited number of patients.
[b] Stage III may be subclassified in stage IV, which includes cases with advanced pulmonary fibrosis (hilar retraction, coarse linear opacities, honeycombing, bullae, emphysematous changes, architectural distortion, and pulmonary hypertension).

Skin

Granulomatous skin lesions are present in 15–25% of patients with sarcoidosis. The most common are maculopapular eruptions, infiltration of old scars and tattoos, subcutaneous nodules, plaques, and lupus pernio. The last two are associated with chronic sarcoidosis (10).

Eye

Ocular involvement occurs in 15–20% of patients. Because it may be asymptomatic, slit-lamp and ophthalmoscopic examinations should be performed on every patient with sarcoidosis. Fluorescein angiography may be indicated if posterior uveitis is suspected. The most frequent findings are anterior or posterior uveitis, choroidoretinitis, periphlebitis, papiledema, and retinal hemorrhages. Conjunctivitis, lacrimal gland involvement, and keratoconjunctivitis sicca may be present as well (1, 8).

Reticuloendothelial System

Peripheral lymphadenopathy involving the cervical, supraclavicular, epitroclear, axillary, and inguinal nodes may be present. In addition to intrathoracic, mesenteric chain and retroperitoneal lymph nodes may be present as well. Splenic involvement is frequent, although splenomegaly occurs only in 5–10% of cases and may result in pancytopenia. Multiple low-attenuation nodules may be seen in the spleen on CT. Bone marrow involvement is rare (1, 8).

Liver

Although liver involvement at biopsy is very frequent in sarcoidosis, mild hepatomegaly with slight cholestasis occurs in 20–30% of patients. Hepatic sarcoidosis affects the periportal areas. Severe chronic cholestasis syndrome, portal hypertension, and Budd–Chiari syndrome are rare. Multiple low-attenuation nodules in the liver on CT may be observed (1, 8).

Neurosarcoidosis

About 5–10% of patients with sarcoidosis have clinical recognizable neurological involvement. It has a predilection for the basal meninges of the brain, so cranial nerve involvement, particularly facial paralysis, are common. Other central nervous system (CNS) manifestations include aseptic meningitis, seizures, pyramidal tract signs, optic nerve dysfunction, papilledema, hypothalamic and pituitary lesions with diabetes insipidus or hypopituitarism, and cognitive impairment. Spinal cord involvement is rare. Cerebrospinal fluid (CSF) analysis may show lymphocytosis, increased proteins, and oligoclonal bands. Gadolinium-enhanced magnetic resonance imaging (MRI) may reveal nonenhancing multifocal periventricular and subcortical white matter lesions mimicking those of multiple sclerosis, meningeal enhancement, space-occupying lesions, and hydrocephalus. Peripheral axonal polyneuropathy is not frequent. Recently, small fiber neuropathy with autonomic involvement has been reported (11).

Musculoskeletal System

Transient or chronic polyarthralgias are common but frank arthritis is not frequent. Asymptomatic muscle involvement is common, but symptomatic diffuse or nodular myopathy is rare. Bone lesions, usually osteolytic, are not frequent and predominate on the hands and foot, but any bone may be affected (1, 8).

Heart

Clinical heart involvement occurs in 5% of patients. Arrhythmias, complete heart block, sudden death, papillary muscle dysfunction, and congestive heart failure may be present. Cor pulmonale is usually secondary to chronic pulmonary fibrosis. Twenty-four-hour Holter monitoring, Doppler echocardiogram, nuclear imaging techniques, and cardiac Positron emission tomography and MRI are useful for the diagnosis. Endomyocardial biopsy may reveal granulomas although the diagnostic yield may be low (12).

Other Manifestations

Parotid involvement is frequent and may produce parotid enlargement and xerostomia. Transient or persistent hypercalcemia, hypercalciuria, rarely with nephrocalcinosis and nephrolitiasis, may be present. Interstitial lymphocytic and granulomatous nephritis and renal failure have been reported. Sarcoidosis may involve any structure of the upper respiratory tract, causing more frequently nasal stuffiness. Gastrointestinal, genital, and endocrine gland involvement is rare (1, 8).

Ancillary Tests

In addition to the alterations according to the organs involved, lymphopenia, mild eosinophilia, and hyperglobulinemia may be observed. At diagnosis, at least 60% of patients have increased serum angiotensine-converting enzyme (SACE) level, although it is not specific. Pulmonary function tests (PFT) may reveal decreased forced vital capacity (FVC) and Diffusing capacity for carbon monoxide (DLco). Advanced pulmonary fibrosis may cause airways distortion and decreased forced expiratory volume in 1 second (FEV1). Gallium-67 scanning has a limited sensitivity and specificity, and should not be routinely performed. It may be useful in cases with diagnostic difficulties, particularly in patients with normal or doubtful CXR in which extrathoracic sarcoidosis is suspected. The demonstration of the typical *lambda* and *panda* patterns supports the diagnosis and reinforces the indication of histological confirmation. High-resolution thoracic CT (HRCT) is not indicated when the CXR is typical, but is useful in patients with atypical radiological findings, to detect areas of active alveolitis in cases with pulmonary fibrosis, and to detect specific complications in the lung. In addition to the BHL, the most common findings are widespread small nodules with a bronchovascular and subpleural distribution, thickened interlobular septae, ground-glass areas, and confluent nodular opacities with air-bronchograms, with predilection for mid- and upper-lung zones. With advanced fibrosis, architectural distortion, hilar retraction, fibrous bands, bronchiectasis, and bullae may be observed. The demonstration on bronchoalveolar lavage (BAL) of a lymphocytic alveolitis with a proportion of CD4/CD8 >3.5 has a sensitivity of 53% and a specificity of 94%. However, BAL is not routinely performed unless a transbronchial lung biopsy (TLB) is indicated. Tuberculin skin test is negative in more than 80% of patients (1, 9).

Diagnostic Criteria

The diagnosis of sarcoidosis is based on a compatible clinical and radiological picture, demonstration of noncaseating granulomas with negative cultures for mycobacteria and

TABLE 37.2. Recommended basic assessment of patients with sarcoidosis.

History (including occupational and environmental exposures)
Physical examination
Ophthalmologic examination (slit lamp and ophthalmoscopic examination)
CXR
Standard hematological and biochemistry profiles (including urine and serum calcium level, hepatic enzymes, and renal function tests), and serum angiotensine-converting enzyme level
ECG
Pulmonary function tests (including spirometry and DLco)
Tuberculin skin test
Biopsies (including culture for mycobacteria and fungus)

fungus, and exclusion of other granulomatous diseases (1, 8). Table 37.2 summarizes the basic study protocol, and Figure 37.1 provides an algorithm for the diagnostic assessment of sarcoidosis.

The type of biopsy will depend on the involved organ and its accessibility. The most commonly used are TLB,

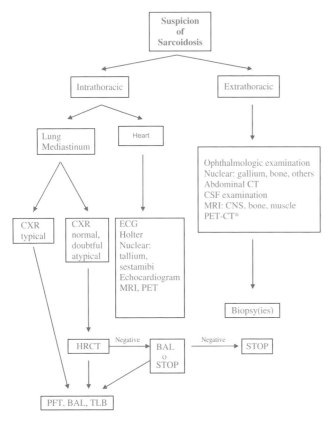

* Combined PET-CT may have a role in the assessment of sarcoidosis in the future

FIGURE 37.1. Algorithm for the diagnostic assessment of sarcoidosis (Adapted from: Mañá J, van Kroonenburg M. Clinical usefulness of nuclear imaging techniques in sarcoidosis. In: Drent M, Costabel U (eds.), Sarcoidosis. Eur Respir Mon 2005; 10(32): 284–300).

mediastinoscopy, and skin and peripheral lymph node biopsies. Less frequently, biopsies of liver, lacrimal and parotid glands, conjunctiva, muscle, upper respiratory tract, scalene lymph node (Daniels biopsy), nervous system, spleen, bone, heart, and kidney may be used as well. When available, the Kveim–Siltzbach test has a sensitivity of 70–90% and a specificity of 97%. Occasionally, granulomatous cells may be seen in cytological specimens obtained by fine needle aspiration, either transbronchial or percutaneous, of mass lesions in patients with suspected sarcoidosis. This may useful in excluding malignancy, and may support the diagnosis, although it is not an absolute proof. Importantly, a biopsy with the typical noncaseating granulomas is non-specific for sarcoidosis, and the differential diagnosis varies according to every organ. Infectious diseases, particularly tuberculosis, and tumor-related sarcoid reactions should always be excluded. When the clinical and radiological findings are not typical, it is recommended to obtain at least two positive biopsies. However, 15–20% of biopsies with granulomas remain without a specific etiology. This has been named as granulomatous lesions of unknown significance (GLUS) syndrome (1). On the contrary, some clinical and radiological pictures, such as LS and asymptomatic patients with a stage I on CXR detected by chance, are so typical of sarcoidosis that histological confirmation may not be necessary. However, these patients must be followed up at least until the hilar adenopathy is completely resolved (7). Once the diagnosis has been established, the work-up for patients with sarcoidosis includes an assessment of the extension and severity of organ involvement, an evaluation to see whether the disease is stable or progressing, and so determine whether therapy is indicated (1, 8).

Prognosis and Therapy

In most patients, particularly those with an acute presentation, the disease resolves spontaneously without sequelae. LS has an excellent prognosis. Rest, nonsteroidal anti-inflammatory drugs, potassium iodide (300 mg/t.i.d. orally), or a short course of low-dose prednisone are useful to treat erythema nodosum (7). In other cases, the disease persists active for long time, or with a tendency to wax and wane, but with minimal organ damage and no significant clinical repercussion. About 10–30% of patients follow a chronic and progressive course despite therapy (1). Occasionally, recurrence of sarcoidosis many years after spontaneous remission may occur (13). Pregnancy is not contraindicated except in severe chronic disease. However, it may be relapsed after parturition. Mortality is less than 5%.

Corticosteroids are the therapy of choice. However, there is a controversy about when to treat a patient with sarcoidosis. Although corticosteroids suppress the inflammatory process, it has not been demonstrated that they alter the long-term outcome of the disease. In consequence, the objective of treatment must be the symptomatic control and prevention of irreversible organ damage, particularly in major organs such as lung, eye, heart, and CNS, trying to cause the minimum secondary effects (14). Alternate-day therapy may be used. Relapses a few months after the suppression of treatment may occur.

Pulmonary Sarcoidosis

In CXR stages II and III treatment should be administered in presence of symptoms, radiological progression, or decreased lung function. In asymptomatic patients with normal lung function, a period of 6-12 months observation is indicated, and treatment should be administered if the patient becomes symptomatic, or there is persistence or progression of radiological findings, or lung function deteriorates. In stage IV, fibrosis may coexist with active alveolitis, and treatment is recommended with a re-assessment of symptoms and lung function 3–6 months later. The recommended therapy is prednisone, 0.5 mg/kg/day, with slow tapering, at least for 1 year. The best way to assess the treatment efficacy in pulmonary sarcoidosis is periodical evaluation of symptoms, CXR, and lung function. Inhaled corticosteroids may be useful if associated bronchial hyperreactivity is present (9).

Extrathoracic Sarcoidosis

The main indications for treatment are posterior uveitis, CNS, and cardiac involvement, and persistent hypercalcemia. Severe cutaneous lesions, hypersplenism, and severe liver, upper respiratory tract and kidney involvement may also require treatment. The recommended therapy is prednisone, 1 mg/kg/day, with slow tapering, at least for 2 years. However, some patients may need more prolonged treatment (15). Severe cases, particularly CNS, may be treated initially with high-dose corticosteroid intravenous pulse therapy. Mild anterior ocular involvement is treated with topical corticosteroids.

Refractory Sarcoidosis

Some cases of sarcoidosis may be refractory to corticosteroid treatment. If the dose of prednisone needed to keep the disease under control is superior to 20 mg/day for prolonged time, various second-line medications may act as steroid-sparing agents. They are usually administered combined with low-dose prednisone. The most used are methotrexate and hydroxychloroquine. Other drugs reported to be useful in uncontrolled reports include azathioprine, cyclophosphamide, pentoxifylline, tetracyclines, and infliximab (Table 37.3) (16, 17). Pacemaker and automatic implantable cardioverter defibrillator may be necessary in cardiac sarcoidosis. Lung and other organ

TABLE 37.3. Commonly used alternative therapies for refractory sarcoidosis.

Intravenous methylprednisolone 500–1000 mg daily for 3 days, and then once a week for 8 weeks (may be combined with some other alternative therapy), and then by other alternative therapy combined with low-dose prednisone

Methotrexate 10–20 mg weekly (cumulative doses 1.5–2.5 g)

Hydroxychloroquine 200–400 mg daily (ocular examinations every 6–12 months)

Azathioprine 50–150 mg daily

Cyclophosphamide oral: 50–150 mg daily; intravenous pulse: 500–2000 mg every 4 weeks during 6 months, and then every 3 months for 2–3 years

Infliximab 3–5 mg/kg intravenous at weeks 0, 2, 6, 12, 18, and 24

Pentoxifyline 400–1200 mg daily

Minocycline 200 mg daily

transplantations have been successfully performed for end-stage disease.

References

1. Hunninghake GW, Costabel U, Ando M, Baughman R, Cordier JF, du Bois R, et al. ATS/ERS/WASOG Statement on sarcoidosis. *Sarcoidosis Vasc Diffuse Lung Dis* 1999; 16: 149–73/*Am J Respir Crit Care Med* 1999; 160: 736–55.
2. Baughman RP, Lower EE, du Bois RM. Sarcoidosis. *Lancet* 2003; 361: 1111–8.
3. Newman LS, Rose CS, Bresnitz EA, Rossman MD, Barnard J, Frederick M, et al. A case control etiologic study of sarcoidosis. Environmental and occupational risk factors. *Am J Respir Crit Care Med* 2004; 170: 1324–30.
4. Barnard J, Rose C, Newman L, Canner M, Martyny J, McCammon C, et al. Job and industry classifications associated with sarcoidosis in a case-control etiologic study of sarcoidosis (ACCESS). *J Occup Environ Med* 2005; 47: 226–34.
5. Spagnolo P, du Bois RM. Genetics of sarcoidosis. *Clin Dermatol* 2007; 25: 242–9.
6. Ziegenhagen MW, Müller-Quernheim J. The cytokine network in sarcoidosis and its clinical relevance. *J Intern Med* 2003; 253: 18–30.
7. Mañá J, Gómez-Vaquero C, Montero A, Salazar A, Marcoval J, Valverde J, et al. Löfgren's syndrome revisited: A study of 186 patients. *Am J Med* 1999; 107: 240–5.
8. Judson MA, Baughman RP, Teirstein AS, Terrin ML, Yeager H Jr, and the ACCESS Research Group. Defining organ involvement in sarcoidosis: The ACCESS proposed instrument. *Sarcoidosis Vasc Diffuse Lung Dis* 1999; 16: 75–86.
9. Lynch JP, White ES. Pulmonary sarcoidosis. *Eur Respir Mon* 2005; 32: 105–29.
10. Mañá J, Marcoval J, Graells J, Salazar A, Peyrí J, Pujol R. Cutaneous involvement in sarcoidosis. Relationship to systemic disease. *Arch Dermatol* 1997; 133: 882–8.
11. Hoitma E, Faber CG, Drent M, Sharma OP. Neurosarcoidosis: A clinical dilemma. *Lancet Neurol* 2004; 3: 397–407.

12. Chapelon-Abric C, de Zuttere D, Duhaut P, Veyssier P, Weschsler B, Huong DLT, et al. Cardiac sarcoidosis. A retrospective study of 41 cases. *Medicine* 2004; 83: 315–34.

13. Mañá J, Montero A, Vidal M, Marcoval J, Pujol R. Recurrent sarcoidosis: A study of 17 cases with 24 episodes of recurrence. *Sarcoidosis Vasc Diffuse Lung Dis* 2003; 20: 212–21.

14. Paramothayan S, Jones PW. Corticosteroid therapy in pulmonary sarcoidosis. A systematic review. *JAMA* 2002; 287: 1301–7.

15. Johns CJ, Michele TM. The clinical management of sarcoidosis. A 50-year experience at the Johns Hopkins Hospital. *Medicine* 1999; 78: 65–111.

16. Baughman RP, Drent M, Kavuru M, Judson MA, Costabel U, du Bois RM, et al. Infliximab therapy in patients with chronic sarcoidosis and pulmonary involvement. *Am J Respir Crit Care Med* 2006; 174: 795–802.

17. Scott TF, Yandora K, Valeri A, Chieffe C, Schramke C. Aggressive therapy for neurosarcoidosis. Long-term follow-up of 48 treated patients. *Arch Neurol* 2007; 64: 691–6.

38
Spondyloarthropathies

Michael Ehrenfeld

Abstract Spondyloarthropathies (SPA) are a group of common inflammatory rheumatic disorders characterized by axial and/or peripheral arthritis, associated with enthesitis, dactylitis, and potential extra-articular manifestations such as uveitis and skin rash. The diseases that comprise the group share a common genetic predisposition, the *HLA-B27* gene; however, this association varies markedly among the various SPAs and among different ethnic groups. Environmental factors seem to be triggering the diseases in the genetically predisposed. The radiographic hallmark of the group is sacroiliitis, which when present is of help in the diagnosis. Various sets of diagnostic and classification criteria were developed over the years with the latest European Spondyloarthropathy Study Group (ESSG) criteria, which are the most widely used. Until recent years, there were no real disease-modifying anti-rheumatic drugs that were able to halt the disease progression. Tumor necrosis factor (TNF)-alfa-blocking agents have now become the mainstream of therapy providing the patients an effective treatment option.

Keywords Spondyloarthritis · spondyloarthropathy · ankylosing spondylitis · psoriatic spondylitis · reactive arthritis · inflammatory bowel disease · spondylitis

The spondyloarthropathies (SPA), now better termed spondyloarthritides, are a group of diverse inter-related inflammatory arthritides that share multiple clinical features as well as common genetic predisposing factors (1, 2, 3). The group includes the prototypical disease ankylosing spondylitis (AS), reactive arthritis (ReA) or spondyloarthritis, psoriatic arthritis (PsA) or spondyloarthritis, SPA associated with inflammatory bowel disease (IBD) (Crohn's disease or ulcerative colitis), undifferentiated SPA (USPA) (3), and juvenile-onset spondyloarthritis.

Spondyloarthritides are characterized by sacroiliitis with inflammatory back pain, peripheral arthropathy, absence of rheumatoid factor and subcutaneous nodules, enthesitis, extra-articular or extra-spinal involvement, including of the eye, heart, lung, and skin. There is a tendency toward familial aggregation as well as varying association with HLA-B27, depending on the population studied. The similarities in clinical manifestations and the genetic predisposition suggest that these disorders share some pathogenic mechanisms. The prevalence of AS is about 0.3–0.8% and the overall prevalence of SPA is similar to that of rheumatoid arthritis (4, 5). Classification criteria for the whole group of the SPA are generally accepted and applied in clinical studies.

Signs and Symptoms

Ankylosing Spondylitis

AS is the most common and most typical form of SPA. It is two to three times more common in men than in women. The initial symptoms, typically in the early adulthood, are usually of dull pain over the buttock and lower lumbar area, accompanied by morning stiffness, relived with exercise and worsened with inactivity. This inflammatory back pain, which usually responds well to NSAIDs, may be unilateral or bilateral and may alternate from side to side. Other initial features include localized pain as a sign of enthesitis depending on the affected location (heels, ischilal tuberosities, costosternal junctions, greater trochanters, and other locations). Frank arthritis may occur in 25–35% of the patients, usually involving large joints in an asymmetrical fashion (shoulder, knee, ankle, hip). Involvement of the cervical spine with neck pain leading to a reduced range of motion, is generally a later manifestation in the course of the disease. Dactylitis, inflammation of an entire digit, commonly termed sausage digit, is another typical feature of the SPA, mainly in PsA and ReA. It is thought to arise from joint and tenosynovial

From: Y. Shoenfeld et al. (eds.): *Diagnostic Criteria in Autoimmune Diseases*, DOI: 10.1007/978-1-60327-285-8_38,
© 2008 Humana Press, Totowa, NJ

inflammation. Other clinical features include recurrent acute anterior uveitis, which occurs in about 30% of the patients and can antedate the spondylitis, cardiovascular manifestations (aortic insufficiency, congestive heart failure, aortitis, angina, pericarditis, and cardiac conduction abnormalities). Dyspnea, cough, or hemoptysis can result from upper lobe pulmonary fibrosis.

Psoriatic Arthritis

PsA develops in 5–40% of psoriasis patients (1, 6). The arthritis is often asymmetric, involving small and large joints. A number of patterns of joint involvement have been described: arthritis mutilans, peripheral oligoarthritis or polyarthritis, spondylitis, and distal interphalangeal joint arthritis (fingers and toes), which are commonly affected (>50%). Cervical spine disease is common (>50%) and usually progresses in severity in parallel with the peripheral joint disease. Psoriasis of the nails (in 83%) or skin may precede or follow joint involvement. The typical psoriatic lesions may be hidden in the scalp, behind the ears, gluteal folds, or umbilicus, occasionally even unnoticed by the patient. Extra-articular features include constitutional symptoms, fatigue, and iritis or uveitis.

Reactive Arthritis

ReA usually manifests itself as arthritis, 2–4 weeks following a urogenital or enteric infection, often in patients bearing the HLA-B27 antigen. Enthesitis, the typical feature of ReA, occurring in 70% of the patients, usually manifesting itself as a calcaneal spur with heel pain or Achilles tendinitis. The knees may be involved with large effusions. Sacroiliitis and spondylitis may occur in almost 50% of the patients. Dactylitis of the fingers or toes is also typical for ReA. A wide range of extra-articular features of ReA include urethritis, cervicitis, vulvovaginitis, salpingitis, and prostatitis. There are also typical dermatological manifestations, oral ulcers, erythema nodosum, conjuncitivitis, as well as cardiac involvement.

IBD

IBD (enteropathic)-associated arthritis is usually a large joint, lower limb asymmetric oligoarthritis. It accompanies IBD in about 10% of patients and occasionally antedates it. As with the other SPA, extra-articular and extra-intestinal features such as uveitis, erythema nodosum, pyoderma gangrenosum, and others, are more common in Crohn's disease than in ulcerative colitis, and occur more often in patients with arthritis. The synovitis runs in parallel with the bowel disease, and may resolve completely following colectomy. The spondyloarthritis and sacroiliitis run however an independent course compared to the bowel disease.

Undifferentiated Spondyloarthropathy

Undifferentiated spondyloarthropathy or spondyloarthritis, is used to describe manifestations of SPA in patients who do not meet criteria for any of the well-defined SPA. There is a female predominance of 1:3 and the clinical manifestations of this type of SPA are basically similar to all other SPAs with fewer extraarticular manifestations. Long-term follow up of these patients shows that even after years of active disease, sacroiliitis and spondylitis are either absent or appear very mildly on routine radiographs. Prognosis is generally good.

Juvenile-onset Spondyloarthropathy

Juvenile-onset spondyloarthropathy is an asymmetric, mostly lower extremity peripheral arthritis, similar to adult AS, that begins most commonly in boys aged 7–16. Enthesitis and dactylitis are prominent features of the disease in children. Systemic manifestations are more frequent in the juvenile SPA than in the adult form.

Laboratory Findings and Serological Markers

There are no specific laboratory tests for the SPAs. The diagnosis is therefore made by combining clinical criteria with radiological findings. Inflammatory disease markers, such as CRP and erythrocyte sedimentation rate (ESR), are generally elevated, though not in all patients, and are therefore less useful for monitoring disease activity of AS. A mild normocytic anemia and thrombocytosis may be present in the more severe cases. Rheumatoid factor and antinuclear antibodies are generally absent in the SPAs. Radiographic changes of the sacroiliac joints are usually symmetric and consist of blurring of the subchondral bone plate, followed by erosions and sclerosis of the adjacent bone. Conventional plain radiographs of the pelvis serve as a good screening tool for evaluation of the sacroiliac joints in patients with inflammatory back pain. Nuclear scanning, computed tomography (CT), or magnetic resonance imaging (MRI) (7) may be employed if the plain X-rays of the pelvis are negative or equivocal.

In most ethnic groups, HLA-B27 is present in approximately 90–95% of patients with AS (2, 8). In the general population AS is likely to develop in up to 6% of HLA-B27-positive adults. Approximately 4–8% of the healthy population is positive for HLA-B27. Sixty percent of psoriatic patients with spondylitis and IBD associated spondylitis are positive for B27, whereas 60–80% of ReA patients and 20–25% of patients with USPA are positive for B27. HLA typing for B27, should however not be used as a routine diagnostic test, and should be only reserved for rare clinical situations in which the presentation is atypical or complex.

Diagnostic Criteria

Table 38.1 describes the older various sets of validated diagnostic criteria which have been proposed over the years for the diagnosis of the SPAs. These criteria starting from the Rome (1961) first diagnostic criteria for AS (9), through the New York (1966) criteria (10), followed by the Modified New York criteria (1984) (11). The Rome criteria, which were developed for AS, carry a sensitivity of 89.2% and a specificity of 96.3%. The New York criteria as well as the modified New York criteria, which were both also developed for AS, carry a sensitivity of 75.8 and 83.4%, respectively, and a specificity of 98.9 and 97.8%, respectively.

Two more validated sets of criteria were later proposed in the early nineties, the first known as the Amor criteria (12) and based on multiple entry criteria, and the second as the European Spondyloarthropathy Study Group (ESSG) criteria, which is based on two entry criteria (13). These sets of more modern criteria are easy to apply in clinical practice, and the moderate level of positive predictive value (73.1 and 60.3%, respectively) and the high level of negative predictive value (99.5 and 99.2%, respectively) of both sets, mean that physicians often use them in daily practice. Tables 38.2 and 38.3 describe these two sets of criteria. A recent attempt to set up even newer candidate classification criteria for young patients with early inflammatory back pain, suggested that fulfilling two of the 4 suggested criteria

(specificity of 81% and a sensitivity of 70%), would be sufficient for the diagnosis of inflammatory back pain (14). Their criteria, which have not been validated so far, include morning stiffness of more than 30 min, improvement in back pain with exercise but not with rest, awakening because of back pain during the second half of the night only, and alternating buttock pain. All criteria developed so far, were developed as classification criteria, although they are often used as diagnostic criteria. Obviously, the use of classification criteria in an attempt to diagnose individual patients leads to an overestimation of the probability of the diagnosis. The modified New York as well as the ESSG criteria have been widely used until now in clinical studies and for diagnosis; however, all criteria sets suffer from limitations due to the fact that they were developed and evaluated in patients with established diagnoses and that they are rather complicated. Furthermore, none of the criteria include MRI interpretations, which carry very high sensitivity and specificity values, as a diagnostic/classification tool (7).

Prognosis

SPA are characterized by mild to moderate flares of active inflammation alternating with periods of little or no inflammation. Proper treatment will result in most patients with minimal or no disability, and in productive life despite back stiffness. A small minority of patients with chronic progressive incapacitating disease will develop disability due to spinal fusion, often with thoracic kyphosis or erosive disease involving peripheral joints, especially of the

TABLE 38.1. Classification criteria for ankylosing spondylitis.

Rome, 1961	New York, 1966	Modified New York, 1984
Clinical criteria	**Clinical criteria**	**Clinical criteria**
1. Low back pain & stiffness for more than 3 months, not relieved by rest	1. Limitation of motion of the lumbar spine in all 3 planes: ant. flexion, lat. flexion, & extension.	1. Low back pain of at least 3 months. Duration improved by exercise and not by rest.
2. Pain and stiffness in the thoracic region.	2. Pain at the dorsolumbar junction or in the lumbar spine.	2. Limitation of lumbar spine in sagittal and frontal planes.
3. Limited motion in the lumbar spine.	3. Limitation of chest expansion to 2.5 cm or less measured at the level of the IV intercostal space.	3. Chest expansion decreased relative to normal values for age and sex.
4. Limited chest expansion.		4. Bilateral sacroiliitis grade 2–4.
5. History or evidence of iritis or its sequelae.		5. Unilateral sacroiliitis grade 3–4.
Radiologic criteria	**Grading of radiographs**	**Definite AS if:**
1. Bilateral sacroiliac changes characteristic of AS (excluding OA).	Normal 0; suspicious 1; minimal sacroiliitis 2; moderate sacroiliitis 3; ankylosis 4.	Unilateral grade 3 or 4, or bilateral grade 2–4 sacroiliitis and any clinical criterion.
Definite AS if:	**Definite AS if:**	
1. Grade 3–4 bilateral sacroiliitis with at least 1 clinical criterion.	1. Grade 3–4 bilateral sacroiliitis with at least one clinical criterion.	
2. At least four clinical criteria.	2. Grade 3–4 unilateral or grade 2 bilateral sacroiliitis with clinical criterion 1 or with both clinical criteria 2 and 3.	
	Probable AS if:	**Probable AS if:**
	Grade 3–4 bilateral sacroiliitis with no clinical criteria.	Three clinical criteria present; or radiologic criterion present with no clinical criteria.

TABLE 38.2. The Amor criteria for the classification of spondyloarthropathy.

Clinical symptoms or past history of:	Criterion value
1. Lumbar and dorsal pain at night ± morning stiffness of lumbar or dorsal area	1
2. Asymmetric oligoarthritis	2
3. Buttock pain (if alternate buttock pain)	1 (2)
4. Dactylitis	2
5. Heel pain or other well defined enthesopathy	2
6. Acute anterior uveitis	2
7. Nongonococcal urethritis or cervicitis within 1 month before the onset of arthritis	1
8. Acute diarrhea within 1 month before the onset of arthritis	1
9. Psoriasis or balanitis or IBD	2
Radiological findings:	
10. Sacroiliitis ≥grade 2 if bilateral, ≥grade 3 if unilateral	2
Genetic background:	
11. Presence of HLA B27 antigen and/or family history of AS, ReA, uveitis, psoriasis, or IBD	2
Response to treatment:	
12. Clear cut improvement within 48 h after taking NSAID or rapid relapse of pain after discontinuation	2

Number of required points = 6; Sensitivity: 93%; Specificity: 89.9%;

TABLE 38.3. The ESSG criteria for the classification of spondyloarthropathy.

Major criteria:

1. Inflammatory spinal pain

History or present symptoms of spinal pain, with four of the five following characteristics: – onset before age 45 years – insidious onset – with morning stiffness – improved by exercise – at least 3 months duration

2. Synovitis

Past/present asymmetric or lower limb predominant arthritis.

Minor criteria:

1. Family history: presence in first-degree or second-degree relatives of any of the following characteristics: – ankylosing spondylitis -psoriasis-acute uveitis -reactive arthritis – inflammatory bowel disease
2. Psoriasis: past/present psoriasis diagnosed by a physician.
3. Inflammatory bowel disease: past/present Crohn's disease or ulcerative colitis, diagnosed by a physician, confirmed by X-ray examination or endoscopy.
4. Alternating buttock pain: past/present pain alternating between right or left gluteal region.
5. Enthesopathy: past/present spontaneous pain or tenderness at examination of the site of the insertion of the Achilles tendon or plantar fascia.
6. Acute diarrhea: episode of diarrhea occurring within 1 month before arthritis.
7. Urethritis: non-gonococcal urethritis or cervicitis occurring within 1 month before arthritis.
8. Sacroiliitis: bilateral grade 2–4 or unilateral grade 3–4 [radiographic grading system: 0 = normal; 1 = possible; 2 = minimal; 3 = moderate; 4 = ankylosis].

Number of required criteria: 1 major + 1 minor criteria. Sensitivity – 93.6%; Specificity – 87%.

hips and shoulders. Apart from this hip involvement and cervical spine disease (associated with earlier age at onset), it is unknown why some patients do better than others. Uveitis is a marker for more severe disease. Poor prognostic indicators include peripheral joint involvement, young age of onset, elevated ESR, and poor response to NSAIDs. Mortality is increased in patients with AS who have severe long-standing disease and significant extra-articular manifestations.

Prevention

Since genetic factors appear to play a role in AS and other SPAs, it is not possible to prevent the disease. Being aware, however, of any personal risk factors for the disease may help in early detection and treatment.

People who have a family member with AS and bear the *HLA-B27* gene, and are younger than 40 years, have a chance of about 20% to develop the disease. If they are however older than 40 years, their chances of getting AS are low. Proper and early treatment can relieve joint pain and help to prevent or delay the onset of physical deformities.

Therapy of the Spondyloarthritides

Nonsteroidal anti-inflammatory drugs (NSAIDs) taken in full anti-inflammatory doses, in combination with physical therapy, were and still are the basic essential therapeutic modality for patients with SPAs, which are aimed only at symptomatic control of the disease. Management of patients with AS should be based on the symptoms and signs, disease activity and severity, and functional status. Sulfasalazine (SZA) is often used in the treatment of AS and other SPAs, mainly for the control of peripheral joint involvement, for which it has been shown to be efficacious. In AS, SZA has demonstrated its efficacy in reducing spinal stiffness, and peripheral arthritis, but not on the enthesitis, the mobility of the spine, or the physical activity. Methotrexate also appears to have some influence on peripheral joint, but studies on its effect on the spine have shown conflicting results. Systemic corticosteroids have been relatively ineffective in controlling the spinal and axial inflammatory process, in contrast to their benefit seen in most other inflammatory arthritides. Bisphosphonates may have a modest effect on both the underlying osteoporosis and the inflammatory disease itself, with a beneficial effect on the spinal symptoms. Extra-articular manifestations of SPAs should be treated based on the clinical setting. Patients might need a total hip arthroplasty, but spinal osteotomy is rarely performed. The Assessment in Ankylosing Spondylitis working group (ASAS) in conjunction with the European League Against Rheumatism (EULAR) task force, have recently set up the first international evidence-based recommendations for the optimal management of AS (15). These recommendations contain 10 key components that provide practice guidelines for appropriate monitoring and treatment of patients, and include functional assessment, pain, stiffness, spinal mobility, patient's global assessment, peripheral joint involvement, enthesitis, acute phase reactants, and radiographs. Until recent years, there were no real disease modifying anti-rheumatic drugs that were able to halt the disease progression. Tumor necrosis factor (TNF)-alfa-blocking agents, which were introduced only few years ago, have now become the mainstream of therapy providing the patients an effective treatment option. All three available anti-TNF inhibitors (Infliximab, etanercept, and adalimumab) have been shown to be remarkably effective in AS without the need to combine them with another disease-modifying drug such as methotrexate (16). Multiple large randomized, placebo-controlled trials of the use of all three TNF blockers in AS and PsA, showed impressive short-term as well as long-term improvements in spinal pain, stiffness, physical function, quality of life, as well as in inflammatory markers and MRI inflammation (17). Several studies have demonstrated that active inflammation of the sacroiliac joint or spine, as shown by MRI, is significantly reduced by all three TNF-blocking agents (18, 19). It has also been recently shown that survival of TNF antagonists in SPA is better than in rheumatoid arthritis (20). Thus, though TNF antagonists seem so far to be a safe and effective option for long-term treatment of patients with SPA, it is meanwhile believed that they should only be introduced in patients who are uncontrollable with conventional therapy, because their long-term safety and effect on the prevention of structural damage have yet to be evaluated and demonstrated in prospective randomized controlled trials.

References

1. Gladman DD. Psoriatic arthritis. *Rheum Dis Clin North Am* 1998; 24: 829–44.
2. De Keyser F, Elewaut D, De Vos M, *et al*. Bowel inflammation and the spondyloarthropathies. *Rheum Dis Clin North Am* 1998; 24: 785–813.
3. Zochling J, Brandt J, Braun J. The current concept of spondyloarthritis with special emphasis on undifferentiated spondyloarthritis. *Rheumatology* 2005; 44: 1483–91.
4. Braun J, Bollow M, Remlinger G, *et al*. Prevalence of spondyloarthropathies in HLA-B27 positive and negative blood donors. *Arthritis Rheum* 1998; 41: 58–67.
5. Saraux A, Guillemin F, Guggenbuhl P, *et al*. Prevalence of the spondyloarthropathies in France: 2001; *Ann Rheum Dis* 2005; 64: 1431–35.
6. Kane D, Stafford L, Bresnihan B, *et al*. A prospective clinical and radiological study of early psoriatic arthritis: an early synovitis clinic experience. *Rheumatology* 2003; 42: 1460–68.
7. Bollow M, Braun J, Hamm B, *et al*. Early sacroiliitis in patients with spondyloarthropathy: Evaluation with dynamic Gadolinium-enhanced MR imaging. *Radiology* 1995; 194: 529–36.
8. Gladman DD, Farewell VT, Kopciuk KA, *et al*. HLA markers and progression in psoriatic arthritis. *J Rheumatol* 1998; 25: 730–33.
9. Bennett PH, and Wood PHN (eds; 1968) Population studies of the rheumatic diseases, 456–457.
10. van der Linden S, van der Heijde D, Braun J. Ankylosing spondylitis. Harris EJ, *et al*. Eds. Kelley's textbook of rheumatology. 7th ed. Philadelphia: Elsevier Saunders; 2005: 1125–41.
11. van der Linden S, Valkenburg HA, Cats A. Evaluation of diagnostic criteria for ankylosing spondylitis. A proposal for modification of the New York criteria. *Arthritis Rheum* 1984; 27: 361–68.
12. Amor B, Dougados M, Mijiyawa M. Critères de classification des spondyloarthropathies. *Rev Rhum Mal Osteoartic* 1990; 57: 85–9.
13. Dougados M, van der Linden S, Juhlin R, *et al*. The European Spondyloarthropathy Study Group preliminary criteria for the classification of spondyloarthropathy. *Arthritis Rheum* 1991; 34: 1218–27.
14. Rudwaleit M, Metter A, Listing J, *et al*. Inflammatory back pain in ankylosing spondylitis: a reassessment of the clinical history for application as classification and diagnostic criteria. *Arthritis Rheum* 2006; 54: 569–78.
15. van der Heijde D, Calin A, Dougados M, *et al*. Selection of instruments in the core set for DC-ART, SMARD, physical therapy, and clinical record keeping in ankylosing spondylitis. Progress report of the ASAS Working Group Assessment in Ankylosing Spondylitis. *J Rheumatol* 1999; 26: 951–54.
16. Zochling J, van der Heijde D, Burgos-Vargas R, *et al*. ASAS/EULAR recommendations for the management of ankylosing spondylitis. *Ann Rheum Dis* 2006; 65: 442–52.
17. Braun J, Baraliakos X, Brandt J, *et al*. Persistent clinical response to the anti-TNF-alpha antibody infliximab in patients

with ankylosing spondylitis over 3 years. *Rheumatology* 2005; 44: 670–76.

18. Mease PJ, Kivitz AJ, Burch FX, *et al.* Continued inhibition of radiographic progression in patients with psoriatic arthritis following 2 years of treatment with etanercept. *J Rheumatol* 2006; 33: 712–21.

19. Haibel H, Rudwaleit M, Brandt HC, *et al.* Adalimumab reduces spinal symptoms in active ankylosing spondylitis: Clinical and magnetic resonance imaging results of a fifty-two week open-label trial. *Arthritis Rheum* 2006; 54: 678–81.

20. Carmona L, Gómez-Reino JJ, and on behalf of the BIOBADASER Group. Survival of TNF antagonists in spondylarthritis is better than in rheumatoid arthritis. Data from the Spanish registry BIOBADASER. *Arthritis Res Therap* 2006; 8: R72. Epub 2006 April 18.

39
Periodic Fever Syndromes

Shai Padeh and Yackov Berkun

Abstract Human autoinflammatory diseases are a heterogeneous group of genetically determined diseases character-ized by seemingly unprovoked inflammation, in the absence of autoimmune or infective causes. These diseases are caused by proteins that involve in the innate immunity and interact with other proteins to form an inflammasome (1), which acts as an early sensor to detect danger signals and initiates the host defense reactions (2). Members of the "NALP" family of proteins (which includes cryopyrin) are components of the inflammasome. Two types of inflammasomes have now been described: the NALP1 inflammasome and the NALP3, or cryopyrin, inflammasome. The stimulation of cryopyrin triggers a series of reactions, which ultimately result in the activation of the proinflammatory cytokine interleukin-1[3].

The past decade has witnessed tremendous advances in the understanding of these disorders. These advances have allowed for therapeutic interventions, resulting in improvement in the short-term and long-term morbidity of all of these diseases. As these syndromes often have overlapping symptoms, diagnostic criteria are essential.

Keywords Familial mediterranean fever · periodic fever accompanied by aphthous stomatitis · pharyngitis · and cervical adenitis syndrome · tumor necrosis factor receptor–associated periodic syndrome (TRAPS) · hyperimmunoglobulinemia D and periodic fever syndrome · familial cold autoinflammatory syndrome · muckle-wells syndrome · neonatal-onset multisystem inflammatory disease/chronic infantile neurologic cutaneous and articular syndrome

Periodic Fever Syndromes

The term hereditary autoinflammatory disease has been proposed to describe a group of disorders characterized by attacks provoked by no known trigger and no evidence for autoimmunity, such as autoantibodies or autoreactive T cells. All syndromes (with the exception of periodic fever, aphthous stomatitis, pharyngitis, and adenitis (PFAPA)) derive from defects of the innate immunity; nine hereditary autoinflammatory syndromes have been identified in the past 9 years: Familial Mediterranean fever (FMF); Tumor necro-sis factor (TNF) receptor–associated periodic syndrome (TRAPS); Hyperimmunoglobulinemia D and periodic fever syndrome (HIDS); Familial cold autoinflammatory syn-drome (FCAS)/familial cold urticaria syndrome (FCUS); Muckle-Wells syndrome (MWS); Neonatal-onset multi-system inflammatory disease (NOMID)/chronic infantile neurologic cutaneous and articular (CINCA) syndrome; Blau syndrome; PAPA (Pyogenic sterile Arthritis, Pyoderma gangrenosum, and Acne) syndrome; and Chronic recurrent

multifocal osteomyelitis (CRMO) (Mageed syndrome). This chapter discusses those syndromes that are associated with recurrent fevers. The growing list of mutations of these Mendelian disorders (544 so far) is routinely updated in INFEVERS (3), run by Toitou et al., a mutational database accessible on the World Wide Web at http://fmf.igh.cnrs.fr/infevers. The proteins coded by these genes participate in the inflammasome, a complex of proteins that have distinct roles in the innate defense system and acts as an early sensor to detect danger signals and initiates the host defense reactions (2).

Familial Mediterranean Fever

FMF is an autosomal recessive disease mainly affecting ethnic groups living around the Mediterranean basin: Sephardic and Ashkenazi Jews, Armenians, Turks, Arabs, and Druze. Scattered cases of FMF have been reported throughout the world. FMF was first described as a separate

From: Y. Shoenfeld et al. (eds.): *Diagnostic Criteria in Autoimmune Diseases*, DOI: 10.1007/978-1-60327-285-8_39,
© 2008 Humana Press, Totowa, NJ

TABLE 39.1. Symptoms and signs of FMF.

Symptoms & signs	Prevalence	
Fever	96%	38.5 to 40°C, 1 to 3 days, resolve without treatment
Sterile peritonitis	91%	The hallmark of the disease, generalized abdominal pain, guarding, rebound, tenderness, and distention, mimicking acute appendicitis. May result in fibrous adhesions, at times the cause of sterility or ileus.
Pleurisy	57%	Acute one-sided febrile, painful breathing, diminished breath sounds, small pleural effusion or mild pleural thickening.
Arthritis, arthralgia	45%	Monoarticular, large joints, lower extremities, lasts longer, often precipitated by minor trauma or effort, leaving no residua. Synovial fluid varies in appearance from cloudy to purulent, large numbers of neutrophils.
Pericarditis	3%	Signs of pericarditis.
Erysipelas like erythema	22–30%	Tender, hot, swollen, sharply bordered red lesions on skin of lower extremities. Edema of the superficial dermis and sparse perivascular infiltrate without vasculitis, deposits of C3 in the wall of the small vessels of the superficial vascular plexus.
Headache	90%	
Proteinuria	Variable in different populations	Frequently in untreated patients, mostly affecting the kidneys, begins with persistent heavy proteinuria leading to nephrotic syndrome. Prevalence in the colchicine era is unknown, and
Amyloidosis	Variable in different populations	different magnitude has been reported in different centers. Derived from circulating acute-phase reactant serum amyloid A protein (SAA). Median SAA concentration >10 mg per liter correlates with poor outcome.
Acute scrotum	2%	Inflammation of the tunica vaginalis testis may mimic episodes of torsion of the testis.
Myalgia	10%	Severe debilitating myalgia, prolonged fever (6–8 weeks), a higher ESR than commonly found, leukocytosis, and hyperglobulinemia.
Henoch Schonlein Purpura	3–11%	HSP in up to 11% of FMF patients. Polyarteritis nodosa (PAN) more commonly, with a younger age of onset (13).
Splenomegaly	3%	
Glomerulonephritis	Sporadic	Various types of glomerulonephritis

nosologic entity in 1945. The benefit of prophylactic treatment with colchicine was first suggested by Goldfinger (4), and was later assessed by double-blind studies. The gene responsible for FMF, *MEFV*, was identified in 1997 (5) that encodes pyrin/Marenostrin, which is present almost exclusively in neutrophils and their precursors (6).

Clinical Manifestations

Repeated attacks at irregular intervals and in an unpredicted sequence, rather than truly periodic attacks, are typical of the disease. In children, about 50% of the cases have symptoms before the age of 6 years, and 80% have symptoms before the age of 10 years (7). The symptoms and signs characteristic of this disease are summarized in Table 39.1.

Biochemical Features

Leukocytosis and elevated acute-phase reactants, including accelerated erythrocyte sedimentation rate (ESR) and elevated levels of C-reactive protein (CRP), fibrinogen, haptoglobin, C3, C4, and serum amyloid A (SAA) are characteristic (8). CRP correlates better with FMF attacks, with levels much higher than that in other inflammatory conditions.

Pathological Features

The MEFV gene. In 1992, the gene responsible for FMF, MEFV, was found to reside on the short arm of chromosome 16 (6). Five years later, the MEFV gene locus was discovered (6). MEFV codes a protein, pyrin (from the Greek word for fire and fever, or marenostrin by French FMF Consortium, the Latin for "our sea"), which plays a role in mitigating an inflammatory response (3). To date, more than 100 disease-causing mutations have been described (2). Molecular diagnosis fails to confirm the diagnosis of FMF in a large number of patients with typical presentation, even after the entire gene has been sequenced (9). Most laboratories providing routine genetic testing of FMF screen for at least the five most frequent mutations (M694 V, V726A, V680I, E148Q, and M694I), because other mutations are found in less than 1% of FMF alleles. One specific mutation, M694 V, has been implicated as a risk factor for amyloidosis.

Diagnostic Criteria

Until 1997, the diagnosis of FMF was based on clinical grounds alone. A short time before the discovery of MEFV gene, diagnostic criteria for FMF were proposed (Table 39.2). Today there is a need to add the MEFV genotype to diagnostic criteria. We suggest homozygosity or compound heterozygosity to MEFV mutations to be

TABLE 39.2. Simplified criteria set for diagnosis of familial Mediterranean fever (FMF) (9).

Major criteria 1–4. Typical attacks	Minor criteria
1. Peritonitis (generalized)	1–2. Incomplete attacks involving one or more of the following sites:
2. Pleuritis (unilateral) or pericarditis	
3. Monoarthritis (hip, knee, ankle)	1. Chest
4. Fever alone	2. Joint
5. Incomplete abdominal attack	3. Exertional leg pain
	4. Favorable response to colchicine

Diagnosis of FMF if ≥1 major criteria, or ≥2 minor criteria. Typical attacks are recurrent (≥3 of the same type), febrile (≥38°C), and short (12 hours and 3 days). Incomplete attacks differ from typical attacks in 1 or 2 features, as follows: 1) < 38°C; 2) longer or shorter attacks; 3) no signs of peritonitis; 4) localized abdominal attacks; 5) atypical joints.

included as major criterion. Because only one or no known MEFV mutations are found in 50–60% of FMF patients, heterozygous state is suggested as minor criteria.

The most common differential diagnosis of FMF is functional abdominal pain, irritable bowel syndrome, and recurrent (intercurrent) infections in young children, in addition to all other disorders that belong to the auto-inflammatory periodic diseases.

Therapy

Until 1973, the treatment of FMF was restricted to alleviating pain. Daily prophylactic treatment with colchicine was suggested by Goldfinger, and assessed by double-blind studies (10). Treatment is started with 1 mg colchicine per day regardless of age or body weight. This dose is increased to 1.5 or 2 mg until remission is achieved.

Periodic Fever Accompanied by Aphthous Stomatitis, Pharyngitis, and Cervical Adenitis Syndrome

First described in 1987 (11), PFAPA syndrome is a chronic disease of unknown cause characterized by periodic episodes of high fever accompanied by aphthous stomatitis, pharyngitis, and cervical adenitis, often associated with headache or abdominal or joint pain (11).

Clinical Manifestations

Typically, patients present with febrile attacks, which last for 3–6 days, and recur every 3–8 weeks, with fever, chills, sweats, headache, and muscle and bone pain. The affected children had no long-term sequelae. Episodes of fevers begin at the age of 4.2 ± 2.7 years. General malaise, resembling streptococcal pharyngitis, tonsillitis with negative throat

TABLE 39.3. Clinical presentation of patients with PFAPA of PFAPA in two large series.

Symptom	Thomas et al (%)(22)	Padeh et al (%)(23)
Fever	100	100
Exudative tonsillitis	72[a]	100
Malaise	NA	100
Cervical adenopathy	88	100
Aphthae	70	68
Headache	60	18
Abdominal pain	49	18
Arthralgia	79	11
Chills	80	NA
Cough	13	NA
Nausea	32	NA
Diarrhea	16	NA
Rash	9	NA

Abbreviations: NA, not available; [a]Pharyngitis rather than exudative tonsillitis

cultures, and cervical adenopathy are typical of the syndrome. The clinical presentation of patients with PFAPA in two large series is summarized in Table 39.3.

Diagnostic Criteria

The differences between the two series probably derive from the differences in the diagnostic criteria of the two centers (Table 39.4).

Pathological Features

The cause of PFAPA is unknown. Long (12) has hypothesized that the periodicity of the PFAPA syndrome derives from intermittent expression or suppression of antigens or epitopes of infectious agents or an alteration in the nature or kinetics of immunological response.

TABLE 39.4. Diagnostic criteria for PFAPA syndrome from two centers.

Thomas et al (%)	Padeh et al (%)
Regularly recurring fevers with an early age of onset (<5 years of age)	Monthly fevers—cyclic fever at any age group
Constitutional symptoms in the absence of upper respiratory infection with at least one of the following clinical signs:	
Aphthous stomatitis	Possibly aphthous stomatitis
Cervical lymphadenitis	Cervical lymphadenitis
Pharyngitis	Exudative tonsillitis + negative throat culture
Exclusion of cyclic neutropenia	
Completely asymptomatic interval between episodes	Completely asymptomatic interval between episodes
Normal growth and development	Rapid response to a single dose of corticosteroids

Therapy

Most patients who are given one dose of corticosteroid (2 mg/kg/day prednisone or prednisolone or, preferably, 0.3 mg/kg of bethamethasone) report a dramatic resolution of fever within 2 to 4 hours after the ingestion of the corticosteroid.

Tumor Necrosis Factor Receptor–Associated Periodic Syndrome (TRAPS)

TRAPS, formerly known as familial Hibernian fever (FHF), is an autosomal dominant periodic disease characterized by recurrent attacks of fever, abdominal pain, localized tender skin lesions, and myalgia, first described in persons of Irish-Scottish ancestry. Pleurisy, leukocytosis, and high ESR are other features. A germline mutation in the TNFRSF1A gene causes the disease (13). The type 1 receptor (the p55 TNF receptor) is encoded by a gene located on chromosome 12p13.2. (14). More than 82 mutations in TNFRSF1A have been associated with TRAPS so far (2). TNFRSF1A is expressed in various cells (15) and has been shown to induce cytokine secretion, expression of adhesion molecules leukocyte activation, host resistance to intracellular pathogens, pyrexia, and cachexia.

Clinical Manifestations

The median age of onset is 3 years. Attacks last for 21 days on average and occur every 5–6 weeks. Attacks begin with a subtle onset of deep muscle cramping that crescendo over the course of 1–3 days. Myalgia, typically affecting only a single area of the body, is waxing and waning throughout the course of the attack. The rash is a centrifugal, migratory, erythematous patch, most typically overlying a local area of myalgia. Abdominal pain, often mimicking acute appendicitis, occurs in 92% of patients. Conjunctivitis, periorbital edema, or periorbital pain is reported in 82% of patients. Chest pain (57%) may be either musculoskeletal or pleural in origin.

Biochemical Features

Elevation of ESR, CRP, haptoglobin, fibrinogen, and ferritin is the rule. Diagnostic criteria. No valid criteria has been published. Suggested criteria are summarized in Table 39.5.

Therapy

Unlike in FMF, glucocorticoids decrease the severity of symptoms but not the frequency of attacks. Colchicine, azathioprine, cyclosporine, thalidomide, cyclophosphamide, chlorambucil, intravenous immunoglobulin, dapsone, and

TABLE 39.5. TRAPS should be considered when:

1. A combination of the inflammatory symptoms, as described previously, recurs in episodes lasting >5 days.
2. Myalgia is associated with an overlying erythematous rash that together displays a centrifugal migratory pattern over the course of days and occur on the limbs or trunk.
3. There is ocular involvement with attacks.
4. Symptoms respond to glucocorticosteroids but not to colchicine.
5. Symptoms segregate in the patient's family in an autosomal dominant pattern.
6. Mutations in the TNFRSF1A gene on mutation analysis.

methotrexate have been tried but have not been found to be beneficial. Etanercept, resulted in 66% response rate, and more recently, Anakinra has been reported beneficial in a patient with TRAPS.

Hyper-IgD and Periodic Fever Syndrome (HIDS)

HIDS is a syndrome characterized by periodic febrile attacks occurring every 4–8 weeks with an intense inflammatory reaction accompanied by lymphadenopathy, abdominal pain, diarrhea, joint pain, hepatosplenomegaly, and cutaneous signs. HIDS was originally described by Van der Meer (16) in 1984. In 1995, by consensus, the acronym of HIDS was selected to designate the hyper-IgD syndrome (17). Mutations in the mevalonate kinase (MVK) gene are responsible for this syndrome. MVK deficit has also been reported in mevalonic aciduria, a rare inherited disorder that is characterized by developmental delay, failure to thrive, hypotonia, ataxia, and myopathy, which is a completely different disease (18). Most patients originated from Europe, namely the Netherlands (28 cases, 56%), France (10 cases, 20%), and Italy (3 cases, 6%). One patient was from Japan. Patients present as early as 0.5 year of age and have a life-long persistence of periodic fever.

Clinical Manifestations

The clinical manifestations are summarized in Table 39.6.

TABLE 39.6. Clinical presentation of HIDS.

High spiking fever, preceded by chills	76%
Lymphadenopathy	94%
Abdominal pain	72%
Vomiting	56%
Diarrhea	82%
Headache	52%
Skin lesions (erythematous macules, papules, nodules, urticarial lesions)	82%
Polyarthralgia	80%
Nondestructive arthritis large joints (knee and ankle),	68%
Serositis	Rare
Amyloidosis	Not reported

Biochemical Features

During an attack, there is a brisk acute-phase response, with leukocytosis, and high levels of CRP and serum amyloid A. The serum IgD level is persistently elevated (>100U/mL). In 82% of cases, the serum IgA is likewise elevated (≥2.6 g/L). Mevalonate kinase is an important enzyme in the cholesterol metabolic pathway and follows 3-hydroxy-3-methylglutaryl–coenzyme A reductase. In classic HIDS, the activity of mevalonate kinase is reduced to 5% to 15% of normal.

Pathological Features

Most patients are compound heterozygotes for missense mutations in the MVK gene. More than 100 mutations have been reported (2). How a deficiency of mevalonate kinase is linked to an inflammatory periodic fever syndrome remains known.

Diagnostic Criteria

The diagnostic criteria are summarized in Table 39.7.

Therapy

No effective treatment is known. Thalidomide and simvastatine had a limited effect. Favorable experiences with etanercept in three patients, and anakinra in one patient have been reported.

TABLE 39.7. Diagnostic criteria for HIDS.

The diagnosis is established by
1. Detection of elevated excretion MVA in urine.
2. Increased immunoglobulin (Ig) D (> 100 U/mL and A (≥ 2.6 g/L).
3. Elevated excretion of mevalonic acid.
4. The diagnosis is confirmed by demonstration of deficient MVK enzyme activity or by identification of two disease-causing mutations in the MVK gene.

Cryopyrin-Associated Periodic Syndromes (CAPS)

The CIAS1 (Cold-Induced Autoinflammatory Syndrome) gene, located on chromosome 1p44, encodes a pyrin-like protein, cryopyrin, expressed predominantly in peripheral blood leukocytes. CIAS1-related autoinflammatory syndromes (CRAS) are three different diseases caused by mutation in the CIAS1 gene: familial cold autoinflammatory syndrome (FCAS), Muckle–Wells syndrome (MWS), and neonatal-onset multisystem inflammatory disease (NOMID, also called chronic infantile neurologic cutaneous and articular syndrome or CINCA syndrome). FCAS, MWS, and NOMID/CINCA syndrome appear to represent a spectrum of diseases, with FCAS being the mildest and NOMID/CINCA syndrome being the most severe. Over time, the number of mutations in CIAS1 is growing (up to 90), with a spectrum of diseases ranging from FCUS to MWS to OMID/CINCA syndrome (2). A summary of the clinical and genetic characterization of these syndromes is presented in Table 39.8.

TABLE 39.8. A summary of the clinical and genetic characterization of the autoinflammatory fevers syndromes.

Syndrome	Abbreviation	Distinguishing clinical findings	Inheritance pattern	Gene	Protein
Familial Mediterranean Fever	FMF	Episodes 1–3 days, polyserositis, amyloidosis common	Autosomal recessive	MEFV	Pyrin (Marenostrin)
TNF-receptor associated periodic syndrome	TRAPS	Long episodes (often >1 week), periorbital edema, migratory myalgia and rash	Autosomal dominant	TNFRSF1A	TNF-receptor type 1 (p55, CD120a, TNFR1)
Hyper-IgD syndrome	HIDS	Lymphadenopathy, starts in first year, high IgD, attack after immunization	Autosomal recessive	Mevalonate kinase (MVK)	Mevalonate kinase (MK)
Syndrome of pyogenic arthritis, pyoderma gangrenosum, acne	PAPA	Pyogenic arthritis, Pyoderma gangrenosum	Autosomal dominant	PSTPIP1 (CD2BP1)	PSTPIP1 (CD2BP1)
Blau syndrome	BS	Granulomatous Inflammation	Autosomal dominant	NOD2 (CARD15)	NOD2/CARD15
Cryopyrin-associated periodic syndrome (CAPS)					
Familial Cold Autoinflammatory syndrome	FCAS	Provoked by cold exposure, brief episodes (hours)		CIAS1/ NALP3/ PYPAF1	
Muckle-Wells syndrome	MWS	Hearing loss, amyloidosis common		CIAS1/ NALP3/ PYPAF1	
Neonatal onset multisystemic inflammatory disease	NOMID/ CINCA	Almost continuous, chronic aseptic meningitis, hearing loss, arthropathy	Autosomal dominant	CIAS1/ NALP3/ PYPAF1	Cryopyrin (NALP3, PYPAF1)

NOMID/CINCA Syndrome

The triad of cutaneous rash, chronic meningitis, and arthropathy characterizes CINCA syndrome. First described in 1981, it is a disease of chronic inflammation, often starting at birth, which lasts the entire lifetime. Only recently, it has been linked to mutations in the CIAS1 gene on chromosome 1q44.

Clinical Manifestations

Fever and rash are dominant symptoms; lymphadenopathy and hepatosplenomegaly are often present during flares. Headaches, seizures, transient episodes of hemiplegia, and spasticity of the legs reflect chronic aseptic meningitis. Skull anomalies include increased cranial volume, frontal bossing, and late closure of the anterior fontanelle. Progressive visual defect evolving to blindness in the most severe cases, progressive perceptive deafness, hoarseness and saddle-nose deformity are other features of the disease. Shortening of the hands and feet, clubbing of the fingers, patellar overgrowth, and wrinkled palms and soles are characteristic of the disease.

Biochemical Features

High levels of acute-phase reactants, anemia, and high platelet counts are often found.

Diagnostic Criteria

No diagnostic criteria has been suggested so far as only 100 cases have been identified worldwide (2). Diagnosis is suggested when the above clinical signs are presented in a patient. Genetic analysis confirms the diagnosis in only 50% of the cases.

Therapy

No effective treatment is known, but recently success with the IL-1 receptor antagonist Anakinra was reported (19).

Muckle–Wells Syndrome (MWS); Urticaria-Deafness-Amyloidosis Syndrome

In 1962, Muckle and Wells described a dominantly inherited syndrome of urticaria, progressive perceptive deafness, and amyloidosis (20). First symptoms usually start in infancy and consist of nonpruritic urticaria, low-grade fever, and often arthritis and conjunctivitis. Neurosensory hearing loss begins during adolescence and slowly evolves

into deafness. Absent organ of Corti, atrophy of the cochlear nerve, and amyloid infiltration of the kidneys have been found on autopsy. The severity of the disease resides in the development of AA amyloidosis (20). No diagnostic criteria are available, and the diagnosis is confirmed in clinically suspected cases by genetic analysis.

Familial Cold Autoinflammatory Syndrome (FCAS)

FCAS, formerly known as familial cold urticaria, is a rare autosomal dominant syndrome characterized by fever, rash, and arthralgia brought about by exposure to cold. After exposure to cold (0.5 to 6 hours), patients develop urticarial wheals, pain and swelling of joints, chills, and fever (21). Systemic amyloidosis with nephropathy is a frequent cause of death. The clinical phenotype varies largely, and some patients report a very regular periodic fever, irregular severe febrile episodes, relatively mild arthralgia, dry cough, inflammatory cardiomyopathy and nephropathy, and euthyroid thyroiditis (21).

Diagnostic Criteria

No diagnostic criteria are available, and the diagnosis is confirmed in clinically suspected cases by genetic analysis.

Therapy

Therapy includes educating the patients, movement to warmer climates, and warming treatments. Anti-inflammatory agents, anabolic steroids, high-dose corticosteroids, and colchicine have variable effect in these patients. Antihistamines are generally not effective. Stanozolol and anakinra have also been reported to be effective (19).

Summary

Human autoinflammatory diseases (except for PFAPA) are a heterogeneous group of genetically determined diseases characterized by seemingly unprovoked inflammation, in the absence of autoimmune or infective causes, and are caused by defect in proteins of the innate immunity.

References

1. Drenth JPH, W.M. van der Meer JWM The Inflammasome — A Linebacker of Innate Defense. *N Engl J Med.* 2006;355:730–732.
2. Stehlik C, Reed JC,. The PYRIN connection: novel players in innate immunity and inflammation. *J Exp Med.* 2004 [2];200(5):551–558.
3. Touitou I e. INFEVERS: the repertory of Familial Mediterranean Fever (FMF) and hereditary autoinflammatory

disorders mutations. 2007:Available at: http://fmf.igh.cnrs.fr/infevers. Accessed July 10, 2007.

4. Goldfinger SE. Colchicine for familial Mediterranean fever. *N Engl J Med.* 1972;287(25):1302.

5. Pras E, Aksentijevich I, Gruberg L, et al. Mapping of a gene causing familial Mediterranean fever to the short arm of chromosome 16. *N Engl J Med.* 1992;329:1509–1513.

6. Consortium. TFF. A candidate gene for familial Mediterranean fever. *Nat Genet.* 1997;17:25–31.

7. Padeh S. Periodic fever syndromes. *Pediatr Clin North Am.* 2005;52(2):577–609, vii.

8. Berkun Y, Padeh S, Reichman B, Zaks N, Rabinovich E, Lidar M, Shainberg B, Livneh A. A Single Testing of serum amyloid a levels as a tool for diagnosis and treatment dilemmas in familial mediterranean fever. *Semin Arthritis Rheum.* 2007;37(3):182–8.

9. Cazeneuve C, Sarkisian T, Pecheux C, et al. MEFV-gene analysis in Armenian patients with familial Mediterranean fever: diagnostic value and unfavorable renal prognosis of the M694 V homozygous genotype—genetic and therapeutic implications. *Am J Hum Genet.* 1999;65:88–97.

10. Zemer D, Revach M, Pras M, et al. A controlled trial of colchicine in preventing attacks of familial Mediterranean fever. *N Engl J Med.* 1974;291:932–944.

11. Marshall GS, Edwards KM, Butler J, et al. Syndrome of periodic fever, pharyngitis, and aphthous stomatitis. *J Pediatr.* 1987;110:43–46.

12. Long SS. Syndrome of periodic fever, aphthous stomatitis, pharyngitis, and adenitis (PFAPA)—what it isn't. What is it? *J Pediatr.* 1999;135(1):1–5.

13. McDermott MF, Aksentijevich I, Galon J, et al. Germline mutations in the extracellular domains of the 55 kDa TNF receptor, TNFR1, define a family of dominantly inherited autoinflammatory syndromes. *Cell.* 1999;97:133–144.

14. Derre J, Kemper O, Cherif D, et al. The gene for the type 1 tumor necrosis factor receptor (TNF-R1) is localized on band 12p13. *Hum Genet.* 1991;87:231–233.

15. Smith CA, Davis T, Anderson D, et al. A receptor for tumor necrosis factor defines an unusual family of cellular and viral proteins. *Science.* 1990;248(4958):1019–1023.

16. Van der Meer JWM, , Vossen JM, Radl J, et al. Hyperimmunoglobulinemia D and periodic fever: a new syndrome. *Lancet.* 1984;i:1087–1090.

17. Drenth JPH, Powell RJ. Hyperimmunoglobulinemia D syndrome: conference. *Lancet.* 1995;345:445–446.

18. Drenth JP, Cuisset L, Grateau G, et al. Mutations in the gene encoding mevalonate kinase cause hyper-IgD and periodic fever syndrome. International Hyper-IgD Study Group. *Nat Genet.* 1999;22:178–181.

19. Frenkel J, Wulffraat NM, Kuis W. Anakinra in mutation-negative NOMID/CINCA syndrome: comment on the articles by Hawkins et al and Hoffman and Patel. *Arthritis Rheum.* 1994;50(11):3738–3739.

20. Dode C, Le Du N, Cuisset L, et al. New mutations of CIAS1 that are responsible for Muckle-Wells syndrome and familial cold urticaria: a novel mutation underlies both syndromes. *Am J Hum Genet.* 2002;70:1498–1506.

21. Porksen G, Lohse P, Rosen-Wolff A, et al. Periodic fever, mild arthralgias, and reversible moderate and severe organ inflammation associated with the V 198 M mutation in the CIAS1 gene in three German patients—expanding phenotype of CIAS1 related autoinflammatory syndrome. *Eur J Haematol.* 2004;73(2):123–127.

40
Fibromyalgia Syndrome

Arnson Yoav, Dvorish Zamir, Amital Daniela and Amital Howard

Abstract   Not many disorders raise debate and questioning as fibromyalgia (FM).

Although FM has classification criteria many physicians worldwide doubt the existence of FM as a distinct clinical entity. This pain syndrome characterized by diffuse symmetric muscular pain has no distinct biological marker, coexist with multiple psychiatric and organic disorders and often develops secondary or subsequent to another established disease.

The following review will elaborate on the basic clinical characteristics of FM, will cover and question the considerations behind the currently used classification criteria and discuss the various scales and scoring systems that are used in order to assess the severity of this syndrome.

Keywords   Fibromyalgia · tender points · disability · pain · tenderness

Introduction

FM is a common cause of chronic musculoskeletal pain. It is a disease that affects muscles and soft tissues such as tendons and ligaments. The condition is not associated with tissue inflammation and the etiology of the disease is not yet fully understood. Clinical descriptions of what we now call FM have been reported since the mid-1800s. Various terms, including "neurosthenia" and "muscular rheumatism" had originally been applied. In 1904, Gowers was the first to use the term "fibrositis," which was used until the mid)1980s.

The estimated prevalence of FM in the general community is 2% for both sexes, 3.4% for women and 0.5% for men. The prevalence increases with age, reaching greater than 7% in women aged 60–79 years (1). The cardinal manifestation of FM is diffuse musculoskeletal pain. Although the pain may initially be localized, often in the neck and shoulders, it eventually involves many muscle groups. Patients typically complain of diffuse pain over the neck, middle and lower back, chest wall, and upper and lower limbs. The pain is chronic and persistent, although it usually varies in intensity. Patients often have difficulty distinguishing joint from muscle pain and also report a sensation of swelling; however, the joints do not appear swollen or inflamed on examination. Pain is often aggravated by exertion, stress, lack of sleep, and weather changes. Sensations of numbness, tingling, burning, or a crawling perception are often described (1, 2).

Patients also may have a variety of poorly understood pain symptoms, including abdominal and chest wall pain and symptoms suggestive of irritable bowel syndrome, pelvic pain, and bladder symptoms of frequency and urgency suggestive of the female urethral syndrome or of interstitial cystitis (3).

Signs and Symptoms

Fatigue is present in more than 90% of cases and is occasionally the chief complaint. Most patients report light sleep and feeling unrefreshed in the morning whereas others report symptoms suggestive of pathologic sleep disturbances such as sleep apnea or nocturnal myoclonus. Light-headedness, dizziness, and feeling faint are common symptoms. Headaches (either muscular or migraine-type) are present in a majority of patients (3). Psychiatric features presented including mood disturbances, especially depression, anxiety, post-traumatic stress disorder and heightened somatic concern, and cognitive dysfunction especially short-term memory loss (2, 3, 4, 5, 6).

Additional symptoms and clinical manifestations may include complaints of ocular dryness, multiple

From: Y. Shoenfeld et al. (eds.): *Diagnostic Criteria in Autoimmune Diseases*, DOI: 10.1007/978-1-60327-285-8_40,
© 2008 Humana Press, Totowa, NJ

chemical sensitivity and "allergic" symptoms, palpitations, dyspnea, vulvodynia, dysmenorrhea, nondermatomal paresthesias, weight fluctuations, night sweats, dysphagia, dysgeusia, glosodynia, and weakness.

FM is often accompanied by other diseases. As many as 80% of patients with FM also fulfill criteria for chronic fatigue syndrome, up to 80% have headaches, 75% have temporomandibular disorders, and up to 60% may have irritable bowel syndrome (2, 5, 7, 8).

Diagnosis

Diagnosing FM is based on the combination of patient history, physical examination, laboratory evaluations, and exclusion of other causes for symptoms attributed to FM. The clinical diagnosis of FM is based largely upon the patient's history of chronic, generalized pain and associated features. The features include fatigue, sleep disturbances, headache, cognitive difficulty, and mood disturbances (Table 40.1).

TABLE 40.1. Clinical characteristics of fibromyalgia.

Cardinal signs:
Generalized pain
Tender points sensitive to pressure
Characteristic manifestations (more than 75% of the patients):
Fatigue
Non-restorative sleep
Sleeping disorders
Stiffness (especially in the morning)
Common manifestation (More than 25% of the patients):
Irritable colon
Raynaud's Phenomena
Headache
Sensation of swelling
Parastesia
Functional impotence
Psychiatric comorbidities (e.g. anxiety, depression)
Symptomatic sensitivity (e.g. cold or stress)

FM is currently diagnosed using the American College of Rheumatology (ACR) classification criteria from 1990 (Table 40.2). The diagnostic criteria are widespread musculoskeletal pain and excess tenderness in at least 11 of 18 predefined anatomic sites (Figure 40.1). The existence of both criteria confers an 80% sensitivity and specificity differentiating patients with FM from patients with other chronic pain disorders.

A thorough general physical examination is valuable to assess existing concomitant disorders. Musculoskeletal and neurological examination should routinely be performed to help exclude any obvious arthritis, connective tissue disorder, or neurological condition from FM. Nevertheless, existing secondary FM to another primary rheumatic or other illness should be considered.

Tender Point Examination

To establish the diagnosis, a tender point examination should be done, Applying pressure equivalent to about 4 kg/cm to selected anatomic locations. This can be accurately measured with a dolorimeter or estimated by palpation with a finger. An easy bedside test may be applied by pressing examiner's fingers strong enough to whiten the fingernail bed, this degree of pressure is approximately equivalent to 4 kg/cm. The pressure should be applied gradually over a few seconds and to both right and left sides of the body. Control locations, such as over the thumbnail or the mid-forearm, should also be examined and should not be as tender as the predefined tender points.

The sensitivity and specificity of a threshold of 11 tender points were approximately 50% and 95%, respectively. Using pain diagrams, rather than a tender point examination, provides similar diagnostic utility.

TABLE 40.2. The American College of Rheumatology 1990 Classification Criteria for FM (9).

History of widespread pain. Pain is considered widespread when all of the following are present: pain in the left side of the body, pain in the right side of the body, pain above the waist, and pain below the waist. In addition, axial skeletal pain (cervical spine or anterior chest or thoracic spine or low back) must be present. In this definition shoulder and buttock pain is considered as pain for each involved side. "Low back" pain is considered lower segment pain
Pain in 11 of 18 tender point sites on digital palpation
Pain on digital palpation must be present in at least 11 of the following 18 tender point sites:
Occiput: Bilateral, at the sub-occipital muscle insertions
Low cervical: Bilateral at the anterior aspects of the intertransverse spaces at C5–C7
Trapezius: Bilateral at the midpoint of the upper border
Supraspinatus: Bilateral, at origins above the scapula spine near the medial border
Second rib: Bilateral, at the second costochondral junctions just lateral to the junctions on upper surfaces
Lateral epicondyle: Bilateral, 2 cm distal to the epicondyles
Gluteal: Bilateral, in upper outer quadrant of buttocks in anterior fold of muscle
Greater trochanter: Bilateral, posterior to the trochanteric prominence
Knee: Bilateral, at the medial fat pad proximal to the joint line
Digital palpation should be performed with an approximate force of 4 kg. For a tender point to be considered "positive," the subject must state that the palpation was "painful." "Tender" is not to be considered painful. For classification purposes, patients will be said to have FM if both criteria are satisfied. Widespread pain must have been present for at least 3 months. The presence of a second clinical disorder does not exclude the diagnosis of FM

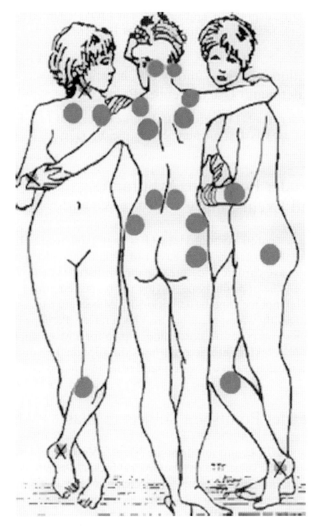

FIGURE 40.1. Illustration demonstrating the anatomical location of the tender points assessed in Fibromyalgia.

Laboratory Testing

Extensive laboratory testing is unnecessary for diagnostic purposes. There are no biomarkers or serologic tests that are specific or of diagnostic value in FM. The pathophysiology of FM is considered to be related to aberrant central pain mechanisms. Various central nervous system processes in the brain and spinal cord manifest abnormalities in patients with FM (Table 40.3). Fluctuations of

TABLE 40.3. Central nervous system anomalies reported in fibromyalgia (10,11,9).

Reduced levels of serotonin and 5-hydroxyindole acetic acid (5-HIAA) in plasma and cerebrospinal fluid.
Elevated levels of substance P in cerebrospinal fluid.
Reduced plasma levels of Somatomedin C.
Elevated plasma levels of Prolactin.
Anomalies of the Hypothalamic-pituitary-adrenal axis (mainly hyporeactivity to CRH).
Hypoperfusion of certain regions of the brain (particularly in the caudate nucleus and the thalamus).

arious neurotransmitters concentrations were reported in FM, especially serotonin and substance P; however, it is far from being clear whether these changes are causative or consequential. The hypothalamic-pituitary-adrenal axis, which is responsible for stress response exhibits mostly diminished response to TRH (3, 4, 10).

Functional Assessment

The assessment of the FMS patients consists on various clinical scores borrowed from psychology, neurology, rheumatology, and pain. The various trials are required because of the disease versatile nature. No single scoring system has been validated specifically for tracking FM progression and response. The key features that are meaningful while assessing the disease severity, the clinical course and the response to treatment are pain, fatigue, sleep quality, quality of life, and psychiatric assessment.

Pain Assessment

Pain assessment of chronic generalized pain is a core feature of FM. Several tools are available for the assessment of pain, including the daily pain diary, the *Short Form-McGill Pain Questionnaire* (SF-MPQ), the Brief Pain Inventory, and the *Leeds Assessment of Neuropathic Symptoms and Signs* (LANSS).

A daily diary has been used to assess the impact of pain on patients with FM and has been reported to be useful for demonstrating the manner by which pain influences activities of daily living in these individuals.

The McGill Pain Questionnaire provides detailed information on the characteristics of pain in FM. It includes 78 pain adjectives that are divided into four major categories (sensory, affective, evaluative, and miscellaneous sensory). The SF-MPQ consists of 15 adjectives (11 sensory, 4 affective) taken from the full MPQ.

The Brief Pain Inventory, originally developed for the assessment of cancer pain but currently is validated and commonly used in chronic pain states. It comprises multiple questions regarding pain intensity, the role of pain in interference in the patient's life, pain relief, pain quality, and patient perception of the cause of pain (12).

The LANSS Pain Scale is an instrument developed to diagnose neuropathic pain and to differentiate it from nociceptive pain. The LANSS Pain Scale items may be particularly useful for differentiation of FM pain from pain present in RA and other arthritic diseases. *Tender point assessment* is a useful part of the official ACR criteria for the diagnosis of FM. However, tender points are not unique to the syndrome. In addition to tender point count, tender point intensity has been developed as an assessment tool. The FM Intensity Score (FIS) is obtained by averaging the pain intensity scores (on a 0–10 scale) for the 18 sites assessed in the Manual Tender Point Survey. It has been suggested that the FIS might be helpful when patients are followed through serial examinations over time and for making comparisons among patients. Tender point count only partially correlates to the over all disability patients report (5, 13).

Fatigue and Sleep Quality

Fatigue and sleep quality Fatigue is one of the core features of FM, and its measurement is important in both the research and clinical settings. The *Multidimensional Assessment of Fatigue index* is a 16-item instrument developed to provide information about this symptom (14). The *Fatigue Severity Scale*, originally developed for multiple sclerosis and lupus fatigue assessment, may also prove useful.

Sleep quality can be assessed on a 100 mm linear scale with "sleep is no problem" at one extreme and "sleep is a major problem" at the other extreme. Similar scales can be used to rate number of awakenings, and "restedness" on awakening in the morning.

Quality of Life and Functional Assessment

Quality of Life and Functional Assessment-Measurement of global sense of well being, quality of life, and functional capacity in multiple dimensions (physical, vocational, social, emotional) is a key area of assessment and is considered essential by regulatory agencies when contemplating approval of medications for chronic pain states.

The MOS *Short Form-36* (SF-36) Health Survey is a generic instrument with 8 subscales (15). Assessment with the SF-36 has shown that patients with FM have reduced physical functioning, physical role functioning, body pain, general health, vitality, and social functioning versus healthy subjects.

The *FM Impact Questionnaire* (FIQ) is a simple instrument specifically designed to reflect changes in the FM patient's general status over time. It includes 10 questions and takes about 5 minutes to complete. The questions are designed to quantify functional disability, pain intensity, sleep disorder, muscular stiffness, anxiety, depression, and overall sense of well being; visual analog scales (VAS) are used to evaluate pain, fatigue, morning stiffness, stiffness

severity, depression, and anxiety. The FIQ is regarded as a reliable tool assessing the severity of FM (16).

Critiques to the Validity of Classification Criteria and Use of Tender Points

Tender points (TP) are central to the concept of FM, but their use has drawn a number of criticisms (17):

Tender Points are Arbitrary and Exclusionary

When a cutoff point of 11/18 TP is used, those who fail to meet that criterion don't have FM. What, then, do those who have chronic widespread pain but fewer than 11 TP have? The opposite issue, having the requisite number of TP but not meeting the definition of FM because pain isn't sufficiently widespread, has also been raised. Perhaps for clinical purposes a "borderline" range for FM could be defined, taking into account both variation in TP counts and the definition of "widespread pain."

Tender Points are Subject to Bias

Manual TP counts and to some extent, dolorimetry-based counts, are subject to psychophysical biases. As such, they are an imperfect measure of mechanical pain threshold. Patients may also learn where the TP are and become "expectant," such that the number of TP is overestimated. Similar biases may also occur on the part of the examiner. For example, if the first few points are positive the examiner may be biased toward positive findings for remaining points. Nevertheless, the extent to which such biases lead to a misdiagnosis remains undocumented. Interestingly, in one study in which blinded observers were asked to distinguish FM patients from simulators and healthy controls, they did so with 80% accuracy (18).

TP Counts do not Reflect the Complexity of FM

Although TP are used to classify patients who have a syndrome that is complex ill defined, TP do not reliably reflect its severity. An alternative would be to redefine FM by either the degree of disability or the combination of underlying pathophysiological processes (i.e., pain threshold, affective distress, fatigue). Undoubtedly, this would be a difficult undertaking, given the range and variation in symptoms in FM. An advantage of such an approach would be direct evaluation and consideration of symptoms that now seem only incidentally related to TP, such as fatigue, sleep disturbance, and mood disturbance.

The Relationship of Tender Points to Underlying Pathology is Unclear

The significance of TP is still undetermined. These anatomical locations are more sensitive in healthy controls as well as patients with FM. Peripheral tissue abnormalities such as muscle hypoxia and sympathetic nervous activation can lead to stimulation of nociceptors that, in turn, leads to CNS sensitization and chronic pain (11). It is possible that TP represent such areas of increased nociceptor activation.

Treatment

Many patients with FM benefit from a multidisciplinary approach in clinical practice. The range of pharmacologic therapies that have efficacy in relieving at least some symptoms in subsets of patients with FM and the fact that no single treatment is completely effective in all patients suggest that multiple pathogenic mechanisms may contribute to FM, and that their influence may differ from one patient to another. The complex nature of FM suggests that multimodal, individualized treatment programs that combine pharmacologic and nonpharmacologic therapies as well may be necessary to achieve optimal outcomes in patients with this syndrome.

Pharmacotherapy

A wide range of agents have been employed in the treatment of patients with FM. However, only a small number of these medications have demonstrated effectiveness in controlled clinical trials. Antidepressants, primarily tricyclics, are effective, but they have a relatively narrow therapeutic index, and their use may be limited by poor tolerability. SSRI have better tolerability than tricyclics, but do not appear to be as effective in relieving the wide range of FM-associated symptoms. Medications that inhibit reuptake of both norepinephrine and serotonin (SNRI) show promise in treating both pain of FM and associated symptoms of sleep disturbance and fatigue, yet with fewer side effects than traditional tricyclics (19). The new antiepileptic pregabalin has been shown to be effective for reducing many of the symptoms associated with FM and is well tolerated (20). Recently this drug was granted an FDA approval for the indication of FM.

Non-pharmacologic Treatment

A variety of non-pharmacologic treatments have been demonstrated to have at least modest efficacy in patients with FM. A 2004 systematic review found strong evidence for effectiveness of cardiovascular exercise, cognitive behavioral therapy (CBT), patient education, and multidisciplinary interventions that combined elements of aerobic exercise, CBT, and patient education (2). The same review found moderate evidence for efficacy of strength training, hypnotherapy, biofeedback, and mineral springs or salt baths (balneotherapy). Weak evidence exists for manipulative and manual therapies (chiropractic, massage) and physical modalities including electrotherapy and therapeutic ultrasound, whereas moderate evidence was also found for acupuncture.

Multidisciplinary Treatment

There is strong evidence that multidisciplinary treatment is effective in treating FMS. Five studies of multidisciplinary treatment that combined education, CBT, or both with exercise found beneficial effects on patient self efficacy and overall FMS impact as measured by the FIQ.

The current guidelines for treating FM are that FMS diagnosis must first be confirmed and the condition explained to the patient and family. Any comorbid illness, such as mood disturbances or primary sleep disturbances, should be identified and treated. Medications to consider initially are low doses of tricyclic antidepressants or cyclobenzaprine. Some SSRIs, SNRIs, or anticonvulsants may become first-line FMS medications as more trials are reported.

All patients with FM should begin a cardiovascular exercise program. Most patients will benefit from CBT or stress reduction with relaxation training. A multidisciplinary approach combining each of these modalities may be the most beneficial. Patients with FM not responding well to these steps should be referred to a rheumatologist, physiatrist, psychiatrist, or pain management specialist.

References

1. Wolfe F, Ross K, Anderson J, Russell IJ, Hebert L. The prevalence and characteristics of fibromyalgia in the general population. *Arthritis Rheum* 1995; 38(1): 19–28.
2. Goldenberg DL, Burckhardt C, Crofford L. Management of fibromyalgia syndrome. *JAMA* 2004; 292(19): 2388–95.
3. Buskila D. Fibromyalgia, chronic fatigue syndrome, and myofascial pain syndrome 4. *Curr Opin Rheumatol* 1999; 11(2): 119–26.
4. Abeles AM, Pillinger MH, Solitar BM, Abeles M. Narrative review: The pathophysiology of fibromyalgia. *Ann Intern Med* 2007; 146(10): 726–34.

5. Amital D, Fostick L, Polliack ML et al. Posttraumatic stress disorder, tenderness, and fibromyalgia syndrome: Are they different entities? 1. *J Psychosom Res* 2006; 61(5): 663–9.

6. Clauw DJ. Fibromyalgia: Update on mechanisms and management. *J Clin Rheumatol* 2007; 13(2): 102–9.

7. Anderberg UM, Marteinsdottir I, Theorell T, von KL. The impact of life events in female patients with fibromyalgia and in female healthy controls 75. *Eur Psychiatry* 2000; 15(5): 295–301.

8. Goldenberg DL. Fibromyalgia syndrome. An emerging but controversial condition. *JAMA* 1987; 257(20): 2782–7.

9. Wolfe F, Smythe HA, Yunus MB et al. The American College of Rheumatology 1990 Criteria for the Classification of Fibromyalgia. Report of the Multicenter Criteria Committee. *Arthritis Rheum* 1990; 33(2): 160–72.

10. Stratz T, Fiebich B, Haus U, Muller W. Influence of tropisetron on the serum substance P levels in fibromyalgia patients 7. *Scand J Rheumatol* Suppl 2004; (119): 41–3.

11. Vierck CJ, Jr. Mechanisms underlying development of spatially distributed chronic pain (fibromyalgia). Pain 2006; 124(3): 242–263.

12. Cleeland CS, Ryan KM. Pain assessment: Global use of the Brief Pain Inventory. *Ann Acad Med* Singapore 1994; 23(2): 129–38.

13. Perrot S, Dumont D, Guillemin F, Pouchot J, Coste J. Quality of life in women with fibromyalgia syndrome: Validation of the QIF, the French version of the fibromyalgia impact questionnaire. *J Rheumatol* 2003; 30(5): 1054–9.

14. Littlejohn GO. A database for fibromyalgia. *Rheum Dis Clin North Am* 1995; 21(2): 527–57.

15. Ware JE, Jr., Sherbourne CD. The MOS 36-item short-form health survey (SF-36). I. Conceptual framework and item selection. *Med Care* 1992; 30(6): 473–83.

16. Burckhardt CS, Clark SR, Bennett RM. The fibromyalgia impact questionnaire: Development and validation. *J Rheumatol* 1991; 18(5): 728–33.

17. Harth M, Nielson WR. The fibromyalgia tender points: Use them or lose them? A brief review of the controversy. *J Rheumatol* 2007; 34(5): 914–22.

18. Khostanteen I, Tunks ER, Goldsmith CH, Ennis J. Fibromyalgia: can one distinguish it from simulation? An observer-blind controlled study. *J Rheumatol* 2000; 27(11): 2671–6.

19. Arnold LM, Lu Y, Crofford LJ et al. A double-blind, multicenter trial comparing duloxetine with placebo in the treatment of fibromyalgia patients with or without major depressive disorder 11. *Arthritis Rheum* 2004; 50(9): 2974–84.

20. Arnold LM, Goldenberg DL, Stanford SB et al. Gabapentin in the treatment of fibromyalgia: A randomized, double-blind, placebo-controlled, multicenter trial 2. *Arthritis Rheum* 2007; 56(4): 1336–44.

Part V
Endocrine and Reproductive Autoimmune Diseases

41
Hashimoto Thyroiditis

Roberto Rocchi, Noel R. Rose and Patrizio Caturegli

Abstract   Hashimoto thyroiditis is one of the most common autoimmune diseases in humans. It is characterized by a marked lympocytic infiltration of the thyroid gland, which ultimately results in loss of function and hypothyroidism. This chapter reviews the major clinical and therapeutic features of Hashimoto's thyroiditis.

Keywords   Thyroiditis · autoimmunity · thyroxine

Definition

Hashimoto thyroiditis (HT), also known as chronic lymphocitic thyroiditis, is one of the most common autoimmune diseases in humans (1). HT comprises several clinicopathological types: the goitrous (or classic) form, the atrophic form (also known as idiopathic myxedema), post-partum thyroiditis, and the hyperthyroid "Hashitoxicosis". Clinically, the most prevalent goitrous HT form is characterized by a diffuse enlargement of the thyroid (goiter), with or without hypothyroidism. Pathologically, all HT variants feature a marked lymphocytic infiltration of the thyroid. HT is a prototypic example of organ-specific autoimmune diseases mediated by CD4+ T cells, and often associates with other autoimmune diseases, such as atrophic gastritis, type 1 diabetes, Addison's disease, and hypophysitis.

Epidemiology

HT is frequent, representing the most frequent cause of spontaneously acquired hypothyroidism in industrialized countries. Its prevalence is estimated to be about 1 in 1000 people (1); its incidence is 0.2, 1, and 1.3% in regions with low (mean urinary iodine excretion <50 μg/l), normal, or high iodine intake (>150 μg/l), respectively (2). Accurate epidemiological data are scanty, however, because definition of HT can vary (3). HT affects significantly more women than men: the female-to-male ratio is about 18:1, with a peak frequency during the fourth decade of life.

History

The first description of chronic autoimmune thyroiditis belongs to Hakaru Hashimoto, a surgeon who described in 1912 four women with a chronic disorder of the thyroid gland. He named the condition *struma lymphomatosa* because of a diffuse lymphocytic infiltration of the gland with fibrosis and parenchymal atrophy. In 1956, Rose and Witebsky first proved that HT was caused by an autoimmune response to thyroglobulin, inducing the disease in rabbits by immunization with homologous thyroid extract and *Freund's* adjuvant (4). In the same year, Roitt and Doniach reported that patients with HT had high serum concentrations of thyroglobulin antibodies (5). In 1957, the microsomal fraction of thyroid homogenates was identified as second thyroid autoantigen, subsequently proved to be thyroperoxidase. These observations opened a new view on HT, focusing the interest of researchers on autoimmunity as the actual cause of the disease.

Pathological Features

The pathological lesions of all HT types involve both the interstitium around the thyroid follicles, and the thyroid follicular cells (thyrocytes). Interstitial lesions are characterized by a marked infiltration of hematopoietic cells, mainly composed of lymphocytes, dendritic cells, and some plasma cells. Lymphocytes organize into true lymphoid follicles (called tertiary or ectopic lymphoid follicles), with topological compartmentalization of T cells in

From: Y. Shoenfeld et al. (eds.): *Diagnostic Criteria in Autoimmune Diseases*, DOI: 10.1007/978-1-60327-285-8_41,
© 2008 Humana Press, Totowa, NJ

the cortex and B cells in the center, often with clear germinal centers. Lymphocytes come in close contact with the thyrocytes, and are believed to be the direct mediators of thyrocyte destruction. Occasionally, lymphocytes are seen to penetrate the cytoplasm of the thyrocyte, a phenomenon known as emperipolesis. Thyrocyte lesions vary in intensity from one part of the gland to another. In some areas, thyrocytes are hyperplastic and encircle small follicles containing minimal colloid. In other areas, thyrocytes acquire a striking appearance; hence, they have been named Hürthle cells (or oxyphilic cells or oncocytes). Hürthle cells are thyrocytes that have increased size, hyperchromatic nucleus and, most characteristically, a cytoplasm that stains intensely pink with eosin and is filled with eosinophilic granules (6).

In the goitrous variant, the thyroid is enlarged, has a rubber-like consistency, and a pale gray appearance. In the atrophic variant, the thyroid is markedly reduced in size, often not detectable when palpating the neck, and has an intense deposition of fibrous tissue in the interstitium, with almost complete disappearance of the thyroid follicles. The post-partum and Hashitoxicosis variants resemble pathologically the goitrous variant.

Clinical Manifestations

The goitrous HT form with hypothyroidism and the atrophic form are clinically characterized by the signs and symptoms of hypothyroidism. These typically have an insidious onset and can go unrecognized for prolonged periods. Thyroid hormones affect the metabolic status of practically all organs and tissues, and therefore a lack of thyroid hormones has systemic consequences, which are summarized in Table 41.1. The most typical clinical manifestations are described below.

a. **Skin and appendages:** skin alterations are due to intradermal accumulation of *hydrophilic mucoproteins* with consequent *edema* (*myxedema*). The skin is usually dry, cold, pale, yellowish, and thickened. The face is swollen and the tongue thickened. Hairs are coarse, the nails thin and frail, and the patients often refer hair loss.

b. **Cardiovascular system:** *bradycardia* is the most common cardiac symptom, along with reduced systolic output and low voltage at electrocardiogram. Cardiomegaly may be present and accompanied by pericardial effusion. Severe hypothyroidism leads to *hypercholesterolemia* and *hypertriglyceridemia*, with increased risk of coronary *atherosclerosis* and increased risk of *angina* and myocardial infarction.

c. **Skeletal muscles and bones:** muscle contraction and relaxation are delayed. Owing to myxedematous infiltration of connective tissue, muscles can appear falsely hypertrophic (pseudohypertrophy). Muscle cramps

TABLE 41.1. Symptoms and signs of overt hypothyroidism.

Symptom or Sign	Frequency
Adynamia	Up to 99%
Dry and pale skin	Up to 97%
Sleepiness	90%
Slow discourse	90%
Palpebral edema	90%
Macroglossia	80%
Edema of the face	80%
Hair fragility	75%
Cardiomegaly	65%
Constipation	60%
Weight gain	55%
Peripheral edema	55%
Dyspnea	55%
Hoarse voice	50%
Memory impairment	50%

and pain can be observed. Joints pain is sometimes reported.

d. **Neuropsychiatric system:** aphasy, sleepiness, and memory impairment are common. Less common is depression. Carpal tunnel syndrome may occur.

e. **Gastroenteric tract:** severe constipation is the most common gastrointestinal symptom. *Atrophic gastritis* with a defect in iron absorption can occur in patients with HT and antibodies against gastric cells.

f. **Hemopoietic system:** *anaemia* is frequent. It can be *normocitic* (because of a reduction in the renal secretion of erythropoietin), *hypochromic* and *microcytic* (because of a defect in iron absorption), or *megaloblastic* (because of gastric atrophy with vitamin B_{12} malabsorption).

g. **Endocrine system:** *oligomenorrhea* and/or *menometrorrhagia* are frequent, and HT can sometimes co-occur with other endocrine autoimmune diseases such as primary cortical adrenal insufficiency and insulin-dependent type I diabetes.

h. **Urogenital system:** the bladder can be atonic with consequent urine retention.

In the goitrous form without hypothyroidism, the clinical manifestations are limited to the presence of a small goiter, usually not associated with significant compression symptoms of major anatomical structures in the neck, such as dyspnea (from compression of the trachea), dysphagia (from compression of the esophagus), and dysphonia (from involvement of the laryngeal nerves). Often patients develop a so-called subclinical hypothyroidism, characterized by normal serum thyroid hormone levels but increased serum thyrotropin (TSH) levels. These patients often are asymptomatic but may complain of fatigue and cold intolerance.

HT rarely presents with hyperthyroidism, a condition sometimes termed Hashitoxicosis that is almost indistinguishable from Graves' disease.

Postpartum thyroiditis occurs after pregnancy. It is found in about 7% of women during the first 6 months after delivery (7). It can cause hypothyroidism and/or hyperthyroidism that are usually transient but can be seriously symptomatic (8). Postpartum thyroiditis increases the risk of developing later permanent hypothyroidism, and is often misdiagnosed as postpartum depression (9).

Laboratory Findings

Laboratory tests most commonly performed in HT patients include serum levels of thyroid stimulating hormone (TSH), free thyroxine (fT4), and thyroperoxidase (TPO) antibodies. Detectable TPO antibodies are found in 90 to 95% of HT patients, depending on the presence of the atrophic or classical types. Serum thyroglobulin antibodies are positive in 60–80% of patients with HT, and they are not considered a good clinical marker of autoimmune thyroiditis as the TPO antibodies, although they may have predictive value. Some patients with the atrophic form of HT develop antibodies that block the TSH receptor, contributing to the induction of hypothyroidism. Thyroid antibodies are also found in Graves' disease, and in a small percentage of patients with nodular goiter, thyroid cancer, and even in normal individuals.

Overt hypothyroidism can induce severe alterations of the lipid profile, increasing the serum levels of triglycerides and cholesterol.

Ultrasound scan of the thyroid gland in HT shows a peculiar pattern characterized by a diffusely reduced echogenicity. Ultrasound scan of atrophic variant reveals a thyroid gland smaller than normal with hyperechogenic striae due to parenchymal fibrosis.

Radioiodine uptake (RAIU) and radionuclide scan do not provide fundamental information for the diagnosis of HT. RAIU can be normal, reduced, or increased in HT depending on the functional phase of the disease. Radionuclide scan shows diffuse or irregular distribution of the tracer, sometimes mimicking hypo-hyperfunctioning nodules (Table 41.2).

Fine needle aspiration (FNAB) is usually not performed for the diagnosis of HT. It can be helpful, however, in the presence of thyroid nodules and primary hypothyroidism with negative thyroid autoantibody tests. A FNAB positive for HT reveals the presence of lymphocytes and Hürthle cells.

Functional evaluation of the thyroid gland is performed by TSH and fT4 measurement. The hypothalamic-pituitary-thyroid axis is very sensitive to even minimal variations of circulating thyroid hormones, adjusting the TSH secretion accordingly. Therefore, serum TSH is the most important index to monitor the thyroid function. Increased TSH levels can occur before any reduction in fT4 levels, a condition called subclinical hypothyroidism. Overt hypothyroidism is characterized by increased levels of TSH, reduced levels of fT4 and sometimes of free triiodothyronine (fT3) (Table 41.1). Low levels of fT3 (and fT4) with normal TSH levels direct the diagnosis to a nonthyroidal illness syndrome (central hypothyroidism). Although thyroid hormone fluctuations are described, HT usually follows a chronic downward course from a functional point of view. In most cases, once hypothyroidism appears, no recovery is observed but rather a progressive loss of thyroid function.

Therapy

The therapy of permanent primary hypothyroidism is based on the daily, lifelong oral administration of synthetic T4 (levo-thyoxine, L-T4) (10). Immunosuppressive agents such as corticosteroids are not required in a disease such as HT that can be easily, safely, and economically treated with L-T4.

Replacement therapy in adult patients with overt hypothyroidism requires a mean dose of 1.6-1.8 µg/kg body weight of L-T4. Therefore, daily doses usually range from 75 to 125 µg/day and 100-175 µg/day for men. The goal of L-T4 replacement therapy is to return TSH levels to the normal range. Elderly patients usually require 20-30% lower doses to normalize serum TSH. In severe, long-lasting hypothyroid L-T4 treatment should be administered starting from very low doses (12.5 µg/day), and then reaching the full substitutive dose in several weeks. This regimen is designed to avoid angina, myocardial infarction, and/or atrial fibrillation.

Replacement therapy with L-T4 in subclinical hypothyroidism is debated, although the trend among clinical endocrinologists is to treat patients with borderline high levels of TSH (cutoff levels ranging from 4 to 10 mU/L have been conventionally used to define an elevated TSH serum concentration) (11), and high titers of thyroid antibodies, because they are likely to develop overt hypothyroidism.

L-T4 therapy for treatment of goiter in patients with euthyroid HT is controversial. L-T4 administration may prevent goiter growth and protect patients from the possible evolution to hypothyroidism but there is no universal consensus on this issue. Owing to differences in the half-life

TABLE 41.2. Biochemical and instrumental features of overt hypothyroidism.

Parameter	Changes
fT4	Reduced
fT3	Normal or reduced
TSH	Increased
TgAb	Highly positive
TPOAb	Highly positive
Total cholesterol	Increased
Triglycerides	Increased
Ultrasound echogenicity	Reduced
Radionuclide thyroid scan	Usually irregularly distributed
Radioiodine thyroid uptake	Normal, increased, or reduced

of thyroid hormones (that of T4 is about a week, whereas T3 half-life is only a few hours), and the fact that T4 is entirely produced by the thyroid gland whereas most of T3 (80%) comes from the peripheral enzymatic conversion of T4 to T3, addition of T3 to the administration of T4 does not provide advantage for treating overt hypothyroidism. Once euthyroidism is restored by L-T4 therapy, annual thyroid hormones and TSH monitoring is recommended.

Acknowledgment. The work was supported by NIH grant DK 55670 P.C.

References

1. Jacobson, D. L., S. J. Gange, N. Rose, and N. M. H. Graham. 1997. Epidemiology and estimated population burden of selected autoimmune diseases in the United States. *Clin Immunol Immunopathol* 84:223–243.
2. Teng, W., Z. Shan, X. Teng, H. Guan, Y. Li, D. Teng, Y. Jin, X. Yu, C. Fan, W. Chong, F. Yang, H. Dai, Y. Yu, J. Li, Y. Chen, D. Zhao, X. Shi, F. Hu, J. Mao, X. Gu, R. Yang, Y. Tong, W. Wang, T. Gao, and C. Li. 2006. Effect of iodine intake on thyroid diseases in China. *N Engl J Med* 354:2783–2793.
3. Vanderpump, M. P., W. M. Tunbridge, J. M. French, D. Appleton, D. Bates, F. Clark, J. Grimley Evans, D. M. Hasan, H. Rodgers, F. Tunbridge, and et al. 1995. The incidence of thyroid disorders in the community: a twenty-year follow-up of the Whickham Survey. *Clin Endocrinol (Oxf)* 43:55–68.
4. Rose, N. R., and E. Witebsky. 1956. Studies on organ specificity. V. Changes in the thyroid glands of rabbits following active immunization with rabbit thyroid extracts. *J Immunol* 76:417–427.
5. Roitt, I. M., D. Doniach, P. N. Campbell, and R. V. Hudson. 1956. Auto-antibodies in Hashimoto's disease (lymphadenoid goitre). *Lancet* 271:820–821.
6. Caturegli, P., and C. Ruggere. 2005. Karl Hurthle! Now, who was he? *Thyroid* 15:121–123.
7. Man, E. B., W. S. Jones, R. H. Holden, and E. D. Mellits. 1971. Thyroid function in human pregnancy. 8. Retardation of progeny aged 7 years; relationships to maternal age and maternal thyroid function. *Am J Obstet Gynecol* 111:905–916.
8. Haddow, J. E., G. E. Palomaki, W. C. Allan, J. R. Williams, G. J. Knight, J. Gagnon, C. E. O'Heir, M. L. Mitchell, R. J. Hermos, S. E. Waisbren, J. D. Faix, and R. Z. Klein. 1999. Maternal thyroid deficiency during pregnancy and subsequent neuropsychological development of the child. *N Engl J Med* 341:549–555.
9. Glinoer, D., and F. Delange. 2000. The potential repercussions of maternal, fetal, and neonatal hypothyroxinemia on the progeny. *Thyroid* 10:871–887.
10. Wiersinga, W. M. 2001. Thyroid hormone replacement therapy. *Horm Res* 56 Suppl1:74–81.
11. Brabant, G., P. Beck-Peccoz, B. Jarzab, P. Laurberg, J. Orgiazzi, I. Szabolcs, A. P. Weetman, and W. M. Wiersinga. 2006. Is there a need to redefine the upper normal limit of TSH? *Eur J Endocrinol* 154:633–637.

42
Atrophic Thyroiditis

Luis J. Jara, Olga Vera-Lastra and Gabriela Medina

Abstract   Atrophic thyroiditis is an organ-specific autoimmune disease characterized by thyroid autoantibodies, functional hypothyroidism, and absence of goiter. Atrophic thyroiditis is a rare entity, which occurs between the ages of 40–60 years especially in elderly women. Immunogenetical analysis suggests that atrophic thyroiditis may be a distinct entity from Hashimoto's disease. Genetic and environmental factors appear to interact leading to appearance of autoantigens with autoantibody formation. The frequency of HLA-DR8 and HLA-DQB1*0302 is significantly increased in AT patients positive for TSH-binding inhibitor immunoglobulin compare with controls and goitrous autoimmune thyroiditis. Atrophic thyroiditis is a Th2 disease with blocking anti-TSH receptor antibodies. It has been suggested that Hashimoto's thyroiditis, primary myxedema or AT, and Graves' disease are different expressions of a basically similar autoimmune process, and that the clinical appearance reflects the spectrum of the immune response in the particular patient. This response may include cytotoxic antibodies, stimulatory antibodies, blocking antibodies, or cell-mediated immunity. The clinical presentation varies from asymptomatic AT, overt hypothyroidism, and myxedema. The pathological features are atrophic thyroid gland with lymphocytic infiltration and fibrous tissue replacing normal thyroid parenchyma. There are no current diagnostic criteria for AT. We propose the following bases for AT diagnosis: clinic or subclinic hypothyroidism, positive thyroid stimulation blocking antibodies and thyroid ultrasound with diffuse low thyroid echogenicity associated with a reduced thyroid volume.

In asymptomatic AT, preventive thyroid replacement therapy is indicated in patients with elevated basal TSH levels. Overt hypothyroidism always requires hormonal substitution.

Keywords   Atrophic thyroiditis · antithyroid antibodies

Atrophic thyroiditis (AT) is an organ-specific autoimmune disease characterized by thyroid autoantibodies, functional hypothyroidism, and absence of goiter. Patients with autoimmune overt hypothyroidism may present with goitrous Hashimoto's disease, postpartum thyroiditis, or AT. The available evidence is not enough to prove that the goitrous precedes the atrophic form, but immunogenetical analysis suggest that AT may be a distinct entity (1, 2).

History

The initial report of autoimmune thyroid disease (AITD) dates back to 1912, when Hakira Hashimoto described four women in whom the thyroid gland was enlarged and appeared to have transformed into lymphoid tissue ("struma lymphomatosa") as an organ-specific autoimmune disease with diffuse infiltration of lymphoid cells and parenchymal atrophy. There is controversy on whether AT is considered the end-stage of goitrous disease because little histological progression has been observed in patients up to 20 years of follow-up (1).

Epidemiology

AITD is the most common of all autoimmune diseases affecting 1.5% of the population, mainly women; however, AT is not very frequent. AT is, after ablation hypothyroidism, the most common cause of thyroid failure in adults and it usually occurs between the ages of 40 and 60 years. In Tunisia, AT was present in 32.2% of a cohort of 1079 patients (3). In Germany, AITD usually manifests as AT with functional hypothyroidism affecting elderly women in particular (4).

From: Y. Shoenfeld et al. (eds.): *Diagnostic Criteria in Autoimmune Diseases*, DOI: 10.1007/978-1-60327-285-8_42,
© 2008 Humana Press, Totowa, NJ

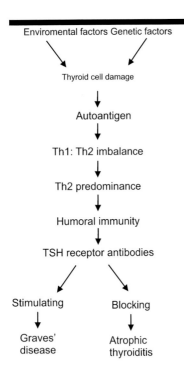

FIGURE 42. 1. The proposed pathogenic mechanisms of AT include the interaction between environmental and genetic factors. The consequence is thyroid cell damage with expression of neoantigens and stimulation of immune response leading to Th2 cytokines production and consequently blocking autoantibody formation. These cytotoxic autoantibodies (anti-TRBAb) seem to be responsible for autoimmune thyrocyte depletion (adapted from Fountoulakis and Tsatsoulis, Ref. (5)).

Pathogenesis

Antagonist antibodies to the TSH receptor are present in 20–50% of patients with AT. In contrast, these antibodies are also found in up to 10% of patients with goitrous thyroiditis and overt hypothyroidism. AT with blocking anti-TSH receptor antibodies may be regarded as the opposite end to that of Graves' disease. Here again, predominance of humoral immunity may enhance production of anti-TSH receptor antibodies. In fact, AT is a Th2 disease (Figure 42.1) (5). Genetic and environmental factors appear to interact leading to appearance of autoantigens, and T lymphocytes are crucial in the pathogenesis of autoimmune thyroiditis.

Genetic Factors

HLA associations with AT have been described since the 1970 s. Subsequent studies found that HLA-DR3 increased in patients with AT, and HLA-DR5 in patients with goitrous autoimmune (Hashimoto's), compared with controls.

These findings stress the immunogenetic heterogeneity between goitrous thyroiditis and AT (6). HLA A, B, C, DR, and DQ alloantigens serologically and HLA-DQ by gene analysis were determined in patients with AT and randomly chosen controls. The genetic susceptibility to AT was closely associated to HLA-DR5 and DQ7 and was not distinct from goitrous disease. Factors other than genetic ones explain the different immunological and clinical manifestations of chronic lymphocytic thyroiditis (7). In contrast, using the same methods, Cho et al (8) investigated in Korean patients whether the associations between HLA alleles of patients with autoimmune hypothyroidism varied according to the presence or absence of TSH receptor-blocking antibody (TRBab). The frequency of HLA-DR8 and HLA-DQB1*0302 was significantly increased in AT patients who were significantly positive for TSH-binding inhibitor immunoglobulin compared with controls and those with goitrous autoimmune thyroiditis. This study concluded that TRBab-positive AT is immunogenetically different from goitrous autoimmune and TRBab-negative AT.

The localization and functional characteristics of tumor necrosis factor (TNF) beta gene (short arm of chromosome 6) raise the possibility that it may be involved in the susceptibility to AITD. Chung et al (9) analyzed the TNF beta gene polymorphism with the restriction enzyme NcoI in Korean AT patients with and without TRBab, goitrous autoimmune thyroiditis, and healthy controls. The frequency of HLA-DR8 antigens was significantly increased in patients with TRBab-positive AT compared with control subjects. The DR8-positive patients with TRBab-positive AT had more homozygotes for the TNF beta* 1 allele compared with the DR8-negative patients with TBRab-positive AT and DR8-positive controls. This association may be related to susceptibility markers responsible for the production of TRBab in AT patients. Recently, Zantut-Wittmann et al (2) demonstrated that DRB1*04 and DQB1*03 alleles are associated with AT only, supporting the concept that there are genotypic differences between goitrous and atrophic forms.

Immunological Factors

Immunological mechanisms have been sequentially proposed to be responsible for autoimmune thyrocyte depletion in AT.

Early reports showed that AT is associated with the production of antibodies that block the thyroid-growth-promoting activity of TSH. The effects of IgG from patients with AT on cAMP responses and iodine metabolism (post-receptor processes), using cultured thyroid cells, were examined. Two types of thyroid function-blocking antibodies in AT were found: TSH-binding blocking antibodies and antibodies which block post-receptor processes.

These antibodies might be responsible for thyroid dysfunction in AT and may induce AT. The frequency of TSH-binding inhibitory immunoglobulins (TBII), TSH-stimulated cAMP response inhibitory immunoglobulins (TSII), and TSH-stimulated cell growth inhibitory immunoglobulins (TGII) in patients with AT was higher than in patients with autoimmune goitrous thyroiditis. These antibodies block not only TSH-induced cAMP production but also TSH-induced DNA synthesis and iodine uptake in cultured thyroid cells (10). Antithyroid stimulation blocking antibodies are detectable in 46% of AT patients and almost exclusively in overt hypothyroid patients (11). Their prevalence is higher in hypothyroid patients with AT than in Hashimoto's disease suggesting a role in the development of hypothyroidism and AT (12). Analysis of cytotoxicity regarding thyroid size showed a higher incidence of cytotoxic antibodies in AT vs. goitrous disease. The specific lysis in AT patients was significantly higher than in goitrous patients (13). The histopathological features of AT with TBII antibodies were carried out using immunohistochemical procedures. Significant follicular atrophy with epithelial flattening including decreased positive staining of the follicular epithelial cells for thyroglobulin in AT was characteristically observed. These results suggest that the mechanism for the development of hypothyroidism in AT with TBII might be because of suppression of thyroid cell function through the inhibition of endogenous TSH stimulation by the blocking antibody with subsequent epithelial degenerative destruction (14).

Autoimmune destructive mechanisms, such as antibody-dependent cytotoxicity, K and NK cytotoxicity, T-lymphocyte cytotoxicity, lymphokine cytotoxicity, and apoptosis have been proposed to be responsible for autoimmune thyrocyte depletion in Hashimoto's thyroiditis and Graves' disease (15). However, there are scarce studies in AT. It has been suggested that Hashimoto's thyroiditis, primary myxedema or AT, and Graves' disease are different expressions of a basically similar autoimmune process, and that the clinical appearance reflects the spectrum of the immune response in the particular patient. This response may include cytotoxic antibodies, stimulatory antibodies, blocking antibodies, or cell-mediated immunity. Thyrotoxicosis is viewed as an expression of the effect of circulating thyroid stimulatory antibodies. Hashimoto's thyroiditis is predominantly the clinical expression of cell-mediated immunity leading to destruction of thyroid cells, which in its severest form produces thyroid failure and idiopathic myxedema or AT (16).

Clinical Manifestations

The clinical presentation of AT varies from asymptomatic AT, overt hypothyroidism, and myxedema. Asymptomatic AT is characterized by the presence of serum

TABLE 42.1 Differential diagnosis in AITD.

Characteristic	Subclinical autoimmune thyroiditis	Classic Hashimoto's thyroiditis	Atrophic Thyroiditis
Stage	Early	Advanced	Final
Antithyroid antibodies	Positive	Positive	Positive
Goiter	None or very small	Large	None
	Soft to firm	Firme	
Thyroid function	Euthyroid	Euthyroid Hypothyroid Destructive thyrotoxicosis	Hypothyroid

antithyroid antibodies in good correlation with thyroid lymphoplasmocytic infiltrations. Asymptomatic AT affects 5–15% of the general population, especially elderly women. Patients with asymptomatic AT have no goiter and are clinically euthyroid. While circulating thyroid hormones are always in the normal range, peak TSH and TRH and basal TSH values are increased in two-third of the cases (17). There is a familial aggregation of asymptomatic AT and a frequent association with other autoimmune diseases such as Sjögren's syndrome, autoimmune hepatitis, atrophic gastritis, type I diabetes mellitus, adrenal insufficiency, and vitiligo (4). Development of overt hypothyroidism with classic symptoms/signs (lethargy, constipation, cold intolerance, and myxedematous facies) in these patients is common (17). Occasionally, patients with AT may present asthenia, diffuse myalgia, notable hair loss, and sinus bradycardia. Young patients with muscular fatigability, myalgia, cramps, or proximal weakness, of uncertain origin, may have AT, and the evaluation of thyroid function is appropriate (16).

The rare AT mostly presents as primary myxedema and is discovered less frequently during the exploration of an unclear hypercholesterolemia. It is generally admitted that primary myxedema in adults is the outcome of autoimmune AT. Other rare manifestations of AT and associations include myxedema pericarditis, cardiac tamponade, dissecting aneurysm of the aorta, neuropsychological deficits, multiple sclerosis, and myocardial infarction (1). The differential diagnosis of AT is showed in Table 42.1.

Pathological Features

AT is characterized by atrophic thyroid gland with lymphocytic infiltration and fibrous tissue replacing normal thyroid parenchyma.

To investigate the histopathological features of AT with blocking type-TSH-binding inhibitor immunoglobulins (TBII), morphological observations were carried out using additional immunohistochemical procedures. There

TABLE 42.2. Diagnostic studies in AT.

AT clinical picture	TSH	TRH	T3	T4	Anti-TRBAb	Anti-TPOAb	Ultrasound/ Scintiscan
Subclinical hypothyroidism	↑	↑	N	N	↑↑	↑-Negative	↓ volume/ N or ↓ uptake
Overt hypothyroidism	↑	↑	↓↓	↓↓	↑↑	↑-Negative	↓↓ volume/ ↓↓ uptake

N = Normal

exist apparent differences between AT and Hashimoto's thyroiditis. Significant follicular atrophy with epithelial flattening including decreased positive staining of the follicular epithelial cells for thyroglobulin in AT was characteristically observed. These results suggest that the mechanism for the development of hypothyroidism in AT with blocking type-TBII might be due to suppression of thyroid cell function through the inhibition of endogenous TSH stimulation by the blocking antibody with subsequent epithelial degenerative destruction (14).

Diagnostic Studies

The main laboratory abnormalities and image findings observed in AT are summarized in Table 42.2. An abnormal thyroid echographic pattern characterized by a diffuse low thyroid echogenicity associated with a reduced thyroid volume was found in 96% of patients with AT. Of interest, in 18% of patients, the scintiscan was normal. Thyroid echography can be considered the first morphological study in AT with high specificity and sensitivity (18). Other studies are necessary to define the positive and negative predictive value of antibodies in AT.

Treatment

In asymptomatic AT, preventive thyroid replacement therapy is indicate in patients with elevated basal TSH levels. Overt hypothyroidism always requires hormonal substitution (1, 16).

Diagnostic Criteria

There are no current diagnostic criteria for AT. Therefore, we propose the following bases for AT diagnosis:

1. Clinic or subclinic hypothyroidism: Clinical picture of overt hypothyroidism or increase of TSH and TRH values without symptoms.
2. Positive thyroid autoantibodies: Positive thyroid stimulation blocking antibodies (TRBAb).
3. Thyroid ultrasonographic characteristic: Abnormal thyroid echographic pattern characterized by diffuse

low thyroid echogenicity associated with a reduced thyroid volume.

References

1. Dayan CM, Daniels GH. Chronic autoimmune thyroiditis. N Engl J Med 1996 11; 335:99–107.
2. Zantut-Wittmann DE, Persoli L, Tambascia MA, Fischer E, Franco Maldonado D, Costa AM, Joao Pavin E. HLA-DRB1*04 and HLA-DQB1*03 association with the atrophic but not with the goitrous form of chronic autoimmune thyroiditis in a Brazilian population. Horm Metab Res 2004; 36:492–500.
3. Chabchoub G, Mnif M, Maalej A, Charfi N, Ayadi H, Abid M. Epidemiologic study of autoimmune thyroid disease in south Tunisia. Ann Endocrinol (Paris) 2006; 67:591–5.
4. Lahner H, Quadbeck B, Janssen OE, Mann K. Diagnosis and treatment of autoimmune thyroiditis. MMW Fortschr Med 2004; 146: 28–30.
5. Fountoulakis S, Tsatsoulis A. On The pathogenesis of autoimmune thyroid disease: A unifying hypothesis. Clin Endocrinol 2004; 60:397–409.
6. Farid NR, Sampson L, Moens H, Barnard JM. The association of goitrous autoimmune thyroiditis with HLA-DR5. Tissue Antigens 1981; 17:265–8.
7. Bogner U, Badenhoop K, Peters H, Schmieg D, Mayr WR, Usadel KH, Schleusener H. HLA-DR/DQ gene variation in nongoitrous autoimmune thyroiditis at the serological and molecular level. Autoimmunity 1992; 14:155–8.
8. Cho BY, Chung JH, Shong YK, Chang YB, Han H, Lee JB, Lee HK, Koh CS. A strong association between thyrotropin receptor-blocking antibody-positive atrophic autoimmune thyroiditis and HLA-DR8 and HLA-DQB1*0302 in Koreans. J Clin Endocrinol Metab 1993; 77:611–5.
9. Chung JH, Cho BY, Lee HK, Kim TG, Han H, Koh CS. The tumor necrosis factor beta * 1 allele is linked significantly to HLA-DR8 in Koreans with atrophic autoimmune thyroiditis who are positive for thyrotropin receptor blocking antibody. J Korean Med Sci 1994; 9:155–61.
10. Takasu N, Yamada T, Katakura M, Yamauchi K, Shimizu Y, Ishizuki Y. Evidence for thyrotropin (TSH)-blocking activity in goitrous Hashimoto's thyroiditis with assays measuring inhibition of TSH receptor binding and TSH-stimulated thyroid adenosine 3',5'-monophosphate responses/cell growth by immunoglobulins. J Clin Endocrinol Metab 1987; 64:239–45.
11. Chiovato L, Vitti P, Santini F, Lopez G, Mammoli C, Bassi P, Giusti L, Tonacchera M, Fenzi G, Pinchera A. Incidence of antibodies blocking thyrotropin effect in vitro in patients with euthyroid or hypothyroid autoimmune thyroiditis. J Clin Endocrinol Metab 1990; 71:40–5.

12. Amino N. Autoimmunity and hypothyroidism. Baillieres Clin Endocrinol Metab. 1988; 2:591–617.

13. Bogner U, Hegedüs L, Hansen JM, Finke R, Schleusener H. Thyroid cytotoxic antibodies in atrophic and goitrous autoimmune thyroiditis. *Eur J Endocrinol* 1995; 132:69–74.

14. Sugenoya A, Itoh N, Kasuga Y, Kobayashi S, Ohhashi T, Nagai N, Iida F. Histopathological features of atrophic thyroiditis with blocking type-TSH binding inhibitor immunoglobulins. *Endocr J* 1995; 42:277–81.

15. Stassi G, De Maria R. Autoimmune thyroid disease: new models of cell death in autoimmunity. *Nat Rev Immunol* 2002; 2:195–204.

16. Akamizu T, Amino N, J De Groot LJ. Hashimoto's Thyroiditis. 2007. http://www.thyroidmanager.org

17. Bonnyns M, Vanhaelst L, Bastenie PA. Asymptomatic atrophic thyroiditis. *Horm Res* 1982; 16:338–44.

18. Vitti P, Lampis M, Piga M, Loviselli A, Brogioni S, Rago T, et al. Diagnostic usefulness of thyroid ultrasonography in atrophic thyroiditis. *Clin Ultrasound* 1994; 22: 375–9.

43
Subacute Thyroiditis

Yemil Atisha-Fregoso and Mario Garcia-Carrasco

Abstract   Subacute thyroiditis (SAT), also known as giant cell thyroiditis, subacute granulomatous thyroiditis, de Quervain's thyroiditis or pseudogranulomatous thyroiditis, is the most common cause of thyroid pain.

It is a self-limiting inflammatory disorder associated with many viral infections, although there is not an established role for them in the pathogenesis of SAT. Autoantibodies may be present, but their importance is probably negligible. The classical course of the disease includes an initial stage of hyperthyroidism followed by a second stage of hypothyroidism, usually transitory. Treatment is for support only and consists of non-steroidal anti-inflammatory drugs and, in more severe cases, corticosteroids. Symptoms of hyperthyroidism should be treated with beta-blockers.

Keywords   Subacute thyroiditis · De Quervain's thyroiditis · thyrotoxicosis

Epidemiology

The estimated incidence is four to five cases per 100,000 persons. It affects four times more women than men, and occurs most often at 40–50 years of age (1); it is rare in childhood and in the elderly. A tendency to a seasonal and geographical aggregation of cases has been noted, being more frequent in summer, and so there has been a suggested linkage with certain viruses such as echovirus and coxsackievirus groups A and B (2); also, an association with other viruses such as measles virus and Epstein–Barr virus has been reported (3).

History

The first description of cases of subacute thyroiditis (SAT) was made by Mygind in 1895 who described 18 cases defined as "thyroiditis acute simplex." In 1904 De Quervain described the entity formally, as well as the association with the granulomatous changes and giant cells in thyroid tissue (4).

Pathogenesis

The cause of the clinical picture seen in SAT is the destruction of the follicular epithelium, mainly by apoptosis, which releases the preformed hormone stored inside the gland. What triggers this phenomenon is still unknown.

As previously mentioned, SAT has been usually attributed to a viral infection, but currently there is not enough evidence to establish a cause-effect pattern.

A genetic predisposition has also been suggested, and it is recognized that there is a higher incidence of SAT in those with the HLA-Bw35 haplotype, and a family aggregation has been proposed (5).

Autoantibodies are found in low titers and probably have only a secondary role after initial tissue alteration. T-lymphocytes sensitized against thyroid antigens may be found, and tissue samples contain large numbers of antigen-reactive T cells (6), but these alterations, not unlike the found antibodies, are probably part of the inflammatory process after thyroid destruction.

Clinical Manifestations

The clinical picture begins with a prodrome of generalized myalgias, pharyngitis, low-grade fever, and fatigue. After that, the patients develop pain in the anterior region of the neck, and it must be distinguished from other disorders that may arise from the same area. On palpation, the gland is exquisitely tender and is usually affected asymmetrically. In some cases thyroid nodules can be found on examination.

From: Y. Shoenfeld et al. (eds.): *Diagnostic Criteria in Autoimmune Diseases*, DOI: 10.1007/978-1-60327-285-8_43,

Up to 50% of patients have thyrotoxicosis, and they usually complain of palpitation and nervousness. Even though the elevation of thyroid hormones and clinical picture is mild, in most extreme cases thyroid storm caused by SAT has been described (7).

After depletion of thyroid hormones storages, there is a characteristic second phase of the disease consisting of hypothyroidism; this state could be considered a recuperation period that usually lasts from 6–12 months; in its latter part, the thyroid architecture and function are restored and most patients return to euthyroidism without sequels of the disease.

Pathological Features

The follicular lesions seen in SAT are characterized by a central core of colloid surrounded by multinucleate giant cells; these lesions progress to form granulomas. With progression of the disease, there are areas with a variable degree of fibrosis and areas of follicular regeneration. Usually, the biopsy material shows various stages distributed irregularly. At a late stage, when the disease remits, the normal architecture of the gland is restored.

Biochemical Features

At the initial stages of the disease, the first change seen is an increase in thyroglobulin concentration (8). The erythrocyte sedimentation rate and the C-reactive protein levels are increased. In accordance with the clinical evolution, there is an increment in thyroid hormones, with a T4 : T3 ratio greater than 20 (9), that reflects the proportion of stored hormones, and helps to differentiate from the real hyperthyroideum states (e.g., Graves' disease, where the gland is hyper-functional). Initially, when the hypothyroidism develops, the thyroid-stimulating hormone (TSH) levels remain suppressed and if the first studies are taken by this time it could be misdiagnosed as a central hypothyroidism. Later, there is a compensatory response with high TSH.

Serological Features

Thyroid autoantibodies (including thyroid-stimulating antibodies) may be found in SAT (10) but these are usually transitory, and have no correlation with the thyroid function (11). In one study, TSH receptor-blocking antibodies were found more frequently in SAT patients with a prolonged hypothyroidism than in patients with a faster recovery (20 versus 3%) (12).

Diagnostic Criteria

Usually, there is a preceding upper tract viral infection. The levels of thyroid hormones vary with time; during the first stages, there is a temporary increase of free T4, but later the levels decline, even though hypothyroidism usually develops later in the course of disease. The radioactive iodine uptake at 24 h is less than 5%. The Doppler ultrasonography shows a heterogeneous parenchyma with flow reduction in the hypoechoic areas and a normal or only slightly increased flow in the rest of the gland. The results obtained in diagnostic tests in SAT are summarized in Table 43.1.

Prognosis

Painful SAT recurs in only about 2% of individuals (13). When hypothyroidism presents itself, it usually persists for less than 6 months, but this state may persist for a year and in 10–15% of cases it requires substitution treatment for the long term.

Prediction

There are not an established prediction score.

TABLE 43.1. Main characteristics of subacute thyroiditis.

Diagnostic test	Expected result in SAT
TSH levels	Suppressed at initial stages, posterior increase
RAIU at 24 h	Less than 5%
Anti-TPO antibodies	Absent, if positive low titer
CRP and ESR	High
Vascularity in Doppler ultrasonography	Low to normal
T4 and T3 levels	Initially high, posterior depletion

Anti-TPO: antithyroid peroxidase; CRP: C-reactive protein; ESR: erythrocyte sedimentation rate; RAIU: radioactive iodine uptake test; T3: triiodothyronine; T4: thyroxine; TSH: Thyroid stimulating hormone.

Therapy

The first line of treatment for SAT consists of nonsteroidal anti-inflammatory drugs. The median time from start of therapy to complete relief of pain is 5 weeks. If after one week of treatment no improvement occurs, prednisone may be added in a dosage of 40–60 mg daily tapered to complete discontinuation over 4–6 weeks (14); symptoms may reappear after withdrawal of treatment, but in these cases response is obtained with the reinstitution of treatment. Both the medications previously mentioned are only tried to provide pain relief. Symptoms of hyperthyroidism are treated with beta-blockers until the free T4 concentration returns to normal.

References

1. Fatourechi V, Aniszewski JP, Fatourechi GZ, et al. Clinical features and outcome of subacute thyroiditis in an incidence cohort: Olmstead County, Minnesota, study. *J Clin Endocrinol Metab* 2003; 88: 2100–5.
2. Martino E, Buratti L, Bartalena L, et al. High prevalence of subacute thyroiditis during summer season in Italy. *J Endocrinol Invest* 1987; 10: 321–3.
3. Espino-Montoro A, Medina-Perez M, González-Martín MC, et al. Subacute tiroiditis associated with positive antibodies to the Espstein-Barr virus. *An Med Interna* 2000; 17: 546–8.
4. De Quervain F. Die akute nicht Eiterige Thereoiditis und die Beteiligung der Schilddruse an akuten intoxikationen und infektionen Uberhaupt. *Mitt Grenz Med Chir* 1936; 44: 538–90.
5. Zein EF, Karaa SE, Megarbane A. *Presse Med* 2007; 36: 808–9.
6. Totterman TH. Distribution of T, B and thyroglobulin binding lymphocytes infiltrating the thyroid gland in Graves' disease, Hashimoto thyroiditis and de Quervain's thyroiditis. *Clin Immunol Immunopathol* 1978; 10: 270–7.
7. Swinburne JL, Kreisman SH. A rare case of subacute thyroiditis causing thyroid storm. *Thyroid* 2007; 17: 73–6.
8. Pearce EN, Farwell AP, Braverman LE. Thyroiditis. *N Engl J Med* 2003; 348: 2646–55.
9. Amino N, Yabu Y, Miki T, et al. Serum ratio of triiodothyronine to thyroxine, and thyroxine-binding globulin and calcitonin concentrations in Graves' disease and destruction-induced thyrotoxicosis. *J Clin Endocrinol Metab* 1981; 53: 113–6.
10. Mitani Y, Shigesmasa C, Kouchi T, et al. Detection of thyroid stimulating antibody in patients with inflammatory thyrotoxicosis. *Horm Res* 1992; 37: 196–201.
11. Strakosch CR, Joyner D, Wall JR. Thyroid stimulating antibodies in patients with subacute thyroiditis. *J Clin Endocrinol Metab* 1978; 46: 345–8.
12. Tamai H, Nozaki T, Mukuta T, et al. The incidence of thyroid stimulating blocking antibodies during the hypothyroid phase in patients with subacute thyroiditis. *J Clin Endocrinol Metab* 1991; 73: 245–50.
13. Iitaka M, Momotani N, Ishii J, Ito K. Incidence of subacute thyroiditis recurrences after a prolonged latency: 24-year survey. *J Clin Endocrinol Metab* 1996; 81: 466–9.
14. Bindra A, Braunstein GD. Thyroiditis. *Am Fam Physician* 2006; 73: 1769–76.

44
Graves Disease

Francesca Menconi, Yael L. Oppenheim and Yaron Tomer

Abstract   Graves disease (GD) is an autoimmune thyroid disease characterized by the formation of thyrotropin receptor-stimulating antibodies that activate the thyrotropin receptor causing thyrotoxicosis. Although the etiology of GD is unknown, it is believed to be a complex autoimmune disease caused by an interaction between susceptibility genes and environmental triggers, such as iodine and infection. GD is diagnosed mainly by demonstrating the presence of thyrotoxicosis and the pathognomonic thyrotropin stimulating antibodies. GD is associated with two main complications, Graves' ophthalmopathy and dermopathy. The etiology of these complications is unknown, but is believed to be due to a cross-over autoimmune response. Therapy of GD is directed at the thyrotoxicosis and not at the autoimmune mechanisms causing the disease, which are still not fully understood. The thyrotoxicosis is treated by either suppressing the production of thyroid hormones with anti-thyroid medications, or removing/ablating the thyroid gland by surgery or radioactive iodine.

Keywords   Thyroid · Graves disease · autoimmunity · thyrotoxicosis · ophthalmopathy

Graves disease (GD) is an autoimmune thyroid disease characterized clinically by the presence of hyperthyroidism, diffuse goiter, and, in some patients, ophthalmopathy and dermopathy. GD is caused by circulating antibodies directed against the thyrotropin receptor (TSHR). These antibodies mimic the effect of pituitary thyrotropin (TSH), and induce thyroid hormone over-production and hypersecretion, as well as hypertrophy and hyperplasia of the thyroid follicles, resulting in diffuse goiter. The cause of Graves ophthalmopathy (GO) and dermopathy is still unknown, but a cross-reaction between thyroidal and orbital and/or connective tissue antigens has been postulated.

Epidemiology

GD is the most common cause of hyperthyroidism in iodine-sufficient areas, accounting for 70–80% of all cases of hyperthyroidism. According to some estimates, it is the most prevalent autoimmune disorder in the USA [reviewed in ref (1)]. Epidemiological surveys from various, mostly iodine sufficient, regions have shown an annual incidence of GD of approximately 20–25 per 100,000, in

Caucasian populations (2). The prevalence of GD is similar among Caucasians and Asians, but it is lower among Africans [reviewed in (1)]. GD typically affects women at ages 30–50 years. The incidence of GD is 5–10 times greater in women than in men, and GD is uncommon in children.

History

GD is named after the Irish physician Robert Graves who first described the association of palpitations, goiter, and proptosis of the eyes in 1835. In 1840, the same constellation of symptoms was described by the German physician von Basedow. Therefore, in continental Europe, GD is sometimes referred to as Basedow disease. The eponym GD is more commonly used in the USA. In 1956, Adams and Purves identified in the serum of patients with GD a thyroid-stimulating factor that was not thyrotropin (TSH), which they called long-acting thyroid stimulator (LATS) because of its sustained activity. The LATS were later identified as immunoglobulin G antibodies that can bind to and stimulate the TSH receptor on the thyroid cell membranes (TSH receptor antibodies, TRAb) (3). The

From: Y. Shoenfeld et al. (eds.): *Diagnostic Criteria in Autoimmune Diseases*, DOI: 10.1007/978-1-60327-285-8_44,
© 2008 Humana Press, Totowa, NJ

TRAb were later shown to compete with TSH for binding to thyroid membranes, forming the basis for the commonly used assay to detect TRAb.

Pathogenesis

GD is a complex disease caused by an interaction between susceptibility genes and environmental triggers (e.g., dietary iodine, infection) (2). When genetically susceptible individuals are exposed to certain environmental triggers, thyroid-specific T cells are formed that infiltrate the thyroid gland and activate B cells to produce TSH receptor (TSHR)-stimulating antibodies. TSHR-stimulating antibodies stimulate thyroid cells to proliferate and secrete excess thyroid hormones causing goiter and hyperthyroidism. It is not known what causes the production of thyroid specific T cells. The current paradigm is that certain genes, such as CTLA-4 and CD40, induce a state of hyperactivity of T cells and antigen-presenting cells, whereas additional genes, such as HLA-DR alleles containing arginine at position 74 of the DRB1 chain, direct the thyroid specificity of the immune response (2). The trigger of the autoimmune response to thyroid antigens is believed to be an environmental insult, likely an infectious agent. Infectious agents can trigger an autoimmune response to the thyroid either by molecular mimicry or by bystander activation. Molecular mimicry occurs when sequence or structural similarity exists between infectious agents and thyroidal antigens resulting in the formation of thyroid-specific T cells and/or antibodies because of cross-over specificity. However, so far no specific infectious agent protein has been conclusively linked to GD. Bystander mechanisms can lead to thyroid autoimmunity when thyroidal injury, such as caused by infection or excess iodine, stimulates thyroid inflammation and infiltration by T cells because of secretion of cytokines and chemokines. This can lead to exposure of cryptic epitopes of thyroidal proteins resulting in an autoimmune response to thyroid antigens. Through epitope spreading, the autoimmune response can focus on the TSHR. Thyroid-specific T cells can then stimulate B cells to produce TSHR-stimulating antibodies (4). Because GD is characterized by thyrocyte proliferation while Hashimoto's thyroiditis is characterized by thyrocyte apoptosis, it is believed that the thyroid infiltrating T cells in GD activate anti-apoptotic pathways.

Up to 10–20% of GD patients develop severe form of GO. The cause of GO is still unknown, but GO is believed to result from a cross-over autoimmune response to eye antigens. Several studies have shown expression of the TSHR and insulin-like growth factor (IGF)-1 receptor in orbital fibroblasts and adipocytes. Stimulation of the TSHR and IGF-1 receptor on orbital fibroblasts can lead to the production of hyaluronic acid and cytokines/chemokines which trigger infiltration of the orbits by T cells, thereby leading to GO (5).

Clinical Manifestations

Signs and symptoms of GD can be divided into those caused by the excess circulating thyroid hormones (hyperthyroid symptoms) and those that are specific to GD. Typical symptoms of hyperthyroidism are present in most patients with GD, and are summarized in Table 44.1. Patients can present with various combinations of these symptoms, but the most common presenting symptoms are nervousness, heat intolerance, weight loss, and palpitations (6). In the elderly these classical symptoms may not be present, and GD may be asymptomatic (the so-called *apathetic* hyperthyroidism), or may present only with fatigue and weight loss. In other cases, mostly in older individuals, the presenting signs are cardiac, such as atrial

TABLE 44.1. Symptoms and signs of Graves' disease.

General	In females	In elderly	Specific to GD
Palpitations/Tachycardia	Oligomenorrhea	Apathetic Hyperthyroidism	Diffuse goiter
Nervousness	Amenorrhea	Atrial Fibrillation	Bruit over thyroid
Tremor			Ophthalmopathy
Weight loss			Swelling of legs
Goiter			Dermopathy
Heat sensitivity			Splenomegaly
Perspiration			Acropachy
Fatigue			
Dyspnea			
Diarrhea			
Supra-ventricular tachycardias			
Increased appetite			
Gynecomastia			

fibrillation, or, more rarely, congestive heart failure. Besides symptoms caused by thyroid hyperfunction one or more of the following characteristic signs of GD may be present:

- *Goiter*: a diffuse enlargement of thyroid gland that ranges from minimal to marked. It is more common in young people but can be present also in older patients. Often a loud bruit can be heard over the thyroid with a stethoscope because of the increased blood flow to the thyroid.

- *Ophthalmopathy*: it is clinically evident in up to 50% of GD patients (1), whereas severe ophthalmopathy is seen in 5–10% of patients. Ophthalmopathy usually appears within a year before or after the onset of hyperthyroidism. Orbital involvement is, in most cases, bilateral, but it can be unilateral (in up to 15% of cases) (reviewed in ref 7). The majority of GD patients have a mild and non-progressive ocular involvement, but in its most severe form ophthalmopathy can be disfiguring, and it is associated with significant visual impairment that can lead to visual loss (reviewed in ref 7). The clinical features of ophthalmopathy are summarized in Table 44.2.

- *Dermopathy*: it is present in 1–2% of GD patients, most commonly in those affected by severe ophthalmopathy. Graves' dermopathy usually manifests by non-pitting edema with occasional raised, hyperpigmented papules, and it is commonly localized over the anterior shins (pretibial mixedema). In severe cases it can lead to elephantiasis.

- *Thyroid acropachy*: it is a very rare manifestation of GD. It is usually associated with pretibial mixedema and ophthalmopathy. It is characterized by soft tissue swelling and periosteal bone changes in the fingers and toes, causing clubbing.

TABLE 44.2. Symptoms and signs of ophthalmopathy.

Symptoms
   Burning sensation in the eyes
   Retroocular pressure
   Excessive tearing
   Photophobia
   Ocular pain, related or unrelated to eye movement
   Diplopia
   Blurred vision
Signs
   Redness of the eyelids
   Redness of the conjunctiva
   Swelling of periorbital tissue
   Inflammation of caruncle and/or plica
   Conjunctival edema (chemosis)
   Eyelid retraction
   Protrusion of the eyes (proptosis)
   Extra-ocular muscle dysfunction
   Visual loss (rare)

Pathological Features

Grossly the thyroid gland can be enlarged. Microscopic evaluation reveals hypertrophy and hyperplasia of thyroid follicular cells. There is lymphocytic infiltration, and colloid is sparse. The thyroid follicular cells have an elongated columnar appearance, are folded over in papillary configurations, and they protrude into the lumen of the follicle (8).

Biochemical and Serological Features

Blood counts and chemistries do not show specific changes in patients with GD. In some patients, mild abnormalities in liver functions and hypercalcemia can be observed. All patients exhibit low or undetectable TSH levels accompanied by increased serum concentrations of thyroxine (T4) and/or triiodothyronine (T3), demonstrating primary hyperthyroidism. In some patients only T3 levels are elevated (T3 toxicosis). To avoid diagnostic difficulties caused by changes in thyroid-binding proteins, free thyroxine (fT4) and free triiodothyronine (fT3) levels should be measured (reviewed in ref 6). Serum TRAb are measured using assays that test for inhibition of binding of labeled TSH to thyroid membranes or cells. When measured with high-sensitivity assays, TRAb are positive in >95% of GD patients. The serum levels of thyroid peroxidase (TPO) antibodies are elevated in about 75% of GD patients whereas thyroglobulin antibodies are detectable in about 50% of GD patients (reviewed in ref 9).

Diagnostic Criteria

Clinical and/or biochemical features of hyperthyroidism are present in nearly all GD patients. The findings of high-serum fT4 and/or fT3 levels, in combination with low or undetectable TSH concentrations, are necessary to confirm the diagnosis of primary hyperthyroidism. As summarized in Table 44.3, the diagnosis of GD is confirmed in a patient with primary hyperthyroidism based on the presence of one or more of the following: (a) ophthalmopathy and/or dermopathy; (b) detectable TRAb in the serum; and (c) diffuse radioactive iodine uptake. TRAb are

TABLE 44.3. Diagnostic criteria for GD. For diagnosis the major criterion and at least one of the three minor criteria should be positive.

Major criterion
   Hyperthyroidism (clinical and/or biochemical)
Minor criteria
   Clinical manifestation of ophthalmopathy
   Positive serum TRAb
   Diffuse radioactive iodine uptake

pathognomonic for GD, and their levels correlate with disease severity. Measurement of TRAb is mandatory in pregnant women with a past or present history of GD, because TRAb can cross the placenta, stimulate the fetal thyroid gland, and cause neonatal hyperthyroidism (10). Measurement of TRAb is also helpful in predicting remission of GD after a course of anti-thyroid drugs (reviewed in ref 6). Twenty-four-hour radioactive iodine uptake is increased in GD as in most hyperthyroid states and is not generally needed to make the diagnosis. However, it can be helpful for ruling out destructive thyroiditis (painless thyroiditis or post-partum thyroiditis), conditions in which hyperthyroidism is associated with a low 24-h radioactive iodine uptake.

Prediction

Currently, there is no algorithm to predict GD. However, there are well-known risk factors that can give some estimate of the risk of developing disease. Known risk factors for GD include genetic susceptibility (2), the presence of thyroid antibodies, female gender, dietary iodine, pregnancy, and infection. Abundant epidemiological data demonstrate a strong genetic predisposition to the development of GD. It is well known that GD clusters in families. Our group has recently calculated the sibling risk ratio for GD, i.e. the ratio of the prevalence of GD in siblings of affected individuals to the prevalence of GD in the general population, to be 11.6 (reviewed in ref 2). Moreover, twin studies have shown a 35% concordance rate in monzygotic twins compared with 3% in dizygotic twins, demonstrating a strong genetic predisposition to GD (reviewed in ref 2). So far six genes have been shown to contribute to the etiology of GD, including immune-modulating genes and thyroid-specific genes. The first group includes the *HLA-DR, CD40, CTLA-4,* and *PTPN22* genes, whereas the second group includes the thyroglobulin and TSHR genes. It is clear that additional genes contribute to the genetic susceptibility to GD and that these genes interact. Indeed, we have recently shown a 16-fold increased risk for GD in individuals carrying HLA-DR alleles containing arginine at position 74 of the DRB1 chain and a certain thyroglobulin gene amino acid variant. However, we do not anticipate being able to predict GD with high predictive values based on gene polymorphisms (2).

Therapy

Treatment options for Graves' hyperthyroidism include medical therapy, radioactive iodine, and surgery. Therapy should be targeted to the specific individual, based on severity of thyrotoxicosis, the presence of goiter and ophthalmopathy, and individual patient concerns and preferences. Medical therapy consists primarily of suppressing the hyperthyroid symptoms with beta blockers, and blocking thyroid hormone synthesis with thionamides (e.g. Tapazole, propylthiouracil). Beta blockers are often used initially as they can alleviate the symptoms and allow time for more definitive therapy.

Thionamides are often used as the initial treatment of hyperthyroidism of any cause, as response rate is high. Potential toxicities of thionamides include bone marrow toxicity (agranulocytosis) and hepatotoxicity, both of which can be potentially life threatening. Thionamides are considered the treatment of choice in children, adolescents, and pregnant women with GD (6). However, the rates of persistent remission after thionamides are discontinued are reported to be 20–50%. In the USA, persistent remission rates after 1–2 years of thionamide treatment are about 20–30% (11). In those patients who do not achieve long-term remission, most physicians prefer definitive treatment with radioactive iodine ablation (most commonly) or surgery. In severe cases of hyperthyroidism, steroids and iodine such as Lugol's iodine or potassium iodide (SSKI) are given in addition to high doses of thionamides.

Radioactive iodine therapy is an alternate effective means of treating Grave's disease. This modality can take several months to fully treat the hyperthyroidism. In the interim, some patients require thionamide treatment. Most patients receiving radioactive iodine therapy become hypothyroid and require life-long thyroid hormone replacement. Although radioactive iodine is a relatively safe therapy, it can worsen GO. In patients with ophthalmopathy who are treated with radioactive iodine, a 4- to 5-week course of steroids, starting at the day of radioactive iodine therapy, is recommended.

Surgery to remove the thyroid can also be used to treat Grave's disease. Total thyroidectomy will cure the hyperthyroidism, but render the patient hypothyroid, requiring life-long levothyroxine replacement therapy. Patients should receive beta blockers, and their thyroid functions should be normalized with thionamide treatment before surgery to avoid complications of accelerated hyperthyroidism during surgery. None of the above-mentioned modalities specifically targets the autoimmune mechanisms causing GD.

GO is treated with steroids, orbital irradiation, or surgery, but all these therapies do not cure the disease. Recently, anti-CD20 monoclonal antibodies have been successfully tried in GO.

References

1. Weetman AP. Graves' Disease. *N Engl J Med* 2000; 343(17): 1236–48.
2. Tomer Y, Davies TF. Searching for the autoimmune thyroid disease susceptibility genes: From gene mapping to gene function. *Endocr Rev* 2003; 24: 694–717.

3. Volpè R. Graves' disease. Braverman LE, Utiger RD (eds.), *Werner and Ingbar's The Thyroid a Fundamental Clinical Text*. Lippincott Williams & Wilkens, Philidelphia; 1991: 648–57.

4. Prabhakar BS, Bahn RS, Smith TJ. Current perspective on the pathogenesis of Graves' disease and ophthalmopathy. *Endocr Rev* 2003; 24(6): 802–35.

5. Garrity JA, Bahn RS. Pathogenesis of graves ophthalmopathy: Implications for prediction, prevention, and treatment. *Am J Ophthalmol* 2006; 142(1): 147–53.

6. Cooper DS. Hyperthyroidism. *Lancet* 2003; 362: 459–68.

7. Bartalena L, Pinchera A, Marcocci C. Management of Graves' ophthalmopathy: Reality and perspectives. *Endocr Rev* 2000; 21: 168–99.

8. Oertel JE, LiVolsi VA. Pathology of thyroid diseases. Braverman LE, Utiger RD (eds.), *Werner and Ingbar's The Thyroid a Fundamental Clinical Text*. Lippincott Williams & Wilkens, Philidelphia; 1991: 603–42.

9. McLachlan SM, Rapoport B. Why measure thyroglobulin autoantibodies rather than thyroid peroxidase autoantibodies? *Thyroid* 2004; 14(7): 510–20.

10. Lazarus JH. Hyperthyroidism. *Lancet* 1997; 349: 339–43.

11. Ross DS. Management of the various causes of thyrotoxicosis. Braverman LE (ed.), *Diseases of the Thyroid*, Humana Press, Totowa, NJ; 2003: 177–98.

45
Postpartum Thyroiditis

Alex Stagnaro-Green

Abstract   Postpartum thyroiditis is an autoimmune condition marked by hormonal abnormalities in the first postpartum year in women who were euthryoid before conception. The presence of thyroid antibodies in the first trimester of pregnancy is associated with a 33–50% chance of developing postpartum thyroiditis. Treatment is rarely needed in the hyperthyroid phase of postpartum thyroiditis whereas levothyroxine therapy is frequently required in the hypothyroid phase. Most women are euthyroid by the end of the first postpartum year. Nevertheless, the majority of women who have had postpartum thyroiditis develop permanent primary hypothyroidism within 10 years.

Keywords   Postpartum thyroiditis · thyroid peroxidase antibodies

Description of the Disease

Postpartum thyroiditis (PPT) is an autoimmune disorder that occurs in the first postpartum year in women with no history of thyroid disease before pregnancy. The classical form, which occurs in 25% of women, consists of a hyperthyroid phase followed by a hypothyroid phase, with a return to euthyroidism before the end of the first postpartum year. Thirty-two percent of women have a hyperthyroid phase in isolation and 43% present solely with a hypothyroid phase (1). Although the majority of women are euthyroid by the end of the first postpartum year, a small percentage of women remain permanently hypothyroid.

Epidemiology

The incidence of postpartum thyroiditis varies between 1 and 16% with most studies indicating an incidence between 5 and 10%. Women with a history of type 1 diabetes mellitus, another autoimmune disorder, have a threefold increase in the incidence of postpartum thyroiditis. Specifically, the incidence of PPT in the general population of women in the New York metropolitan area was 8.8% (2), whereas it increased to 25% in women with type 1 diabetes (3).

History

In 1948, Roberton described the first series of women with thyroid disease after pregnancy (4). Evaluation of 483 pregnancies revealed 114 women with symptoms of an underactive thyroid and who responded to thyroid extract. Amino and colleagues published a seminal article on PPT in 1982 in the *New England Journal of Medicine* (5). In a prospective study, 507 women were evaluated postpartum for thyroid disorders, of whom 5.5% developed abnormal thyroid function tests in the postpartum period.

Pathogenesis

Postpartum thyroiditis is an autoimmune disorder triggered by the immune changes which occur during pregnancy and postpartum. Multiple lines of evidence support the autoimmune nature of PPT. First, 33–50% of women who are thyroid antibody positive in the first trimester (thyroid peroxidase antibody and/or thyroglobulin antibody) develop PPT, whereas PPT is extremely rare in thyroid antibody negative women. Second, the higher the titer of the thyroid antibody, the more likely that PPT will occur. Third, there are specific HLA predilections for PPT, namely HLA-DR 3, 4, and 5 (6). Finally, a prospective study has demonstrated distinct immune changes, specifically an elevation in the CD4+/CD8+ ratio in women who develop PPT (2). On the basis of the overwhelming evidence of the autoimmune nature of PPT, Muller et al. concluded that, "The natural course of thyroid autoimmune disease often encompasses a long subclinical prodromal phase... From this perspective, postpartum thyroiditis is 'just' an aggravation of an existing thyroiditis after an amelioration of the inflammation during pregnancy" (7).

From: Y. Shoenfeld et al. (eds.): *Diagnostic Criteria in Autoimmune Diseases*, DOI: 10.1007/978-1-60327-285-8_45,

Clinical Manifestations

The clinical manifestations can vary from a complete lack of symptoms, to mild hyperthyroidism, to profound hypothyroidism. The presence and degree of symptoms depends on a number of factors, including the severity of the thyroid hormonal dysfunction and probably the rapidity with which the hormonal changes occur. Furthermore, it is often difficult to distinguish the symptoms of PPT from the normal physiological changes that occur during the postpartum period. Table 45.1 presents four studies that have documented increased symptoms in women with PPT, in either the hyperthyroid or hypothyroid phase, compared with a control group of postpartum euthyroid women (5, 8, 9, 10).

Pathological Features

Table 45.2 presents the findings of 15 thyroid biopsies in women with clinical and laboratory-confirmed PPT. Eight of the specimens were obtained while the patient was hypothyroid, four were collected during the early euthyroid recovery phase, and three were obtained during late recovery (11).

Biochemical Features

The biochemical features of PPT depend upon which phase of PPT the patient is in, or if the hormonal status of the patient is in transition. During the hyperthyroid phase, which typically lasts less than 3 months, TSH is suppressed and is often accompanied by a minor elevation of T3 and T4. The hypothyroid phase, which is typically more severe and longer lasting, can present with a mild to marked elevation of the TSH and a moderate to dramatic decrease in T4. During transition times, thyroid function

TABLE 45.2. Thyroid biopsy results of women with Postpartum Thyroiditis.

Hypothyroid Phase and early recovery (n = 12)
-lymphocytic infiltration—diffuse and focal thyroiditis
-follicular destruction in various degrees
-hyperplastic follicular changes in various degrees
-7 of 12 showed an oxyphilic change of the follicular cells
Late recovery (n = 3)
-lymphocytic infiltration—only focal thyroiditis
-no follicular destruction

tests may be misleading. For example, it is feasible to have perfectly normal thyroid hormonal levels during the transition period from hyperthyroidism to hypothyroidism, as hormone levels pass through the normal range.

Serological Features

The immune marker for PPT is the presence of thyroid peroxidase antibody and/or thyroglobulin antibody. Thyroid antibodies decrease in titer throughout pregnancy, often becoming undetectable by the third trimester. In the postpartum period, once released from the immunosuppressive effect of pregnancy, antibody titers rebound, often reaching levels that surpass those detected in the first trimester (2). Although there are rare cases in which PPT develops in the absence of thyroid antibody positivity, it typically reflects an insensitivity of the assay used.

Diagnostic Criteria

The diagnosis of PPT is based on an elevated or suppressed TSH in the first postpartum year in women without a pre-pregnancy history of thyroid disease. It is important to differentiate PPT from the de novo presentation of

TABLE 45.1. Symptoms documented to be statistically more common in women with postpartum thyroiditis as compared with a control group.

First author	Year	Country	Hyperthyroid symptoms	Hypothyroid symptoms
Amino (1)	1982	Japan	Fatigue Palpitations	Not reported
Hayslip (8)	1988	USA	No increase in symptoms	Impaired concentration Carelessness Depression
Lazarus (9)	1999	UK	Lack of energy Irritability	Lack of energy Poor memory Dry skin Cold intolerance Aches and pains
Walfish (10)	1992	Canada	Palpitations Heat intolerance Nervousness	Hypothyroid phase reported as more symptomatic than the thyrotoxic phase

Reprinted with permission from the *J Clin Endocrinol Metab* 1992; 74: 645–653.

Graves' disease. From an epidemiological perspective, new onset hyperthyroidism in the postpartum period is 40 times more likely to be PPT than Graves' disease. Classical stigmata of Graves' disease, such as a bruit or exophthalmos, confirm the diagnosis of Graves'. In some cases, a radionuclide scan is needed to differentiate PPT (low-uptake scan) from Graves' disease (high-uptake scan).

Prognosis

The vast majority of women who develop PPT return to the euthyroid state by one year postpartum. Long-term studies of women who have had PPT reveal a 23–63% incidence of developing permanent hypothyroidism (12, 13). Women who have had an initial episode of PPT resolve have a 67% chance of developing PPT in a subsequent pregnancy (14).

Prevention

Earlier attempts to prevent the occurrence of PPT through the administration of either iodine or levothyroxine have been unsuccessful (15). Negro et al., in 2007, demonstrated a decrease in the incidence of PPT through selenium administration (16). Women who were thyroid antibody positive in the first trimester were given selenium after the 11th week of pregnancy and into the postpartum. Women receiving selenium had a 29% incidence of PPT compared with 49% in women who received placebo (p < 0.01).

Treatment

Treatment of the hyperthyroid phase of PPT is typically unnecessary as the symptoms are usually mild and the time course sufficiently short. When treatment is required a limited course of beta blockers, titrated to control the symptoms of hyperthyroidism, is all that is required. Treatment of the hypothyroid phase depends on the severity of the symptoms, the degree of elevation of the TSH, and whether a subsequent pregnancy is being planned. Intervention with levothyroxine is recommended if the TSH exceeds 10 µU/ml or if the TSH is between 4 and 10 µU/ml and the patient is symptomatic. Asymptomatic women with TSH levels between 4 and 10 µU/ml, and who are planning to conceive in the near future, also require levothyroxine therapy because of the risk of miscarriage and impaired neurological function in the developing fetus. Once levothyroxine is initiated, I recommend maintaining

treatment until the mother has completed her child bearing. One year after the birth of the final child, I halve the dose of levothyroxine to determine whether permanent hypothyroidism has developed (1). Women who have been successfully weaned from thyroid hormone replacement require annual thyroid hormone testing to screen for permanent hypothyroidism, which is dramatically increased in women who have had an episode of PPT (14).

References

1. Stagnaro-Green, A. (2002) Clinical Review 152: Postpartum thyroiditis, *J Clin Endocrinol Metab* **87 (9)**, 4042–4047.
2. Stagnaro-Green, A., Roman, S.H., Cobin, R.H., El-Harazy, E., Wallenstein S., Davis, T.F. (1992) A prospective study of lymphocyte-initiated immunosuppression in normal pregnancy: Evidence of a T-cell etiology for postpartum thyroid dysfunction, *J Clin Endocrinol Metab* **74**, 645–653.
3. Alvarez-Marfany, M., Roman, S.H., Drexler, A.J., Robertson, C., Stagnaro-Green, A.S. (1994) Long-term prospective study of postpartum thyroid dysfunction in women with insulin dependent diabetes mellitus *J Clin Endocrinol Metab* **79**, 10–16.
4. Roberton, H.E.W. (1948) Lassitude, coldness, and hair changes following pregnancy, and their response to treatment with thyroid extract *British Med J* **94**, 2275–2276.
5. Amino, N., Mori, H., Iwatani, Y., Tanizawa, O., Kawashima, M., Tsuge, I., Ibaragi, K., Kumahara, Y., Miyai, K. (1982) High prevalence of transient post-partum thyrotoxicosis and hypothyroidism *N Eng J Med* **306**, 849–852.
6. Vargas, M.T., Briones-Urbina, R., Gladman, D., Papsin, F.R., Walfish, P.G. (1988) Antithyroid microsomal autoantibodies and HLA-DR5 are associated with postpartum thyroid dysfunction: Evidence supporting an autoimmune pathogenesis *J Clin Endocrinol Metab* **67**, 327–333.
7. Muller, A.F., Dexhage, H.A., Berghout, A. (2001) Postpartum thyroiditis and autoimmune thyroiditis in women of childbearing age: recent insights and consequences for antenatal and postnatal care *Endocr. Rev.* **22**, 605–630.
8. Hayslip, C.C., Fein, H.G., O'Donnell, V.M., Friedman, D.S., Klein, T.A., Smallridge, R.C. (1988) The value of serum antimicrosomal antibody testing in screening for symptomatic postpartum thyroid dysfunction *Am J Obstet Gynecol* **159**, 203–209.
9. Lazarus, J.H. (1999) Clinical manifestations of postpartum thyroid disease *Thyroid* **9**, 685–689.
10. Walfish, P.G., Meyerson, J., Provias, J.P., Vargas, M.T., Papsin, F.R. (1992) Prevalence and characteristics of postpartum thyroid dysfunction: results of a survey from Toronto, Canada. *J Endocrinol Invest* **15**, 265–272.
11. Mizukami, Y., Michigishi, T., Nonomura, A., Hashimoto, T., Nakamura, S., Tonami, N., Takazakura, E. (1993) Postpartum thyroiditis: A clinical, histologic, and immunopathologic study of 15 cases *Anatomic Path* **100**, 200–205.
12. Othman, S., Phillips, D.I.W., Parkes, A.B., Richards, C.J., Harris, B., Fung, H., Darke, C., John, R., Hall, R.,

Lazarus, J.H. (1990) A long-term follow-up of postpartum thyroiditis *Clin Endocrinol* **32,** 559–564.

13. Azizi, F. (2004) Age as a predictor of recurrent hypothyroidism in patients with postpartum thyroid dysfunction *J Endocrinol Invest* **27,** 996–1002.

14. Lazarus, J.H., Ammari, F., Oretti, R., Parkes, A.B., Richards, C.J., Harris B. (1997) Clinical aspects of recurrent postpartum thyroiditis *Br J Gen Prac* **47,** 305–308.

15. Kampe, O., Jansson, R., Karlsson, F.A. (1990) Effects of L-thyroxine and iodide on the development of autoimmune postpartum thyroiditis *J Clin Endocrinol Metab* **70,** 1014–1018.

16. Negro, R., Greco, G., Mangieri, T., Pezzarossa, A., Dazzi, D., Hassan H. (2007) The influence of selenium supplementation on postpartum thyroid status in pregnant women with thyroid peroxidase autoantibodies *J Clin Endocrinol Metab* **92,** 1263–1268.

46
Autoimmune Diabetes Mellitus

Felicia Hanzu and Ramon Gomis

Abstract Diabetes mellitus is a metabolic disorder characterized by chronic hyperglycemia and following lifelong complications in which exogenous insulin is required for surviving and prevention of ketosis. Clinical and experimental data indicate that in genetically predisposed individuals, possibly triggered by exposure to certain environment factors, there is primarily a cellular (through auto-aggressive lymphocytes T) and thereafter a humoral (by selective anti-islet antibodies)-mediated destruction of pancreatic beta cells. Specific biochemical assayed auto-antibodies (anti-GAD65, anti-insulin, and anti-IA-2) are the essential markers used for diagnostics and prediction. Treatment consists in daily administration of exogenous insulin under self-monitoring conditions of blood glucose and diet; new non-invasive insulin products are now available. Concomitant pancreas and kidney transplant can be performed in patients with end-stage renal disease. Future goals include beta-cell substitution by islets transplant or stem cell therapy and prevention therapy in order to permit early prophylaxis for persons at risk. Global immunosuppressant protocols carry an unacceptable morbidity. Trials with non-Fc-binding anti-CD3 monoclonal antibodies and concomitant antigenic immunization are in course.

Keywords Autoimmune diabetes · beta cell · insulin · auto-antibodies · anti-insulin · anti-GAD65 · anti-IA-2

Description of the Disease

Diabetes mellitus (DM) is a group of metabolic disorders characterized by chronic hyperglycemia (from glucose intolerance in early stage to franc hyperglycemia), with disturbances of carbohydrate, fat, and protein metabolism resulting from defects in insulin secretion, action, or both, as result of three fundamental processes, which variably accelerate the loss of beta cells through apoptosis: constitution, insulin resistance, and autoimmunity (accelerator hypothesis) regardless of specific etiology (1). This include long-term complications of distinct organs, especially eyes, nerve fibers, kidney, and blood vessels (ADA classification of DM in Table 46.1) (2).

Type 1A DM is the major form of DM requiring exogenous insulin for survival and preventing ketosis as a consequence of beta-cell destruction and also the principal autoimmune DM form because of a cellular-mediated, organ-specific, progressive beta-cell destruction. Autoimmunity is described by the presence of more than one of specific auto-antibodies: anti-GAD65, anti-insulin, and anti-IA-2 (ICA512), IA-2β. Other rare forms of autoimmune DM have been described (stiff-man syndrome, syndrome type B). Autoimmune DM can be associated with other autoimmune diseases singular or as a part of the autoimmune polyglandular syndrome type 1 and 2 (APS-I and APS-II) (6).

Etiopathogenesis

DM type 1A is an autoimmune organ-specific chronic disease in genetically predisposed individuals possibly initiated (triggered) by exposure to certain environmental factors. There is primary a cellular destruction mainly from auto-reactive and auto-aggressive effector T-cell-mediated process, a selective infiltration of beta cells and insulitis (infiltrate with CD4, CD8 T lymphocytes, B lymphocytes, macrophages), and destruction through perforin- and cytokine-mediated cytotoxic mechanisms. A secondary immune response is marked by the generation of auto-antibodies, humoral markers of immune destruction [anti-glutamic acid decarboxylase-65 (GAD65), insulinoma-associated antigen IA-2(ICA512), and IA-2ß and anti-insulin], and progressive destruction

From: Y. Shoenfeld et al. (eds.): *Diagnostic Criteria in Autoimmune Diseases*, DOI: 10.1007/978-1-60327-285-8_46,

of the pancreas. This process progresses silently through the years, the first metabolic evidence of beta-cell decline being the alteration of first-phase insulin response to intravenous glucose, followed by the impairment of glucose dynamics (alternate glucose tolerance and fasting hyperglycemia), and finally overt hyperglycemia and DM when the great part of beta cells are destroyed (Figure 46.1).

TABLE 46.1. Diabetes mellitus classification (2).

I. Type 1 diabetes (ß-cell destruction, usually leading to absolute insulin deficiency)
  a) Immune mediated
  b) Idiopathic, non-autoimmune and non-HLA dependent
II. Type 2 diabetes (from predom. insulin resistance with relative insulin deficiency to a predom. secretory defect with insulin resistance)
III. Other specific types
  A. Genetic defects of beta cell function
    1. Chrs 12, HNF-1α (MODY3)
    2. Chrs 7, glucokinase (MODY2)
    3. Chrs 20, HNF-4α (MODY1)
    4. Chrs 13, insulin promoter factor-1 (IPF-1; MODY4)
    5. Chrs 17, HNF-1ß (MODY5)
    6. Chrs 2, Neuro*D1* (MODY6)
    7. Mitochondrial DNA
  B. Genetic defects in insulin action: Type A insulin resistance, Leprechaunism, Rabson-Mendenhall sdr, Lipoatrophic diabetes, etc
  C. Diseases of the exocrine pancreas: Trauma, Pancreatectomy, Neoplasia p., Cystic fibrosis Hemochromatosis, pancreatopathy, etc
  D. Endocrinopathies: Acromegaly, Cushing's sdr., Glucagonoma, Pheochromocytoma Hyperthyroidism, Somatostatinoma, Aldosteronoma,
  E. Drug- or chemical-induced: Vacor, Streptazocina, Pentamidine , Nicotinic ac., Thyroid hormone, Glucocorticoids , Diazoxide, ß-adr. Agonists, Dilantin, Thiazides, α-Interferon, etc
  F. Infections: congenital rubéola, cytomegalovirus, etc
  G. Uncommon forms of immune-mediated diabetes: 'Stiff-man' sdr, Anti–insulin receptor antibodies, etc.
  H. Other genetic syndromes: Down's sdr, Klinefelter, Prader-Willi, Turner, Wolfram, Friedreich ataxia, Huntington chorea, Laurence-Moon-Biedl, Myotonic dystrophy, Porphyria
IV. Gestational diabetes mellitus (GDM)

Immune-inflammation markers are present since the onset of autoimmune cascade through the entire evolution of DM 1 (3, 4). Although in children, beta-cell destruction is accelerated during rapid onset of overt hyperglycemia and ketoacidosis, in adults there remains a residual cell function for some years, form denominated "latent auto-immune diabetes" (LADA) (5, 6).

Epidemiology

Incidence rate of DM type 1 varies with age (DM 1A can appear at any age but have a high incidence under the age of 15 years: 3/4 before 18 years of age; little known about the determinants occurring in adult type 1 diabetes), race (the risk is higher among white population), and countries [highest frequency is according to recent studies in Nordic countries but also in Portugal and Sardinia: ranging from 21.2 to 36.8 per 100,000 per year; the lowest frequency in Asia and Latin America: ranging from 0.1 to 3.5 per 100,000 per year (4, 5)]. The Eurodiab study, a register involving 44 countries in Europe, indicates annual rates of increase in incidence of DM 1A, the larger increase being noted in children 3–4 years of age. Range of variations within white population is almost as great as between races, suggesting the concomitant involvement of genetic and environmental factors (6). Environmental trigger factors that could initiate the autoimmune process are in discussion: common viruses (large seasonal character peak in winter, only proven association for congenital rubella, contradictory results from animal experiments), nutrition (exposure to cow milk proteins and absence of breast feeding in new born) (6). Genetic susceptibility: DM 1A is a complex genetic disorder with strong genetic association to certain human leukocyte antigen (HLA) alleles at the DQ (A and B) and DR (3 and 4) loci on chromosome 6

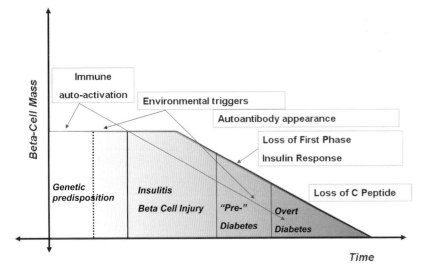

FIGURE 46.1. Model of pathogenesis and natural history of DM type 1A. (Modified after Eisenbarth GS, ed. Type 1A diabetes: cellular, molecular and clinical immunology, available in teaching slides http://www.Barbaradaviscenter.org).

TABLE 46.2. Criteria for the diagnosis of autoimmune diabetes mellitus (2).

1. Symptoms of diabetes plus casual plasma glucose concentration ≥200 mg/dl (11.1 mmol/l).
   Casual is defined as any time of day without regard to time since last meal. The classic symptoms of diabetes include polyuria, polydipsia, and unexplained weight loss.
   or
2. FPG ≥126 mg/dl (7.0 mmol/l). Fasting is defined as no caloric intake for at least 8 h.
   or
3. 2-h postload glucose ≥200 mg/dl (11.1 mmol/l) during an OGTT. The test should be performed as described by WHO, using a glucose load containing the equivalent of 75 g anhydrous glucose dissolved in water.
   >one biochemically assayed selective islet antibody (anti-GAD65, anti-insulin, anti-IA-2 (ICA512), IA-2β) set at ≥99th percentile of normal individuals)

Note: In the absence of unequivocal hyperglycemia, these criteria should be confirmed by repeat testing on a different day. The third measure (OGTT) is not recommended for routine clinical use. The use of the hemoglobin A1c (A1C) for the diagnosis of diabetes is not recommended at this time. IFG, IGT, and TTGO are defined as prediabetes (IFG: a jeun glucose:100–125 mg/dl, IGT: glucose at 2 h: 140–199 mg/dl). Histological confirmation of pancreas insulitis is not routinely demanded.

(pathogenic HLA alleles: DQA1*0501, DQB1*0201 in linkage disequilibrium with DR3; DQA1*0301, DQB1*0302 with DR4; protective association for DQA1*0102 and DQB1*0602). HLA is responsible for half of the familial clustering of DM 1A, the rest is presumably because of other genetic factors or shared family environment. Overall, risk of DM of a sibling of a patient with DM 1A is 6% and the general population risk is of 0.4%. Genetic risk is estimated in general population with unknown HLA at 0.3%, for identical twins 50%, for heterozygote for HLA DR3/4, DQ2/8 in general population 6%, for identical twins 70%, for sibling 20%. Twins and family studies have demonstrated that DM type 1 family clustering depends from DM onset age and sex of affected parent and has a 20 times higher recurrence risk ratio (regarding normal population) in sibling. Some other important genetic associations between DM 1A and other polymorphic markers as class I VNTR marker of the 5'-region of the insulin gene on chromosome 11 have been described (6).

History/Classification

Descriptions of DM symptoms are present since antiquity. Marking events are in 1674, Willis first mentioned the term of sweetness in relationship with diabetes (sweet urine); in 1797, Rollo introduced the low-carbohydrate diet; in 1880, Lanceroux and Bouchardat grouped DM in diabete maigre and diabete gras; in 1889, Minkovsky and Mering established the role of pancreas; in 1893, Langerhans described the islet organization of pancreas; in 1921–1922, together with the development of the concept of endocrine secretion, insulin is discovered and synthesized concomitantly from Banting, Best, Collip, Paulescu, and Macload. After 1922, DM enters in the insulin era treatment beginning with the first animal crystal product to the actual inhalator and synthetic insulin and insulin analogous (IA). Insulin treatment has totally modified the life expectancy of DM 1 patients and leads over time to the actually multidisciplinary complications and treatment

approach. In 1979, the first general institutionalized classification of DM in which the pathologic value of insulin resistance is standed is accepted from ADA (American Diabetes Association), EASD (European Association for the Study of Diabetes), and NIH (National Institutes of Health). The IDDM (insulin-dependent DM) and NON-IDDM (non-insulin-dependent DM) forms of DM became accepted. In 1997, 1999, 2003, and 2006, ADA and EASD expert committee updated the classification by changing to DM type 1 and 2 and created the prediabetes IFG and IGT diagnostic stages (Tables 46.1 and 46.2). Diabetes research was accelerated by the development of molecular biology, biochemistry, and cell biology. Insulin radioimmunoassay (1960), detection of auto-antibodies, discovery of proinsulin and peptide C, and cloning of insulin gene (1970) are only some of the marking events (6).

Diagnostics Criteria

Diagnostics criteria for DM are yearly revised by ADA, EASD, NIH, and WHO. Complete diagnostics of DM1A include DM and autoimmunity criteria as follows: (a) general diagnostics criteria of DM (Table 46.2) (2); (b) serological markers of the autoimmune etiology: the presence of >1 of biochemical-assayed specific antigen auto-antibodies: anti-IA-2 (ICA512) and IA-2 β (phogrin), anti-GAD65 (only GAD65+ are slow progressors), and anti-insulin (appears first in children, false positive in patients who have previously received treatment with insulin) considering the set point values at ≥99th percentile of normal individuals. Intracitoplasmatic antibody (ICA) screening is less used (low specificity and selectivity) (7). Patients with adult late onset of autoimmune DM (LADA) present frequently only anti-GAD65 antibodies (5). (3) Additional serum residual markers of beta-cell destruction: the absence of serum peptide C and proinsulin. Biopsy and histology of the endocrine pancreas (beta-cell islets) are not rutinary necessary for the confirmation of autoimmunity (2).

Laboratory Features

Laboratory features used in DM 1A include a large spectrum of biochemical, serological markers for (a) prediction of DM 1A: serological autoimmune markers, ±insulin secretion dynamics with ICARUS protocol, and ±GTT (glucose tolerance test) (8); (b) diagnostics of DM 1A (Table 46.2) (2); (c) metabolic follow-up (guidelines for adults and children in Tables 46.3 and 46.4) and self-monitoring of blood glucose (10); (d) diagnostics and treatment of acute complication (Table 46.6) (6); and (e) screening and follow-up of chronic complications: DM-specific and autoimmune-specific (Table 46.6)(10).

Prediction (Screening)

The presence of a long prodromal autoimmune activity and of serologic autoimmune markers permit the prediction of autoimmune diabetes. Prediction would be useful for relatives of patients with DM or for vigilance to escape ketoacidotic coma at onset and cerebral edema and death if we would have treatment. Best current predictor is the presence of one of the specific autoimmunity serologic

markers biochemically assayed (auto-antibodies for insulin, GAD65, ICA512) with the set point at ≥99th percentile of normal individuals. Auto-antibodies are present in 80% of DM; 1/300 from general population present >2 antibodies; the number of antibodies is positively correlated with the evolution rate of the autoimmune destruction. The prediction dual-parameter model inglobates concomitant multiple islet auto-antibody detection and insulin secretion dynamics. Identification of adults with autoimmune serologic markers (in particular present are anti-GAD65) through the presumed DM 2 (5–30% of patients thought to have DM type 2 have DM type 1) marked the necessity of early insulin therapy and the underlying autoimmune etiology (8).

Prevention of Beta-Cell Destruction

Prevention of beta-cell destruction at primary (to prevent the development of autoimmunity), secondary (to prevent beta-cell destruction), and tertiary (after the onset of DM or pancreas transplant) levels is an attractive but at times not a large-scale applicable measure regarding the toxicity and side effects of efficient available medical

TABLE 46.3. Metabolic control recommendations for adults with diabetes (10).

Glycemic control	
Hb A1C	<7.0 %[*]
Preprandial capillary plasma glucose adolescents and adults	90–130 mg/dl (5.0–7.2 mmol/l)
Peak postprandial capillary plasma glucose	<180 mg/dl (<10.0 mmol/l)
Blood pressure (TA)	<130/80 mmHg
Lipids	
LDL	<100 mg/dl (<2.6 mmol/l)
Triglycerides	<150 mg/dl (<1.7 mmol/l)
HDL	>40 mg/dl (>1.0 mmol/l)[♂,] >50 mg/dl[♀]

Key concepts in setting glycemic goals:
- A1C is the primary target for glycemic control[*] (Referenced to a non-diabetic range of 4.0–6.0% using a DCCT-based assay)
- Goals should be individualized
- Certain populations (children, pregnant women, and elderly) require special considerations
- More stringent glycemic goals (i.e., a normal A1C, <6%) may further reduce complications at the cost of increased risk of hypoglycemia
- Less intensive glycemic goals may be indicated in patients with severe or frequent hypoglycemia
- Postprandial glucose (at 1–2 h after beginning of the meal)may be targeted if A1C goals are not met despite reaching preprandial glucose goals

TABLE 46.4. Plasma blood glucose and A1C goals for DM for children (10).

Age (years)	Plasma blood glucose goal range (mg/dl)			Rationale
	Before meals	Bedtime/overnight	HbA1C	
Toddlers and preschoolers (0–6)	100–180	110–200	<8.5% (but >7.5%)	High risk and vulnerability to hypoglycemia
School age (6–12)	90–180	100–180	<8%	Risks of hypoglycemia and relatively low risk of complications prior to puberty Developmental and psychological issues
Adolescents and young adults (13–19)	90–130	90–150	<7.5%	

- Blood glucose goals should be higher than those listed above in children with frequent hypoglycemia or hypoglycemia unawareness.
- A lower goal is reasonable based on benefit-risk assessment.

TABLE 46.5. Clinical features at diagnosis of DM1 (6).

$\frac{3}{4}$ onset before 18 years age
Polyuria and thirst, weakness or fatigue, polyphagia with weight loss
Other children-specific symptoms: nocturnal enuresis, growth retardation
Acute complication at diagnosis: diabetic ketoacidosis (mort. 2,5–9%), mortality through cerebral edema especially in children

therapy. None of the prevention trials performed till now [cyclosporine, metrotrexate, nicotinamide (ENDIT), insulin (DPT-1)] has been useful. Immunosuppressive therapies have important side effects. Anti-CD3 mono-clonal antibodies are currently in trials (8, 9).

Clinical Manifestations

Symptoms at diagnostic varies in severity after acuteness of insulin deficiency (Table 46.5). The rate of beta-cell destruction is quite variable, being rapid in some individuals (mainly infants and children) and slow in others (mainly adults). Others have modest fasting hyperglycemia that can rapidly change to severe hyperglycemia and/or ketoacidosis in the presence of infection or other stress. Particularly, adults may retain residual beta-cell function sufficient to prevent ketoacidosis for many years; such individuals eventually become dependent on insulin for survival and are at risk for ketoacidosis. At this latter stage of the disease, there is little or no insulin secretion, as manifested by low or undetectable levels of plasma C-peptide (6).

Acute and Chronic Complications

Acute and chronic complications of DM are summarized in Table 46.6. Acute DM 1-specific complications (diabetic ketoacidosis, hypoglycemia) can appear at any moment along evolution of DM and can be triggered from intercurrent infection, intensive insulin treatment, insufficient treatment, or other pathological conditions. Along the years of evolution, the natural history of diabetes includes long-term complications of distinct organs, especially eyes, kidney, nerve fibers, and blood vessel (micro- and macropathology) with important social, life quality, and morbidity and mortality consequences. The mechanism of these alterations relies on disturbance of carbohydrate, fat and protein metabolism, and toxic accumulation of end products as cause of insulin deficiency and chronic hyperglycemia. As a particularity regarding the characteristic autoimmune active state, DM 1A associates frequently with autoimmune diseases. The immune etiology of diabetes marks an inherited failure in the maintenance of self-tolerance, the presence of DM 1A being a marker of specific HLA alleles; therefore, patients with DM 1A are predisposed to autoimmune diseases. The most important are thyroid autoimmunity, Addison's disease, celiac disease, vitiligo, pernicious anemia, and auto-immune hepatitis – alone or as a part of the autoimmune polyglandular syndrome type 1 and 2 (APS-I and APS-II) (6).

Management

The basic treatment of DM 1 consists in lifelong individualized daily exogenous insulin substitution (dose: 0.5–1.0 UI/kg/24 h) required for survival and prevention of ketosis, balanced with medical nutrition therapy. Physical exercise and control of weight slows the development of complications. All chronic complications necessitate regular follow-up and lifelong treatment. Tight metabolic control through intensificate insulin replacement treatment which consist in prandial rapid (bolus) insulin (minimum three injections daily), a basal lent insulin (1 injection), and correction-dose insulin is today a consensus in DM therapy (10, 11). After an initial slow-down in the development of insulin products with the successful implementation of human recombinant insulin and decrease of insulin allergy and other immune-mediated reactions to pork insulin, today new rapid absorbable insulin analogs (IA) are in development, some of them being already in clinical practice (Table 46.7). Insulin rapid analogous, used as prandial bolus, present the advantage of a rapid action and better control of postprandial glycemia. Insulin long-acting analogos bind to serum albumin and maintain a basal insulin, mimicking better the physiological response. Both types of IA diminished the risk of hypoglycemia. There is no significant improvement in HbA1c using IA but development of chronic complications seems to be diminished by a better control of glycemic peri-prandial variation, phenomena not well described by HbA1c. IA permit patients a greater flexibility in timing of meals, snacks, exercise, but still there is no perfect insulin treatment available. CSII (continuous subcutaneous insulin infusion pumps) using rapid IA are at times also in use (12, 13). The inhalable dry-powder formulation-packaged human recombinant insulin with a pharmacokinetics close to IA recently approved in both the United States and the European Union represents a new attractive non-invasive therapy option (14).

TABLE 46.6. Complications of Diabetes mellitus (6).

Complications of DM 1	Screening/Follow-up	Therapeutic approaches	Special considerations
Acute complications in DM 1A			
• **Diabetic ketoacidosis** (*Hyperglycemic hyperosmolar coma*)	-urine and serum: -high glucose, acidosis, ketones, high osmolality, electrolyte disturbances	Intensive Care Unit (ICU)	-mortality in children at DM onset through cerebral edema -search associated infection, other pathologies
• **Hypoglycemia** (*neuroglicopenia to coma*) (±contrareglatory awareness signs)	-blood glucose <70mg/dl	-in function of severity 15–20 g CH, glucagon, ICU	
Chronic complications:			
• **Ocular disease** Retinopathy: (Microvascular complication) **A.** *Non-proliferativ* (NPR) **B.** *Proliferativ* (PDR) ±*Macular edema* *Severe vision loss and blindness* Cataract Cornea ulcerations, conjunctivitis	-detailed dilated eye examination by ophtalmolog within 3–5 years after the onset ore at puberty (general evaluation is not necessary before 10 years age)	-blood pressure therapy -therapy of nephropathy -photocoagulation	-aspirin (AAS) and aldose reductase inhibitors haven't proved their use in therapy. -established risk factors are nephropathy , high blood pressure, pregnancy, puberty -perspective therapy with inhibitors/ antagonists of growth factors (VEGF, GH, IGF) -DM retinopathy remains the primer cause of blindness in adults
• **Kidney disease:** (Microvascular complication) Intercapilar diffuse or nodular glomerulosclerosis: -*Microalbuminuria*: 30–299 µg/ mg creatinine -*Macroalbuminuria* ≥300 µg/mg creatinine -*arterial hypertension* (HTA) -*Renal failure and dialysis* (ESRD)	-annual screening of patients with diabetes duration of ≥5 years -albuminuria in spot collection (µg/mg creatinine); or 24 h/ time course collection -creatinine clearance (for GFR)	-ACE inhibitors or ARBs (reduce albuminuria, HTA control) -reduction of protein ingestion to 0,8/kg/24 h	-best prediction marker of evolution to ESRD remains persistent (microalbuminuria) in spot collection -nephropathy occurs in 20–40% of patients with DM and is the single leading cause of end stage renal disease (ESRD) -Renal failure is the major cause of mortality in DM 1A.
• **Macrovascular affectation** -*accelerated, systemic atherosclerosis* -*cardiovascular, cerebrovascular, peripheral disease* • **Cardiovascular disease** -*diabetic cardiomiopathy* -*macrovascular, atherosclerotic disease* -*arterial hypertension (HTA)*	-lipoprotein profile -eco Doppler and carotid intimae media thickness -invasive selective investigation/ treatment		-weight control -smoking cessation -low dietary -antiplatelet agents -management of dietary Na -TA≤130/80 mmHg (therapy of choice: ACE inhibitors,angiotensine receptor blockers ARBs), -pharmacological therapy of disliproteinemias -PTCA/stent

-proteinkinase C 1, 2β isoforms selective inhibitors and inhibitors of advanced glycated products are new therapeutic perspectives of diabetic micro- and macrovascular disease

• **Neuropathy (NP)** Generalized symmetric polyNP: *Chronic distal sensor motor DPN (freq.)* *Acute sensory (rare)* *Autonomic (freq.)* orthostatic hypotension, resting tachycardia, loss of sweetness, gastrointestinal (gastroparesis, constipation, diarrhea), urinary bladder atony, impotence, sexual feminine disturbances	-exclusion of other treatable NP - clinical examination -screening 5 years after onset of DM for autonomic NP -yearly screening for NP -organ selective probes for autonomic neuropathy	-inspection/self-care -corticoids (focal, multifocal NP) -midodrine, 9-alfa- fluorohidrocortisone, metoclopramid, -tricyclic drugs anticonvulsants paracetamol with codeine, capsaicin	-autonomic neuropathy should be always treated for symptoms relief

TABLE 46.6. (Continued)

Complications of DM 1	Screening/Follow-up	Therapeutic approaches	Special considerations
Focal and multifocal NP: *Cranial, Truncal, Focal limb,* *Proximal motor* **• Diabetic feet** (vascular and neuropathy mechanism) *-bones and joint deformation,* *osteomielitis* *-foot and leg ulcers, gangrene,* *osteomielitis*		-self-care/medical inspection each 3–6 month -podcare if case	
• Others: Unusual frequent infection Diabetic dermopathy	-recurrent pielonefritis, papillary renal necrosis, necrotizing fasciitis/myositis, cholecystitis emphysematous	-hospitalization	

TABLE 46.7. Pharmacokinetics and bioavaibility of actual used insulin products (12, 13, 14).

	Name and type	Onset	Peak	Duration	Observations	Application form
Rapid-acting Insulin analogs	-aspart, -glulisine -lispro	10–30′	30′–3 h	3–5 h	Absorbed more quickly than short-acting insulin, but effects wear off sooner -permit a rapid control of glycemy -less hypoglycemic events	inj.
Short-acting Insulin	-regular (human)	30–60°	2– 5 h	up to 8 h	Works quickly, but effects doesn't last as long as intermediate-acting insulin	inj.
Intermediate-acting Insulin	-NPH (human)	1–2 h	4–12 h	16–24 h	Starts working later than short-acting insulin, but effects last longer	inj.
Long-acting Insulin analogs	-glargine -detemir	1–5 h	No clear peak	up to 24 h	-takes several hours to work, but provides insulin at a steady level for up to 24 h < nocturnal hypoglycemia's -dismininushed weight gain	inj.
Pre-mixed	Combination of intermediate-acting and short- or rapid-acting insulin					inj.
Inhaled insulin -human rDNA insulin	-exubera	10–20′	30–90′	6 h	-starts working faster than regular injected insulin and lasts as long -short acting insulin -produce transitory decrease of respiratory capacity -pharmacokinetic and absorption depend from airway and pulmonary permeability (1 mg correspond to 3 UI insulin)	inh.

Self-Monitoring, Patients' Education, and Metabolic Follow-up

Self-monitoring, patients' education, and metabolic follow-up are the three basic conditions for the management of a multiple insulin injection regimen in DM type 1. ADA guidelines suggest blood glucose measuring for three or more times a day. Table 46.3 presents a summary of goals for the principal laboratory parameters used as metabolic markers (10). Treatment programs should take into consideration age, sex, school or work, cultural factors, and presence of complications. Glycemic control is best judged by combination of the patient's self-testing results (as performed) and the current HbA1C result (HbA1C should be measured: 2/year in stable glycemic control and 4/year in therapy changes) (10, 15).

Treatment Monitoring in Children and Adolescents

As the incidence of DM is increasing and the majority (3/4) of DM 1A patients are diagnosticated before 18 years, there is a need to adapt ADA adult therapy goal criteria taking into account the different age-related

physical and social aspects as risk of hypoglycemia
because of increased insulin sensitivity, theoretical
absence of complications before puberty, physical and
psychical growth, neurological vulnerability and inability to provide complete self-care and family dynamics,
and physiologic differences related to sexual maturity
(Table 46.4). A flexible therapy, with smaller hypogly-
cemic risk and less weight gain as permitted from IA or
CSII using rapid-acting IA, seems to better satisfy this
particular metabolic needs. A special attention should
be given to the correct diagnostics of the potential
associated autoimmune celiac disease which can be a
cause of growth retardation in apparently well-treated
DM children (10).

Complication/Adverse Effects of Insulin Therapy

All insulin users should carry medical identification.
Insulin pens facilitate the multi-injection treatment.
Hypoglycemia and weight gain, classic side effects, less
frequent for IA and maybe for inhalator insulin, are still
the most common complication of a tight metabolic
control (12, 16). Other side effects regarding insulin purity and immunogenicity are decreasing. Inhalator human
insulin seems to present an unexpected production of
auto-antibodies and determines a transitory reduction
of pulmonary capacity. CSII potential complications
remain ketosis episodes from pump malfunction, infections, or inflammation at the needle site. Good weight
control and metabolic control were reported by adding
Metformin to insulin substitution (10).

New Therapy Perspectives

New Therapy Perspectives consist in the replacement (substitution) of beta cells by pancreas, islet, and finally stem
cell therapy.

Pancreas/islet transplant/stem cell therapy

The pancreas transplant may be done excepting a very
good defined patient subcategory simultaneous to, or
subsequent to, a kidney transplant (17). Pancreatic islet
cell transplants despite significant potential advantages
over whole-gland transplants remain a procedure performed only within the setting of controlled research
studies (18). New no-corticoid systemic immunosuppressant regimens with fewer side effects are in study. Stem
cell therapy remains an important future goal therapy in
pancreas substitution: recently, encouraging results have
been obtained with an autologous non-myeloablative

hematopoietic stem cell transplantation (AHST) protocol
in newly diagnosed type 1 DM (19).

Global Immunosuppressant Protocols

Global immunosuppressant protocols of the types used for
transplant recipients clearly carry an unacceptable morbidity. Immunologists caring for patients with autoimmune diseases have a need to establish organ-specific
immunological tolerance that is just as pressing as that
facing transplant surgeons. The lack of surrogate markers
for the desired therapeutic T-cell effects complicates interpretation. Trials with non-Fc-binding anti-CD3 monoclonal antibodies and concomitant antigenic immunization
with promising results in animals are in course for primary
and secondary prevention before complete destruction of
beta cells (20).

References

1. Wilkin TJ. The accelerator hypothesis: Weight gain as the missing link between Type I and Type II diabetes. *Diabetologia* 2001; 44(7): 914–22.
2. American Diabetes Association. Report of the Expert Comittee on the Diagnosis and Classification of Diabetes Mellitus. *Diabetes Care* 1997; 20: 1183–1197, and *Diabetes Care* 2003; 26: 3160–7.
3. Gianani R, Eisenbarth GS. The stages of type 1A diabetes. *Immunol Rev.* 2005; 04: 232–49.
4. Nicoletti F, Conget I, Di Marco R, Mazzarino MC, Bendtzen K, Messina A, Gomis R. Serum concentrations of the interferon-gamma-inducible chemokine IP-10/CXCL10 are augmented in both newly diagnosed Type I diabetes mel patients and subjects at risk of developing the disease. *Diabetologia* 2002; 45: 1107–10.
5. Aguilera E, Casamitjana R, Ercilla G, Oriola J, Gomis R, Conget I. Adult-onset atypical (type 1) diabetes: Additional insights and differences with type 1A diabetes in a European Mediterranean population. *Diabetes Care* 2004; 27: 1108–14.
6. Barnett MD, Krall LP. The history of Diabetes; Warram JH, Krolewski AS. Epidemiology of Diabetes mellitus; Reijonen H, Concannon P. Genetics of Type 1 Diabetes; Diabetic com-plications, clinical aspects; Eisenbarth GS. Type 1 Diabetes Mellitus in 14th edition of *Joslin's Diabetes Mellitus* ed. By Kahn RC., Weir GC, King GL, Jacobson AM, Moses AC, Smith RJ, 2005.
7. Wasserfall CH, Atkinson MA. Autoantibody markers for the diagnosis and prediction of type 1 diabetes. *Autoimmun Rev* 2006; 5(6): 424–8.
8. Skyler JS. Prediction and prevention of type 1 diabetes: pro-gress, problems, and prospects. (Rev). *Clin Pharmacol Ther* 2007; 81(5): 768–71.
9. Flores L, Naf S, Hernaez R, Conget I, Gomis R, Esmatjes E. Transforming growth factor beta at clinical onset of Type 1 diabetes mellitus. Is there a case for pharmacologic interven-tion? A pilot study. *Diabet Med* 2004; 21: 818–22.
10. American Diabetes Association. Standars of medical care in Diabetes-2007. *Diabetes Care* 2007; 30(Suppl. 1); Care of

children and adolescents with type 1 diabetes: A statement of the American Diabetes Association. *Diabetes Care* 2005; 28: 186–212.

11. Gomis R, Page SR. New emergent concepts in type 1 diabetes mellitus, The Year in Diabetes. ed by *Clinical Publishing Services* 2003: 119–65.

12. Hirsch I B. Insulin analougues (Rev). *MD N engl J Med* 2005; 352: 174–83.

13. Gomis R, Storms F, Conget I, Sinnassamy P, Davies M, on behalf of the AT. Lantus Study Group. Improving metabolic control in suboptimally controlled subjects with type 1 diabetes: Comparasion of two treatment algorithms using insulin glarigine. *Diabetes Res Clin Pract* 2007; 77: 84–91.

14. Skyler JS, Jovanovic L, Klioze S, Reis J, Duggan W, Inhaled Human Insulin Type 1 Diabetes Study Group. Two-year safety and efficacy of inhaled human insulin (Exubera) in adult patients with type 1 diabetes. *Diabetes Care* 2007; 30(3): 579–85.

15. Jansa M, Vidal M, Viaplana J, Levy I, Conget I, Gomis R, Esmatjes E. Telecare in a structured therapeutic education programme addressed to patients with type 1 diabetes and poor metabolic control. *Diabetes Res Clin Pract* 2006; 74(1): 26–32.

16. Gomis R, Esmatjes E. Asymptomatic hypoglicemia: Identification and impact. *Diabetes Metab Res (Rev)* 2004; 20(Suppl. 2): S47–9.

17. Smets YF, Westendorp RG, van der Pijl JW, de Charro FT, Ringers J, de Fijter JW, Lemkes HH. Effect of simultaneous pancreas-kidney transplantation on mortality of patients with type-1 diabetes mellitus and end-stage renal failure. *Lancet* 1999; 5; 353(9168): 1915–9.

18. Conget I, Piquer S, Julia M, Gomis R, Esmatjes E, Garcia-Pagan JC, Bosch J, Gilabert R, Ricart MJ, Fernandez-Cruz L, Manyalich M. Feasibility and safety of pancreatic islet transplantation in the liver by portal vein catheterization using the transjugular route. *Transplantation* 2006; 81: 1220–1.

19. Voltarelli JC, Couri CE, Stracieri AB, Oliveira MC, Moraes DA, Pieroni F, Coutinho M, Malmegrim KC, Foss-Freitas MC, Simões BP, Foss MC, Squiers E, Burt RK. Autologous nonmyeloablative hematopoietic stem cell transplantation in newly diagnosed type 1 diabetes mellitus. *JAMA* 2007; 297(14): 1568–76.

20. Bresson D, von Herrath M. Moving towards efficient therapies in type 1 diabetes: To combine or not to combine? *Autoimmun Rev* 2007; 6(5): 315–22.

47

Autoimmune Addison Disease or Autoimmune Adrenalitis

Jozélio Freire de Carvalho and Rodrigo Antonio Brandão Neto

Abstract   Autoimmune adrenalitis is the most common cause of adrenal failure in developed countries, accounting for about 70% of the cases, characterized by primary adrenal failure and circulating antibodies against enzymes of adrenal cortex. The clinical manifestations are similar to other causes of Addison disease and adrenal glands are usually small and atrophic. This chapter discusses the clinical manifestations, pathology, diagnosis, and treatment of this condition and proposes a diagnostic criteria for the disease.

Keywords   Addison disease · adrenal · adrenal insufficiency · diagnostic criteria · adrenalitis

Epidemiology

Addison disease is a rare disorder; however, it is more common now than how it was 30 years ago because its prevalence in the general population has increased three times since 1970 (1). Male patients are affected with isolated AAD predominately (70%) during the first two decades of life; there is no predominance during the third decade, and thereafter a female preponderance (81%). The female gender is also more frequently affected, when AAD is part of the clinical picture of polyglandular autoimmune syndrome (70%) (2). Primary adrenal insufficiency is clinically evident in 1 in 8000 individuals in Western countries (3, 4) and AAD is the most common cause in these countries, accounting for 68–94% of cases in different studies (1), but the real prevalence of the disease is unknown. A survey of patients with Addison's disease and who are members of the National Adrenal Disease Foundation revealed that 60% had sought the medical attention of two or more physicians before the correct diagnosis was ever made (5). No statistics is available on the number of undiagnosed patients succumbing to adrenal insufficiency.

Pathogenesis

Humoral and cellular immunities play a role in the pathogenesis of AAD. The role of autoantibodies is described in a later section. On cellular immunity, decreased suppressor T-cell function and increased number of circulating Ia-positive T cells have been described in AAD patients (6). With regard to genetic susceptibility, an association with HLA B8, DR3, and DR4 alleles has been observed, except in cases of polyglandular syndrome, in which no specific HLA association has been found (7).

Clinical Manifestations

The symptoms and signs of adrenal insufficiency depend upon the rate and extent of loss of adrenal function. In the acute scenario, nausea, vomiting, anorexia, abdominal pain, fever, weakness, fatigue, lethargy, confusion, and coma may appear. Shock not responsive to volume and vasoconstrictor agents is a typical finding. In the case of chronic disease, the usual complaints center on weakness, fatigue, and weight loss. There are frequent gastrointestinal problems such as nausea and severe abdominal pain, possibly related to loss of gut motility. Dizziness is also a frequent complaint and appears when patients are standing; patients may present with darkening of the skin, hair, and nails, but the symptoms could be so vague that the patient may survive without diagnosis for many years until a minor infection leads to cardiovascular collapse (8). The major findings of the disease are described in Table 47.1.

From: Y. Shoenfeld et al. (eds.): *Diagnostic Criteria in Autoimmune Diseases*, DOI: 10.1007/978-1-60327-285-8_47,
© 2008 Humana Press, Totowa, NJ

TABLE 47.1. Clinical manifestations of Addison disease.

Symptoms	Frequency
Weakness and fatigue	95–100%
Anorexia	95–100%
Loss of weight	95–100%
Dehydration	80%
Hypotension and tachycardia	88–94%
Abdominal pain or cramps	31%
Nausea, vomiting	75–86%
Diarrhea	16%
Salt craving	16%
Postural symptoms	15%
Skin or mucosal hyperpigmentation	90–94%
Listlessness	90%
Amenorrhea and reduced libido	(frequency not reported in most series)

Pathological Features

The adrenal glands are usually small, in contrast to larger volumes observed in tuberculosis or neoplasias. Histopathology reveals a widespread mononuclear cell infiltrate with lymphocytes, plasma cells, and macrophages during active phase. The normal three-layer histological structure is not more distinguishable, and there is peliomorphism and necrosis of the adrenocortical cells. Subsequently, fibrous tissue can replace the cortex. Adrenal insufficiency manifestations appear only after at least 90% of the cortex has been destroyed (9).

Laboratory Features

Table 47.2 summarizes the laboratory findings in AAD. Levels of cortisol, measured between 8 and 9 am, <3 µg/dL confirm the diagnosis of adrenal insufficiency. On the contrary, levels >19 µg/dL exclude this diagnosis. Levels between 3 and 19 µg/dL require additional tests. Alternatively, a short ACTH stimulation test can be performed using intravenous 250 µg of synthetic ACTH. If after 30 or

TABLE 47.2. Laboratory and image findings in Addison disease.

Hypoglycemia
Hyponatremia
Hyperkalemia
Increasing of BUN and creatinine
Hypercalcemia
Mild acidosis
Normocytic and normochromic anemia
Neutropenia, lymphocytosis, and eosinophilia
Low cortisol levels
High ACTH levels
Computed tomography or magnetic resonance image with drenal alterations

60 min of this injection there is an increase in serum cortisol level to a peak <18 µg/dL (500 nmol/L), the diagnosis of adrenal insufficiency is established (Table 47.3).

Autoantibodies

For many years, the best marker for identifying AAD has been high titers of cortex adrenal cortex autoantibodies (ACAs), detected by indirect immunofluorescence on cryostatic sections of adrenal glands (1). These antibodies bind all three zones of the adrenal cortex. Low titers of ACA have been described in unequivocal post tuberculosis adrenalitis. More recently, the identification of the enzyme steroid-21-hydroxylase as the antigen allowed the development of highly sensitive and specific radiobinding assays for steroid-21-hydroxylase (CYP21A2 or P450c21) autoantibodies detection (10) The antigen targets are the steroidogenic enzymes: P450scc (CYP11A1, side-chain cleavage enzyme), P450c17 (CYP17, 17-alpha-hydroxylase), and P450c21 (CYP21A2, 21-hydroxylase). These antibodies may be present in 80% of the cases (1). Anti-adrenal antibodies are more common in women and in patients with autoimmune disorders who have these autoantibodies develop adrenal insufficiency at a rate of up to 19% per year (11). In fact, the presence of ACA in polyglandular autoimmune syndrome type 1 patients has a predictive value for the development of adrenal insufficiency of 92% in this population.

Diagnostic Criteria

First, it is necessary to diagnose adrenal insufficiency (Table 47.3).

The second step is to define the autoimmune nature of this process; however, there are no diagnostic criteria available. We therefore suggest in this chapter some elements that can lead to AAD diagnosis. The main point in the differential diagnosis is to exclude secondary conditions that can cause adrenal insufficiency, such as tuberculosis, HIV, drugs, and genetic disorders. After excluding these conditions, it is important to have an image of adrenal glands; the finding of an enlarged gland makes the autoimmune process less probable. On the contrary, the presence of autoantibodies to adrenal tissue or against steroid enzymes practically confirms the diagnosis of autoimmune adrenal insufficiency. Alternatively, in the absence of these antibodies and with concomitant autoimmune conditions, the probable diagnosis can also be supported (Table 47.3).

TABLE 47.3. Proposed diagnostic criteria for autoimmune Addison disease.

1. Basal cortisol <3 μg/dL (83 nmol/L) and/or ACTH >100 pg/mL (22 pmol/L), at 8 to 9 am
   or
   Serum cortisol is less than 18 mcg/dL (500 nmol/L) after 30 or 60 min of intravenous injection of 250 μg of synthetic ACTH
2. Normal or reduced adrenal gland volume on computed tomography (CT) and magnetic resonance image (MRI) and absence of calcifications on abdominal X-ray or CT.
3. Anti-cortex adrenal antibodies or high titers of anti-21-hydroxylase antibodies
4. Exclusion of other causes of primary adrenal insufficiency: genetic (clinical signs or symptoms: achalasia, alacrimia, deafness, or hypogonadotropic hypogonadism in males or genotyping); adrenoleukodystrophy (levels of very long-chain fatty acids within normal range); infectious diseases (tuberculosis, paracoccidiomycosis, histoplasmosis, HIV, CMV); drugs (mitotane, ketoconazoles, rifampin, etc); adrenal hemorrhage or thrombosis; neoplasias; infiltrative (sarcoidosis, amyloidosis, hemochromatosis).
5. Other(s) concomitant autoimmune condition(s) (Hashimoto thyroiditis, pernicious anemia, rheumatological autoimmune disease, autoimmune hemocytopenia, and others)

Definitive diagnosis 1, 2, 3, and 4
Probable diagnosis 1, 2, 4, and 5

Differential Diagnosis

There are some conditions that may mimic adrenal insufficiency shock such as sepsis, hypovolemia cardiogenic shock, exogenous intoxication, hyperkalemia from renal failure, and abdominal pain from porphyria. Malignancy is an important differential diagnosis for those presenting with gastrointestinal complaints and weight loss. Clinical conditions that induce hyperpigmentation (antimalarial, antineoplastic, tetracyclines, phenothiazines, zidovudine, hemochromatosis, porphyria cutanea tarda, heavy metals) should be also excluded. About 50% of the patients have isolated autoimmune adrenal failure; the rest present an autoimmune polyendocrinopathy (APS) including adrenal failure (5). This syndrome has two forms, namely types I and II. APS-1 is defined by the presence of three principle components of the disease: chronic mucocutaneous candidiasis or moniliasis, acquired hypoparathyroidism, and autoimmune Addison disease positive Addison disease. APS-2 is defined by autoimmune Addison disease together with autoimmune thyroid disease (Schmidt syndrome) and/or IMD (Carpenter syndrome)

Prognosis

The survival of patients adequately diagnosed and treated is the same as the normal population. Before steroid replacement, the survival rate was usually 2 years or less.

Treatment

The standard initial therapy is replacement with corticosteroids. During an acute crisis, therapy should not be delayed owing to performing diagnostic studies or awaiting laboratories results. Hydrocortisone, 100 mg intravenous every 6 hours for 24 hours, should be given for all patients with strong clinical suspicions of AAD, associated with physiological saline (1 L in the first hour is appropriated in most cases). After cardiovascular stabilization, the hydrocortisone dose should be reduced to 50 mg every 6 h and subsequently tapered to oral maintenance in 4–5 days. In case of complications of persistence, maintain or increase dose to 200 to 400 mg/day. The correction of hem dynamical and metabolic disturbances with large volumes of intravenous saline and glucose is mandatory. Looking for precipitating factors is recommended, particularly infections.

The glucocorticoid chronic replacement is usually given in two to three doses, with a half to two-thirds of the dose in the early morning in order to mimic the physiologic secretion pattern. Studies indicate that the daily cortisol secretion is between 5 and 10 mg/m² (12, 13). It is equivalent to the oral administration of 15–25 mg of hydrocortisone or 25–37.5 mg of cortisone acetate. Mineralocorticoid replacement is done using accomplished with fluorohydrocortisone (florinef, 0.05–0.2 mg daily). Hypertension, bradycardia, suppressed renin levels, and retardation in growth rate are clinical signs of over-treatment with mineralocorticoids; this reposition is usually not necessary when high doses of cortisol are used. However it should be given if a synthetic glucocorticoid (prednisolone or dexamethasone) is used and when the cortisol dose has been tapered to near-maintenance levels. Weight, blood pressure, and electrolytes should be checked periodically.

"Education about the disease, use of personal card or bracelet/necklace containing the diagnosis are strongly recommended for all patients with adrenal insufficiency. Additionally, in stress periods…" to increase cortisol dosage are strongly recommended for all patients, patients who are to undergo surgery also need to adjust the glucocorticoid dose. For major surgeries, administration of intravenous hydrocortisone 100 mg/m² per day is necessary for 24 h perioperatively and postoperatively, before tapering over several days to a maintenance dose (5). Patients should also learn when and how to inject dexamethasone during emergencies.

References

1. Betterle C, Dal Pra C, MAntero F, Zanchetta R. Autoimmune adrenal insufficiency and autoimmune polyendocrine syndromes: Autoantibodies, autoantigens, and their applicability in diagnosis and disease prediction. *Endocr Rev* 2002; 23: 327–64.

2. Spinner MW, Blizzard RM, Childs B. Clinical and genetic heterogeneity in idiopathic Addison's disease and hyperparathyroidism. *J Clin Endocrinol Metab* 1968; 28: 795.

3. Kong MF, Jeffcoate W. Eighty-six cases of Addison's disease. *Clin Endocrinol (Oxf)* 1994; 41: 757–61.

4. Lovas K, Husbye ES. High prevalence and increasing incidence of Addison's disease in western Norway. *Clin Endocrinol* 2002; 56: 787–91.

5. Ten S, New M, Maclaren N. Clinical Review 130: Addison's Disease. *J Clin Endocrinol Metab* 2001; 86: 2909–22.

6. Rabinowe SL, Jackson RA, Dluhy RG, Williams GH. Ia-positive T lymphocytes in recently diagnosed idiopathic Addison's disease. *Am J Med* 1984; 77: 597.

7. Farid NR, Bear JC. The human major histocompatibility complex and endocrine disease. *Endocr Rev* 1981; 2: 50.

8. Stewart PM. The adrenal cortex. *In*: Larsen PR, Kronenber HM, Melmed S, Polonsky KS, editors. William's textbook of endocrinology. 10th ed. Saunders: Philadelphia; 2002. p. 491–551.

9. Betterle C, Scalici C, Presotto F, et al. The natural history of adrenal function in autoimmune patients with adrenal autoantibodies. *J Endocrinol* 1988; 117: 467.

10. Falorni A, Nikoshkov A, LAureti S, Grenbäch E, Hulting AL, Casucci G, Santeusanio F, Brunetti P, Luthman H, Lernmark A. High diagnostic accuracy for idiopathic Addison's disease with a sensitive radiobinding assay for autoantibodies against recombinant human 21-hydroxylase. *J Clin Endocrinol Metab* 1995; 80: 2752–5.

11. Barker NW. The pathologic anatomy in twenty-eight cases of Addison's disease. *Arch Pathol* 1929; 8: 432.

12. Aerlt W, Allolio B. Adrenal Insufficiency. *Lancet* 2003; 361:1881–93.

13. Esteban NV, Loughlin T, Yergei AL et al. Daily cortisol production rate in man determined by stable isotope dilution mass spectrometry. *J Clin Endocrinol Metab* 1991; 72: 39–45.

48
Autoimmune Hypophysitis

Daria La Torre, Alberto Falorni, Elena Bartoloni Bocci and Roberto Gerli

Abstract   Autoimmmune hypophysitis (AH) is due to an immune-mediated inflammation of the pituitary gland. The tissue damage proceeds through different stages: the initial pituitary enlargement, secondary to infiltration and oedema, can evolve to remission for spontaneous or pharmacological resolution of the inflammation, or evolve to progressive diffuse destruction with gland atrophy for fibrotic replacement, thus leading to various degrees of pituitary dysfunction.

The autoimmune process against the pituitary gland is made evident by the appearance of circulating anti-pituitary autoantibodies (APAs), mainly detected by indirect immunofluorescence on cryostatic sections of human or primate pituitary. Among the target autoantigens recognized by APA are alpha-enolase, gamma-enolase, and the pituitary gland-specific factors (PGSFs) 1a and 1b. However, the low diagnostic sensitivity and specificity of APA for AH strongly limits the clinical use of this marker.

Despite its low incidence, AH should be considered in the differential diagnosis of non-secreting space-occupying lesions of sella turcica, to avoid misdiagnosis that may lead to an aggressive surgery approach, as endocrine dysfunction and the compressive effect may be transient.

Keywords   Anti-pituitary autoantibodies · lymphocytic hypophysitis · hypopituitarism · hyperprolactinemia

Lymphocytic Hypophysitis (LH) is an inflammatory disorder primarily affecting anterior (Lymphocytic Adenohypophysitis, LAH), posterior (Lymphocytic Infundibuloneurohypophysitis, LINH), or both (Lymphocytic Panhypophysitis, LPH) pituitary lobes. It is commonly referred to as "Autoimmune Hypophysitis" (AH), because its epidemiological, histomorphological, and clinical features are suggestive of an autoimmune pathogenesis. The inflammatory destruction can be self-limiting or can result in permanent endocrine/neurological dysfunction, and even in potentially life-threatening complications.

Epidemiology

AH is rare, although reported with increasing frequency in the past years. The extrapolated incidence on overall population is low, approximately 1 in 9 million/year (1), but probably underestimated. LAH is more common in women and has an established strong association with late pregnancy and postpartum (from 30 to 70% of cases) (1, 2, 3). Mean age is third to fourth decade. No strict female predisposition is reported for LINH and LPH, though a weak female predisposition has been reported for LPH (1).

History

AH was first described in 1962 (4), as post-mortem finding of extensive lymphocytic infiltrate of anterior pituitary in a young woman affected by Hashimoto's thyroiditis, dead for circulatory shock one year after her second delivery. The demonstration of the existence of pituitary autoantibodies was first provided in 1965 (5) in sera from patients with Sheehan's syndrome, by using a complement consumption test. From 1970, several case reports have documented the same histopathological features, though limited to the infundibulum stem and neurohypophyseal tissue, in patients presenting with diabetes insipidus. Although evidence of global glandular involvement has been documented from 1991, to consider LAH and LINH as aspects of the same nosologic entity with a common pathogenesis is challenging, because of their different structural, histological, and ontogenetical characteristics.

From: Y. Shoenfeld et al. (eds.): *Diagnostic Criteria in Autoimmune Diseases*, DOI: 10.1007/978-1-60327-285-8_48,
© 2008 Humana Press, Totowa, NJ

Pathogenesis

The autoimmune process probably targets specific pituitary cell sub-types, with early selective loss of ACTH, FSH/LH, or TSH-secreting cells and subsequent triggering of an unselective destruction of the gland.

On the association with pregnancy, changes in both immunologic system modulation and pituitary volume or its blood supply may play a major role (1).

Clinical Manifestations

Clinical findings can be divided into three groups, as reported in Table 48.1. Their relative frequency varies depending on the involvement of anterior, posterior, or both pituitary lobes. Most patients present with symptoms related to compressive and inflammatory effects of enlarged pituitary on sellar and parasellar structures, as headache, described in >50% of cases at diagnosis (2, 3, 6). Among the symptoms of hypopituitarism, those attributable to hypogonadism and hyperprolactinemia are reported with different frequency (1, 2). With the exception of lactating women, hyperprolactinemia does not occur commonly and may be secondary to stalk compression, impaired dopamine effect for inflammation, immunological destruction of lactotrophs with prolactin (PRL) release, or supposed PRL-secretion stimulating autoantibodies. Symptoms of hypocortisolism are also frequently reported. Symptoms related to diabetes insipidus, reported with an overall frequency that varies from 20 to 48% (2, 3), are constantly present in LINH and LPH, due to direct

Table 48.2. Autoimmune diseases associated with AH.

Disease	Frequency (%)
Hashimoto's thyroiditis	7.4
Autoimmune polyglandular syndrome 2	1.8
Graves' disease	1.6
Systemic lupus erythematosus	1.3
Sjögren's syndrome	0.8
Type 1 diabetes mellitus	0.8
Optic neuritis	0.8
Autoimmune gastritis	0.5
Addison's disease	0.5
Sarcoidosis	0.5
Primary biliary cirrhosis	0.3
Myocarditis	0.3
Temporal arteritis	0.3
Beçhet's disease	0.3
Erythema nodosum	0.3
Rheumatoid arthritis	0.3
Idiopathic thrombocytopenic purpura	0.3

From ref. (1) (adapted)

infundibulo-neurohypophyseal damage, but can also occur in LAH as a consequence of stalk compression and impaired vasopressin transport. The coexistence of other autoimmune diseases (Table 48.2), mainly Hashimoto's thyroiditis, is reported consistently at about 25% of cases.

Pathological Features

Histological examination with immunohistochemistry shows polyclonal lympho-plasmacytic infiltrate with plasma cells, rarely eosinophils and occasionally neutrophils and macrophages; aspects of focal or diffuse destruction of glandular acines and evolution to fibrosis are common (3). More recently, mast-zellen and folliculo-stellate cells, with chemotactic and antigen-presenting role, have been described (1), supporting the role of immune response. Documented neurohypophyseal, infundibular or pituitary stalk tissue involvement is reported with varying frequency ranging from 20 to 62% (1, 2).

Biochemical Features

Partial or complete impairment of one or more hormonal axes is almost invariably present in all cases: more often basal hypocortisolism, reduced gonadotrophins with or without low levels of testosterone and estrogens, and hypothyroidism. A transient hyperthyroidism during the early stage of Hashimoto's thyroiditis is possible. Mono-hormonal deficits are rare and affect, in descending order of frequency: ACTH, FSH-LH, TSH, PRL, and GH (1, 2, 3).

Table 48.1. Clinical manifestations of AH.

	Effects	Symptoms
Pituitary enlargement		
	Distension of dura madre	Headache
	Compression of optic chiasm	Visual field, acuity reduction
	Expansion in cavernous sinus	Cranial nerves palsy (rare)
	Hypocortisolism	Hypotension, hypoglycaemia
Anterior pituitary defects		
	Hypothyroidism	Fatigue, myxedema, bradycardia
	Hypogonadism	Impotence, decreased libido
	Hypoprolactinemia	Impaired lactation
Infundibulum/Posterior pituitary defect		
	Diabetes insipidus	Polyuria, polydipsia
Stalk impairment		
	Hyperprolactinemia	Amenorrhea/galactorrhea

Serological Features

Currently, the most widely used method for detecting anti-pituitary autoantibodies (APA) is indirect immunofluorescence on cryostatic sections of human or primate pituitary. However, the clinical use of this assay type is strongly limited by low diagnostic sensitivity and specificity, APA being detected also in healthy control subjects, in patients with pituitary adenomas, and in patients with endocrine autoimmune diseases with no clinical or imaging signs of lymphocytic hypophysitis. The use of a four-layer immunofluorescence technique has enabled the first demonstration of prolactin cell-specific autoantibodies (7). Subsequently, ACTH cell-specific autoantibodies were also demonstrated, especially in patients with Cushing's disease or isolated ACTH deficiency. In these latter patients, ACTH-cell autoantibodies seem to be directed against aspartil protease (8). GH-secreting cell autoantibodies have been detected in some patients with Turner's syndrome and partial or idiopathic GH deficiency (9), but their role is still controversial. The use of an immunoblotting method has led to the identification of α-enolase as the first pituitary autoantigen recognized by human autoantibodies (10). However, α-enolase is widely expressed in several human tissues and α-enolase autoantibodies have a very low diagnostic specificity for lymphocytic hypophysitis. More recently, enolase has also been recognized as a target of pituitary autoantibodies (11). Interestingly, gamma-enolase is expressed in both the pituitary and the placenta, thus providing a theoretical basis for the strong association between pituitary autoimmunity and pregnancy. Finally, the use of radioligand-binding assays has shown the presence of autoantibodies against GH, pituitary gland-specific factor 1a (PGSF1a), and/or pituitary gland-specific factor 1b (PGSF1b) in 18% of lymphocytic hypophysitis patients with gland enlargement and in 36% of lymphocytic hypophysitis patients with no pituitary enlargement, as well as in 10% of patients with other autoimmune diseases (12). Although the research on pituitary autoantibodies is constantly growing, at present the clinical applicability of these immune markers in the routine diagnosis and management of patients with lymphocytic hypophysitis is limited by a very low diagnostic sensitivity and specificity and by conflicting results generated by different methods.

Diagnostic Criteria

AH should be suspected in females presenting with pituitary enlargement in the peri-partum or with pituitary dysfunction and underlying autoimmunity and in all patients with a rapidly growing pituitary mass. Although definitive diagnosis can be achieved only by histology on trans-

TABLE 48.3. Differential imaging features in AH and pituitary adenoma.

	AH	Adenoma
Pre-contrast mass aspect	Symmetric enlargement	Asymmetric enlargement
Cystic aspect	Rare	Frequent
Anterohypophyseal post-contrast enhancement	Rapid – Uniform Intense	Slow Less intense
Sellar floor	Intact	Depressed – Eroded
Pituitary stalk	Thickened	Displaced

sphenoidal biopsy specimen, non-invasive diagnosis can be putatively assessed by MRI and endocrine deficit pattern. Distinctive radiological characteristics of AH are summarized in Table 48.3. In LAH, the mass, typically isointense in T1-weighted sequences, is shaped as a triangle or dumbbell, and often has a suprasellar extension. In cases presenting with diabetes insipidus, MRI can be negative at first stages. Common features are posterior lobe swelling and stalk thickening (2, 13), associated with loss of neurohypophyseal pre-contrast hyperintensity and alteration of early enhancement pattern, that are probably due to vascular alterations (13). Atrophy with empty sella is not uncommon.

Prognosis

Natural history of AH is unpredictable, from spontaneous recovery with remission of clinical, laboratory, and imaging data (1, 14, 15) to permanent hormonal/neurological impairment or even death, mostly because of adrenal insufficiency. Some authors report recurrence after pharmacological improvement (6, 16), and biochemical and imaging long-term follow-up is recommended. LINH is often self-limiting (13).

Prediction

Pregnancy and occurrence of other autoimmune diseases are the major risk factors for the development of AH, though lymphocytic hypophysitis is extremely rare. Because of the rarity of the condition and the low diagnostic sensitivity and specificity of pituitary autoantibodies, no information is currently available on the predictive value of these markers for AH. In a recent study of patients with idiopathic hyperprolactinemia (17), APA were detected in 26% of cases and a partial anterior pituitary hormone impairment was detected in 35% of APA-positive individuals, which paves the way to future studies aimed at testing the ability of APA in identifying forms of subclinical lymphocytic hypophysitis.

Therapy

Most patients require therapy. Available treatment strategies are symptomatic, aiming at reducing pituitary size. Neurosurgery has been the most common treatment so far (1). It provides a definitive histological diagnosis and promptly relieves compressive symptoms that are the primary indication for surgical approach. It is rarely effective in resolving endocrine dysfunctions, with the exception of hyperprolactinemia-related hypogonadism (2). So far, post-surgical follow-up reports have been short term and have shown both recovery and recurrences (6, 16), with significant incidence of iatrogenic hypopituitarism, especially diabetes insipidus (1, 3, 6). For these reasons, most authors suggest to limit its indications, favouring a more conservative treatment (2, 6). Among pharmacologic therapies, high-dose glucocorticoids are reported both as a first line (e.g. 20–60 mg/d prednisone (16, 18), 120 mg/d methylprednisolone (19)) and as second instance after neurosurgery, effective in reducing pituitary size in 75% of cases (2) and in improving endocrine dysfunction (19). Other reported pharmacological treatments include azathioprine, used in a patient with a recurring, inoperable mass (20), and metothrexate (6, 18). Efficacy of radiotherapy is controversial (1). In conclusion, conservative management could consist of steroidal treatment, monitoring for endocrine status (with possible hormonal replacement and dopaminergic treatment of hyperprolactinemia) and MRI, leaving surgery in case of lack of response and worsening of symptoms.

References

1. Caturegli P, Newschaffer C, Olivi A, Pomper MG, Burger PC, Rose NR. Autoimmune hypophysitis. *Endocr Rev* 2005; 26: 599–614.
2. Gutenberg A, Hans V, Puchner MJA, Kreuzer J, Brück W., Caturegli P., Buchfelder M. Primary hypophysitis: Clinical-pathological correlations. *Eur J Endocrinol* 2006; 155: 101–107.
3. Thodou E, Asa SL, Kontogeorgos G, Kovacs K, Horvath E, Ezzat S. Clinical case seminar: lymphocytic hypophysitis: Clinicopathological findings. *J Clin Endocrinol Metab* 1995; 80: 2302–2311.
4. Goudie RB, Pinkerton PH. Anterior hypophisitis and Hashimoto's disease in a woman. *J Pathol Bacteriol* 1962; 83: 584–585.
5. Engelberth O, Jezkova Z. Autoantibodies in Sheehan's syndrome. *Lancet* 1965; i: 1075.
6. Leung GK, Lopes MB, Thorner MO, Vance ML, Laws ER Jr. Primary Hypophysitis: A single-center experiences in 16 cases. *J Neurosurg* 2004; 101: 286–271.
7. Bottazzo GF, Pouplard A, Florin-Christensen A, Doniach D. Autoantibodies to prolactin-secreting cells of human pituitary. *Lancet* 1975; 2: 97–101.
8. Sauter NP, Toni R, McLaughlin CD, Dyess EM, Kritzman J, Lechan RM. Isolated adrenocorticotropin deficiency associated with an autoantibody to a corticotroph antigen that is not adrenocorticotropin or other proopiomelanocortin-derived peptides. *J Clin Endocrinol Metab* 1990; 70: 1391–1397.
9. Bottazzo GF, McIntosh C, Stanford W, Preece M. Growth hormone cell antibodies and partial growth hormone deficiency in a girl with Turner's syndrome. *Clin Endocrinol* 1980; 12: 1–9.
10. O'Dwyer DT, Smith AI, Matthew ML, Andronicos NM, Ranson M, Robinson PJ et al. Identification of the 49-kDa autoantigen associated with lymphocytic hypophysitis as α-enolase. *J Clin Endocrinol Metab* 2002; 87: 752–757.
11. O'Dwyer DT, Clifton V, Hall A, Smith R, Robinson PJ, Crock PA. Pituitary autoantibodies in lymphocytic hypophysitis target both gamma- and alpha-enolase – a link with pregnancy? *Arch Physiol Biochem* 2002; 110: 94–98.
12. Tanaka S, Tatsumi KI, Takano T, Murakami Y, Takao T, Hashimoto K, Kato Y, Amino N. Detection of autoantibodies against the pituitary – specific proteins in patients with lymphocytic hypophysitis. *Eur J Endocrinol.* 2002; 147: 767–775.
13. Imura H, Nakao K, Shimatsu A, Ogawa Y, Sando T, Fujisawa I, Yamabe H. Lymphocytic infundibuloneurohypophysitis as a case of central diabetes insipidus. *N Engl L Med* 1993; 329: 683–689.
14. Gagneja H, Arafah B, Taylor HC. Histologically proven lymphocytic hypophysitis: Spontaneous resolution and subsequent pregnancy. *Mayo Clin Proc* 1999; 74: 548–552.
15. Bevan JS, Othman S, Lazarus JH, Parkes AB, Hall R. Reversible adrenocorticotropin deficiency due to probable autoimmune hypophysitis in a woman with post-partum thyroiditis. *J Clin Endocrinol Metab* 1992; 74: 548–552.
16. Nishioka H, Ito H, Fukushima C. Recurrent lymphocytic hypophysitis: case report. *Neurosugery* 1997; 41: 684–686.
17. De Bellis A, Colao A, Pivonello R, Savoia A, Battaglia M, Ruocco G, Tirelli G, Lombardi G, Bellastella A, Bizzarro A. Antipituitary antibodies in idiopathic hyperprolactinemic patients. *Ann N Y Acad Sci.* 2007; 1107: 129–135.
18. Tubridy N, Saunders D, Thom M, Asa SL, Powell M, Plant GT, Howard R. Infundibulohypophysitis in a man presenting with diabetes insipidus cavernous sinus involvement. *J Neurol Neurosurg Psychiatr* 2001; 71: 798–801.
19. Kristof RA, Van Roost D, Klingmüller D, Springer W, Schramm J. Lymphocytic hypophysitis: non-invasive diagnosis and treatment by high dose methylprednisolone pulse therapy? *J Neurol Neurosurg Psychiatr* 1999; 67: 398–402.
20. Lecube A, Francisco G, Roderiguez D, Ortega A, Codina A, Hernandez C, Simo R. Lymphocytic hypophysitis successfully treated with azathioprine: first case report. *J Neurol Neurosurg Psychiatr* 2003; 74: 1581–1583.

49
Autoimmune Parathyroid Disease

Corrado Betterle

Abstract   The chapter takes into consideration the clinical manifestations, genetic patterns, histopathology, animal models, cellular immunity, circulating autoantibodies, target autoantigens, laboratory diagnostic criteria, and the therapy of the autoimmune parathyroid diseases. Much of these data satisfy the criteria for autoimmune diseases.

The mechanism of damage of the parathyroid glands in autoimmune parathyroid diseases may be related to a cell-mediated immune response against parathyroid antigens. Ca-SRAbs appear to be serological markers of the disease; however, the possible effect of the autoantibodies on the Ca-SR activity needs to be confirmed.

Keywords   Chronic hypoparathyroidism · normocalciuric hyperparathyroidism · calcium sensing receptor antibodies · autoimmune polyglandular syndromes · experimental parathyroiditis

Anatomy and Physiology of Parathyroid

The parathyroid glands (usually four glands) are located behind the thyroid gland and contain chief and oxypil cells. The chief cells produce the parathyroid hormone (PTH), which controls the homeostasis of the calcium and phosphate concentration of the extracellular fluids and expresses on the cell surface the calcium sensing receptor (Ca-SR), a member of the G-protein-coupled receptor family consisting of 1085 amino acids (AA) (1). The Ca-SR is involved in detecting variations in ionized calcium serum concentrations and modulation of the production of PTH. Secretion of PTH is inversely correlated to the serum concentration of ionized calcium. PTH itself has the effects (a) on bone—it regulates calcium exchange at osteocytic sites and enhances osteoclast-mediated bone reabsorption; (b) on distal tubules of the kidney—it increases the reabsorption of calcium, decreases the reabsorption of phosphate and stimulates the conversion of 25-hydroxyvitamin D to its active metabolite, 1,25-dihydroxyvitamin D (calcitriol). Calcitrol is important for enhancing calcium bone reabsorption and absorption of dietary calcium. The combined actions of PTH and calcitriol on target tissues regulate the serum levels of calcium and phosphate (1).

Definition, Classification, and Epidemiology of Hypoparathyroidism

The term "hypoparathyroidism" describes a group of disorders characterized by hypocalcemia and hyperphosphatemia resulting from either the destruction of the parathyroid glands and low levels of PTH or an inability of PTH to act on target tissues and high PTH levels (1). Table 49.1 summarizes the main causes of hypoparathyroidism. Spontaneous hypoparathyroidism due to genetic, infiltrative, or autoimmune diseases is very rare, and the most frequent cause of acquired hypoparathyroidism is due to complications of thyroid surgery.

Parathyroid Autoimmune Disease

The original criteria for defining autoimmune diseases proposed in 1957 included: (a) demonstration of serum autoantibodies, (b) demonstration of lymphoplasmacellular infiltration in the target organs, (c) inducing the disease experimentally by immunization with autoantigens or passive transfer of the disease by serum or lymphocytes (2).

Autoimmune parathyroid disease is a chronic inflammatory disorder of parathyroid glands which usually is manifested as chronic hypoparathyroidism (CHP), although presentation in a form of hyperparathyroidism has been

From: Y. Shoenfeld et al. (eds.): *Diagnostic Criteria in Autoimmune Diseases*, DOI: 10.1007/978-1-60327-285-8_49,
© 2008 Humana Press, Totowa, NJ

TABLE 49.1. Causes of hypoparathyroidism.

1. Surgery	• Complications of the neck surgery (most commonly thyroid surgery)
2. Radiation of the neck	• For lymphomas or ^{131}I therapy for thyroid diseases
3. Infiltrative processes	• Wilson's disease
	• Hemochromatosis
	• Thalassemia
	• Amyloidosis
	• Cancers
	• Granulomatous diseases
4. Autoimmunity	• Isolated
	• Associated with type 1 autoimmune polyglandular syndrome (type 1 APS)
	• Associated with other autoimmune diseases
5. Genetic (Idiopathic)	• Autosomal recessive
	• X-linked
	• Barakat's syndrome
6. Embryologic defects	• Di George's syndrome
	• Parathyroid agenesis
7. Defective production of PTH	• Hypomagnesiemia
	• Hypermagnesiemia
	• Alcohol
	• Maternal hypercalcemia
8. Resistance to PTH	• Type 1a,b,c pseudohypoparathyroidism

recently described (see later). Features of autoimmune parathyroid disease and analysis of published studies are reviewed in this chapter.

Animal Models

It has been observed that rats immunized with parathyroid tissue in Freund's adjuvant developed parathyroid atrophy, with disaggregation of the parathyroid glands followed by hypoparathyroidism, although parathyroid autoantibodies were not detectable (3).

A spontaneous acquired hypoparathyroidism was described in dogs; Saint Bernard, Cross-bred, German Shepherd, and Terrier breeds were the most commonly affected. The pathogenesis of primary hypoparathyroidism in dogs is not clear but the presence of lymphocytic infiltration and parathyroid gland atrophy suggest an autoimmune background (4).

In non-obese diabetic (NOD) mouse developing type 1 diabetes mellitus, infiltration of parathyroid glands with lymphocytes of helper/inducer phenotype was sometimes observed (5).

However, to date, an experimental animal model of autoimmune CHP has not been yet developed.

Histopathology

The few studies of parathyroid glands obtained at autopsy from patients with CHP (either isolated or associated with type 1 APS) show parathyroid atrophy with mononuclear cell infiltration, but in many cases parathyroid tissue was undetectable (6). Recently, a form of CHP associated with the presence of autoantibodies to the Ca-SR (Ca-SRAbs)

that were able to mimic calcium and inhibit PTH production in normal parathyroid tissue was also described (7). Furthermore, patients with hypocalciuric hypercalcemia associated with the presence of Ca-SRAbs that inhibit the function of Ca-SR and induce production of PTH together with parathyroid lymphocytic infiltration have been reported (8). But these reports refer to a relatively small number of cases.

Cellular Immunity

Peripheral blood lymphocyte subset phenotypes in patients with adult-onset CHP show significantly higher prevalence of CD4 (helper T cells), CD29/CD4 (inducer of helper T cells), CD16 and CD56 (natural killer cells), and CD3/DR (activated T cells) compared with lymphocyte subsets found in normal controls (9). In two of the patients, the mitogenic response of peripheral lymphocytes to parathyroid cell membranes was also studied, but proliferation response was not observed. To date, there is no available information on the phenotype of lymphocytes infiltrating the parathyroid tissue in CHP.

Parathyroid Autoantibodies

The history of parathyroid autoantibodies is very complex and the data from 1966–1986 were reviewed by Betterle in 2006 (10). Parathyroid autoantibodies were first found by Blizzard in 1966 using indirect immunofluorescence (IIF) on human parathyroid adenoma or normal tissue sections in 38% of the patients with CHP, mostly those affected by type 1 APS; in 26% of CHP patients with autoimmune Addison's disease; in 12% of CHP patients with Hashimoto's thyroiditis, and in 6% of controls. However, the parathyroid cells involved were not specified.

Furthermore, autoantibodies reacting with both oxyphil and chief cells were found by Irvine in 1969 using IIF in 11% of the patients with CHP and in 11% of the controls, and this reactivity was not absorbed by rat liver extracts.

In 1985, it was revealed by Swana that the parathyroid antibodies detected using IIF were reactive with human mitochondria present in the oxyphil cells and the antigen identified by Betterle with a 46-kDa molecular weight.

Autoantibodies reacting with the surface of human parathyroid cells (or parathyroid sections) by IIF and able to inhibit PTH secretion were reported in patients with CHP in 1986. These autoantibodies were able to mediate a complement-dependent cytotoxity in cultured bovine parathyroid cells, but they lost their reactivity after absorption with parathyroid endothelial cells.

In 1996, Li et al. (11) identified autoantibodies against a human parathyroid membrane-antigen of 120–140kDa molecular weight (the size of the Ca-SR) by immunoblot in 5 of 25 patients (20%) with CHP (2 of 17 = 12% of type 1 APS and 3 of 8 = 37.5% of CHP associated with chronic thyroiditis) and reported to be specific for Ca-SR

(Ca-SRAbs). In immunoblotting analysis using a membrane fraction of HEK-293 cells expressing the recombinant human Ca-SR, Ca-SRAbs, were found in 8 of 25 (32%) patients with CHP (3 of 17 = 17.6% type 1 APS and 5 of 8 = 62.5% CHP associated with thyroiditis) (11). The higher prevalence of Ca-SrAbs found with the second method might have been related to overexpression of the Ca-SR in HEK-293 cells. In order to identify the autoepitopes involved, two fragments of the Ca-SR cDNA coding for the extracellular or the intracellular parts were transcribed and translated in vitro and the sera of 14 of 25 (56%) patients with CHP (6 of 17 = 35% with type 1 APS and 8 of 8 = 100% with chronic thyroiditis) immunoprecipitated the extracellular domain of the Ca-SR. In contrast, no reactivity with the extracellular or intracellular domain of the receptor was found with the sera from patients with other autoimmune diseases or from the normal controls (11).

Subsequently, using Western blotting analysis and preparations of parathyroid adenomas, Ca-SRAbs were found in 25 of 51 patients (49%) with CHP (45 with isolated CHP and 6 with CHP associated with chronic thyroiditis, or type 1 diabetes mellitus, or alopecia). However, the Ca-SRAbs were also found in 13% of the normal controls in the same study (12).

In a different study, using recombinant extracellular domain of the human Ca-SR in an immunoblotting assay, Ca-SRAbs were found in 7 of 31 (23%) patients with CHP (6 of 17 isolated = 35%, 1 of 6 type 1 APS = 17%, 0 of 8 with other autoimmune diseases) (13).

In contrast, in an immunoprecipitation assay using ^{35}S-labelled recombinant Ca-SR antigen, Ca-SRAbs could not be detected in any of 90 type 1 APS patients, 73 of whom had CHP (14).

More recently, however, using an immunoprecipitation assay with the Ca-SR expressed in HEK 293 cells, Ca-SRAbs were found in CHP sera from 12 of 14 (86%) patients with type 1 APS and in 2 of 28 (7%) patients with Graves' disease (15).

In endocrine autoimmunity, it is well known that the existence of autoantibodies to cell surface receptors can cause hyper- or hypofunction of the receptors by mimicking or blocking the actions of the respective hormones or mediators (such as TSH-receptor autoantibodies, acetylcholine receptor autoantibodies, or insulin receptor autoantibodies). Also, the ability of Ca-SRAbs to either block or stimulate the Ca-SR and induce hyper- or hypoparathyroidism in some patients has been described.

For example, two families with four members presenting with a syndrome mimicking the genetic familial hypocalciuria hypercalcemic and autoimmune diseases (one with celiac disease and three with thyroid antibodies) were reported (16). Antibodies reacting with the Ca-SR were detected in serum samples from these patients, and these Ca-SRAbs appeared to induce the secretion of PTH in dispersed human parathyroid cells, in vitro (16).

TABLE 49.2. Parathyroid autoantigens and autoantibody profiles.

Autoantibodies(Abs):	Autoantigen target
Parathyroid cytoplasmic Abs	Not known
Oxyphilic Cells Abs	Human mitochondria
Parathyroid Surface Abs	Endothelial cells
Ca-SR Abs	Ca-SR
NALP5 Abs	NALP5

In addition, a Ca-SRAb-positive patient who manifested hypercalcemic hypocalciuria associated with multiple autoimmune diseases (hypophysitis, bollous pemphigoid, rheumatoid arthritis) was described (8). Serum Ca-SRAbs of IgG$_4$ class in this patient were reported to have ability to inhibit Ca-SR activity and induce the secretion of PTH. This patient did not benefit from parathyroidectomy (lymphocytic parathyroiditis was found on histopathological examination) and the symptoms were controlled only by high doses of corticosteroids (8).

In contrast, the familial hypocalciuric hypercalcemia is an autosomal dominant inherited syndrome as a result of inactivating mutations in the extracellular Ca-SR gene on chromosome 3 and is characterized by mild-to-moderate hypercalcemia with relative hypocalciuria and normal or slightly elevated circulating levels of PTH and no evidence of autoimmunity (16).

Ca-SRAbs activating the receptors and inhibiting the secretion of PTH were also described in two patients with a hypoparathyroid syndrome with low levels of PTH and normal parathyroid tissue (7).

The autoantibodies and autoantigen profiles of parathyroid tissue are summarized in Table 49.2.

Addendum: on March 6, 2008 (358, 1018–28) a paper appeared on N. Engl. J. Med. where immunoscreening of a human parathyroid cDNA library with sera from APS-1 patients with hypoparathyroidism identified reactivity to the NACHT leucine rich repeat 5 (NALP5). Sera from 87 APS-1 patients and 257 controls, were subsequently used to determine the frequency and specificity of autoantibodies against NALP5. NALP5-specific autoantibodies were detected in 49% of APS-1 patients with hypoparathyroidism but were absent in ABS-1 patients without hypoparathyroidism, in patients with Hypoparathyroidism isolated or associated to other autoimmune disorders and in healthy controls. NALP5 is predominantly expressed in the cytoplasm of parathyroid chief cells. NALP5 is the first tissue-specific autoantigen identified for hypoparathyroidism in APS-1. Autoantibodies against NALP5 are highly specific and diagnostic for this prominent component of this autoimmune syndrome.

Genetics of Parathyroid Autoimmune Diseases

CHP in the context of type 1APS is a recessive inherited disease associated with mutations in the AIRE

(AutoImmune REgulator) gene (17, 18). The AIRE gene maps to chromosome 21q22.3, consists of 14 exons and encodes a 545-amino acid protein of 58 kDa. To date more than 58 mutations in AIRE gene associated with type 1 APS have been described (18). The most frequent mutation is *R257X,* present in exon 6 and found in 82% of the alleles of Finnish patients with type 1 APS, but also frequent in other central and eastern European populations. The second frequent mutation described is *del13,* present in exon 8, the most common mutation observed in Caucasian-American, British and Irish patients. A *Y85C* mutation in exon 2 was the mutation detected in Iranian-Jewish patients.

In Italy there are three hot spot areas for APS-1, one in north east of Italy where the *R257X* in homozygous or heterozygous combinations with *del13* are the most frequently found mutations. Another hot spot is in Sardinia where *R139X* on exon 3 is the typical mutation and the third is in Apulia where the mutation *W78R* on exon 2 and *Q358X* on exon 9 are the two typically found mutations. APS-1 is the first autoimmune disease that appears to be caused by identified mutations in a single gene. The genetic mutations observed in APS-1 may be responsible for the break-down in immunotolerance in humans.

The identification of the main AIRE gene mutations should be helpful in identifying healthy carriers of the mutations in high-risk populations and in the screening of unaffected family members of APS-1 patients.

In terms of HLA markers, HLA-DRB1*01 and/or DRB1*09 were found to be significantly increased in patients with isolated CHP or CHP associated with thyroid or other autoimmune diseases but excluding Addison's disease or chronic candidiasis compared with controls (12).

In patients with idiopathic sporadic hypoparathyroidism, no differences were found between the frequencies of parathyroid gene polymorphisms and normal controls (19).

CHP and Type 1 APS

APS type 1, also called APECED (autoimmune-polyendocrine-candidiasis-ectodermal-dystrophy), usually presents at first in childhood, with chronic candidiasis, followed by CHP and Addison's disease (17, 18). The estimated prevalence of type 1 APS worldwide is very low, ranging from 1 in 4400 in Veneto (Italy), 1 in 9000 among the Iranian-Jewish community, 1 in 14.4.000 in Sardinia (Italy), 1 in 25,000 in Finland, 1 in 35,000 in Apulia (Italy), 1 in 43,000 in Slovenia, 1 in 80,000 in Norway, 1 in 129,000 in Poland, and 1 in 10,000.000 in Japan (20). The observed female/male ratio ranged from 0.8 to 2.4 (17, 18).

Other autoimmune and non-autoimmune diseases often appear in patients with APS-1: (a) *autoimmune endocrinopathies:* hypergonadotropic hypogonadism (18–60%) marked by the presence of steroid-producing cell antibodies, Type 1 diabetes mellitus (0–12%)

characterized by islet-cell and glutamic acid decarboxylase autoantibodies (GADAbs), chronic thyroiditis (4–36%) marked by thyroid autoantibodies and lymphocytic hypophysitis (7%); (b) *autoimmune gastrointestinal and liver diseases:* chronic atrophic gastritis (13–27%) with parietal cell autoantibodies (PCA), pernicious anemia (0–15%) with PCA and intrinsic factor autoantibodies; coeliac disease, with endomysium autoantibodies or tissue transglutaminase autoantibodies; autoimmune hepatitis (5–31%), marked by liver–kidney microsomal autoantibodies (LKM) recognizing the cytochrome P450 CYPIA2 and CYP2A6, or aromatic L-amino acid decarboxylase, (c) *autoimmune skin diseases:* vitiligo (0–25%) associated with complement-fixing melanocyte autoantibodies, or antibodies to SOX9 and SOX10 and alopecia areata (13–72%), marked by anti-tyrosine hydroxylase antibodies; (d) *autoimmune exocrinopathies:* Sjögren's syndrome (12–18%) associated with autoantibodies to extractable nuclear antigens (ENAs); (e) rheumatic diseases (f) *malabsorption* (6–22%) due to intestinal lymphangiectasia, exocrine pancreatic insufficiency, cystic fibrosis, intestinal infections, deficiency in cholecystokinin, or autoimmune gastrointestinal dysfunctions marked by either tryptophan hydroxylase or histidine decarboxylase autoantibodies, (g) cholelitiasis (44%); (h) *ectodermal dystrophy:* (10–52%) characterized by keratoconjunctivitis, nail dystrophy, defective dental enamel formation, and faulty teeth; (i) *immunological deficiencies:* T-cell defect to *Candida albicans,* IgA deficiency, polyclonal hypergammaglobulinemia; acquired asplenia; (j) *cancer* of the oral mucosa, esophagus, and stomach; (k) *calcifications of* basal ganglia, tympanic membranes and subcapsular lens opacities, and nephrocalcinosis; (l) *vasculitis:* (3%); and (m) ectodermal dystrophy (17, 18).

Among 60 patients with CHP in the context of type 1 APS, we have observed that the mean age at onset of CHP was 7 years and the female/male ratio was 1.8.

CHP Associated with Other Autoimmune Diseases

CHP can occur in association with other autoimmune diseases excluding Addison's disease and chronic candidiasis, such as thyroid autoimmune diseases where CHP contributes to APS type 3; or vitiligo, alopecia, type 1 diabetes, gastric autoimmunity or celiac disease where CHP contributes to APS type 4.

In these cases, CHP appears at a more advanced age. In general, no mutations in the AIRE gene are present, but the disease may be correlated with DRB1*01 or DRB1*09 class II HLA genes (12).

In our observation, the mean age at onset in 7 patients with CHP associated with APS type 3 or APS type 4 was 20 years, and the female/male ratio was 6/1.

TABLE 49.3. Different clinical forms of autoimmune parathyroid disease.

	CHP in context of type 1 APS	CHP in context of type 3 or 4 APS	CHP isolated	Hyperparathyroidism
Associated Diseases	Chronic candidiasis and/ or Addison's disease	ATD, vitiligo, alopecia, type 1 diabetes, celiac disease, pernicious anemia.	None	Other autoimmune diseases
Mean age at onset	7 years	20 years	27 years	Nd
Female/Males	2/1	6/1	2/1	
AIRE Gene mutation	In homozygosis	No	No	Nd
Class II HLA	No	DRB1*01 or DRB1*09	DRB1*01 or DRB1*09	Nd
Ca-SRAb	0–86%	17–62.5% some with ability to stimulate the Ca-SR	35–37.5% some with ability to stimulate the Ca-SR	With ability to block the Ca-SR
PTH levels	Low	Low	low	High
Histopathology	Lymphocytic parathyroiditis	Lymphocytic parathyroiditis	Lymphocytic parathyroiditis	Normal tissue

ATD = Autoimmune Thyroid Diseases, Nd = Not Defined.

Isolated CHP

CHP can present as isolated disease and generally occurs in adults and may be related to DRB1*01 or DRB1*09 class II HLA genes (12).

We have observed 41 patients with isolated CHP and the mean age at onset was 27 years and the female/male ratio was 1.5/1.

Table 49.3 summarizes the profile of the main clinical forms and features of autoimmune parathyroid disease.

Clinical Features

Clinical or latent hypocalcaemia is the main manifestation of CHP. The clinical hypocalcaemia manifests with paresthesias, laryngospasm and seizures, circumoral numbness, and carpopedal spasms. The latent hypocalcaemia is characterized by Chvostek's and Trousseau's signs. The Chvostek's sign is elicited by tapping the facial nerve anterior to the ear to produce homolateral contraction of the facial muscles. The Trousseau's sign is characterized by adduction of the digits, flexion of the wrist and the meta-carpopharingeal joints after inducing limb ischemia by inflating the cuff of a blood pressure-measuring instrument fitted on the upper arm to 20 mm Hg above the systolic blood pressure for 3–5 min. Anxiety, depression, confusion, and psychosis can also be present. Cataracts and calcifications of the basal ganglia are also common in patients with all the forms of CHP. EEG can reveal non-specific changes, and ECG prolonged QT intervals (1).

Laboratory Diagnosis

The laboratory diagnosis of autoimmune parathyroid disease is based on low serum calcium levels, elevated serum phosphate levels and low plasma PTH concentrations. However, occasionally the laboratory tests show the calcium levels elevated, while the phosphate levels are low with the elevated PTH and low calciuria (1).

Therapy

In patients with severe hypocalcemia, therapy consists of intravenous infusion of calcium; to obtain the desired serum calcium levels, it may be necessary to give 1–3 g of calcium gluconate (10 to 30 mL of 10% calcium gluconate) in 10 min followed by a continuous infusion of calcium using, for example, a solution of 5% dextrose in water containing 100 mL of 10% calcium gluconate per liter.

Oral calcium and vitamin D therapy should be started as soon as possible in patients diagnosed with CHP. Calcitriol, the active form of vitamin D, is a physiological treatment and the doses required vary from 0.25 μg twice a day to 0.5 μg 3–4 times a day. In addition, 1–2 g of oral calcium citrate or calcium carbonate per day in divided doses should be given. The goal of the therapy is to maintain the serum ionized calcium levels in the lower limit of the normal range to avoid hypercalciuria (1).

Concluding Remarks

In general, autoimmune parathyroid disease presents as chronic acquired hypoparathyroidism; however, some patients may present with hyperparathyroidism with low calciuria. The autoimmune parathyroid disease satisfies many of the proposed criteria for classification of autoimmune diseases (2). Specifically: (a) atrophy and presence of lymphocytic infiltration of the parathyroid glands; (b) the disease can be reproduced in experimental animals by injection of parathyroid extracts; (c) specific autoantibodies reactive with parathyroid preparations are detectable in patients sera and the extracellular domain of the Ca-SR has been identified as the putative autoantigen; (d) CHP can be associated with other autoimmune diseases, and; (e) there is a genetic predisposition linked to AIRE gene mutations when associated with type 1 APS or to class II HLA genes when isolated or associated with other autoimmune diseases (25).

The mechanism of autoimmune damage of the parathyroid glands is not clear at present; however, experimental and histopathological evidences suggest that a cell-mediated immune response against the parathyroid tissue is involved. Ca-SRAbs appear to be serological markers of the disease; however, the possible effect of the autoantibodies on the Ca-SR activity needs to be confirmed.

Acknowledgments. This study was supported in part by the EU Research Project EurAPS: Autoimmune polyendocrine syndrome type I—a rare disorder of childhood as a model for autoimmunity (contract number LSHM-CT 2005–005223).

References

1. Levine, M.A. (2001) Hypoparathyroidism and pseudohypoparathyroidism. In: *Endocrinology*, Vol. 2. De Groot, L.J., Jameson, L.J., (eds). Elsevier Saunders, Philadelphia PA, pp. 1611–36.
2. Witebsky, E., Rose, N.R., Terplan, K., Paine, J.R., Egan, R.W. (1957) Chronic thyroiditis and autoimmunization, *JAMA* **164**, 1439–47.
3. Lupulescu, A., Pop, A., Merculiev, A., Neascu, C., Heitmanek, C. (1965) Experimental iso-immune hypoparathyroidism in rats, *Nature (London)* **206**, 415–16.
4. Russel, N.J., Bond, K.A., Robertson, I.D., Parry, B.W., Irwin, P.J. (2006) Primary Hypoparathyroidism in dogs: A retrospective study of 17 cases, *AustVetJ* **84**, 285–90.
5. Krug, J., Williams, A.J.K., Beales, P.E., Doniach, I., Gale, E.A.M., Pozzilli, P. (1991) Parathyroiditis in the non obese diabetic mouse-a new finding, *J Endocrinol* **131**, 193–6.
6. McIntyre, Gass, J.D. (1962) The syndrome of keratokonjunctivitis superficial moniliasis idiopathic hypoparathyroidism and Addison's disease, *Am J Ophthalmol* **54**, 660–74.
7. Kifor, O., Mcelduff, A., Leboff, M.S., Moore F.D., Butters, R., Gao, P., Cantor, T.L., Kifor, I., Brown. M.E. (2004) Activating antibodies to the calcium-sensing receptor in two patients with autoimmune hypoparathyroidism, *J Clin Endocrinol Metab* **89**, 548–56.
8. Pallais, J.C., Kifor, O., Chen, Y.B., Slovik, D., Brown, E.M. (2003) Acquired hypocalciuric hypercalcemia due to autoantibodies against the calcium-sensing receptor, *N Engl J Med* **351**, 362–9.
9. Wortsman, J., McConnachie, P., Baker, J.R., Mallette, L.E. (1992) T-lymphocyte activation in adult-onset idiopathic hypoparathyroidism, *Am J Med* **92(4)**, 352–6.
10. Betterle, C. (2006) Parathyroid and autoimmunity, *Ann Endocrinol (Paris)* **67**, 147–54.
11. Li, Y., Song, Y.H., Rais, N., Connor, E., Schatz, D., Muir, A., Maclaren, N. (1996) Autoantibodies to the extracellular domain of the calcium sensing receptor in patients with acquired hypoparathyroidism, *J Clin Invest* **97**, 910–14.
12. Goswami, R., Brown, E.M., Kochupillai, N, Gupta, N., Rani, R., Kifor, O., Chattopadhyay, N. (2004) Prevalence of calcium sensing receptor autoantibodies in patients with sporadic idiopathic hypoparathyroidism, *Eur J Endocrinol* **150**, 9–18.
13. Mayer, A., Ploix, C., Orgiazzi, J., Desbos, A., Moreira, A., Vidal, H., Monier, J.C., Bienvenu, J., Fabien, N. (2004) Calcium-sensing receptor autoantibodies are relevant markers of acquired hypoparathyroidism, *J Clin Endocrinol Metab* **89**, 4484–8.
14. Soderberg, A., Myhre, A.G., Gebre-Medhin, G., Hedstrand, H., Landgren, E., Miettinen, A., Eskelin, P., Halonen, M., Tuomi, T., Gustafsson, J., Husebye, E.S., Perheentupa, J., Gylling, M., Manns, M.P., Rorsman, F., Kampe, O., Nilsson, T. (2004) Prevalence and clinical associations of 10 defined autoantibodies in autoimmune polyendocrine syndrome type I, *J Clin Endocrinol Metab* **89**, 557–62.
15. Gavalas, N.G., Kemp, E.H., Krohn, K.J., Brown, E.M., Watson, P.F., Weetman, A.P. (2007) The calcium-sensing receptor is a target of autoantibodies in patients with autoimmune polyendocrine syndrome type 1, *J Clin Endocrinol Metab* **92**, 2107–14.
16. Kifor, O., Moore, F.D., Delaney, M., Delaney, M., Garber, J., Hendy, G.N., Butters, R., Gao, P., Cantor T.L., Kifor, I., Brown E.M., Wysolmerski, J. (2003) Syndrome of hypocalciuric hypercalcemia caused by autoantibodies directed at the calcium-sensing receptor, *J Clin Endocrinol Metab* **88**, 60–72.
17. Betterle, C., Greggio, N.A., Volpato, M. (1998) Autoimmune polyglandular disease type 1, *J Clin Endocrinol Metab* **83**, 1049–55.
18. Perheentupa, J. (2006) Autoimmune Polyendocrinopathy-candidiasis-ectodermal dystrophy, *J Clin Endocrinol Metab* **91**, 2843–50.
19. Goswani, R., Mohapatra, T., Gupta, N., Rani, R., Tomar, N., Dikshit, A., Sharma, R.K. (2004) Parathyroid hormone gene polymorphism and sporadic idiopathic hypoparathyroidism *J Clin Endocrinol Metab* **89**, 4840–5.

50
Autoimmune Polyendocrine Syndromes

Angela Tincani, Angela Ceribelli, Ilaria Cavazzana, Franco Franceschini, Alberto Sulli and Maurizio Cutolo

Abstract Autoimmune polyendocrine syndromes (APSs) are defined as a multiple autoimmune-mediated endocrine gland failure. The currently used classification criteria of APS, based on clinical data only, propose four main clinical presentations.

APS-1 is characterised by three main clinical features: chronic candidiasis, chronic hypoparathyroidism and Addison's disease. APS-2 (or Schmidt syndrome) is a combination of Addison disease (AD), autoimmune thyroid disease (TAD) and/or Type 1 Diabetes Mellitus. APS-3 is defined as an association between TAD and another systemic or organ-specific autoimmune disease. Because TAD is the most prevalent autoimmune condition in the general population, APS-3 is the most frequently observed autoimmune polyendocrine syndrome. APS-4 includes other combinations of the autoimmune disorders previously described, which cannot be allocated in other APS definitions.

Most of the autoimmune endocrine diseases of APS are characterised and preceded by the development of organ-specific autoantibodies, usually directed to antigens expressed by endocrine cells. Different authors have suggested a common pathogenesis, basing on a similar mononuclear leukocyte infiltration and the detection of organ-specific autoantibodies.

Keywords Autoimmune polyendocrine syndromes (APS) · Addison disease · diabetes mellitus · thyroid autoimmune disease · chronic candidiasis · chronic hypoparathyroidism · autoantibodies · AIRE gene

Nowadays, the concept of "shared autoimmunity" is widely used to define situations in which, because of genetic or environmental factors, several complete or incomplete features of autoimmune disease are simultaneously detected in the same patient. This is the case of autoimmune polyendocrine syndromes (APSs) that are defined as a multiple autoimmune-mediated endocrine gland failure (1). The first case-report was originally described in 1855 as a combination of pernicious anaemia, vitiligo and idiopathic adrenal insufficiency, but a systematic classification of the different association of endocrine diseases was published in 1980, according to Neufeld and Blizzard criteria (2) (Table 50.1).

Clinical Features

In recent years, the study of APS has received a great impulse thanks to improved knowledge of autoimmune diseases and their natural history, and thanks to the discovery of new autoantibodies related to clinical manifestations (1). After a careful clinical observation, Neufeld and Blizzard (2) suggested a classification of APS, based on clinical criteria only, describing four main clinical presentations (Table 50.1).

APS-1

Originally described in 1929, APS-1 is a very rare syndrome (prevalence from 1:9000 to 1:200,000), characterised by three main clinical features: chronic candidiasis, chronic

TABLE 50.1. Classification of different APS (1).

	Disease association
APS-1	Chronic candidiasis, chronic hypoparathyroidism, Addison's disease
APS-2	Addison's disease (*always present*) *with* autoimmune thyroid disease *and/or* Type 1 Diabetes Mellitus
APS-3	Autoimmune thyroid disease associated with other autoimmune diseases (*excluding* Addison's disease and/or hypoparathyroidism)
APS-4	Other combinations of the same autoimmune diseases

From: Y. Shoenfeld et al. (eds.): *Diagnostic Criteria in Autoimmune Diseases*, DOI: 10.1007/978-1-60327-285-8_50,
© 2008 Humana Press, Totowa, NJ

TABLE 50.2. Disease components of APS1 (1, 2).

Disease components	%
Major clinical manifestations	
Hypoparathyroidism	76–100
Addison's disease	22–100
Mucocutaneous candida	18–100
Minor clinical manifestations	
Hypogonadism	24–60
Alopecia areata	13–72
Nail and teeth dystrophy	10–52
Chronic atrophic gastritis	13–27
Autoimmune hepatitis	5–31
Autoimmune thyroid disease	4–36
Vitiligo	0–25
Type 1 Diabetes Mellitus	0–13

hypoparathyroidism and Addison's disease (1). Although two of the three major criteria are sufficient to diagnose it, most patients have all the major clinical components of the syndrome (1). Table 50.2 shows the frequency of major and minor disease components of APS-1. A *chronic Candida infection* can represent the first clinical presentation of APS-1, generally occurring during the first years of life. It involves nails, skin and mucous membranes (oral mucosa, oesophagus), and it is probably due to a selective T-lymphocyte defect against *Candida albicans* (1). In contrast, these patients maintain a normal B-cell response, which prevents the development of a systemic candidiasis (3). *Chronic hypoparathyroidism*, usually present before the 15 years of age, can be clinically recognised by the onset of paresthesias, neuro-muscular hyperexcitability (sometimes with tetany), hypotension and malabsorption (with steatorrhca), and always associated with hypocalceamia and hyperphosphoremia.

The third clinical component of APS1 (Addison's disease) can develop between 6 months to 40 years of age, with clinical manifestations of a combined deficiency of mineralocorticoids, glucocorticoids and androgens. Aspecific symptoms, such as generalised weakness, fatigue, weight loss and anorexia, are usually insidious. However, a full-blown adrenal failure could lead to gastrointestinal involvement (nausea, vomiting, abdominal pain), cardiovascular symptoms (hypotension or syncope), hypoglycaemia and sexual dysfunctions, such as secondary amenorrhea (detectable in 25% of patients) and hypergonadotropic hypogonadism (25–60% of cases) (1).

Other clinical features are reported in patients affected by APS-1, and they are defined as *minor clinical manifestations*. In brief, skin involvement, detectable in 13–72% of cases, is represented by alopecia areata, localised at scalp or spread to axillary and pubic hair (universal alopecia), or nail and teeth dystrophy. Autoimmune thyroiditis and autoimmune liver diseases are reported in 4–36% of cases (1), while Type I Diabetes Mellitus, atrophic gastritis or vitiligo are more rarely described (0–20%).

APS-2

APS-2 (or Schmidt's syndrome) is characterised by a combination of Addison's disease (AD), autoimmune thyroid disease (TAD) and/or Type 1 Diabetes Mellitus (1) (Table 50.3). It usually affects adults, with a predominant female prevalence (3:1) and a mean age of presentation of 35 years (1). All the patients show a classical AD, associated to TAD in 70–82% of cases (1). Most of them develop Graves' disease, generally before AD, or chronic thyroiditis, that can occur before or after the diagnosis of AD. Diabetes Mellitus can be present in about 30–50% of patients. Moreover, different authors have reported an incomplete APS-2, characterised by only one constitutive disease of the syndrome with only positive serology for other APS-2 components (1). Minor clinical manifestations of APS-2 are also shown in Table 50.3.

APS-3

APS-3 is defined as an association between TAD and another systemic or organ-specific autoimmune disease (2). Because TAD is the most prevalent autoimmune condition in the general population, APS-3 is the most frequently observed autoimmune polyendocrine syndrome. Recently, given the wide spectrum of different autoimmune disorders involved, some authors have suggested a new classification of APS-3 (1). TAD can be classified in to four groups of different disorders, according to the main systems involved such as endocrine, gastrointestinal, skin/haematopoietic/nervous system and connective tissue diseases/vasculitis, as shown in Table 50.4 (4). Analysing a wide series of patients with TAD, authors have suggested that about 52% of the subjects with TAD could show an APS-3, as complete (TAD with another autoimmune disease) or incomplete type (TAD with organ and non-organ specific autoantibodies) (1). Moreover, TAD could be detected in about 10% of the

TABLE 50.3. Disease components of APS2 (modified from 1).

Disease components	%
Major clinical manifestations	
Addison's disease	100
Thyroid Autoimmune Disease	70–82
Type 1 Diabetes Mellitus	30–50
Minor clinical manifestations	
Vitiligo	4.5–11
Pernicious anaemia	4.5–11
Chronic atrophic gastritis	4.5–11
Hypogonadism	4–9
Autoimmune hepatitis	4
Alopecia	1–4

TABLE 50.4. Classification of APS3 according to Betterle 2001 (4).

Autoimmune thyroid diseases
Hashimoto's thyroiditis, idiopathic myxoedema, asymptomatic thyroiditis Endocrine exophtalmus Graves' disease

+

3 A Endocrine diseases	3 B Gastrointestinal apparatus	3 C Skin/Hemopoietic/Nervous system	3 D Connective tissue diseases/vasculitis
Type 1 Diabetes Mellitus Hirata's Syndrome	Atrophic gastritis Pernicious anaemia Celiac disease	Vitiligo Alopecia	SLE Discoid Lupus Erythematosus
	Chronic inflammatory bowel disease	Autoimmune hemol. Anemia Autoimmune thrombocytopenia Anti-phospholipid syndrome	MCTD RA Systemic sclerosis Sjogren's S.
Premature ovarian failure Lymphocytic neurohypophysitis	Autoimmune hepatitis Primary biliary cirrhosis Sclerosing cholangitis	Myasthenia gravis Multiple sclerosis Stiff-man syndrome	Systemic vasculitis

patients affected by Type 1 Diabetes Mellitus (DM) and it is a very common finding also in patients affected by systemic autoimmune diseases (5), such as Systemic Lupus Erythematosus (SLE) (6), Mixed Connective Tissue Disease (MCTD) (5), Sjögren's syndrome (SS) (5, 7) and Psoriatic and Rheumatoid arthritis (RA) (7).

APS-4

APS-4 includes other combinations of the autoimmune disorders previously described, which cannot be allocated in other APS definitions, for instance AD with hypogonadism, celiac disease or myasthenia gravis (2).

Diagnosis

A diagnosis of APS-1, where chronic candidiasis, hypoparathyroidism and Addison's disease are usually present, can be assessed performing several laboratory tests, in order to analyse calcium/phosphorus metabolism, serum electrolytes and hormonal dosage. Chronic hypoparathyroidism is always characterised by hypocalcaemia, hyperphosphoremia and low urine levels of calcium, with increased urinary phosphorus. PTH levels are low or undetectable. A full-blown Addison's disease shows hyponatriemia, hypochloremia, hyperkaliemia and a mild persistent eosinophilia. The correct assessment of serum levels of ACTH and cortisol must be performed early in the morning: ACTH is usually increased, while cortisol is reduced. Aldosterone and dehydroepiandrosterone are frequently reduced. No specific tests are useful to evaluate the spread of Candida infection, even if an esophagogastroscopy or a colonoscopy could be performed in selected cases. Autoimmune thyroid disease, detected both in APS-2

and APS-3, can be diagnosed analysing thyroid hormones, anti-thyroid autoantibodies (anti-thyreoglobulin and anti-thyreoperoxydase) and thyroid ultrasound.

Immunologic Abnormalities

Most of the autoimmune endocrine diseases of APS are characterised and preceded by the development of organ-specific autoantibodies, usually directed to antigens expressed by endocrine cells. Within APS-1, antibodies directed to parathyroid are described by different authors in 11–38% of patients with chronic hypoparathyroidism (8). More recently, anti-calcium-sensing receptors antibodies were reported in hypoparathyroidism and APS1 (9), but they are not assessed by routine laboratories.

In Addison's disease, a variety of autoantibodies against the adrenal cortex (ACA) intracellular enzymes were reported, especially directed against the antigen 21-hydroxylase (21-OH), side-chain cleavage (SCC) enzyme and 17α-hydroxylase (1). About 84% of Addison's patients show autoantibodies against at least one of these proteins, but only 21-OH and SCC enzyme are considered the major antigens and the more specific autoantibody targets. Moreover, in AD other immunologic alterations can be assessed, such as IgA deficiency or polyclonal hypergammaglobulinemia (1).

Other autoantibodies are described as markers of minor autoimmune features in APS1. Antibodies to GAD65 (glutamic acid decarboxylase 65) and TH (tyrosine hydroxylase) can be associated to intestinal dysfunction in APS1. Anti-GAD65 and anti-IA2 (tyrosine phosphatase-like protein IA2) seem to predict the development of Type 1 Diabetes Mellitus in APS1. In addition, antibodies to pituitary protein 6 (TDRD6) have been detected in patients with GH deficiency in APS1 (10).

Different authors have reported a wide spectrum of organ-specific autoantibodies associated to vitiligo in APS1: antibodies directed to melanin-producing cells (11), anti-aromatic aminoacid decarboxylase (AADC) and, recently, autoantibodies to transcription factors Sox9 and Sox10 (12). Sox10 is involved in the differentiation of tissues derived from the neural crest and its expression seems to be important in the migration process of melanoblasts to dermis during differentiation. A specific reactivity to Sox10 has been found in about 63% of patients with APS1 and vitiligo, while all anti-Sox10-positive sera display a reactivity also to Sox9 (12).

In contrast, autoantibodies associated to Type 1 Diabetes Mellitus (in APS2) are not usually performed routinely: they are represented by anti-islet-cell antibodies (ICA), anti-GAD65 and anti-IA2 antibodies (1). Antibodies to 17-αhydroxylase and anti-SCC enzyme can be considered as markers of increased risk for premature ovarian failure, detected in 4–9% of APS-2 patients (13). Autoimmune thyroid diseases, taking part of both APS2 and APS3, are characterised by specific anti-thyroid antibodies, namely anti-thyreoglobulin and anti-thyreoperoxydase antibodies, which can be tested by most routine laboratories. Non-organ specific autoantibodies, such as antinuclear antibodies (ANAs), can be detected in about one-third of patients affected by TAD, and they represent the hallmark of different systemic autoimmune diseases, taking part of APS-3.

Non-organ autoantibodies, such as ANA, anti-ENA and anti-DNA antibodies, show a pivotal role in the correct diagnosis of systemic autoimmune diseases, as isolated or associated to TAD in APS-3. ANAs are usually positive in 96–100% of patients affected by SLE, MCTD and Systemic sclerosis (SSc). Minor frequencies (50–70%) can be detected in Sjogren's syndrome, Dermatomyositis/Polymyositis and Rheumatoid Arthritis. Some antinuclear specificities can be considered "diagnostic markers" of disease, such as anti-dsDNA and anti-Sm in SLE, anti-Ro/SSA and anti-La/SSB in SS, anti-Scl70 (Topoisomerase I) and anti-centromere in Systemic Sclerosis (SSc) or anti-U1RNP in MCTD. Moreover, in order to define a correct diagnosis of RA, it is mandatory to detect Rheumatoid factor and anti-CCP (cyclic citrullinated peptide), recently known as the best marker of the disease, with high specificity and predictive value.

Pathogenesis

Since their first descriptions in 1912, different authors have suggested a common pathogenesis of the different types of APS, basing on a similar mononuclear leukocyte infiltration observed in some goitrous thyroid glands, in adrenal cortex of Addison's patients and in pancreatic islets of subjects with Type 1 Diabetes Mellitus (1). During the 1950s, other authors suggested a second pathogenetic mechanism, displaying an endocrine dysfunction, due to the detection of organ-specific autoantibodies, such as anti-thyroid antibodies in patients with hypothyroidism and Hashimoto's thyroiditis. The nature of the relationship between anti-thyroid autoimmunity and the pathogenesis of autoimmune diseases is presently unknown. Some authors have shown that anti-thyreoglobulin antibodies can form immune complexes, and anti-microsomal antibodies not only bind to thyroid peroxidase but also modulate natural killer cell activity in autoimmune thyroiditis (14). An alteration of the immune regulation and the occurrence of circulating autoantibodies, directed against antigens expressed in endocrine cells, are nowadays the two major pathogenetic hypotheses explaining the glandular failures in different APS.

APS-1 is an autosomal recessive syndrome that recognises the main pathogenetic role in different mutations of a regulatory gene, called "AIRE", located on chromosome 21 (15). AIRE encodes for a transcription regulatory protein. About 42 different mutations have been identified as missense mutations, insertions and deletions leading to the alteration of functional properties of intracellular proteins. Although the mutation of a single gene is directly responsible for APS1, the clinical expression of the syndrome depends on mutations of both alleles (1). Recently, different authors have reported that AIRE mutations could lead to altered immunological tolerance and abnormal negative selection of self-reactive thymocytes. In animal models, AIRE deletions are responsible for the abolished expression of insulin promoter genes in thymus and, consequently, of an increase of islet-reactive T cells escaping thymic deletion (16).

Additional genes could be responsible for the widespread clinical features of APS, in terms of susceptibility or protection for specific endocrine diseases. APS1 patients show particular HLA aplotypes: HLA A28 is more common than in normal population, and HLA DR5 has increased frequency in Jewish-Persian and Italian APS1 patients (1). Moreover, HLA DQB1 (0602) is considered protective for the development of Type 1 Diabetes Mellitus in APS1 (17). APS2 shows more strict HLA associations: an increased prevalence of HLA-DR3 or DR4 has been found (1), especially in patients with Type 1 Diabetes Mellitus (DR4, DQB10302) (18). These findings have been recently confirmed: the aplotype DR3/DR4 represents a risk factor (relative risk of 2.7–3.2) for the development of APS2, while the presence of other alleles (DR1, DR7, DR13 and DR14) seems to confer a kind of protection against the syndrome (1). A higher frequency of HLA DQA1 (0301) seems to be strictly associated with APS2, with no specific association with any of its components, except for alopecia.

On the contrary, the huge number of organ-specific autoantibodies, mentioned earlier, are always directed to intracellular enzymes of target organs. Nevertheless, in animal models mimicking the clinical features of different APS, the autoimmune destruction of various target organs seems to be a multi-step process where multiple genetic polymorphisms converge to induce local abnormalities (inflammation of the gland) and a specific dysregulation of the immune system (1).

Therapy

Specific hormone replacement represents the first treatment for thyroid and adrenal failure, in APS1, 2 and 3. Chronic hypoparathyroidism is corrected by the administration of calcium and vitamin D, while insulin therapy for type 1 Diabetes Mellitus is mandatory. The chronic candidiasis of APS1 is periodically treated with Itraconazole, although not very effective for mucosal involvement (1).

References

1. Betterle, C., Zanchetta, R. (2003) Update on autoimmune polyendocrine syndromes (APS). *Acta Bio Medica* **74**, 9–33.
2. Neufeld, M., Blizzard, R.M. (1980) Polyglandular autoimmune diseases. In: Symposium on autoimmune aspects of endocrine disorders. Pinchera, A., Doniach, D., Fenzi, G.F., Baschieri, L. (Eds) Academic press, New York, 357–65.
3. Peterson, P., Perheentupa, J., Krohn, K.J. (1995) Detection of candidal antigens in autoimmune polyglandular syndrome type 1. *Clin Diagn Lab Immunol* Suppl **1**, 1–24.
4. Betterle, C., Dalpra, C., Greggio, N., Volpato, M., Zanchetta, R. (2001) Autoimmunity in isolated Addison's disease and in polyglandular autoimmune diseases type 1, 2 and 4. *Ann Endocrinol (Paris)* **62**, 193–201.
5. Bira, E., Szekanecz, Z., Czirjaik, L., Danka, K., Kiss, E., Szaba, N.A., Szucs, G., Zeher, M., Bodolay, E., Szegedi, G., Baka, G. (2006) Association of systemic and thyroid autoimmune diseases. *Clin Rheumatol* **25**, 240–5.
6. Mihailova, D., Grigorova, R., Vassileva, B., Mladenova, G., Ivanova, N., Stephanov, S., Lissitchky, K., Dimova, E. (1999) Autoimmune thyroid disorders in juvenile chronic arthritis and systemic lupus erythematosus *Adv Exp Med Biol* **455**, 55–60.
7. Ruggeri, R.M., Galletti, M., Mandolfino, M.G., Aragona, P., Bartolone, S., Giorgianni, G., Alesci, D., Trimarchi, F., Benvenga, S. (2002) Thyroid hormone autoantibodies in primary Sjogren's syndrome and rheumatoid arthritis are more prevalent than in autoimmune thyroid disease, becoming progressively more frequent in these diseases. *J Endocrinol Invest* **25**, 447–54.
8. Blizzard, R.M., Chee, D., Davis, W. (1966) The incidence of parathyroid and other antibodies in the sera of patients with idiopathic hypoparathyroidism. *Clin Exp Immunol* **1**, 119–28.
9. Gavalas, N.G., Kemp, E.H., Krohn, K.J., Brown, E.M., Watson, P.F., Weetman, A.P. (2007) The calcium-sensing receptor is a target of autoantibodies in patients with autoimmune polyendocrine syndrome type 1. *J Clin Endocrinol Metab* **92**, 2107–14.
10. Bensing, S., Fetissov, S.O., Mulder, J., Perheentupa, J., Gustafsson, J., Husebye, E.S., Oscarson, M., Ekwall, O., Crock, P.A., Hakfelt, T., Kampe, O. (2007) Pituitary autoantibodies in autoimmune polyendocrine syndrome type 1. *Proc Natl Acad Sci USA* **104**, 949–54.
11. Betterle, C., Caretto, A., Pedini, B., Rigon, F., Bertoli, P., Peserico, A. (1992) Complement-fixing activity to melanin-producing cells preceding the onset of vitiligo in a patient with type 1 polyglandular failure. *Arch Dermatol* **128**, 123–4.
12. Hedstrand, H., Ekwall, O., Olsson, M.J., Landgren, E., Kemp, E.H., Weetman, A.P., Perheentupa, J., Husebye, E., Gustafsson, J., Betterle, C., Kampe, O., Rorsman, F. (2001) The transcription factors SOX9 and SOX10 are vitiligo autoantigens in Autoimmune Polyendocrine Syndrome Type I. *J Biol Chem* **276**, 35390–5.
13. Falorni, A., Laureti, S., Santeusanio, F. (2002) Autoantibodies in autoimmune polyendocrine syndrome type II. *Endocrinol Metab Clin North Am* **31**, 369–89.
14. Szyper-Kravitz, M., Marai, I., Shoenfeld, Y. (2005) Coexistence of thyroid autoimmunity with other autoimmune diseases: friend or foe? Additional aspects on the mosaic of autoimmunity. *Autoimmunity* **38**, 247–55.
15. Aaltonen, J., Bjorses, P., Sandkuijl, L., Perheentupa, J., Peltonen, L. (1994) An autosomal locus causing autoimmune disease: autoimmune polyglandular disease type I assigned to chromosome 21. *Nat Genet* **8**, 83–7.
16. Liston, A., Gray, D.H., Lesage, S., Fletcher, A.L., Wilson, J., Webster, K.E., Scott, H.S., Boyd, R.L., Peltonen, L., Goodnow, C.C. (2004) Gene dosage-limiting role of Aire in thymic expression, clonal deletion, and organ-specific autoimmunity *J Exp Med* **200**, 1015–26.
17. Gianani, R., Eisenbarth, G.S. (2003) Autoimmunity to gastrointestinal endocrine cells in autoimmune polyendocrine syndrome Type 1. *J Clin Endocrinol Metab* **88**, 1442–4.
18. Huang, W., Connor, E., Dela Rosa, T., Muir, A., Schatz, D., Silverstein, J., Crockett, S., She, J-X., Maclaren, N. (1996) Although DR3-DQB10201 may be associated with multiple component diseases of the autoimmune polyglandular syndrome, the human leukocyte antigen DR4-DQB10302 haplotype is implicated only in beta-cells autoimmunity. *J Clin Endocrinol Metab* **81**, 2259–63.

51
Endometriosis

Maurizio Cutolo and Simone Ferrero

Abstract   Endometriosis is a benign, estrogen-dependent, gynecological disorder associated with pelvic pain and infertility. It affects between 10 and 47% of women undergoing surgery because of pain symptoms and/or infertility. Pain and infertility represent the major clinical problems of women with endometriosis. Several serum markers have been proposed for the diagnosis of endometriosis (including CA-125, CA-19.9, sICAM-1, PP14, and IL-6), but none of them has been proved to have sufficient accuracy to be used in clinical setting. It is possible to suspect the presence of endometriosis on the basis of patient's history and gynecological examination, but imaging techniques are required to confirm the presence of the lesions and establish the severity of the disease. The gold standard for the diagnosis of endometriosis is the visual inspection of the pelvis at laparoscopy. The treatment of endometriosis may be medical, surgical or combined. Medical therapy aims primarily to decrease the intensity of pain symptoms but there is no evidence that it can reduce the extent of the lesion; exogenous estrogens should be avoided. Surgical excision of endometriotic lesions is associated with improvements not only in pain symptoms but also in quality of life, and it can usually be performed by laparoscopy.

Keywords   Diagnosis · endometriosis · symptoms · treatment

Endometriosis is a benign, estrogen-dependent, chronic gynecological disorder associated with pelvic pain and infertility. It is defined as the presence of endometrial glands and stroma outside the uterus. Endometriotic lesions may have various locations: they are found more frequently on the pelvic peritoneum, on the ovaries, in the rectovaginal septum, on the uterosacral ligaments, and more rarely in the bowel, bladder, ureters, diaphragm, pleura, and lungs (1, 2) (Table 51.1).

Epidemiology

Endometriosis is primarily a disease of the reproductive years, and it is only rarely observed in adolescent and postmenopausal women (estrogen-dependent). The diagnosis is based on surgical visualization of the disease; this criterion has hampered epidemiological investigations aimed at estimating the true prevalence of the disease in women without specific pathology. Prospective studies documented a prevalence of endometriosis of 4–19% in women undergoing laparoscopic tubal sterilization; but it is more frequent in women undergoing surgery because of pain symptoms or infertility (10–47%).

Pathogenesis

Despite years of research, the precise etiology of endometriosis remains unknown. The most widely accepted theory on the pathogenesis of endometriosis is the Sampson's theory proposing that the disorder originates from retrograde menstruation of viable endometrial tissue through the fallopian tubes into the peritoneal cavity where it implants on peritoneal surface or pelvic organs. This theory is supported by three observations: endometrial cells enter the peritoneal cavity through the Fallopian tubes, refluxed endometrial cells are viable in the peritoneal cavity, and the refluxed endometrial cells can adhere to peritoneum and proliferate. However, retrograde menstruation is a common event in almost all cycling women, and therefore, it remains unclear why not all women develop endometriosis. Immunological abnormalities present in women with endometriosis may contribute to the development and persistence of the disease. Several studies proved that macrophages contained in the peritoneal fluid of women with endometriosis are hyperactivated and that they secrete cytokines and growth factors. Ovarian hormones not only have direct effects on endometrial and endometriotic tissue, but also they have indirect

From: Y. Shoenfeld et al. (eds.): *Diagnostic Criteria in Autoimmune Diseases*, DOI: 10.1007/978-1-60327-285-8_51,

TABLE 51.1. Locations of endometriotic lesions in women undergoing surgery.

Location	Estimated prevalence (%)
Cul de sac	35–72
Left ovary	18–44
Right ovary	17–31
Left broad ligament	25–52
Right broad ligament	21–43
Left uterosacral ligament	21–45
Right uterosacral ligament	15–41
Fallopian tubes	5–16
Bowel	5–25
Bladder	1–33
Ureter	0.01–1

Data obtained from Jenkins et al. (1) and Redwine (2)

TABLE 51.2. Presenting symptoms for endometriosis diagnosis.

Symptom	Estimated prevalence (%)
Dysmenorrhea	78.7
Pelvic pain	69.4
Dyspareunia	44.9
Bowel upset (e.g., constipation, diarrhea)	36.4
Bowel pain	29.0
Infertility	26.2
Ovarian mass/tumor	19.5
Dysuria	9.9
Other urinary problems	6.2

Data obtained from a cross-sectional study of self-reported data from 940 women with surgically diagnosed endometriosis (5).

effects on endometriosis through the inflammatory cells present in the peritoneal cavity. Estrogen receptors α and β are overexpressed in macrophages of women with endometriosis when compared with controls (3). Furthermore, there is a correlation between the expression of estrogen receptor β and the proinflammatory cytokines (IL-1β, TNF-α, IL-6) on peritoneal fluid macrophages both in women with and without endometriosis; on the contrary, the expression of estrogen receptor α correlates with cytokine production selectively in women with endometriosis but not in controls (4). These interactions between steroid hormones and peritoneal fluid macrophages suggest that estrogen may promote the progression of endometriosis by acting on the immune system (4).

Clinical Manifestations

Pain represents the major clinical problem of women with endometriosis (Table 51.2) (5). There is no correlation between the severity of pain and the extent of disease; some anatomic locations of endometriotic lesions have been associated with specific symptoms. Deep dyspareunia is typically caused by the presence of endometriotic nodules on the uterosacral ligaments. Bowel endometriotic lesions determine a wide range of gastrointestinal complains ranging from mild symptoms mimicking irritable bowel syndrome to noncyclic chronic pelvic pain and subocclusion. Besides pain symptoms, women with endometriosis may suffer infertility. The mechanisms by which endometriosis causes infertility are still largely not well defined. These include anatomical changes that lead to adhesions or tubal obstruction, potential negative effects of peritoneal and follicular fluid on egg maturation and sperm motility, potential oocyte maturational abnormalities and hormonal variations, and the effects of endometriosis on uterine receptivity for implantation.

Pathological Features

The histological diagnosis of endometriosis is based on the presence of both ectopic endometrial glands and stroma in the specimens removed at surgery. In most of the cases, hematoxylin–eosin staining allows the diagnosis; immunohistochemical staining with CD10 may be of value in confirming a diagnosis of endometriosis when there is a histological doubt.

Serological Features

Table 51.3 lists potential serum markers proposed for the diagnosis of endometriosis. Peripheral levels of CA-125 have been extensively investigated for the diagnosis of endometriosis. Elevated serum levels of CA-125 are not

TABLE 51.3. Potential serum markers for diagnosis of endometriosis.

Tumor markers
  CA125
  CA19.9
Polypeptides
  Glycodelin A (PP14)
  Soluble intercellular adhesions molecule-1 (sICAM-1)
  Vascular cellular adhesion molecule-1 (VCAM-1)
  Angiogenin
Cytokines and growth factors
  Interleukin-6 (IL-6)
  Vascular endothelial growth factor (VEGF)
  Epidermal growth factor (EGF)
  Insulin-like growth factor-1 (IGF-1)
  Hepatocyte growth factor (HGF)
Auto-antibodies (Abs)
  Anti-endometrial Abs
  Antiphospholipid Abs
  Auto-Abs against carbonic anhydrase
  Auto-Abs against transferrin
  Auto-Abs against α2-Heremans-Schmidt glycoprotein
  Auto-Abs against oxidatively modified lipoproteins
  Auto-Abs against laminin-1
  Antithyroid Abs

specific for endometriosis and are also associated with other gynecological and non-gynecological disorders (such as ovarian cancers, adnexitis, pancreatitis). The diagnostic performance of serum CA-125 in detecting endometriosis has been summarized in a meta-analysis of 16 cohort studies and seven case-control studies including women with infertility or chronic pelvic pain (6). The receiver-operating characteristic (ROC) curves showed a poor diagnostic performance. For a specificity of 90%, the sensitivity was only 28%; if the sensitivity was increased to 50%, the specificity decreased to 72%. When the analysis was limited to women with advanced endometriosis, the ROC curve showed a better diagnostic performance. For a specificity of 89%, the sensitivity was 47%; an increase of the sensitivity to 60% resulted in a decrease of the specificity to 81%. Although CA-125 is an inexpensive test, its performance in the detection of endometriosis is low. There are a limited number of reports on the significance of serum CA-19.9 levels in the diagnosis of endometriosis. A retrospective study including 101 women with surgically proven endometriosis and 22 controls showed that the sensitivity of CA-19.9 is significantly lower than that of CA-125 (34 and 49%, respectively) thus limiting the diagnostic value of this marker particularly in the early stages of disease (7). The concomitant dosage of CA-125 and CA-19.9 does not add significant information in respect to the CA-125 test alone in diagnosing endometriosis.

Soluble intercellular adhesions molecule-1 (sICAM-1) is secreted from the endometrium and endometriotic implants; its serum levels may be slightly increased in women with endometriosis however the measurement of this molecule does not allow to discriminate patients with endometriosis from controls. Vascular cellular adhesion molecule-1 (VCAM-1) has been found to have increased serum concentration in women with advanced endometriosis but up to now it has not been largely investigated.

Serum placental protein 14 (PP14) is significantly higher in women with endometriosis than in controls; however, it has limited value in diagnosing the disease because of low sensitivity. Angiogenin, which may promote the establishment of new blood supply for the lesions, has increased serum levels in women with endometriosis during the follicular phase of the menstrual cycle and has recently been proposed as potential blood marker for the diagnosis of endometriosis. Although several authors investigated the value of serum IL-6 measurement in predicting endometriosis, no study has definitely proved that it can be clinically used to discriminate women with and without endometriosis either alone or in combination with other markers. Various growth factors may be involved in the pathogenesis of endometriosis (i.e., vascular endothelial growth factor, epidermal growth factor, insulin-like growth factor I, hepatocyte growth factor); although some of these molecules have been found to have increased peripheral levels in women with endometriosis, none of them has been proved to be useful for predicting the presence of the disease.

Women with endometriosis have increased levels of a variety of auto-antibodies (Abs) that have been investigated for their diagnostic potential. Anti-endometrial Abs have been widely demonstrated to be increased in women with endometriosis; the sensitivity of serum anti-endometrial Abs screening ranges from 71 to 85%, whereas specificity ranges from 67 to 100% (8). The exact antigen remains unknown; therefore, no simple antigen-antibody assay is currently available (8) and the measurement of these Abs is not used in clinical practice. Anti-phospholipid Abs against inositol, cardiolipin, ethanolamine, and beta-2-glycoprotein 1 have increased levels in women with endometriosis but up to now there is no evidence that these Abs can be used in a clinical setting as screening markers or in the follow-up after treatment. Serum protein-containing glycotopes such as sialylated T antigen might induce Abs response in patients with endometriosis. Women with endometriosis have significantly higher levels of Abs to carbonic anhydrase, transferrin and α2-Heremans–Schmidt glycoprotein (α2-HSG). Antibody response to α2-HSG and carbonic anhydrase is against a common carbohydrate epitope, the Thomsen–Friedenreich antigen (Galbeta 1-3 GalNAc), suggesting that autoimmune response might either play a direct role in the disease process or reflect an abnormality of glycosylation in endometriosis. Women with endometriosis have increased serum levels of Abs against oxidatively modified lipoproteins. Aberrant immunological mechanisms including the production of auto-Abs may be involved in the pathogenesis of endometriosis-related infertility. Infertile patients with endometriosis have increased prevalence of auto-Abs against laminin-1, which is a multifunctional glycoprotein of the basement membrane involved in embryogenesis, embryonic implantation, and placentation (9, 10, 11). Thyroid autoimmunity has also been documented in infertile women with endometriosis.

Many cardinal features of endometriosis, such as inflammation and neoangiogenesis, are shared with several other conditions; therefore, it is unlikely that a single biochemical marker will yield sufficient sensitivity and specificity to be used in clinical practice. However, in recent years, proteomic technology has been applied to the research of new markers of endometriosis with promising results (12).

Diagnostic Criteria

The visual inspection of the pelvis at laparoscopy is the gold standard investigation for the diagnosis of endometriosis, unless disease is visible in the vagina or elsewhere (13). As laparoscopy is an invasive procedure, the diagnosis is often combined with surgical treatment. Although positive histology of the specimens excised at surgery confirms the diagnosis of endometriosis, negative histology does not exclude it because a biopsy might be negative because of the surgeon's limited experience, the size of the biopsy, the experience of the pathologist, and the quality of the histological sample. It is controversial whether histology should be obtained if peritoneal disease alone is present; visual inspection is usually adequate but histological confirmation of at least one lesion is ideal. In cases of ovarian endometrioma and in deeply infiltrating disease, histology should be obtained to identify endometriosis and to exclude rare instances of malignancy (13). It is possible to suspect the presence of endometriosis on the basis of symptoms reported by the patients and findings at gynecological examination, but limited information can be obtained on the extent of lesions. Therefore, preoperative imaging is required for determining the location and severity of disease. Transvaginal ultrasound (TVU) is reliable in diagnosing ovarian endometriotic cysts of diameter ≥ 4 cm; in case of smaller cysts, particularly with diameter < 2 cm, the identification by TVU may be less accurate. Pelvic endometriotic nodules can also be diagnosed by TVU; the sensitivity, specificity, and positive and negative predictive values of TVS for the diagnosis of deep pelvic endometriosis are 79, 95, 95, and 78%, respectively (14). Magnetic resonance imaging (MRI) is insensitive in the detection of small peritoneal lesions (≤ 4 mm), but it is increasingly used to determine the presence of larger deep endometriotic nodules. A large prospective study demonstrated that MRI has sensitivity of 90%, specificity of 91%, positive predictive value of 89%, and negative predictive value of 91% in diagnosing deep pelvic endometriosis (15). Recently, multislice-computed tomography combined with colon distension by water enteroclysis has been proved to have high accuracy in determining the presence of bowel endometriotic nodules with sensitivity of 98.7%, specificity of 100%, positive predictive value of 100%, and negative predictive value of 95.7% (16).

Prediction

Endometriosis can easily be suspected by experienced clinicians on the basis of patient's history and clinical examination particularly in advanced stages; in these patients, radiological examination is performed for determining the extent of the lesions and providing adequate informed consent before surgery rather than for confirming the presence of the disease. Minimal lesions are more difficult to diagnose during clinical consultation, and they are usually detected only at the time of laparoscopy.

Therapy

Medical therapy aims primarily to eradicate painful symptoms; there is no evidence that currently available medical therapies can enhance fecundity and reduce the extent of endometriosis. Table 51.4 lists the available medical therapies for endometriosis. Nonsteroidal anti-

TABLE 51.4. Medical therapies for endometriosis.

Nonsteroidal anti-inflammatory drugs
Contraceptives (to be reassessed)
Oral contraceptives
Contraceptive patch
Contraceptive ring
Progestogens
Derivative of progesterone
Medroxyprogesterone acetate
Megestrol acetate
Dydrogesterone
Derivative of 19-nortestosterone
Norethindrone
Norgestrel
Lynestrenol
Levonorgestrel
Gestrinone
Gonadotropin-releasing hormone analogs
Leuprolide
Nafarelin
Buserelin
Goserelin
Danazol
Aromatase inhibitors
Anastrozole
Letrozole

inflammatory drugs are a non-specific but important part of the medical treatment of endometriosis; they are the only medical option available for women attempting to conceive although they may have an anti-ovulatory effect when taken at mid-cycle. Several studies proved that suppression of ovarian function for 6 months reduces endometriosis-associated pain (13). Today, oral contraceptives (OC) are commonly prescribed treatment for endometriosis; however, there is limited scientific evidence to demonstrate the long-term safety of this therapy. No epidemiological study has demonstrated the benefit of OC in preventing endometriosis or reducing its progression. Although OC are often prescribed as first-line treatment when patients present with dysmenorrhea, pain symptoms typically re-emerge once medical treatment is discontinued or when the disease progresses in severity. Therefore, the administration of exogenous estrogens should be avoided in women with endometriosis because of the potential effects on the ectopic lesions and on the immune system (4, 17, 18). Progestogens can be safely used in women with pain symptoms related to the presence of endometriosis; these drugs initially induce decidualization of endometrial tissue followed by atrophy. Both gonadotropin-releasing hormone analogs and danazol have been used in the treatment of endometriosis; however, they may cause several adverse effects. In the last 20 years, our understanding of the pathogenesis of endometriosis at the molecular and cellular levels has significantly improved; this has provided researchers with new molecular targets for the treatment of this disorder. New drugs are currently under development (19), and they may improve our ability to eliminate endometriotic lesions when present or more likely to prevent recurrence of endometriosis after surgical treatment (20).

Surgical therapy may include removal (excision) or destruction (ablation) of endometriotic tissue. Several studies proved that excision of endometriotic lesions is associated with improvements not only in pain symptoms but also in quality of life. Laparoscopy can be used in almost all women with endometriosis, and this technique decreases cost, morbidity, and the risk of adhesions postoperatively. Laparotomy should be reserved for patients with advanced stage disease in whom laparoscopy is judged to be not possible depending on the experience of the surgeon.

Prevention

There is no solid evidence that the development of endometriosis can be prevented. However, prevention of endometriosis must include the reduction in environmental exposure to phytoestrogens or hormone disruptors such as polychlorinated biphenyl (PBC) or dioxin, which may facilitate the development of the disorder. It remains unclear whether lifestyle (regular exercise, cigarette smoking, alcohol use, and caffeine intake) may also affect the risk of developing endometriosis.

References

1. Jenkins S, Olive DL, Haney AF. Endometriosis: Pathogenetic implications of the anatomic distribution. *Obstet Gynecol* 1986; 67(3): 335–8.
2. Redwine DB. Ovarian endometriosis: A marker for more extensive pelvic and intestinal disease. *Fertil Steril* 1999; 72(2): 310–5.
3. Capellino S, Montagna P, Villaggio B, et al. Role of estrogens in inflammatory response: Expression of estrogen receptors in peritoneal fluid macrophages from endometriosis. *Ann N Y Acad Sci* 2006; 1069: 263–7.
4. Montagna P, Capellino S, Villaggio B, et al. Peritoneal fluid macrophages in endometriosis: Correlation between the expression of estrogen receptors and inflammation. *Fertil Steril* 2007 (Epub ahead of print).
5. Sinaii N, Plumb K, Cotton L, et al. Differences in characteristics among 1,000 women with endometriosis based on extent of disease. *Fertil Steril* 2007 (Epub ahead of print).
6. Mol BW, Bayram N, Lijmer JG, et al. The performance of CA-125 measurement in the detection of endometriosis: A meta-analysis. *Fertil Steril* 1998; 70(6): 1101–8.
7. Harada T, Kubota T, Aso T. Usefulness of CA19-9 versus CA125 for the diagnosis of endometriosis. *Fertil Steril* 2002; 78(4): 733–9.
8. Bedaiwy MA, Falcone T. Laboratory testing for endometriosis. *Clin Chim Acta* 2004; 340(1–2): 41–56.
9. Inagaki J, Sugiura-Ogasawara M, Nomizu M, et al. An association of IgG anti-laminin-1 autoantibodies with endometriosis in infertile patients. *Hum Reprod* 2003; 18(3): 544–9.
10. Inagaki J, Kondo A, Lopez LR, Shoenfeld Y, Matsuura E. Anti-laminin-1 autoantibodies, pregnancy loss and endometriosis. *Clin Dev Immunol* 2004; 11(3–4): 261–6.
11. Inagaki J, Kondo A, Lopez LR, Shoenfeld Y, Matsuura E. Pregnancy loss and endometriosis: Pathogenic role of anti-laminin-1 autoantibodies. *Ann N Y Acad Sci* 2005; 1051: 174–84.
12. Ferrero S, Gillott DJ, Remorgida V, et al. Haptoglobin beta chain isoforms in the plasma and peritoneal fluid of women with endometriosis. *Fertil Steril* 2005; 83(5): 1536–43.
13. Kennedy S, Bergqvist A, Chapron C, et al. ESHRE guideline for the diagnosis and treatment of endometriosis. *Hum Reprod* 2005; 20(10): 2698–704.
14. Bazot M, Thomassin I, Hourani R, Cortez A, Darai E. Diagnostic accuracy of transvaginal sonography for deep pelvic endometriosis. *Ultrasound Obstet Gynecol* 2004; 24(2): 180–5.
15. Bazot M, Darai E, Hourani R, et al. Deep pelvic endometriosis: MR imaging for diagnosis and prediction of extension of disease. *Radiology* 2004; 232(2): 379–89.
16. Biscaldi E, Ferrero S, Fulcheri E, Ragni N, Remorgida V, Rollandi GA. Multislice CT enteroclysis in the diagnosis of bowel endometriosis. *Eur Radiol* 2007; 17(1): 211–9.
17. Cutolo M, Capellino S, Sulli A, et al. Estrogens and autoimmune diseases. *Ann N Y Acad Sci* 2006; 1089: 538–47.
18. Cutolo M, Sulli A, Capellino S, et al. Anti-TNF and sex hormones. *Ann N Y Acad Sci* 2006; 1069: 391–400.
19. Ferrero S, Abbamonte LH, Anserini P, Remorgida V, Ragni N. Future perspectives in the medical treatment of endometriosis. *Obstet Gynecol Surv* 2005; 60(12): 817–26.
20. Ferrero S, Ragni N, Remorgida V. Antiangiogenic therapies in endometriosis. *Br J Pharmacol* 2006; 149(2): 133–5.

52
Autoimmune Ovarian Failure

Francisco Carmona

Abstract   Premature ovarian failure (POF) is a complex disease with multiple etiopathogenic mechanisms including autoimmunity. In this chapter the different autoimmunity patterns related with POF are reviewed. Some of these patterns are related with global autoimmune regulation whereas others may be related with inflammatory autoimmunity against ovarian antigens.

Keywords   Autoimmunity · infertility · ovarian failure

Introduction

Premature ovarian failure (POF) is a dramatic disease in which young women lose their ability to became pregnant. POF was defined 40 years ago by Moraes-Ruehsen (1) as the end of menses before 40 years and after menarche. So, such patients will present a hypergonadotropic hypogonadism hormonal profile combined with secondary amenorrhea. In some cases a familial history is present. Fifty percent of patients present hot flushes and some other signs of hypoestrogenism (vaginal atrophy, dyspareunia, etc.). This syndrome (amenorrhea, hot flushes, genital atrophy, infertility) was first described by Atria in 1950. Diagnosis is confirmed when elevated follicle-stimulating hormone (FSH) levels [higher than levels of luteinizing hormone (LH)] are found (usually over 40 m UI/ml) in patients with a compatible clinical picture.

The incidence of POF is lower than 1% (2). There are two histological types of POF. In the first one, there is a complete absence of ovarian follicles, and it is characteristic of congenital forms as gonadal dysgenesis or hermaphroditism. In the second one, some follicles can be found. It must be kept in mind that most cases of the follicular form will develop a complete absence of follicles. Despite many cases of POF have been effectively linked to chromosomal, genetic, enzymatic, toxic, infectious, and iatrogenic causes (3), the underlying etiopathogenic mechanism causing most POF cases remains unresolved. Recently, some studies have suggested that some cases of POF may be the direct result of autoimmune-mediated destruction of the ovaries.

Relationship of POF and Other Autoimmune Diseases

One of the reasons to suspect the autoimmune etiology of POF is its high frequency of association with other autoimmune diseases. The most well-established autoimmune association with POF is the one linked to Addison's disease, a primary autoimmune adrenal insufficiency frequently associated to a multiple endocrine failure and involving high serum levels of antibodies targeted to steroid-producing cells, which is often preceded by POF. Two main types of autoantibodies are detected in patients with Addison's disease: Cy-Ad antibodies, directed against adrenal cells cytoplasm, and St-C antibodies, which also react with a variety of steroid-producing cells, including adrenal cortex, testes, trophoblast and with different types of ovarian cells as follicular and luteal cells. Thus, 60% of patients with Addison's disease and secondary amenorrhea present St-C antibodies, which are also present in just 15–20% of patients with Addison's disease but without amenorrhea. Furthermore, 40% of these patients will develop a POF during the next 10–15 years of follow-up.

Some other features support the idea of autoimmune origin of POF. Histological evidence of inflammatory lymphocytic infiltration of the ovaries was apparent in 11% of POF patients, 78% of which were positive for steroid cell antibodies (4). Furthermore, Hoek et al. (4) described that in all cases of patients with positive St-C antibodies a lymphocytic oophoritis was present and that 78% of patients with lymphocytic oophoritis tested positive for

From: Y. Shoenfeld et al. (eds.): *Diagnostic Criteria in Autoimmune Diseases*, DOI: 10.1007/978-1-60327-285-8_52,

St-C antibodies. Also, the distribution of lymphocytic infiltration, which is more intense in corpus luteum and corpus albicans, clearly shows that steroid-producing cells are the target of autoimmune attack.

There has not been showed any genetic predisposition in cases of POF associated to Addison's disease. This disease has been related with the HLA-B8/DR3 haplotype and particularly with the DR B1 0301 allele (5). POF has been related just with the HLA-A28 haplotype (6).

Some enzymes involved in steroid production may be the target for St-C and Cy-Ad autoantibodies, particularly in case of POF associated with Addison's disease. Such steroid cell autoantibodies show some specificity for p450-17a-hydroxylase and the p450 side chain cleavage product of p450-17α-hydroxylase (7). Antibodies to the FSH receptor have also been found in a small percentage of POF patients, and antibodies from POF patients have been shown to inhibit FSH-induced DNA synthesis in ovarian tissue extracts. These results, however, were not confirmed using cells transgenically expressing human FSH or (LH) receptors (7). Several studies have shown that antibodies to zona pellucida antigens may be implicated preferentially in POF. These studies, however, used immunostaining of porcine oocytes to determine zona pellucida binding, and recognition of porcine oocytes appears to be highly non-specific because it occurs in sera from 60% of healthy fertile women and even occurs in 40% of male serum samples. The actual frequency of zona pellucida autoantibodies may be more in the order of 2.4%, as has been observed in a study involving over 800 infertile women (8).

Isolated POF

Although the frequency of concurrence with other autoimmune conditions varies somewhat between different study populations, and POF often occurs as part of an autoimmune polyglandular syndrome with high frequencies of hypothyroidism, insulin-dependent diabetes mellitus, and adrenal abnormalities (9), POF may also occur as an isolated ovarian-specific disorder independent of any polyglandular or global systemic autoimmune events. Thus, many cases of POF may represent a primary autoimmune ovarian abnormality, whereas other cases may represent secondary effects of a more global endocrine autoimmune dysfunction. As such, POF may have multiple distinct autoimmune manifestations perhaps dependent on the tissue distribution of the targeted autoantigen and/or the underlying specificity or lack thereof of native immune regulatory fsunctions. It should be noted that the pathophysiologic significance of ovarian autoantibodies and the cognate target antigen(s) that they recognize remains unclear.

Similarly, there are some signs of autoimmunity in isolated POF:

a. *Autoantibodies against other endocrine systems:* Autoantibodies against tyroid are the more frequently found (14%) among patients with isolated POF, autoantibodies against gastric wall cells (4%), against Langerhans cells (2%) and against acetyl-choline receptor (2%) are also frequent. However, just antibodies against Langerhans cells and against acetyl-choline receptor are clinically relevant. These antibodies are related with two severe diseases: diabetes mellitus type I and myasthenia gravis, respectively. Furthermore, other autoimmune diseases as systemic lupus erythematosus had been related with POF.

b. *Antinuclear antibodies (ANA):* Patients testing positive for ANA are at increased risk for developing POF; it has been described that 24% of patients positive for ANA will develop a POF, whereas just 5% of patients in the control group testing negative for ANA will present a POF.

c. *Anti-DNA:* Blumenfeld et al. found anti-DNA antibodies in 10.5% of women with POF whereas in a control group of healthy fertile women just 3.3% presented such antibodies.

d. *Antireceptor antibodies:* Antireceptor antibodies are targeted against membrane hormone receptor. These antibodies may act mimicking the physiologic hormonal action or blocking the hormone function depending on their specificity and affinity (10). Some investigators have described the presence of antibodies directed against FSH and LH receptors in patients with POF (11, 12, 13). However, such antibodies have also been detected in patients with iatrogenic ovarian failure (4).

e. *Anti-zona pellucida antibodies:* This type of antibodies have been described in 5.6% of patients with infertility of unknown origin (14) and have been also described in patients with POF. In experimental animal models, these antibodies have been able to inhibit the follicular development (15).

Ovarian Histology in Patients with Isolated POF

In 60% of patients with isolated POF, fibrotic ovaries, without follicular presence, are observed. In the remaining 40% the number of follicles is highly variable, from a few to an almost normal amount. These patients with normal number of ovarian follicles present gonadotrophin resistance syndrome.

Cellular Immunity Alterations in Patients with Isolated POF

Several studies have shown increased activation of T cells in patients with POF (16). However, such an increment has been also described in patients with natural menopause (16), and it has been suggested that estrogen may modulate the T-cell activation arguing that T-cell activation observed in isolated POF is the consequence of the hypoestrogenemia presented by these patients. Furthermore, hormonal replacement therapy may decrease the number of activated T cells (16). The T-killer cells are also diminished in number and function as monocytes are (16). However, neither patients with isolated POF nor menopausal women have increased susceptibility to infectious diseases.

Subclinical Ovarian Failure

There are a special group of patients having infertility of unknown origin and elevated basal levels of FSH (greater than 15 mUI/l). These patients have normal menstrual cycle, but they used to have bad results in in vitro fertilization cycles with high rates of canceled cycles. Wheatcroft et al. (17) studied a group of 14 women with subclinical ovarian failure having normal menstrual cycle and younger than 40 years. They determined a number of autoantibodies including antiovary, antiendometrium, antihypofysis, antiadrenal, antimicrosomal, anticardiolipin, antihistone, antinuclear, and other; they also determined different type of T cells and complement levels. They also included two control groups. The first one included 15 patients with infertility of unknown origin but with basal FSH levels lower than 10 mUI/l and the second control group included 10 fertile women with normal FSH levels and ovarian cycle. There were no differences among the three groups studied. The authors concluded that subclinical ovarian failure is not an autoimmune alteration.

Experimental Animal Models of Autoimmune Oophoritis

Several animal models of experimental autoimmune oophoritis (EAO) have been used in POF studies, with each model providing unique mechanisms for induction of POF. One of the currently available EAO animal models include induction of autoimmune oophoritis by immunization with rat or bovine ovarian homogenate in complete Freund's adjuvant. In this case, inflammatory infiltrates appear in the ovaries within 14 days, and the appearance of germinal centers and increased splenic activity of both B and T cells indicates that cellular and humoral immunity are involved in this form of EAO. Serum ovarian antibodies appear after 28 days and may passively transfer decreased fertility measured by decreased litter size into naïve recipients. It is speculated that the antibodies produced in this form of EAO may mediate disease by

interfering with zona pellucida antigens, thereby disrupting ovulation and/or fertilization (4).

Experimental models of autoimmune oophoritis also include those methods that target zona pellucida; thus, immunization with heterologous zona pellucida antigens results in autoimmune oophoritis characterized by follicle depletion and ovarian failure. Immunization with zona pellucida proteins rapidly induces a marked atretic appearance and reduction, and, eventually disappearance, in the number of primary growing follicles. An inflammatory oophoritis such as that observed following immunization with ovarian homogenate, however, does not occur (18).

Experimental models also include those that develop spontaneously and lead to polyglandular abnormalities as a result of global immune regulatory failure after neonatal thymectomy. Neonatal thymectomized BALB/c and C57BL/6 mice spontaneously develop autoimmune oophoritis along with autoimmune disorders of the thyroid, gut, parotid gland, and lacrimal gland within 3–14 weeks after thymectomy. This polyglandular form of oophoritis is accompanied by a loss of oocytes and elimination of ovarian follicles. Circulating autoantibodies against oocytes, zona pellucid proteins, and steroid-producing cells appear within 4 weeks and reach their highest titers within 7–9 weeks. The inflammation subsides after 14 weeks, and the ovaries become atrophic. This type of experimental oophoritis in mice is similar to that observed in women with POF associated to Addison's disease (19, 20, 21).

Conclusion

POF affects 1% of women in reproductive age. Its etiopathogenic factors remain unclear in most cases but include chromosomal, genetic, enzymatic, toxic, infectious, and iatrogenic causes. An abundance of evidence indicates that autoimmunity is primarily responsible for the symptoms of a substantial cohort of POF patients mainly in cases associated with Addison's disease and oophoritis. These patients present antibodies targeted against steroid-producing cells and also antigens shared by ovarian and adrenal cells. Furthermore, the linphoplasmocitary infiltration observed around these cells in patients with POF associated with Addison's disease strongly suggests an autoimmune origin. Different animal models add further evidence.

In patients with isolated POF, the evidence favoring an autoimmune origin is not so strong. It has been described some alterations on the immune cells, and these patients present a greater incidence of type I diabetes and myasthenia gravis than general population. However, against the autoimmune origin of POF in these patients is the fact that it is very difficult to find oophoritis in cases of isolated POF.

References

1. de Moraes-Ruehsen M, Jones GS. Premature ovarian failure. *Fertil Steril* 1967; 18: 440–61.
2. Coulam CB, Adamson SC, Annegers JF. Incidence of premature ovarian failure. *Obstet Gynecol* 1986; 67: 604–6.
3. Davis SR. Premature ovarian failure. *Maturitas* 1996; 23: 1–8.
4. Hoek A, Schoemaker J, Drexhage HA. Premature ovarian failure and ovarian autoimmunity. *Endocr Rev* 1997; 18: 107–34.
5. Bottazzo GF, Mirakian R, Drexhage HA. Adrenalitis, oöphoritis and autoimmune polyglandular disease. In: Rich RR et al. (eds.) *Clinical Immunology, Principles and Practice*. Mosby, St. Louis, MO (USA), 1996; 1523–36.
6. Ahonen P, Koskimies S, Lokki ML, Tiilikainen A, Perheentupa J. The expression of autoimmune polyglandular disease type I appears associated with several HLA-A antigens but not with HLA-DR. *J Clin Endocrinol Metab* 1988; 66: 1152–7.
7. Forges T, Monnier-Barbarino P, Faure GC, Bene MC. Autoimmunity and antigenic targets in ovarian pathology. *Hum Reprod Update* 2004; 10: 163–75.
8. Van Voorhis BJ, Stovall DW. Autoantibodies and infertility: A review of the literature. *J Reprod Immunol* 1997; 33: 239–56.
9. Kalantaridou SN, Davis SR, Nelson LM. Premature ovarian failure. *Endocrinol Metab Clin North Am* 1998; 27: 989–1006.
10. DeGroot LJ, Quintans J. The causes of autoimmune thyroid disease. *Endocr Rev* 1989; 10: 537–62.
11. van Weissenbruch MM, Hoek A, van Vliet-Bleeker I, Schoemaker J, Drexhage H. Evidence for existence of immunoglobulins that block ovarian granulosa cell growth in vitro. A putative role in resistant ovary syndrome?. *J Clin Endocrinol Metab* 1991; 73: 360–7.
12. Wheatcroft NJ, Toogood AA, Li TC, Cooke ID, Weetman AP. Detection of antibodies to ovarian antigens in women with premature ovarian failure. *Clin Exp Immunol* 1994; 96: 122–8.
13. Anasti JN, Flack MR, Froench J, Nelson LM. The use of human recombinant gonadotropin receptors to search for immunoglobulin G-mediated premature ovarian failure. *J Clin Endocrinol Metab* 1995; 80: 824–8.
14. Kamada M, Daitoh T, Mori K, Maeda N, Hirano K, Irahara M, Aono T, Mori T. Etiological implicition of autoantibodies to zona pellucida in human female infertility. *Am J Reprod Immunol* 1992; 28: 104–9.
15. Smith S, Hosid S. Premature ovarian failure associated with autoantibodies to zona pellucida. *Int J Fertil Menopaus Stud* 1994; 39: 316–9.
16. Hoek A, van Kasteren Y, de Haan-Meulman M, Hooijkaas H, Schoemaker J, Drexhage HA. Analysis of peripheral blood lymphocyte subsets, NK cells, and delayed type hypersensitivity skin test in patients with premature ovarian failure. *Am J Reprod Immunol* 1995; 33: 495–502.
17. Wheatcroft NJ, Rogers CA, Metcalfe RA, Lenton EA, Cooke ID, Weetman AP. Is subclinical ovarian failure an autoimmune disease? *Human Reprod* 1997; 12: 244–9.
18. Dean J. Biology of mammalian fertilization: Role of the zona pellucida. *J Clin Invest* 1992; 89: 1055–9.
19. Tong ZB, Gold L, Pfeifer KE, et al. Mater, a maternal effect gene required for early embryonic development in mice. *Nat Genet* 2000; 26: 267–8.
20. Tong ZB, Gold L, De Pol A, et al. Developmental expression and subcellular localization of mouse MATER, an oocyte-specific protein essential for early development. *Endocrinology* 2004; 145: 1427–34.
21. Sundblad V, Bussmann L, Chiauzzi VA, et al. Alpha-enolase: A novel autoantigen in patients with premature ovarian failure. *Clin Endocrinol* 2006; 65: 745–51.

53
Autoimmune Orchitis

Clovis Artur A. Silva, Eduardo Ferreira Borba, Marcello Cocuzza, Jozélio Freire de Carvalho and Eloísa Bonfá

Abstract   Testicular autoimmune disease may be primary or secondary. The former is characterized by an isolated infertility and autoantibodies directed to sperm, basement membrane, or seminiferous tubules without evidence of a systemic autoimmune disease. An immunologic basis for some cases of infertility has been identified in approximately 10% of infertile men, suggesting that antisperm antibodies (ASAs) may have a harmful effect in fertilization. The secondary form is manifested by orchitis and/or testicular vasculitis, and it is uniformly associated with a systemic autoimmune disease, particularly polyarteritis nodosa (PAN), Behçet's disease, and Schönlein–Henoch purpura. The overall frequency of acute orchitis in rheumatic diseases is low. The pathogenesis of primary or secondary autoimmune orchitis is unknown and probably involves the access of the immune system to the testis due to inflammation, infection, or trauma in response to antigens or microorganism. Corticosteroids and immunosuppressive drugs are indicated in autoimmune orchitis associated active systemic autoimmune diseases. In isolated male infertility associated with ASAs, in vitro fertilization (IVF), and intracytoplasmic sperm injection (ICSI) seem to offer better results than immunosuppressive therapy.

Keywords   Autoimmune orchitis · gonad · sperm · antisperm antibodies

Introduction

The possible deleterious effect of the immune system in male reproductive tract is largely supported by the association of antisperm antibodies (ASAs) and male infertility. In addition, autoimmune systemic diseases may also target the testicles leading to androgen and sperm production failure (1).

The two important functions of the testis, spermatogenesis and androgen synthesis, are accomplished in distinct compartments, the seminiferous tubules and Leydig cells, respectively. Clinically, the term *orchitis* is defined as an acute symptomatic disease following a local or systemic infection (2). The subacute or chronic asymptomatic inflammation of the testis, including those of noninfectious disease etiologies, is hardly ever diagnosed and, for this reason, often unnoticed (2). Orchitis may be classified according to the causal agent such as infections (bacterial/viral) or traumatic events such as testicular torsion. The most common trigger of viral orchitis is mumps (2). Orchitis may also occur in association with prostate infections and sexually transmitted diseases, for example, gonorrhea and *Chlamydia trachomatis* (2).

Epidemiology

ASAs were observed in the serum and/or in the seminal plasma or on the sperm surface in approximately 10% of infertile male partners (3), whereas autoimmune response against the developing germ cells within the human testis has not been studied extensively. Approximately half of the systemic lupus erythematosus (SLE) patients also have ASA antibodies, without a definite clinical association with infertility (4, 5). Testicular involvement occurs in up to 18% of patients with systemic polyarteritis nodosa (PAN), although autopsy frequencies as high as 93% have been reported (6, 7, 8). Acute clinical orchitis was observed in 4–31% of Behçet's disease patients (8) and in 7–9% of Schönlein–Henoch purpura patients (8, 9). There were two reported cases of relapsing polychondritis (8) and single cases of rheumatoid arthritis (8), SLE (10), and dermatomyositis

From: Y. Shoenfeld et al. (eds.): *Diagnostic Criteria in Autoimmune Diseases*, DOI: 10.1007/978-1-60327-285-8_53,
© 2008 Humana Press, Totowa, NJ

TABLE 53.1. Frequency of clinical orchitis in autoimmune diseases.

Disease	Acute clinical orchitis
Behçet's disease	4–31%
Polyarteritis nodosa	2–8%
Schönlein–Henoch purpura	7–9%
Relapsing polychondritis	2 cases
Rheumatoid arthritis	1 case
Systemic lupus erythematosus	1 case
Dermatomyositis	1 case

(10), respectively. Documented orchitis cases due to autoimmune diseases are illustrated in Table 53.1.

Pathogenesis (Figure 53.1)

Testis has a privileged immune condition, but it accessible to the immune system (2). It is believed that the underlying pathogenic mechanism involved in the testicular autoimmune disease is a T-cell response to antigens or microorganisms that have permeated the testis barrier (11). This hypothesis is supported by the immune condition demonstrated in the blood-testis barrier injury during inflammation, infection, and trauma (2). The most likely mechanism for this barrier breakdown during inflammation is an increase in tumor necrosis factor-α (TNF-α) and transforming growth factor-β (TGF-β) levels (12), which may downregulate occludin expression in Sertoli cells (12) with a consequent disassembly of its tight junctions. The studies on experimental autoimmune orchitis (EAO) have helped to partially elucidate not only autoimmune mechanisms but also as the systemic and local regulation that normally prevents disease in the testis (2).

On the contrary, the most consistent evidence for autoimmune orchitis is the presence of ASA. They can be found in seminal fluid and plasma in men, in addition to cervical mucus, oviductal fluid, or follicular fluid in women. The presence of multiple ASA can lead to the immobilization and/or agglutination of spermatozoa, which may significantly impair

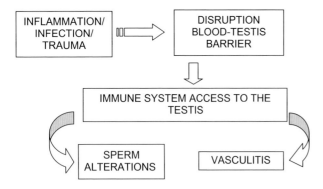

FIGURE 53.1. Pathogenesis of autoimmune orchitis.

sperm motility affecting acrosome reaction, cervical mucus penetration, zona pellucida binding, and sperm–oocyte fusion (2). Also ASA can prevent implantation and/or arrest embryo development. Interestingly, only ASA bound to sperm seems to be relevant for fertility (13), whereas the finding of iso-ASA in men and women's sera does not appear to have clinical implications (13).

Diagnostic Criteria (Table 53.2)

Autoimmune orchitis is defined as autoimmune aggression directed to the testis. There are, however, no diagnostic criteria and autoimmune orchitis may be subdivided into two types:

(a) Primary autoimmune orchitis: isolated infertility and autoantibodies (ASA or antibodies to the basement membrane or the seminiferous tubules) (14) without evidence of a systemic autoimmune disease.
(b) Secondary autoimmune orchitis: orchitis and/or testicular vasculitis associated with a systemic autoimmune disease.

Clinical Manifestations

In the primary form the usual manifestation is isolated infertility. The term *infertility* is used to describe the situation where a couple does not succeed in achieving a spontaneous pregnancy in spite of attempting to conceive during at least 1 year of unprotected intercourse (15). Secondary autoimmune orchitis is rare and mainly associated with PAN, Schönlein –Henoch purpura, and Behçet's disease (8).

The symptoms and signs of clinical orchitis are often difficult to distinguish from those of other acute scrotal processes, mainly acute testicular torsion. Usually, the scrotum is inflamed and swollen, and there may be localized testicular pain during palpation, which may be associate or not with fever.

On the contrary, IgG ASAs were reported in approximately half of 24 SLE patients and were related to anti-DNA titers and disease activity raising the possibility of an

TABLE 53.2. Clinical and serological findings in autoimmune orchitis.

Autoimmune orchitis	Clinical feature	Associated diseases	Antisperm antibodies
Primary	Isolated infertility	None	10%
Secondary	Vasculitis/ inflammation	Behçet's disease; Schönlein–Henoch purpura; polyarteritis nodosa	?

antibody-mediated lesion in this disease (4, 5). We have recently performed a global evaluation of gonadal function in 35 male adolescents and adults with SLE, which confirmed an overall ASA frequency of 40% (5). These antibodies, however, were associated neither with the severity of sperm alterations nor with intravenous cyclophosphamide therapy (5).

Diagnostic Tests for ASA in Males

The direct immunobead binding test detects antibodies on the sperm cell surface (sperm head, mid-piece, and/or tail) using immunobead rabbit antihuman Ig (IgA, IgG, and IgM) kits (Irvine Scientific, Santa Ana, CA, USA). At least 50% of the motile spermatozoa must be coated with immunobeads in order to validate the clinical significance of test. Negative control should have a score <10% bead attachment and positive control a score >20% bead attachment (16). Others methodologies to detect ASA include postcoital test and the hemizona assay (11).

Pathological Features

The histopathology evolution of orchitis can be learned from studies in EAO, and it is characterized in the early stages by peritubular and/or interstitial mixed cellular infiltrates. As the disease progresses, there is infiltration of mononuclear cells into the interstitium and sloughing of germinal cells begins to occur, culminating in granuloma formation, necrosis, and ultimately complete absence of spermatogenesis (17). EAO is a T-cell-mediated disease in which the inflammatory CD4 (Th1) T-cell mechanism is the critical pathway that targets the spermatogenic germ cells for autoimmune attack (17). However, despite the significant progress that has been made in the identification of local, genetic, and immunological factors, the pathology of EAO is still not completely understood (17).

On the contrary, in all autoimmune diseases, the underlying pathological condition in testis is a severe vasculitis leading to inflammation and infarction of affected tissue. Acute and chronic inflammation, fibrinoid necrosis of the vessels, and periarteritis in varying amounts are present (8). Infarction was observed in testicular lesions of PAN and in the single reported case of rheumatoid arthritis (8).

Imaging

Several different imaging techniques can be applied in the diagnosis of orchitis and more importantly in the differential diagnosis with testicular torsion and intrascrotal masses (abscesses, tumors, and hydroceles) such as scrotal ultrasound, color Doppler sonography, duplex sonography, and magnetic resonance imaging. With regard to autoimmune involvement, it has been observed that 22% of serial sections of affected testicles demonstrated lesions, and therefore, a $3 \times 3 \times 3$ mm biopsy should be sufficient to detect testicular manifestations of autoimmune diseases (8). Surgical complications of testicular biopsies are rare as minimal hematomas or infections are detected in <2% of cases. Moreover, the risks for an immune response of clinical significance for fertility after biopsies are also low (8).

Treatment

Symptomatic patients should receive analgesic treatment associated with local cooling, scrotal elevation, and bed rest. Local anesthesia by a nerve block using 5 ml of 1% lidocaine around spermatic vessels may be necessary for those with severe pain (8). The overall success rates of these conservative measures in patients with testicular involvement of autoimmune diseases need to be determined (8) considering the finding of a quarter of azoospermia and one-third of permanent oligospermia 2 years after bacterial epididymo-orchitis (8). Corticosteroids and immunosuppressive drugs are drugs of choice in secondary autoimmune orchitis with testicular vasculitis (10). Dapsone has been reported to be useful in Behçet's disease (8). The impact of untreated testicular vasculitis on fertility is not well-known but seems to be relevant.

The real significance of ASA in infertile men is controversial, and currently, there are no standardized treatment regimens. Oral glucocorticoids are commonly used to suppress antibody production, but to date, no double-blind, randomized trial has confirmed their efficacy. Studies following different protocols report pregnancy rates of approximately 30% (18). Studies in which treatment was continued for more than 3 months reported a significant increase in the number of pregnancies amongst those receiving prednisolone compared with placebo (19). However, a meta-analysis showed no significant improvement in pregnancy rates with prednisolone therapy (18).

Intracytoplasmic sperm injection (ICSI) is considered to be the treatment of choice for patients with severe sperm autoimmunity. Clarke et al. showed no significant differences in fertilization rates (62% versus 58%) or clinical pregnancy rates (19% versus 12%) between sperm antibody-positive and sperm antibody-negative patient groups (20). However, recently, higher fertilization rates during in vitro fertilization (IVF) were reported in patients with ASAs and immunosuppressive therapy compared to IVF alone. Thus, treatment of ASAs using corticosteroids should not be prescribed routinely, but it can be considered in patients with ASAs and previous IVF or ICSI fertilization failure.

References

1. Baker HW. Reproductive effects of nontesticular illness. *Endocrinol Metab Clin North Am* 1998; 27(4): 831–50.

2. Fijak M, Meinhardt A. The testis in immune privilege. *Immunol Rev* 2006; 213: 66–81.

3. Lenzi A, Gandini L, Lombardo F, Rago R, Paoli D, Dondero F. Antisperm antibody detection: 2. Clinical, biological, and statistical correlation between methods. *Am J Reprod Immunol* 1997; 38(3): 224–30.

4. D'Cruz OJ, Haas GG Jr, Reichlin M. Autoantibodies to decondensed sperm nuclear deoxyribonucleic acid in patients with antisperm antibodies and systemic lupus erythematosus detected by immunofluorescence flow cytometry. *Fertil Steril* 1994 October; 62(4): 834–44.

5. Soares PM, Borba EF, Bonfa E, Hallak J, Correa AL, Silva CA. Gonad evaluation in male systemic lupus erythematosus. *Arthritis Rheum* 2007; 56(7): 2352–61.

6. Persellin ST, Menke DM. Isolated polyarteritis nodosa of the male reproductive system. *J Rheumatol* 1992; 19(6): 985–8.

7. Fraenkel-Rubin M, Ergas D, Sthoeger ZM. Limited polyarteritis nodosa of the male and female reproductive systems: Diagnostic and therapeutic approach. *Ann Rheum Dis* 2002; 61(4): 362–4.

8. Pannek J, Haupt G. Orchitis due to vasculitis in autoimmune diseases. *Scand J Rheumatol* 1997; 26: 151–4.

9. de Almeida JL, Campos LM, Paim LB, Leone C, Koch VH, Silva CA. Renal involvement in Schönlein–Henoch purpura: A multivariate analysis of initial prognostic factors. *J Pediatr (Rio J)* 2007; 83(3): 259–66.

10. Walker G, Merry P, Sethia K, Ball RY. A case of testicular lupus. *Lupus* 2000; 9(5): 397–8.

11. Shibahara H, Shiraishi Y, Suzuki M. Diagnosis and treatment of immunologically infertile males with antisperm antibodies. *Reprod Med Biol* 2005; 4: 133–41.

12. Hedger MP, Meinhardt A. Cytokines and the immune-testicular axis. *J Reprod Immunol* 2003; 58(1): 1–26.

13. Eggert-Kruse W, Hofsass A, Haury E, Tilgen W, Gerhard I, Runnebaum B. Relationship between local anti-sperm antibodies and sperm-mucus interaction in vitro and in vivo. *Hum Reprod* 1991; 6(2): 267–76.

14. Griffin JE, Wilson JD. Disorders of the testes and the male reproductive tract. In: Larsen PD, Kronenberg HM, Melmed S, Polonsky KS, editors. *Williams Textbook of Endocrinology*. Philadelphia: Saunders; 2003: 709–69.

15. World Health Organization (WHO). *World Health Organization Manual for the Standardized Investigation, Diagnosis and Management of the Infertile Men*. 1st ed. Cambridge: Cambridge University Press; 2000: 1–86.

16. World Health Organization (WHO). *Laboratory Manual for the Examination of Human Semen and Sperm-Cervical Mucus Interaction*. 4th ed. New York: Cambridge University Press; 1999: 1–128.

17. Fijak M, Iosub R, Schneider E, Linder M, Respondek K, Klug J, Meinhardt A. Identification of immunodominant autoantigens in rat autoimmune orchitis. *J Pathol* 2005; 207(2): 127–38.

18. Kamischke A, Nieschlag E. Analysis of medical treatment of male infertility. *Hum Reprod* 1999; 14(Suppl. 1): 1–23.

19. Hendry WF, Hughes L, Scammell G, Pryor JP, Hargreave TB. Comparison of prednisolone and placebo in subfertile men with antibodies to spermatozoa. *Lancet* 1990; 335: 85–8.

20. Clarke GN, Bourne H, Baker HW. Intracytoplasmic sperm injection for treating infertility associated with sperm autoimmunity. *Fertil. Steril.* 1997; 68: 112–7.

Part VI
Hepatobiliary and Pancreatic Autoimmune Diseases

54
Autoimmune Hepatitis

Miguel Bruguera

Abstract   Autoimmune hepatitis is a chronic liver disease of unknown etiology characterized by hypertransaminasemia, hypergammaglobulinemia and an interface hepatitis in the histological examination of the liver, responsive to the treatment with immunosuppressive drugs. Untreated patients tend to progress to cirrhosis and death. The finding of high titres of autoantibodies in the sera, the efficacy of immunosuppressive therapy and the common association of AIH with autoimmune disorders give support to an autoimmune pathogenesis of the disease.

Keywords: Antinuclear antibodies · smooth muscle antibodies · interface hepatitis · cirrhosis · overlap syndromes · immunosuppression.

Autoimmune hepatitis (AIH) may be defined as a self-perpetuating inflammation of the liver of more than 6 months duration and unknown etiology characterized by the elevation of serum transaminases, hypergammaglobulinemia, high titres of serum autoantibodies and histological changes in the liver mainly consisting in periportal hepatitis associated with variable degree of fibrosis. The disease has a progressive course to cirrhosis without treatment. It is considered to be an autoimmune disease because of its common association with autoimmune extrahepatic disorders and the efficacy of immunosuppressive therapy in inducing clinical, biochemical and histological remission in most cases.

History

Waldenström (1) gave the first description of autoimmune hepatitis in young women in 1950. Mackay et al. (2) proposed in 1956 the term lupoid hepatitis owing to the association of AIH with antinuclear antibodies (ANA) and its similarity with systemic lupus erythematosus. The syndrome has since been described under various names (3). The term autoimmune hepatitis was introduced in 1993 by the International Autoimmune Hepatitis Group, which defined the diagnostic criteria (4). These were reviewed in 1999 by the same group (5).

Epidemiology

In comparison with other liver diseases, such as acute or chronic viral hepatitis or alcoholic and non-alcoholic fatty liver diseases, AIH is an infrequent liver disorder. The prevalence is estimated between 50 and 200 cases per million of inhabitants in Caucasian population of developed countries, similar to the prevalence of other autoimmune liver diseases, such as primary biliary cirrhosis. In Africa and Asia the prevalence is lower than in white populations.

AIH may present at any age in either sex, although it occurs most frequently in women between the ages of 10 and 30 years and during postmenopause (6).

Pathogenesis

The pathogenic mechanisms leading to liver cell destruction in AIH are as yet unknown despite extensive investigation into humoral and cell-mediated immunity. Infectious agents, such as viral agents, and other environmental triggers and host factors (genetic susceptibility) play a role in the development of AIH.

From: Y. Shoenfeld et al. (eds.): *Diagnostic Criteria in Autoimmune Diseases*, DOI: 10.1007/978-1-60327-285-8_54,

Clinical Manifestations

In more than one third of cases the disease has an acute onset, mimicking an acute viral hepatitis, because of the presence of jaundice and a rise of serum transaminases over 1000 UI/L (7). Differential diagnosis with the causes of acute hepatitis should be done in these cases (Table 54.1). A minority of cases with acute clinical presentation develop a fulminant hepatic failure, which may lead to death if a liver transplantation is not urgently carried out.

In the majority of the remaining cases the onset is insidious, and the disease is recognized by the finding of abnormal liver function tests in an asymptomatic patient or by anorexia, pain in the right upper quadrant of the abdomen and easy fatigability. This clinical presentation resembles that of other forms of liver disease, and the diagnosis of AIH requires the exclusion of other causes of chronic liver disease (Table 54.1).

In some cases the disease presents with a complication of an advanced chronic liver disease, which was asymptomatic until this moment, in the form of jaundice, ascites or gastrointestinal bleeding due to the rupture of variceal veins.

Jaundice is a common finding in physical examination, as well as a palpable and tender hepatomegaly.

AIH is associated in about 30% of the cases with extrahepatic manifestations, such as Sjögren syndrome, autoimmune thyroiditis, Coomb's positive haemolytic anemia, allergic capillaritis, idiopathic thrombocytopenic purpura and rheumatoid arthritis.

Biochemical Features

Serum transaminase activity and gamma globulin levels are elevated in nearly all patients. Both parameters are most useful in assessing the activity of the disease. Hypergammaglobulinemia is polyclonal with typical predominance of IgG fraction. Hyperbilirrubinemia

occurs in jaundiced patients. Serum alkaline phosphatase level is frequently increased, but usually below two-fold normal. A value above three-fold normal is unusual and suggests an overlap syndrome with primary biliary cirrhosis (8).

Serological Features

Several autoantibodies, detected by indirect immunofluorescence, are relevant to the diagnosis of AIH. ANA are the earliest serological marker of AIH. They are directed against structural components of the cell nucleus. Subtyping of ANA is not useful for diagnostic purposes. ANA are detected by indirect immunofluorescence on rat liver. The most common immunofluorescence patterns are homogenous and speckled patterns. Smooth muscle antibodies (SMA) are directed against F-actin and equally relevant.

A titre of more than 1:80 of ANA or of SMA is regarded as diagnostically significant for AIH. One or both are present in 90% of patients (9).

Less than 10% of patients with AIH, particularly children, have antibodies to liver/kidney microsomes (anti-LKM) and lacked ANA or SMA. Anti-LKM are antibodies to CYP 2D6, and should be distinguished in the indirect immunofluorescence test from antimitochondrial antibodies (AMA), which are the hallmark of primary biliary cirrhosis. AMA stains the cells of proximal and distal renal tubules, while anti-LKM stains only the cells of proximal renal tubules.

Other autoantibodies, such as antibodies to cytosolic antigens (anti-LC-1 and 2) and antibodies to soluble liver antigens (anti-SLA), may also be found in patients with AIH. AIH has been classified into three types according to the pattern of autoantibodies (Table 54.2). Type 1 AIH is characterized by AMA and/or ANA, type 2 by anti-LKM and type 3 by anti-SLA.

TABLE 54.1 Differential diagnosis of autoimmune hepatitis and diagnostic tests.

Disease	Exclusion by
Acute hepatitis A	Anti-HVA IgM
Acute or chronic hepatitis B	HBsAg, HBV DNA
Acute or chronic hepatitis C	Anti-HCV, HCV RNA
Drug-induced hepatitis	History, drug withdrawal
Primary biliary cirrhosis	Cholestasis, antimitochondrial antibodies
Primary sclerosing cholangitis	Cholangiography
Wilson's disease	Ceruloplasmin, urine copper, copper in the liver
Haemochromatosis ferritin,	Serum iron, transferrin saturation, Iron deposition in the liver

TABLE 54.2 Features of the three subtypes of autoimmune hepatitis.

	AIH tipo 1	AIH tipo 2	AIH tipo 3
Characteristic autoantibodies	ANA, SMA	Anti-LKM	Anti-SLA
Target antigen	Nuclear proteins and actin	Cytochrome P450 (CYP) 2D6	UGA-suppressor associated protein
Prevalence	80%	10–15%	5–10%
Common age of onset	Bimodal (14–30 and > 50 years)	Mainly paediatric	All ages
Extrahepatic manifestations	40%	34%	60%

Pathological Features

The most specific histological lesion of AIH is interface hepatitis with predominant lymphocytes, and plasma cells infiltrate either in portal tracts or in periportal areas. Periportal hepatocytes may be organized forming rosettes surrounded by lymphocytes and plasma cells. A lobular hepatitis may be present. In some patients multinucleated giant hepatic cells may be present. Centrilobular necrosis is rare, but may represent to be an early or acute stage.

There may be variables degrees of portal and periportal fibrosis, and cirrhosis may be present at the time of clinical presentation of the disease.

Diagnosis

The diagnosis of AIH is based on the exclusion of other etiologies of liver diseases (Table 54.1). Criteria for definite and probable diagnosis, established by an international panel of experts, may help to establish the diagnosis (5) (Table 54.3). The diagnosis of AIH should be evoked in patients with high levels of serum transaminases and gamma-globulines, and positive test for serum autoantibodies, when other diagnosis, mainly chronic viral hepatitis, drug-induced, alcoholic and biliary diseases, has been excluded (10).

Clinical Variants

Typically patients with AIH have no cholestasis. The coexistence of biochemical and/or histological features of AIH with those of cholestatic immune-related diseases, such as primary biliary cirrhosis or primary sclerosing cholangitis, is known as overlap syndrome (8, 11). Such patients should receive treatment for each one of their diseases, steroids and ursodeoxycholic acid.

Prognosis

The prognosis of AIH depends on the inflammatory activity, the extent of hepatocellular necrosis and the presence or not of cirrhosis, at the moment of diagnosis. Before the introduction of immunosuppressive therapy survival was reduced, particularly in jaundiced patients. In treated patients the prognosis is good, even in those with cirrhosis, because most of them are good responders. However, cirrhotic patients may develop complications of liver cirrhosis, which may require liver transplantation. In nonresponders patients, in those with suboptimal response and in those with multiple relapses when treatment is withdrawn, the prognosis is not so good, because they have a high probability to develop liver cirrhosis (12).

TABLE 54.3 Scoring system for diagnosis of autoimmune hepatitis of the International Autoimmune Hepatitis Group.

	Parameter	Score
Gender	Female	+2
	Male	0
Ratio of elevation of AP versus ALT	> 3.0	−2
	1.5–3	0
	< 3.0	+2
Total GG or IgG	Times upper normal limit	
	> 2	+3
	1.5-2.0	+2
	1.0–1.5	+1
	< 1.0	0
Autoantibodies ANA, SMA or anti-LKM	> 1:80	+3
	1:80	+2
	1:40	+1
	< 1:40	0
AMA	Positive	−2
	Negative	0
Hepatitis viral markers:		
	Positive	−3
	Negative	+3
Other etiologic factors	Recent hepatotoxic drug usage	
	Yes	−4
	No	+1
	Alcohol (average consumption)	
	< 25 g/day	+2
	> 60 g/day	−2
	Genetic factors: HLA DR3 o DR4,	+1
	Other autoimmune diseases	+2
Response to therapy		
	Complete	+3
	Relapse	+3
Liver histology		
	Interface hepatitis	+1
	Predominant lymphoplasmocytic infiltrate	+1
	None of the above	−3
	Biliary changes	−3

Interpretation of aggregate scores: definite AIH, greater than 15 before treatment and greater than 17 after treatment; probable AIH, 10–15 before treatment and 12–17 after treatment.

Treatment

The treatment of AIH is immunosuppression (13). Standard treatment is either prednisone or prednisolone alone or a combination of prednisone and azathioprine (Table 54.4). Both are effective in inducing remission in 80% of the cases. Prednisone monotherapy is preferred in children and young adults, while combination therapy is preferred in adult and old patients, in order to give lower doses of steroids, and in this way to minimize adverse effects of long-term treatment with steroids (Table 54.5).

TABLE 54.4 Treatment of autoimmune hepatitis.

A. Predniso(lo)ne monotherapy
  – First 2 weeks: 30–60 mg/day (according to the severity of clinical
    presentation)
  – Reduction by 5 mg every 10 days or 10 mg every two weeks until
    normalization of transaminases
  – After remission is reached maintenance dose 10–15 mg/day
  – After several months of remission try maintenance dose of
    5–7.5 mg/day. If transaminases rise above upper normal value
    increase the dose of prednisone to induce remission.
  – If response is suboptimal (transaminases are not normal) after
    several months of treatment introduce azathioprine (50–100 mg/
    day) or another immunosuppressive agent.
  – Cessation of therapy after at least 2 years of remission, and do blood
    tests every 1 or 2 months for 6 months to detect relapse.
  – If relapse occurs, start treatment again (dose of prednisone
    depending on the severity of relapse) and decrease the dose
    progressively.

B. Combination therapy
  – Half dose of predniso(lo)ne associated with 50 mg/day of
    azathioprine.
  – Reduce dose of prednisone in the same way as in the monotherapy
    schedule, but maintain a fixed dose of 50 mg/day of azathioprine

TABLE 54.5 Side effects of predniso(lo)ne.

Cosmetic changes (acne, facial rounding, obesity, hirsutism)
Bone changes (osteoporosis, vertebral compression,
  avascular necrosis of bone)
Weight gain
Diabetes mellitus
Cataract
Hypertension
Psychiatric symptoms (euphoria, psychosis, depression)

Clinical remission is defined by the normalization of serum transaminase value (14). Once remission is achieved a low-dose immunosuppressive treatment (5–10 mg of prednisone or 100 mg of azathioprine) should be continued for at least 2 years to reduce the risk of relapse. Azathioprine monotherapy does not induce remission, but can maintain the remission induced by prednisone or the combination prednisone–azathioprine. Therapy should not be withdrawn in any patient who has not achieved complete normalization in biochemistry (15). In those with normal biochemistry for two years treatment can be abandoned. Despite there being a high risk of relapse, as many as 30% of patients could remain in remission.

The proportion of relapsers is related to the duration of immunosuppressive treatment following remission. If the patient experiences a relapse after withdrawal of immunosuppression a long-term low-dose immunosuppressive treatment should be introduced for the maintenance of remission.

If complete remission (normal transaminase values) is not achieved with the combination of prednisone and azathioprine, the addition of another immunosuppressive drug, such as tacrolimus, cyclosporin A or mycofenolatemophetil, is recommended, since the risk of progression to cirrhosis is very high in patients with suboptimal response (16). Failure to achieve remission requires to assess if the diagnosis of AIH is correct and the patient's compliance to the treatment. The use of other immunosuppressive drugs should also be recommended in patients who developed severe adverse effects with steroids.

Liver transplantation is indicated in patients in the end stage of AIH with cirrhosis and in those who present liver failure at onset. Results of liver transplantation are usually excellent.

During pregnancy steroid treatment should not be abandoned. Pregnant patients with compensated cirrhosis must be submitted to an esophageal examination to assess the size of varices.

References

1. Waldenström J. Leber, Blutproteine und Nahrungseiweib. *Dtsch Gesellsch Verd Stoffw.* 1950; 15: 113–119.
2. Mackay IR, Taft CO, Cowlings DS. Lupoid hepatitis. *Lancet* 1956; 2: 1323–1326.
3. Sherlock S. Diseases of the liver. Seventh ed, 1985, Blackwell, London.
4. Johnson PJ, McFarlane IG Meeting report of the International Autoimmune Hepatitis Group. *Hepatology* 1993; 18: 998–1005.
5. International Autoimmune Hepatitis Group Report. Review of criteria for diagnosis of autoimmune hepatitis. *J Hepatol* 1999; 31: 929–938.
6. Kravitz EL. Autoimmune hepatitis. *N Engl J Med*; 2006; 354: 54–66.
7. Nikias GA, Batts KP, Czaja AJ. The nature and prognostic implications of autoimmune hepatitis with acute presentation. *J Hepatol* 1994; 21: 866–871.
8. Chazouillieres O, Wendum D, Serfaty L, Montembault S, Rosmorduc O, Poupon R. Primary biliary cirrhosis-autoimmune hepatitis overlap syndrome: clinical features and response therapy. *Hepatology* 1998; 28: 296–301.
9. Czaja AJ, Freese DK. Diagnosis and treatment of autoimmune hepatitis. *Hepatology* 2002; 36: 479–497.
10. Czaja AJ, Hamburger HA. Autoantibodies in liver diseases. *Gastroenterology* 2001; 120: 239–249.
11. Washington MK. Autoimmune liver disease: overlap and outliers. Modern Pathol, 2007; 20: S15–S30.
12. Manns MP, Vogel A. Autoimmune hepatitis, from mechanism to therapy. *Hepatology* 2006; 43: S132–S144.
13. Czaja AJ. Treatment strategies in autoimmune hepatitis. *Clin Liver Dis* 2002; 6: 799–824.
14. Al-Chalabi T, Heneghan MA. Remission in autoimmune hepatitis: What is it, and can it ever be achieved?. *Am J Gastroenterol* 2007; 102: 1013–1015.
15. Verma S, Gunuwan B, Mendler M, Govindrajan S, Redeker A. Factors predicting relapse and poor outcome in type I autoimmune hepatitis: role of cirrhosis development, patterns of transaminases during remission, and plasma cell activity in the liver biopsy. *Am J Gastroenterol* 2004; 99: 1510–1516.
16. Montano Loza AJ, Czaja AJ. Current therapy for autoimmune hepatitis. *Nature Clin Pract Gastroenterol Hepatol*, 2007; 4: 202–214.

55
Primary Biliary Cirrhosis

Carlo Selmi and M. Eric Gershwin

Abstract   Primary biliary cirrhosis (PBC) is a chronic cholestatic liver disease of unknown etiology for which an autoimmune pathogenesis is supported by clinical and experimental data, including the presence of autoantibodies and autoreactive T cells. In fact, PBC diagnosis is based mainly on the detection of high titer serum anti-mitochondrial antibodies (AMA) or PBC-specific anti-nuclear antibodies (ANA). Several animal models have been described, whereas multiple candidates have been proposed to initiate disease in a genetically susceptible host by molecular mimicry. The natural history of the disease may vary widely whereas no prognostic indexes are currently accepted. The only established medical treatment is based on ursodeoxycholic acid whereas liver transplantation is required in end stages.

Keywords   Autoimmune cholangitis · bile duct cell · mitochondrial antigens

Primary biliary cirrhosis (PBC) is a chronic cholestatic liver disease of autoimmune pathogenesis in which biliary epithelial cells (BEC) lining the small and medium size intrahepatic bile ducts are targeted by an immune-mediated injury. Progressive destruction of BEC ultimately leads to fibrosis and cirrhosis.

Epidemiology

The most commonly affected demographic group is represented by middle-age women (1). PBC affects members of all races (with a possible protection for African Americans), but epidemiological data suggest a wide geographical variability in disease prevalence rates ranging from 40 to 400 per million in the general population, being more common in Northern Europe and USA (2).

History

In 1851, Addison and Gull first described the clinical picture of prolonged obstructive jaundice without obstruction of major bile ducts that was later coined as the Addison–Gull syndrome (3). The term PBC was first introduced in 1950 by Ahrens and colleagues who described a rare condition characterized by the presence of a progressive chronic liver disease with chronic cholestasis (4). A milestone for the definition of PBC as an autoimmune disease was the discovery of its specific association with high-titer serum anti-mitochondrial antibodies (AMA), found in over 90% of patients. The major AMA autoantigen was identified and cloned for the first time in 1987 as the E2 subunit of the pyruvate dehydrogenase complex (PDC-E2) (5).

Pathogenesis

Although the aetiology of PBC remains unknown, it is well-established that PBC is an organ-specific autoimmune disease in which exposure to environmental factors, possibly bacteria or chemicals, triggers the breakdown of immune tolerance to self-PDC, in a genetically predisposed individual (6). Several immunological phenomena have been described in PBC including abnormalities in innate immune response and the presence of autoreactive anti-self PDC-E2 B and T lymphocytes in the affected liver, thus suggesting a generalized autoimmune process in which both innate and adaptive (humoral and cellular) immune responses are jointly involved in the pathogenesis of the disease. Figure 55.1 shows the proposed xenobiotic theory for the pathogenesis of PBC.

Clinical Manifestations

Following the discovery of serum AMA as diagnostic hallmark, the use of screening tests evolved considerably and led to a significant shift in disease presentation patterns,

From: Y. Shoenfeld et al. (eds.): *Diagnostic Criteria in Autoimmune Diseases*, DOI: 10.1007/978-1-60327-285-8_55,
© 2008, Humana Press, Totowa, NJ

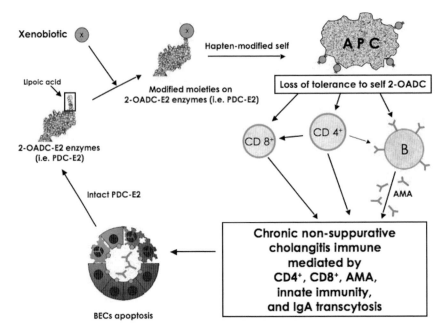

FIGURE 55.1. The proposed theory based on xenobiotics for the induction of PBC. A chemical compound found in the environment substitutes or complexes with the lipoic acid residue attached to the main AMA autoantigen (PDC-E2) liberated by apoptotic bile duct cells. This complex constitutes a modified self that is uptaken by antigen-presenting cells (APC). These cells are critical to the breakdown of tolerance by initiating the autoimmune response by T and B cells that ultimately mediate the onset of the liver injury.

e.g., from being a rare disease associated with jaundice and symptoms of liver failure, to a more common condition diagnosed earlier in its clinical course (1). In fact, up to 60% of the patients are currently diagnosed at asymptomatic stages. Signs and symptoms at presentation are illustrated in Table 55.1. Once disease has progressed to advanced stages, complications can be both metabolic, mainly secondary to long-lasting cholestasis, and related to cirrhosis itself. The latter include malabsorption with steatorrhoea, a reduction in bone density with features of osteopenia and in some cases frank osteoporosis, portal hypertension, and hepatocellular carcinoma. Of note, portal hypertension in PBC may occur early in the course of disease, in some cases before any other sign of cirrhosis. Finally, PBC may be associated in about 30% of the cases with extrahepatic autoimmune disorders mainly Sjögren's syndrome, Raynaud's syndrome, and autoimmune thyroid disease (7).

Pathological Features

Histologically, PBC is characterized by portal inflammation and progressive destruction of intrahepatic bile ducts. Four different stages are recognized according to Ludwig (8) (Table 55.2).

Biochemical Features

The main laboratory abnormalities observed in PBC are summarized in Table 55.3.

Serological Features

Serum AMA represent the immunoserological hallmark of PBC, being detectable in 90–95% of patients with a specificity close to 100%, and they are believed to precede the clinical onset of disease by several years. AMA are

TABLE 55.1. Symptoms and signs of PBC at presentation.

	Prevalence (%)
Asymptomatic	Up to 60
Fatigue	Up to 80
Pruritus	20–70
Hepatomegaly	70
Hyperpigmentation	25
Splenomegaly	15
Jaundice	10
Abdominal pain	10
Xanthelasmas	5–10

TABLE 55.2. Histological stages of PBC according to Ludwig classification (8).

I:	Extensive lymphocytic infiltration around BEC in the portal tract
II:	Progressive loss of normal bile ducts with an involvement of the surrounding parenchyma
III:	Fibrosis
IV:	Cirrhosis with regenerative nodules

TABLE 55.3. Biochemical and serological features of primary biliary cirrhosis (PBC). The semiquantitative ($\uparrow\uparrow$) system indicates the extent of the observed abnormalities.

	Changes
Biochemical feature	
Alkaline phosphatase	$\uparrow\uparrow\uparrow\uparrow$
γ-Glutamyl transferase	$\uparrow\uparrow$
AST/ALT	$\uparrow/\uparrow$
IgM/IgG	$\uparrow\uparrow/=$
Cholesterol	$\uparrow\uparrow$
Total bilirubin	$\uparrow\uparrow$ (late stages)
Serological feature	
AMA	95%
PBC-specific ANA	30–50%

routinely detected by indirect immunofluorescence (IIF) on rat liver/kidney and stomach sections and Hep2 cell lines. Besides IIF, AMA can be detected with more accurate serological assays that are currently not used for routine tests. Of note, neither the titer nor the isotype of AMA are associated with disease severity or predict disease outcome (9). In addition to AMA, 50% of PBC cases are characterized by the presence of highly disease-specific autoantibodies direct to nuclear antigens (ANA). Two distinct ANA patterns at IIF, i.e., rim-like (produced by autoantibodies to the nuclear pore complex proteins gp210 and nucleoporin p62) and multiple nuclear dot (with sp100 and PML proteins as the major targets) patterns are specific for PBC and recent evidence suggests that PBC-specific ANA are associated with a more severe disease (10).

Diagnostic Criteria

The diagnosis of PBC relies on the presence of two of three criteria illustrated in Table 55.4. A liver biopsy is important not only for the diagnosis of some cases (particularly in AMA-negative patients) but for the staging of disease. Different from other autoimmune diseases, diagnostic criteria for PBC are currently accepted and used worldwide despite one line of knowledge that suggests that a "definite" diagnosis should be made when all three criteria are met while the term "probable PBC" is to be used when only two are fulfilled (11). This classification, however, does not

TABLE 55.4. Diagnostic criteria for primary biliary cirrhosis (PBC). The diagnosis is made when two of three criteria are fulfilled. It is of note that the proposed definition of "probable" and "definite" PBC when three or two conditions are met respectively is incomplete.

1. A persistent (>6 months) increase in serum alkaline phosphatase above 1.5 times the upper limit of the normal range
2. Serum AMA >1:40
3. Histological features compatible with PBC

represent the full spectrum of cases because AMA-negative should be regarded as clinically identical to the AMA-positive counterpart (12).

Prognosis

PBC shows a rate of progression that varies widely among patients, ranging from cases with a slow progression of disease over decades to patients having a rapid and fatal course. Approximately 30% of cases show complete biochemical response to medical treatment and 20% a delay of histological progression (13). However, symptomatic patients, those with advanced disease at diagnosis and patients who do not respond to medical treatment, still manifest a markedly elevated risk of dying or undergoing liver transplantation (14).

Prediction

The Mayo score based on age, the presence of ascites, serum bilirubin, albumin, and prothrombin time is the most widely used to predict the natural history and survival of patients (15) although it might prove more helpful in advanced stages. Conversely, it has most recently been suggested that specific ANA patterns correlate with a poor prognosis in patients with early stages of PBC (16).

Therapy

Ursodeoxycholic acid (UDCA), a hydrophilic bile acid, is the only drug currently approved for the treatment of patients with PBC. The adequate dosage range from 13 to 15 mg/kg per day. The efficacy of UDCA in improving liver-related survival is still debated, whereas it has been shown to delay the progression of liver damage particularly in early stages, being ineffective in patients with advanced disease (17) but evidence is still somehow conflicting (18). Immunosuppressants have cumulatively failed to demonstrate real effects on natural history of PBC. Liver transplantation still represents the only effective treatment for the end stage of this disease with good survival rates. Pruritus is currently treated with cholestyramine, but in refractory cases rifampicin can be used for a limited time. The opioid antagonists (naloxone and naltrexone) can lead to symptomatic improvement in selected refractory cases but are poorly tolerated. Cholesterol-lowering agents are usually not needed, but they can be safely used during follow-up. Medical treatment for the metabolic bone loss does not differ from the general practice in these cases.

References

1. Kaplan MM, Gershwin ME. Primary biliary cirrhosis. *N Engl J Med* 2005; 353(12): 1261–73.

2. Selmi C, Invernizzi P, Zuin M, Podda M, Gershwin ME. Genetics and geoepidemiology of primary biliary cirrhosis: Following the footprints to disease etiology. *Semin Liver Dis* 2005; 25(3): 265–80.

3. Addison T, Gull W. On a certain affection of the skin-vitiligoides-alpha planus tuberosa. *Guy's Hosp Rev* 1857; 7: 268.

4. Ahrens EH Jr, Payne MA, Kunkel HG, Eisenmenger WJ, Blondheim SH. Primary biliary cirrhosis. *Medicine (Baltimore)* 1950; 29(4): 299–364.

5. Gershwin ME, Mackay IR, Sturgess A, Coppel RL. Identification and specificity of a cDNA encoding the 70 kd mitochondrial antigen recognized in primary biliary cirrhosis. *J Immunol* 1987; 138(10): 3525–31.

6. Giorgini A, Selmi C, Invernizzi P, Podda M, Zuin M, Gershwin ME. Primary biliary cirrhosis: Solving the enigma. *Ann N Y Acad Sci* 2005; 1051: 185–93.

7. Gershwin ME, Selmi C, Worman HJ, et al. Risk factors and comorbidities in primary biliary cirrhosis: A controlled interview-based study of 1032 patients. *Hepatology* 2005; 42(5): 1194–202.

8. Ludwig J, Dickson ER, McDonald GS. Staging of chronic nonsuppurative destructive cholangitis (syndrome of primary biliary cirrhosis). *Virchows Arch A Pathol Anat Histol* 1978; 379(2): 103–12.

9. Van Norstrand MD, Malinchoc M, Lindor KD, et al. Quantitative measurement of autoantibodies to recombinant mitochondrial antigens in patients with primary biliary cirrhosis: relationship of levels of autoantibodies to disease progression. *Hepatology* 1997; 25(1): 6–11.

10. Invernizzi P, Selmi C, Ranftler C, Podda M, Wesierska-Gadek J. Antinuclear antibodies in primary biliary cirrhosis. *Semin Liver Dis* 2005; 25(3): 298–310.

11. James OF, Bhopal R, Howel D, Gray J, Burt AD, Metcalf JV. Primary biliary cirrhosis once rare, now common in the United Kingdom? *Hepatology* 1999; 30(2): 390–4.

12. Invernizzi P, Crosignani A, Battezzati PM, et al. Comparison of the clinical features and clinical course of antimitochondrial antibody-positive and -negative primary biliary cirrhosis. *Hepatology* 1997; 25(5): 1090–5.

13. Locke GR, III, Therneau TM, Ludwig J, Dickson ER, Lindor KD. Time course of histological progression in primary biliary cirrhosis. *Hepatology* 1996; 23(1): 52–6.

14. Degott C, Zafrani ES, Callard P, Balkau B, Poupon RE, Poupon R. Histopathological study of primary biliary cirrhosis and the effect of ursodeoxycholic acid treatment on histology progression. *Hepatology* 1999; 29(4): 1007–12.

15. Dickson ER, Grambsch PM, Fleming TR, Fisher LD, Langworthy A. Prognosis in primary biliary cirrhosis: model for decision making. *Hepatology* 1989; 10(1): 1–7.

16. Wesierska-Gadek J, Penner E, Battezzati PM, et al. Correlation of initial autoantibody profile and clinical outcome in primary biliary cirrhosis. *Hepatology* 2006; 43(5): 1135–44.

17. Gluud C, Christensen E. Ursodeoxycholic acid for primary biliary cirrhosis. *Cochrane Database Syst Rev* 2002; 1: CD000551.

18. Pares A, Caballeria L, Rodes J. Excellent long-term survival in patients with primary biliary cirrhosis and biochemical response to ursodeoxycholic Acid. *Gastroenterology* 2006; 130(3): 715–20.

56
Primary Sclerosing Cholangitis

Sharonjeet Sangha and Christopher L. Bowlus

Abstract   Primary sclerosing cholangitis (PSC) is a chronic cholestatic liver disease, presenting primarily in adults and affecting men more commonly than women. The etiology of PSC is currently unknown but is thought to be secondary to an autoimmune process. PSC is closely associated with IBD, and an immune-mediated response to either gut microflora or extra-intestinal cell-adhesion molecules has also been implicated in its pathogenesis. Patients are typically asymptomatic at time of presentation with variable laboratory findings. Unlike its sister disease, primary biliary cirrhosis (PBC) in which the antimitochondrial autoantibody is pathognomonic, the atypical peri-nuclear antineutrophil antibody of PSC lacks specificity and sensitivity to make it clinically useful. Rather, diagnosis is established typically by cholangiogram findings and exclusion of secondary causes of sclerosing cholangitis. The clinical course is variable, with most patients progressing to cirrhosis and hepatic failure. The median time of diagnosis to death or liver transplantation is 12–15 years. There is no proven medical therapy for PSC. Ursodeoxycholic acid, which is effective for PBC, has only been shown to improve biochemical cholestasis in PSC leaving liver transplantation as the only option for end-stage PSC.

Keywords   Cholestatic liver disease · inflammatory bowel disease · cholangiocarcinoma · ursodeoxycholic acid · liver transplant

Primary sclerosing cholangitis (PSC) is a cholestatic liver disease characterized by inflammation, destruction, and fibrosis of hepatic biliary ducts. It is a progressive disease, leading to biliary cirrhosis, hepatic failure, and in 6–30% of patients, cholangiocarcinoma (1).

Epidemiology

PSC is more common in men than women with men making up approximately 60% of the cases in most series. The average age at time of diagnosis of PSC is 40 years, but PSC can affect children and mild cases may not be diagnosed until the 7th or 8th decade of life. Approximately 75% of patients with PSC have associated inflammatory bowel disease (IBD); 87% have ulcerative colitis (UC) and 13% have Crohn's disease (2). Conversely, 3–5% of IBD patients will have co-existing PSC. It appears that PSC occurs more frequently in people of Caucasian and Northern European descent, although large epidemiologic studies in other populations are lacking. Studies of predominately Caucasian populations in Olmstead County, Minnesota; Oslo, Norway; Swansea,

Wales; and Manitoba, Canada have estimated annual incidence rates of PSC to be 0.90, 1.3, 0.91, and 0.92 cases per 100,000 person-years (3, 4, 5, 6). Our own experience in a population of over three million members enrolled in a large healthcare system in Northern California of whom only 65% were classified as white is somewhat different with an annual incidence of only 0.59 cases per 100,000 person-years (unpublished data).

History

Sclerosing cholangitis was first documented by French surgeon Delbet in 1924 and described as "irregular fibrosis and stenosis of the biliary tree" (7). Until the 1970 s, the diagnosis of PSC was based largely upon findings at time of laparotomy. PSC was considered a rare disease with less than 100 cases reported in the literature. With the advent of endoscopic retrograde cholangiography (ERC), the diagnosis of PSC became more frequent and characterization of PSC as a distinct liver disease emerged.

From: Y. Shoenfeld et al. (eds.): *Diagnostic Criteria in Autoimmune Diseases*, DOI: 10.1007/978-1-60327-285-8_56,
© 2008 Humana Press, Totowa, NJ

Pathogenesis

The pathophysiology of PSC is unknown with progress in the field hampered by the lack of clinical tools to diagnose PSC in early stages and of adequate animal models of the disease. Associations with autoimmune diseases, HLA haplotypes, and autoantibodies are suggestive of an immune-mediated process. However, features atypical of autoimmune disorders, such as male predominance and the lack of response to immunosuppressive agents, have lead some to challenge the idea that PSC is an autoimmune phenomenon.

On the basis of the association of PSC with IBD, this theory proposes that immune responses to gut microflora within the biliary tree play a primary role in the pathogenesis of PSC (illustrated in Figure 56.1). In the setting of colonic disease, mucosal permeability allows translocation of gut microflora into the portal circulation. Bacteremia within the biliary tree results in T-cell proliferation, release of multiple cytokines and chemokines, as well as activation of B cells and secretion of autoantibodies against biliary epithelial cells. This chronic inflammatory response is responsible for progressive fibrosis, cholestasis, and biliary cirrhosis.

However, this model does not explain the phenomenon of PSC occurring in ulcerative colitis patients after colectomy. More recently, data from David Adams's group has suggested a model of aberrant targeting of autoreactive memory cells in the gut to the liver involving specific adhesion molecules, chemokines, and chemokine receptors (8). Although mucosal address in cell-adhesion molecule (MAdCAM1) is normally restricted to gut-associated lymphoid tissue, hepatic expression has been found in several inflammatory liver diseases and *in vitro* studies support integrin α4β7-mediated adhesion to liver endothelium (9). In addition, vascular adhesion protein 1 (VAP1) may play a role in recruitment of lymphocytes to both the liver and intestine (10). Furthermore, expression of the chemokine CCL25 on PSC liver epithelium appears to recruit T cells expressing the chemokine receptor CCR9 and α4β7. In PSC, these CCR9$^+$α4β7$^+$ cells make up 20% of liver-infiltrating lymphocytes compared with <2% in other liver diseases. CCL21 is also increased in PSC liver and can mediate chemotaxis of CCR7$^+$ liver-infiltrating lymphocytes *in vivo* (11). Genetic evidence supports a role for CCR5 as well. Recently, a 32-bp deletion of the CCR5 gene (CCR5-Δ32) that is found with high frequency in European populations was associated with a decreased susceptibility to PSC but not IBD, suggesting that a functional CCR5 plays a role in the development of PSC but not IBD (12). The factors involved in the specific targeting of lymphocytes to biliary epithelium in PSC are not understood but likely involve CX3CL1, CXCL12 and/or CXCL16.

An underlying genetic predisposition to PSC is well supported. First-degree relatives appear to have a 100-fold increased risk of developing PSC when compared with the general population (13). Further support is gained by the

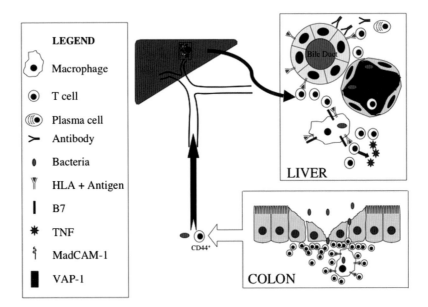

FIGURE 56.1. A model for the immunobiology of PSC. Autoreactive lymphocytes are activated in the colon. Increased permeability of the intestinal mucosa allows bacterial antigens to enter the circulation. Antigens and CD44$^+$ memory cells travel through the portal vein to the liver. Toll-like receptors on biliary epithelium bind bacterial antigens and activate innate immune responses. Memory cells bind to aberrantly expressed adhesion molecules on endothelium of the portal vein. Unknown chemokines and other adhesion molecules lead to migration of inflammatory cells to the bile duct.

increased prevalence of certain Human Leukocyte Antigen (HLA) haplotypes among PSC patients, particularly *DRB1*0301-DQB1*0201*. Interestingly, this HLA haplotype is not associated with IBD and other genetic polymorphisms associated with IBD do not appear to influence susceptibility to PSC. Genome-wide association studies of large, well-characterized cohorts of PSC patients and well-matched controls will hopefully identify the major genetic elements involved in PSC and shed new light on its pathogenesis.

Clinical Manifestations

PSC typically presents with symptoms of cholestasis but may also present with acute cholangitis or complications of advanced liver disease (Table 56.1). Most patients are asymptomatic during early stages of disease, while the development of jaundice, pruritis, fever, fatigue, weight loss, and abdominal pain are signs of advanced disease. Physical exam findings include jaundice, hepatomegaly, and splenomegaly. Complications of chronic cholestasis are vitamin deficiency, steatorrhea, and metabolic bone disease. The most dreaded complication of PSC is cholangiocarcinoma, which has a nearly 1% annual incidence in PSC patients.

The IBD frequently associated with PSC has a unique phenotype and is often asymptomatic. Typical features are pancolitis, "backwash" ileitis, and rectal sparing. Even in the PSC patient without signs or symptoms of IBD, colonoscopy should be performed to rule out occult IBD. This is particularly important given that PSC patients with IBD have a greater risk of colon cancer than IBD patients without PSC.

Pathological Features

The bile duct is the primary site of injury in PSC. Although large intra- and extra-hepatic ducts are typically affected, small bile ducts may also be involved. Segmental strictures with proximal dilation of bile ducts on cholangiogram are

TABLE 56.1. Symptoms and signs of PSC.

Prevalence	
Asymptomatic	15–40%
Fatigue	43–75%
Pruritus	25–70%
Jaundice	30–66%
Hepatomegaly	34–62%
Abdominal pain	16–33%
Splenomegaly	14–30%
Hyperpigmentation	25%
Weight loss	10–20%
Variceal Bleeding	6–14%
Ascites	6–10%

classic findings. Histological features on liver biopsy include bile duct proliferation, periductal fibrosis with pathognomonic "onion-skinning" lesion, periductal inflammation, and bile duct obliteration (14). However, findings may be nonspecific or even normal if only large ducts are involved. Histological features of PSC can be classified into four stages using Ludwig criteria, but prognostic models do not necessarily include liver biopsy (14).

Biochemical Features

In asymptomatic patients, the diagnosis is often based on biochemical features. Serum liver tests are usually consistent with a cholestatic pattern of disease, elevated alkaline phosphatase levels, and mildly elevated serum aminotransferases, but normal liver biochemistries can also be present. PSC should be considered in the differential diagnosis of any patient with cholestatic liver tests, particularly those with IBD or other autoimmune diseases. Serum albumin and bilirubin abnormalities often present during later stages of disease. As with other cholestatic liver diseases, elevated liver and urine copper levels, as well as decreased serum ceruloplasmin may be present.

Serological Features

Multiple autoantibodies have been detected in the serum of PSC patients but none are sufficiently sensitive or specific to have clinical utility. Serum pANCA is the most prevalent, being present in up to 88% of patients (15). Detection of pANCA through indirect immunofluorescence (IIF) reveals an atypical pattern with rim-like staining of the nuclear membrane and staining of intranuclear spots, thought to be invaginations of the nuclear membrane (15). Antinuclear, anticolon, antismooth muscle, anticaridiolipin, thyroperoxidase, and rheumatoid factor autoantibodies are less prevalent. Antimitochondrial antibody is not detected in PSC patients and can be useful in differentiating PSC from PBC. Other serological abnormalities may include hypergammaglobulinemia (30%) and elevated serum IgM (50%) (1).

Diagnostic Criteria

The diagnosis of PSC relies upon clinical assessment, laboratory findings, histopathology, serology, and cholangiography (Table 56.2). In addition, all secondary causes of cholangitis must be excluded. Exclusion criteria include biliary trauma, ischemia, malignancy, and infection. Cholangiography is the most accurate means of PSC diagnosis. Findings include a classic beaded appearance, with diffuse strictures and dilatations of hepatic bile ducts (1, 16).

TABLE 56.2. Biochemical and serological features of PSC.

Biochemical feature	Changes
Alkaline phosphatase	⇑ or normal
AST/ALT	⇑ or normal
Bilirubin	⇑ or normal
	(late stages)
Serological feature	**Frequency**
pANCA	30 – 88%

Magnetic resonance cholangiography (MRC) has recently been shown to be sufficiently sensitive and specific compared with ERC in accurately diagnosing PSC. However, ERC should still be considered if there is a high index of suspicion and the MRC is negative or non-diagnostic. A small number of patients with cholestatic liver tests will have biopsy features consistent with PSC but normal cholangiograms, and should be considered to have small duct PSC. Whether IBD is a prerequisite for this diagnosis remains controversial.

Prognosis

The clinical course of PSC is variable, but is characterized by progressive cholestasis and the eventual development of end-stage liver disease. The average time from diagnosis to death or liver transplant is 12 to 15 years, but the progression is variable. Also, the development of cholangiocarcinoma, which tends to be more frequent early in the course of disease, portends a dismal prognosis.

Prediction

Many models have been developed to prognosticate life expectancy of PSC patients. The Mayo Clinic Revised Natural History Model for PSC is currently the most universally accepted model to predict survival probability (17). Risk score calculation is based on age, bilirubin, albumin, AST, and prior history of variceal bleeding. However, the accuracy of the Mayo model and other systems is poor and should not be applied to individual patients.

Therapy

Currently, there is no proven medical therapy for the treatment of PSC and liver transplant continues to be the only effective treatment for end-stage PSC. Outcomes from liver transplantation are extremely good with 5-year patient survival rates of more than 90%. Numerous clinical studies have looked at various therapeutic agents but usually in small case studies. Immunosuppressive and anti-inflammatory agents, such as methotrexate, cyclosporine, or colchicine, have failed to show clinical benefit. Ursodeoxycholic acid (UDCA), a hydrophilic bile acid, is the only widely used drug that has been studied in large randomized controlled trials. At dose of 15–25 mg/kg/d, it has not been shown to improve the clinical course of PSC, though, in some studies treatment with UDCA leads to improvement in biochemical cholestasis with reductions in AST, ALT, GGT, alkaline phosphatase, and bilirubin (18). Evidence is also suggestive of histological improvement, however, data is limited. UDCA has not been shown to improve survival, symptoms, or the cholangiographic appearance of PSC but may decrease the risk of colon cancer.

Management of the symptoms and complications of cholestasis of PSC are similar to other causes such as primary biliary cirrhosis with exception of the treatment of high-grade biliary strictures with endoscopic dilatation. This has been shown to improve symptoms, serum liver tests, and cholangiographic appearance (19). Whether this alters the natural history of the disease is not known. Often distinguishing a benign stricture from a cholangiocarcinoma can be challenging, but is imperative for the appropriate management of the patient. In light of the poor prognosis of cholangiocarcinoma in all but the earliest stages of disease, we advocate screening of PSC patients with CEA and CA19–9 every 6 months and annual MRC.

References

1. Lee, Y.M. and M.M. Kaplan, *Management of primary sclerosing cholangitis.* Am J Gastroenterol, 2002. 97(3): pp. 528–34.
2. Fausa, O., E. Schrumpf, and K. Elgjo, *Relationship of inflammatory bowel disease and primary sclerosing cholangitis.* Semin Liver Dis, 1991. 11(1): pp. 31–9.
3. Bambha, K., et al., *Incidence, clinical spectrum, and outcomes of primary sclerosing cholangitis in a United States community.* Gastroenterology, 2003. 125(5): pp. 1364–9.
4. Boberg, K.M., et al., *Incidence and prevalence of primary biliary cirrhosis, primary sclerosing cholangitis, and autoimmune hepatitis in a Norwegian population.* Scand J Gastroenterol, 1998. 33(1): pp. 99–103.
5. Kingham, J.G., N. Kochar, and M.B. Gravenor, *Incidence, clinical patterns, and outcomes of primary sclerosing cholangitis in South Wales, United Kingdom.* Gastroenterology, 2004. 126(7): pp. 1929–30.
6. Bernstein, C.N., et al., *The prevalence of extraintestinal diseases in inflammatory bowel disease: a population-based study.* Am J Gastroenterol, 2001. 96(4): pp. 1116–22.
7. Delbet, M., *Retrecissement du choledoque. Cholecysto-duodenostomie.* Bull Mem Soc Chir Paris, 1924. 50: pp. 1144–6.
8. Adams, D.H. and B. Eksteen, *Aberrant homing of mucosal T cells and extra-intestinal manifestations of inflammatory bowel disease.* Nat Rev Immunol, 2006. 6(3): pp. 244–51.
9. Grant, A.J., et al., *MAdCAM-1 expressed in chronic inflammatory liver disease supports mucosal lymphocyte adhesion to*

hepatic endothelium (*MAdCAM-1 in chronic inflammatory liver disease*). Hepatology, 2001. 33(5): pp. 1065–72.

10. Grant, A.J., et al., *Homing of mucosal lymphocytes to the liver in the pathogenesis of hepatic complications of inflammatory bowel disease.* Lancet, 2002. 359(9301): pp. 150–7.

11. Grant, A.J., et al., *Hepatic expression of secondary lymphoid chemokine (CCL21) promotes the development of portal-associated lymphoid tissue in chronic inflammatory liver disease.* Am J Pathol, 2002. 160(4): pp. 1445–55.

12. Henckaerts, L., et al., *CC-type chemokine receptor 5-Delta32 mutation protects against primary sclerosing cholangitis.* Inflamm Bowel Dis, 2006. 12(4): pp. 272–7.

13. Bergquist, A., et al., *Increased prevalence of primary sclerosing cholangitis among first-degree relatives.* J Hepatol, 2005. 42(2): pp. 252–6.

14. Ludwig, J., et al., *Morphologic features of chronic hepatitis associated with primary sclerosing cholangitis and chronic ulcerative colitis.* Hepatology, 1981. 1(6): pp. 632–40.

15. Terjung, B. and H.J. Worman, *Anti-neutrophil antibodies in primary sclerosing cholangitis.* Best Pract Res Clin Gastroenterol, 2001. 15(4): pp. 629–42.

16. Zakim D, B.T., *Hepatology.* 4th edn. Philadelphia, PA: Elsevier Science; 2003.

17. Kim, W.R., et al., *A revised natural history model for primary sclerosing cholangitis.* Mayo Clin Proc, 2000. 75(7): pp. 688–94.

18. Chen, W. and C. Gluud, *Bile acids for primary sclerosing cholangitis.* Cochrane Database Syst Rev, 2003(2): p. CD003626.

19. Lee, J.G., et al., *Endoscopic therapy of sclerosing cholangitis.* Hepatology, 1995. 21(3): pp. 661–7.

57
Extrahepatic Manifestations in Patients with Chronic Hepatitis C Virus Infection

Pilar Brito-Zerón, Albert Bové and Manuel Ramos-Casals

Abstract Patients with chronic hepatitis C virus (HCV) infection often present autoimmune clinical and analytical features, which are often called extrahepatic manifestations. Earlier studies described the association of HCV with several organ-specific manifestations including pulmonary, renal, cutaneous or articular processes and as with the presence of circulating autoantibodies. There is increasing evidence of a close association of HCV with autoimmune and hematological processes, and this may be related to the extrahepatic tropism of the virus. The sialotropism of HCV may explain the close association with SS, whereas its lymphotropism links the virus to cryoglobulinemia, autoimmune cytopenias and lymphoma. The substantial overlap between cryoglobulinemic features and the classification criteria for some systemic autoimmune diseases (SAD) (SLE, RA and PAN) make the differentiation between mimicking and coexistence difficult. This review analyses recent data on the close association of chronic HCV infection with autoimmune (either systemic or organ-specific) and lymphoproliferative processes.

Keywords Hepatitis C virus · extrahepatic manifestations · lymphoma · cryoglobulinemia · Sjögren's syndrome · rheumatoid arthritis · antiphospholipid syndrome · sarcoidosis

Introduction

The hepatitis C virus (HCV), a linear, single-stranded RNA virus identified in 1989, is recognized as one of the viruses most often associated with autoimmune features. A decade ago, various authors described the association of HCV infection with a heterogeneous group of extrahepatic conditions, such as pulmonary fibrosis, cutaneous vasculitis, glomerulonephritis, Mooren ulcers, porphyria cutanea tarda or lichen planus, although it is currently accepted that a weak degree of association exists in some of them (1). More recently, there has been growing interest in the association of chronic HCV infection with circulating autoantibodies, lymphoproliferative processes and autoimmune (both systemic and organ-specific) diseases.

Autoantibodies Associated with Chronic HCV Infection

Circulating autoantibodies are often detected in patients with chronic HCV infection (2, 3). Antinuclear antibodies, rheumatoid factor and anti-smooth muscle antibodies are the most frequently found, whereas other autoantibodies (such as anti-dsDNA, anti-ENA, AMA or antiLKM-1) are infrequent (Table 57.1). ANA have been detected in 589 (18.6%) of 3169 unselected HCV patients included in 16 studies (Table 57.1), although the geographic prevalence varied significantly. Yee et al. reported a three-fold higher prevalence of ANA in HCV females compared with that in males, with no correlation between ANA and the response to antiviral therapy, whereas Stroffolini et al. found no correlation between non-organ-specific autoantibodies (NOSA) and the main HCV-related epidemiological, biochemical and histological features, or the response to antiviral treatment. This suggests that the presence of ANA or NOSA in HCV patients should not be considered a contraindication for antiviral treatment. With respect to other immunological markers, Watt et al. found a correlation between serum immunoglobulin levels in HCV patients (IgA, IgG, and total Ig) and histological progression to liver fibrosis. These results are consistent with our findings in 321 patients with HCV-related cryoglobulinemia, in whom hypergammaglobulinemia was observed more frequently in cirrhotic than in non-cirrhotic patients.

From: Y. Shoenfeld et al. (eds.): *Diagnostic Criteria in Autoimmune Diseases*, DOI: 10.1007/978-1-60327-285-8_57,
© 2008 Humana Press, Totowa, NJ

TABLE 57.1. Meta-analysis of the main studies analysing prevalence of autoantibodies in unselected series of patients with chronic HCV infection.

Author	HCV patients (n)	Cryoglobulins	RF	ANA	DNA	ENA	AMA
Fried et al. (4)	62	–	–	13	–	–	–
Abuaf et al. (5)	272	–	–	50	–	–	0
Borotto et al. (6)	97	–	–	20	–	–	0
Rolachon et al. (7)	93	–	–	14	–	–	0
Pawlotsky et al. (8)	61	21	43	13	–	0	0
McFarlane et al. (9)	101	–	–	0	–	–	0
Richardet et al. (10)	156	–	–	18	–	–	2
Clifford et al. (11)	92	9/68	35/46	13	–	–	–
Czaja et al. (12)	75	–	21/72	24	0	–	–
Cassani et al. (13)	290	–	–	26	–	–	–
Buskila et al. (14)	90	–	36	31	4	1	–
Rivera et al. (15)	189	64	39	43	–	–	–
Cacoub et al. (16)	321	110/196	107/280	123/302	8/299	10/293	1/288
Drygiannakis et al. (17)	142	–	–	72	4	–	1
Stroffolini et al. (18)	502	–	–	79	–	–	–
Yee et al. (19)	645	–	–	50	–	–	–
Total number	3188	204/514	281/738	589/3169	16/606	11/444	4/1210
Percentage		**39.7%**	**38.1%**	**18.6%**	**2.6%**	**2.5%**	**0.3%**

AMA: antimitochondrial antibodies; ANA: antinuclear antibodies; Cryog: cryoglobulins; ENA: ant-extractable nuclear antigens (anti-Ro/SS-A, anti-La/SS-B, anti-RNP, anti-Sm); HCV: hepatitis C virus; RF: rheumatoid factor.

Organ-Specific Autoimmune Diseases and HCV

Recent studies have analyzed the association of HCV with some organ-specific autoimmune diseases such as thyroiditis or diabetes mellitus (DM).

Thyroiditis and HCV

Bini and Mehandru (4) described the development of thyroid disease (overt or subclinical) in 11% of 225 male HCV-infected patients treated with combined antiviral therapy, although the thyroid disease responded well to specific treatment and was reversible in most cases. Antonelli et al. reported a higher frequency of hypothyroidism (13%) and anti-thyroid antibodies (21%) in 630 treatment-naïve HCV patients compared with that in normal controls, and also found similar results in a subset of these HCV patients with associated mixed cryoglobulinemia (MC). However, other studies, performed in the same geographical area, did not find this close association.

DM and HCV

Antonelli et al. have also reported that the prevalence of type 2 diabetes is higher in patients with MC-HCV than in controls, with diabetic MC-HCV+ patients having a more pronounced autoimmune reactivity than non-HCV patients with classical type 2 diabetes. Metabolic disorders in HCV patients may be related to the development of steatosis, whose clinical significance in HCV patients has recently been emphasized.

Overlap between Systemic Autoimmune Diseases and HCV

The association between HCV and systemic autoimmune diseases (SAD) has generated growing interest in recent years. The extrahepatic manifestations often observed in patients with chronic HCV infection (both clinical and immunological) may lead to the fulfilment of the current classification criteria for some SAD (Table 57.2). Recent research has focused on Sjögren's syndrome (SS), rheumatoid arthritis (RA), antiphospholipid syndrome (APS), cryoglobulinemic vasculitis, and sarcoidosis.

Sjogren's Syndrome

Recent experimental, virological, and clinical evidence has revealed a close association between HCV and SS (5, 6). In 2002, we formed the SS-HCV Study Group, a multicenter international collaboration that has, so far, recruited 137 SS-HCV patients (7). We have found that HCV-associated SS is indistinguishable in most cases from the primary form using the most recent set of classification criteria, and we have proposed the term "SS secondary to HCV" in those HCV patients who fulfill the 2002 Classification Criteria. Chronic HCV infection should be considered an exclusion criterion for the classification of primary SS, not because it mimics primary SS, but because the virus may be implicated in the

TABLE 57.2. Different degrees of association between HCV and systemic autoimmune diseases.

Degree of association	Extrahepatic HCV features overlapping with the classification criteria
HIGH	
– *Sjögren's syndrome*	1. Xerostomia,
	2. Xerophthalmia
	3. Ocular tests (+)
	4. Salivary biopsy (+)
	5. ANA, RF
– *Rheumatoid arthritis*	1. Arthritis of 3 or more joint areas,
	2. Arthritis of hand joints
	3. Symmetric arthritis
	4. RF
– *Systemic lupus erythematosus*	1. Arthritis
	2. Glomerulonephritis
	3. ANA, aPL
	4. Cytopenias
INTERMEDIATE	
– *Polyarteritis nodosa*	1. Weakness
	2. Peripheral neuropathy
	3. Raised creatinine
	4. Positive HBV markers
– *Antiphospholipid syndrome*	1. Positive aPL
	2. Atypical thrombotic events
– *Sarcoidosis*	1. Pulmonary fibrosis
– *Inflammatory myopathies*	1. Weakness
	2. Elevated GOT,GPT
LOW	
– *Systemic sclerosis*	1. Pulmonary fibrosis
– *Wegener granulomatosis*	1. Renal involvement
– *Giant cell arteritis*	1. Age > 50 years
– *Polymyalgia rheumatica*	–
– *Ankylosing spondylitis*	–

development of SS in a specific subset of patients. The main differential aspect between primary and HCV-related SS is the immunological pattern, with a predominance of cryoglobulinemic related markers (mixed cryoglobulins, RF, hypocomplementemia) over SS-related markers (anti-Ro/SS-A and anti-La/SS-B autoantibodies) in HCV-related SS (7). We have found a three-fold higher prevalence of hypocomplementemia in SS-HCV patients compared with patients with primary SS. Cryoglobulinemia seems to be the key immunological marker of SS associated with HCV, having a close association with RF activity and complement activation.

Rheumatoid Arthritis

It is understandable that HCV patients with polyarthritis and positive RF may be clinically classified as having RA. Of the 1988 revised ACR criteria, there are four (arthritis of three or more joint areas, arthritis of hand joints, symmetric arthritis, and RF) that some HCV patients may present. Rosner et al. (8) reviewed the prevalence and clinical characteristics of the HCV-related arthritis exhaustively and also analyzed the significant overlap with RA.

The most frequent clinical presentation of HCV-related arthritis is chronic inflammatory polyarthrtis, which may lead to the fulfillment of the ACR classification criteria for RA in more than 50% of cases.

The existence of morning stiffness, rheumatoid nodules, and erosive arthritis (rarely described in the setting of HCV infection and the presence of antibodies to cyclic citrullinated peptide (CCP) may be useful to diagnose a true coexistence of RA and HCV. Wener et al. found no anti-CCP antibodies in HCV patients, although some false-positive results were observed in patients with MC, whereas Bombardieri et al. found anti-CCP antibodies in 76% of patients with RA and in 60% of those with coexisting RA and HCV, but not in HCV patients, irrespective of their articular involvement. This suggests that anti-CCP antibodies may be useful in discriminating HCV patients with a true RA from those with HCV-associated arthropathy.

Systemic Lupus Erythematosus

Viruses have been postulated as potential etiologic or triggering agents in the pathogenesis of SLE. Chronic HCV infection can induce clinical and serologic features (arthritis, nephropathy, haemocytopenias, and low titers of ANA or anti-dsDNA) which, in combination, may meet the ACR 1982 criteria for SLE. In this context of autoimmunity related to HCV, some reports have suggested that HCV infection may mimic or coexist with SLE. These studies suggest that HCV testing should be considered in the diagnosis of SLE, especially in patients without typical SLE cutaneous features and with low titers of autoantibodies (ANA and anti-dsDNA), liver involvement, or cryoglobulinemia. Conversely, patients with chronic HCV infection and extrahepatic features mimicking SLE should be tested for the presence of ANA and anti-dsDNA.

Antiphospholipid Syndrome

The association between HCV and APS is controversial. We have recently analyzed the clinical features of 45 APS-HCV patients (9). In comparison with unselected APS patients, APS-HCV patients had a lower frequency of typical APS features such as peripheral thrombosis or neurological features but a higher prevalence of some atypical or infrequent features such as myocardial infarction or intraabdominal thrombotic events. In addition, a higher frequency of positive immunological markers was observed in patients with APS-HCV, including ANA, cryoglobulins, hypocomplementemia, and RF. Infectious agents may play a diverse etiopathogenic role in the clinical expression of APS, with bacterial infections probably acting as acute triggering agents of a devastating, multiorganic form of APS (catastrophic APS), whereas chronic viral infections (such as HCV and HIV) may trigger a heterogeneous, atypical presentation of APS (10).

Cryoglobulinemic Vasculitis

Two studies have analyzed the clinical characteristics of HCV-related cryoglobulinemia in large series of patients. Sene et al. (11) studied 125 patients with MC retrospectively and found that cryoglobulinemic vasculitis was associated with advanced age, longer duration of HCV infection, type II MC, and a higher MC serum level. Ferri et al. (12) analyzed demographic, clinical, and serologic features and survival in 231 patients with MC. One hundred and sixty-eight patients were tested for HCV infection, with 155 (92%) being positive. Malignancies were observed in 15% of patients, mainly non-Hodgkin's lymphoma (NHL) and hepatocellular carcinoma, and the main causes of death were related to MC (64%), NHL (13%), and liver involvement (13%).

Sarcoidosis

Since the first case reported in 1993, the number of cases of sarcoidosis associated with HCV reported annually has increased significantly, related or not to antiviral therapy. We reviewed the clinical characteristics of 59 patients with sarcoidosis associated with HCV infection (13) and found that sarcoidosis was triggered by antiviral therapy (mainly by IFN) in 75% of cases. Clinicians should be aware of the possibility that sarcoidosis may initially manifest or reactivate during or shortly after treatment with antiviral therapy in patients with chronic HCV infection.

Autoimmune Cytopenias

Although HCV-related cytopenias are not uncommon, they are usually considered as mild laboratory abnormalities with no clinical significance, especially in patients with hypersplenism. The most frequent is thrombocytopenia, which has a chronic clinical course with severe bleeding being uncommon. De Almeida et al. found no association between HCV genotypes and thrombocytopenia, although HCV-RNA was detected more frequently in the platelets of thrombocytopenic patients than in those with a normal platelet count. Wang et al. (72) described a 10-fold higher frequency of thrombocytopenia in HCV patients compared with HCV-negative controls. Thrombocytopenia correlated with the severity of HCV-related liver disease.

Severe cytopenias are observed in some HCV patients, related or not to antiviral therapy. Thrombocytopenia may be severe ($<30 \times 10^9$/L) in treatment-naïve HCV patients, and in some is associated with concomitant autoimmune diseases, cryoglobulinemia and HIV coinfection (14). Two cases of severe Coombs-positive autoimmune hemolytic anemia (AHA) have recently been reported in patients not treated with IFN. Previously, 17 cases of HCV-related AHA had been reported (14), frequently associated with autoimmune diseases, with cryoglobulinemia being the most frequent immunologic marker.

B-Cell Lymphoproliferative Processes and HCV

The specific tropism of HCV for many extrahepatic cell types, especially for circulating blood cells, has recently been demonstrated by several studies (15, 16), providing a clear link between HCV and the development of autoimmune and neoplasic hematological processes. The susceptibility of blood cells to HCV infection might be enhanced by coexisting additional chronic viral infections.

Recent studies have found a higher prevalence of lymphoproliferative disorders in HCV patients. Matsuo et al. (17) performed an elegant meta-analysis of 23 epidemiological studies on the association between HCV and NHL, including 4049 NHL patients. The summary odds ratio (OR) for NHL in HCV patients was 5.70, being 5.04 for B-cell and 2.51 for T-cell NHL. The prevalence of HCV infection in NHL patients may be higher, since Paydas et al. have described false negative results in the ELISA detection of antiHCV antibodies in 8 (72%) out of 11 patients with NHL, in whom the presence of HCV-RNA was confirmed in paraffin-embedded lymphomatous tissues. This occult HCV infection has also been described in some patients with an altered liver profile of unknown origin, in whom the virus was isolated from liver tissue and circulating mononuclear cells, and was not detectable by ELISA and PCR techniques in serum.

Lymphomagenesis in HCV patients might be initiated by the chronic stimulation of polyclonal B cells by the virus, with the posterior development of specific B-cell clonal expansions and pro-carcinogenic mutations. The close relationship between autoimmunity, viruses and cancer is demonstrated by the description of patients with HCV infection, SAD and B-cell lymphoma, who had a high prevalence of cryoglobulinemia, a high frequency of primary extranodal NHL involvement and a poor prognosis (18). The clearest example is the development of NHL in patients with SS-HCV (19). We recommend a careful evaluation of patients with B-cell NHL in order to detect silent autoimmune or chronic viral diseases.

Conclusion

Evidence for a close association of HCV with autoimmune and haematological processes is increasingly demonstrated. The extrahepatic tropism of HCV shows a close etiopathogenic link with some of these processes. The sialotropism of HCV may explain the close association with SS, while its lymphotropism links the virus with cryoglobulinemia, autoimmune cytopenias and lymphoma. It should be noted the important overlap between cryoglobulinemic features and several classification criteria for some SAD like SLE, RA and PAN, making difficult the differentiation between mimic and coexistence situations. However, antiviral therapies are also associated with the development of autoimmune manifestations such as sarcoidosis or cytopenia. The therapeutic management of the HCV-related autoimmune features is a very difficult issue, and recent studies have evaluated the role of new immunosuppressive and biological agents.

References

1. Gumber SC, Chopra S. (1995). Hepatitis C: A multifaceted disease. Review of extrahepatic manifestations. *Ann Intern Med* 123: 615–20.
2. Buskila D, Shnaider A, Neumann L, et al. (1998). Musculoskeletal manifestations and autoantibody profile in 90 hepatitis C virus infected Israeli patients. *Semin Arthritis Rheum* 28: 107–13.
3. Cacoub P, Renou C, Rosenthal E et al. (2000). Extrahepatic manifestations associated with hepatitis C virus infection. A prospective multicenter study of 321 patients. The GERMIVIC. Groupe d'Etude et de Recherche en Medecine Interne et Maladies Infectieuses sur le Virus de l'Hepatite C. *Medicine (Baltimore)* 79: 47–56.
4. Bini EJ, Mehandru S. (2004). Incidence of thyroid dysfunction during interferon alfa-2b and ribavirin therapy in men with chronic hepatitis C: A prospective cohort study. *Arch Intern Med* 164: 2371–6.
5. De Vita S, Sansonno D, Dolcetti R, et al. (1995). Hepatitis C virus infection within a malignant lymphoma lesion in the course of type II mixed cryoglobulinemia. *Blood* 86: 1887–92.
6. Arrieta JJ, Rodriguez-Inigo E, Ortiz-Movilla N, et al. (2001). In situ detection of hepatitis C virus RNA in salivary glands. *Am J Pathol* 158: 259–64.
7. Ramos-Casals M, Loustaud-Ratti V, De Vita S, et al. (2005). Sjögren syndrome associated with hepatitis C virus. A Multicenter Analysis of 137 Cases. *Medicine (Baltimore)* 84: 81–9.
8. Rosner I, Rozenbaum M, Toubi E, Kessel A, Naschitz JE, Zuckerman E. (2004). The case for hepatitis C arthritis. *Semin Arthritis Rheum* 33: 375–87.
9. Ramos-Casals M, Cervera R, Lagrutta M, et al. (2004); Hispanoamerican Study Group of Autoimmune Manifestations of Chronic Viral Disease (HISPAMEC). Clinical features related to antiphospholipid syndrome in patients with chronic viral infections (hepatitis C virus/HIV infection): Description of 82 cases. *Clin Infect Dis* 38: 1009–16.
10. Asherson RA, Shoenfeld Y. (2003). Human immunodeficiency virus infection, antiphospholipid antibodies, and the antiphospholipid syndrome. *J Rheumatol* 30: 214–9.
11. Sene D, Ghillani-Dalbin P, Thibault V, et al. (2004). Long-term course of mixed cryoglobulinemia in patients infected with hepatitis C virus. *J Rheumatol* 31: 2199–206.
12. Ferri C, Sebastiani M, Giuggioli D, et al. (2004). Mixed cryoglobulinemia: demographic, clinical, and serologic features and survival in 231 patients. *Semin Arthritis Rheum* 33: 355–74.
13. Ramos-Casals M, Maña J, Nardi N, et al. (2005). Sarcoidosis in patients with chronic hepatitis C virus infection. Analysis of 68 cases. *Medicine (Baltimore)* 84(2): 69–80.
14. Ramos-Casals M, Garcia-Carrasco M, Lopez-Medrano F, et al. (2003). Severe autoimmune cytopenias in treatment-naive hepatitis C virus infection: clinical description of 35 cases. *Medicine (Baltimore)* 82: 87–96.
15. De Vita S, De Re V, Sansonno D et al. (2000). Gastric mucosa as an additional extrahepatic loxalization of hepatitis C virus: Viral detection in gastric low-grade lymphoma associated with autoimmune disease and in chronic gastritis. *Hepatology* 31: 182–9.
16. Ducoulombier D, Roque-Afonso AM, Di Liberto G, et al. (2004). Frequent compartmentalization of hepatitis C virus variants in circulating B cells and monocytes. *Hepatology* 39: 817–25.
17. Matsuo K, Kusano A, Sugumar A, Nakamura S, Tajima K, Mueller NE. (2004). Effect of hepatitis C virus infection on the risk of non-Hodgkin's lymphoma: a meta-analysis of epidemiological studies. *Cancer Sci* 95: 745–52.
18. Ramos-Casals M, Trejo O, Garcia-Carrasco M, et al. (2004). Triple association between hepatitis C virus infection, systemic autoimmune diseases, and B cell lymphoma. *J Rheumatol* 31: 495–9.
19. Ramos-Casals M, la Civita L, de Vita S, et al.; the SS-HCV Study Group. (2007). Characterization of B cell lymphoma in patients with Sjogren's syndrome and hepatitis C virus infection. *Arthritis Rheum* 57: 161–70.

58
Autoimmune Pancreatitis

Salvador Navarro and Francesc Balaguer

Abstract   Autoimmune pancreatitis (AIP) is a type of chronic pancreatitis characterized by an autoimmune inflammatory process in which lymphocyte infiltration associated with pancreas fibrosis causes organ dysfunction. AIP can manifest as focal or diffuse enlargement of the pancreas with associated strictures of the pancreato-biliary tree giving rise to symptoms including abdominal pain, weight loss and obstructive jaundice, associated with favourable response to corticosteroid treatment. Although AIP is increasingly being recognized to be a worldwide identity, the diagnosis is still challenging. Different groups have defined different criteria for AIP diagnosis. Nevertheless, the absence of integrated criteria makes it difficult to compare studies from different centres, judge relevance of comparisons and establish evidence about this disorder.

Keywords   Autoimmune pancreatitis · IgG4 · lymphoplasmacytic sclerosing pancreatitis · pancreatic fibrosis · anticarbonic anhydrase II antibodies

Autoimmune pancreatitis (AIP) is a type of chronic pancreatitis characterized by an autoimmune inflammatory process in which lymphocyte infiltration associated with pancreas fibrosis causes organ dysfunction. For the past decades, various morphologic descriptions have been proposed to characterize this disease: non-alcoholic duct-destructive chronic pancreatitis, lymphoplasmacytic sclerosing pancreatitis with cholangitis, pseudotumorous pancreatitis, and recently, the term AIP has become widely accepted (1), although it is apparent that AIP is a heterogeneous disease.

AIP is a rare disorder. Although there have been an increase number of reports in the medical literature in the past 10 years, the overall number of patients is still relatively small. Although the incidence has yet to be determined (2), three series have reported the prevalence of AIP as between 5 and 6% of all patients with chronic pancreatitis (3). Patients vary widely in age; however, most are older than 50 years. The disease is at least twice as common in men as in women (3).

Clinically, AIP can manifest as focal or diffuse enlargement of the pancreas with associated strictures of the pancreato-biliary tree giving rise to symptoms including abdominal pain, weight loss and obstructive jaundice, associated with favourable response to corticosteroid treatment (4) (Table 58.1). Serologically, elevation of IgG4 is the most remarkable characteristic (5) (Table 58.2). Owing

TABLE 58.1. Clinical features.

Signs and symptoms	Frequency
Painless jaundice	65% (3)
Non-specific mild abdominal pain	35% (3)
Weight loss	35% (3)
Associated diseases	
Autoimmune disorders	12–50% (3)
Diabetes mellitus	42–76% (3)
Inflammatory bowel disease	17% (3)
Sjögren's syndrome	25% (17)
Primary sclerosing cholangitis	13% (18)
Retroperitoneal fibrosis	? (19)

TABLE 58.2. Laboratory findings and serological markers.

Laboratory findings	
Mild elevation in serum amylase or lipase (<3 times)	87% (3)
Cholestasis profile	>90% (3)
Hypergammaglobulinemia and/or elevated IgG	37–76% (19)
Elevated IgG4	63%-70% (3, 13,14)
Autoantibodies	10–100% (3,19,20)
- Antinuclear antibodies	10–83%
- Antilactoferrin antibodies	76%
- Anticarbonic anhydrase II antibodies	57–100%
- Rheumatoid factor	22–33%

From: Y. Shoenfeld et al. (eds.): *Diagnostic Criteria in Autoimmune Diseases*, DOI: 10.1007/978-1-60327-285-8_58,
© 2008 Humana Press, Totowa, NJ

to its morphological characteristics, it can be extremely difficult to distinguish from pancreatic carcinoma (6). The absence of consistent and uniform criteria has made comparison of different cases diagnosed under various guidelines difficult.

Diagnostic Criteria

Although AIP is increasingly being recognized to be a worldwide identity (7,8,9), the diagnosis is still challenging. Many groups have accepted the diagnostic criteria proposed by the Japan Pancreas Society (JPS), whereas some groups have used their own criteria in reporting AIP. This absence of integrated criteria makes it difficult to compare studies from different centres, judge relevance of comparisons and establish evidence about this disorder.

This chapter will review the current sets of criteria from three different groups: the JPS criteria (10), the Kim criteria (11) and the HISORt criteria (12) from the Mayo Clinic in the United States.

The JPS criteria, published in 2002, cover three procedures: (a) pancreatic imaging, which shows diffuse narrowing of the main pancreatic duct with irregular walls (>1/3 of the length of the entire pancreas) and diffuse enlargement of the pancreas; (b) laboratory data, which show elevated levels of serum gammaglobulin and/or IgG, or the presence of autoantibodies; and (c) histopathological findings, which show marked lymphoplasmacytic infiltration and fibrosis (Table 58.3). Radiological imaging is the essential component of the JPS, usually requiring both an endoscopic retrograde cholangiopancreatography (ERCP) and computed tomography (CT), associated with laboratory or histopathological data. However, these criteria do not include the response to steroids or the association with other autoimmune disorders.

The Kim criteria involve four procedures: (a) imaging; (b) laboratory findings; (c) histological findings; and (d) response to steroids (Table 58.4). Similar to the JPS criteria, imaging criterion must be present for diagnosis,

TABLE 58.3. Japan Pancreas Society diagnostic criteria for autoimmune pancreatitis.

Criteria	Description
Imaging	Diffuse or segmental narrowing of the main pancreatic duct with irregular wall and diffuse or localized enlargement of the pancreas
Laboratory findings	High serum gammaglobulin, IgG or IgG4, or the presence of autoantibodies
Histopathology	Marked interlobular fibrosis and prominent infiltration of lymphocytes and plasma cells

For a diagnosis: Criterion I must be present, together with criterion II and/or III

TABLE 58.4. Kim diagnostic criteria for autoimmune pancreatitis.

Diagnostic criteria	Description
Criterion I. Pancreatic imaging (essential)	1. Diffuse enlargement (swelling) of the pancreas, and 2. diffuse or segmental irregular narrowing of the main pancreatic duct
Criterion II. Laboratory finding	1. Elevated levels of IgG or IgG4, or 2. detected autoantibodies
Criterion III. Histopathology	Fibrosis and lymphoplasmacytic infiltration
Criterion IV. Response to steroid	

For diagnosis, criterion I must be present, together with any of criterions II to IV

along with any one of the other criteria. One important feature of these criteria is that a diagnosis of AIP can be made with typical imaging findings and a response to steroids.

The HISORt criteria consist of five categories: (a) histology, (b) imaging, (c) serology, (d) the presence of organ involvement, and (e) response to steroids (Table 58.5). One of the main features of the HISORt criteria is the need for having tissue specimens, and in fact is the only set of criteria that can establish the diagnosis of AIP only by histological findings. Another particular characteristic is that even when atypical imaging is present (i.e. focal pancreatic mass, focal pancreatic duct stricture), a case which responds to steroids can be diagnosed as AIP. Finally, the presence of high serum IgG4 levels as well as other organ involvement (biliary tract, parotid/lacrimal glands, mediastinal lymphadenopathy, retroperitoneal fibrosis) are also included in the diagnostic criteria.

Comparison of Diagnostic Criteria

The imaging criterion is the cornerstone of both the Kim and the JPS criteria, whereas the HISORt criteria emphasize histological features (Table 58.6). For this reason, the Kim and JPS criteria are considered to be more practical, given the availability of pancreatic imaging in comparison with pancreatic biopsy. The Kim and JPS criteria require the performance of a CT scan and a direct pancreatogram by means of ERCP. This last technique is not seen as a problem, despite its invasivity, because most patients with AIP show obstructive jaundice, and ERCP is usually necessary (3). Although the role of magnetic resonance cholangiopancreatography is not yet well established in the diagnosis of AIP, it could constitute a valuable technique to evaluate the pancreatic tree in cases where ERCP is not mandatory. Both the Kim and the JPS imaging

TABLE 58.5. HISORt diagnostic criteria for autoimmune pancreatitis.

Category	Criteria
A. Histology	1. Diagnostic (any one)
	- Pancreatic histology showing lymphoplasmacytic sclerosing pancreatitis (LPSP).
	- Lymphoplasmacytic infiltrate with abundant (>10 cells/HPF) IgG4-positive cells in the pancreas
	2. Supportive (any one)
	- Lymphoplasmacytic infiltrate with abundant (>10 cells/HPF) IgG4-positive cells in the involved extrapancreatic organ
	- Lymphoplasmacytic infiltrate with fibrosis in the pancreas
B. Imaging	*Typical imaging features*
	1. CT/MRI: diffusely enlarged gland with delayed (rim) enhancement
	2. ERCP: diffusely irregular and attenuated main pancreatic duct
	Atypical imaging features
	- Pancreatitis, focal pancreatic mass, focal pancreatic duct stricture, pancreatic atrophy, pancreatic calcification.
C. Serology	Elevated serum IgG4 level
D. Other organ involvement	Hiliar/intrahepatic biliary strictures, persistent distal biliary stricture, parotid/lacrimal gland involvement, mediastinal lymphadenopathy, retroperitoneal fibrosis.
E. Response to steroid therapy	Resolution/marked improvement of pancreatic/extrapancreatic manifestation with steroid therapy
Diagnosis	1. Group A, diagnostic histology alone
	2. Group B, typical imaging features and elevated serum IgG4.
	3. Group C, unexplained pancreatic disease with serology or other organ involvement and response to steroid.

CT: computed tomography; MRI: magnetic resonance imaging; ERCP: endoscopic retrograde cholangiopancreatography; HPF: high power field.

criterion concurs on the point that the typical features are a diffuse enlargement of the pancreas and a diffuse segmental irregular narrowing of the main pancreatic duct (with a difference in the extent of the main pancreatic duct involvement necessary for diagnosis). In contrast, the HISORt imaging criteria comprises typical and atypical features, such as the focal type of AIP, the tumoral form resembling a pancreatic mass, or even the presence of pancreatic calcification or pancreas atrophy. This atypical imaging criterion of the HISORt criteria may represent an attempt to incorporate these different forms of AIP which are not covered by the current Kim and JPS criteria.

Regarding the serological markers, the current JPS criteria include measurements of serum gammaglobulin, IgG, and autoantibodies. In contrast, the measurement of the serum level of IgG4, a subtype of IgG, is used in the Kim and HISORt criteria. The inclusion of serum IgG4 in the serological criterion is based on reports demonstrating the superior sensitivity of the serum IgG4 level, compared with IgG or gammaglobulin level, for the diagnosis of AIP (3, 13). The HISORt criteria rely exclusively on serum IgG4 level alone as serological criteria. The basis of this reliance on IgG4 levels is supported by a report stating that the overall sensitivity of combined gammaglobulin, IgG and autoantibodies was comparable to that of IgG4 alone. However, the incidence of elevated serum IgG4 in AIP has recently been reported to be around 70%, which is much lower than the results of initial studies (90%) (14). Moreover, there is concern about the specificity of serum IgG4 levels. Elevated levels have been shown to be characteristic of AIP, although mild elevations are seen in up to 10% of subjects without AIP including pancreatic cancer (14). In the Kim criteria, the rationale for the additional inclusion of an autoantibody measurement is based on the improved diagnostic sensitivity when using a combination of serum

TABLE 58.6. Comparison of each diagnostic criterion for autoimmune pancreatitis (6).

	HISORt criteria	JPS criteria	Kim criteria
I. Imaging criterion	- Not essential	- Essential	- Essential
	- Typical and atypical features	- Duct involvement of more than 1/3 of the length of the main pancreatic duct	- No lower limit to the extent of duct involvement
II. Laboratory criterion	- Elevated level of IgG4	- Elevated levels of serum gammaglobulin and/or IgG, or autoantibodies detected	- Elevated levels of serum IgG or IgG4, or autoantibodies detected
	- No measurement of autoantibodies		
III. Histopathological criterion	- Lymphoplasmacytic sclerosing pancreatitis (LPSP)	- "Marked" lymphoplasmacytic infiltration and fibrosis	- Lymphoplasmacytic infiltration and fibrosis
	- Immunostaining of IgG4-+ plasma cells		
IV. Response to steroid therapy	Included	Not included	Included
V. Association with other autoimmune diseases	Included	Not included	Not included
Definite diagnosis	Diagnosis from the histology alone	Criterion I together with criterion II and/or III	Criterion I and any of criteria II-IV

immunoglobulin (IgG or IgG4) and autoantibody levels (5). In conclusion, in the diagnosis of AIP, the simultaneous measurement of autoantibodies and serum immunoglobulin levels may play a complementary role.

Regarding the histological criteria, in the Kim and JPS models, the characteristic features of AIP are fibrosis and lymphoplasmacytic infiltration of the pancreas. These histological features can be present in alcoholic chronic pancreatitis, and may not be specific to AIP (15). Therefore, the diagnosis of AIP is not made from histological findings alone, but can be made in combination with the imaging criteria. In contrast, in the HISORt criteria, AIP can be diagnosed on histological findings alone, where the primary histological finding is lymphoplasmacytic sclerosing pancreatitis (LPSP), which is characterized by dense periductal lymphoplasmacytic infiltration, marked perilobular and intralobular fibrosis and obliterative phlebitis, with no features of chronic pancreatitis (duct dilatation, stones). Despite the high specificity of LPSP, this criterion has some limitations from a practical point of view. The histological diagnosis of LPSP usually require larger specimens (surgical resection) than the obtained by pancreatic biopsy, and in addition, correct pathological diagnosis of LPSP requires a skilled pathologist. Interestingly, in those cases in which pancreatic resection is made without any suspicious of AIP, it would be impossible to establish a diagnosis of AIP based on both the Kim and the JPS criteria (usual omission of direct pancreatogram and serological markers). However, the diagnosis is still possible with the HISORt criteria, in which AIP can be diagnosed with typical histology alone. In clinical practice, the role of a histopathological examination of the pancreas in patients with suspected AIP may help to exclude cancer rather than to provide definitive evidence for a diagnosis of AIP.

The response to oral steroids may provide evidence of an underlying autoimmune disorder. The improvement of pancreatic ductal stenosis by steroid administration may be a unique and specific finding that cannot be seen in other chronic pancreatitis or pancreatic cancer. Moreover, a marked improvement of pancreatic ductal narrowing can be seen as early as 2 weeks after the initiation of treatment. So, steroid response can be used as a diagnostic tool as well as therapeutic one. The JPS criteria are the only criteria that do not include the response to steroid therapy, probably owing to the possible improvement in diffuse pancreatic swelling in patients with pancreatic cancer when treated with steroids. When cancer is suspected, there is also a concern about the delay in the diagnosis of malignancy. Although pancreatic swelling developed in cases with pancreatic cancer may improve with treatment, pancreatic ductal narrowing associated with ductal adenocarcinoma is not relieved even with steroid therapy (6).

Treatment

Although the dramatic response to steroid is a well-known phenomenon in AIP, a detailed steroid schedule has not been not fully established currently (16). Prednisolone is usually initiated at 30–40 mg/day for 1–2 months, and tapered by 5 mg every 2–4 weeks. Some recommend a maintenance dose of 5–10 mg/day of prednisolone to prevent relapses without complete discontinuation of therapy.

The response to therapy can be observed on imaging studies within 2–4 weeks of treatment (16). If follow-up images do not reveal evident improvement, the diagnosis of AIP should be revaluated and the possibility of exploratory laparotomy should be considered.

In patients with AIP, stents are usually inserted into the bile duct to treat obstructive jaundice associated with stenosis of intrapancreatic common bile duct. While stenosis of common bile duct associated to other causes (chronic pancreatitis, cancer) show poor response to endoscopic intervention, patients with AIP show resolution of the bile duct stenosis and allows the biliary prosthesis to be removed within a couple of months.

Finally, laboratory findings also improve with steroid therapy, with normalization of serum IgG, IgG4 and autoantibodies (13, 16).

Conclusion

Although AIP is a rare disorder, an integrated diagnostic set of criteria is strongly needed so that more patients can have the opportunity to receive medical treatment which can avoid any unnecessary invasive procedure.

References

1. Deshpande V, Mino-Kenudson M, Brugge W, Lauwers GY. Autoimmune pancreatitis: more than just a pancreatic disease? A contemporary review of its pathology. Arch Pathol Lab Med 2005;129(9):1148–54.
2. Nishimori I, Tamakoshi A, Otsuki M. Prevalence of autoimmune pancreatitis in Japan from a nationwide survey in 2002. J Gastroenterol 2007;42 Suppl. 18:6–8.
3. Kim KP, Kim MH, Song MH, Lee SS, Seo DW, Lee SK. Autoimmune chronic pancreatitis. Am J Gastroenterol 2004;99(8):1605–16.
4. Finkelberg DL, Sahani D, Deshpande V, Brugge WR. Autoimmune pancreatitis. N Engl J Med 2006;355 (25):2670–6.
5. Choi EK, Kim MH, Lee TY, et al. The Sensitivity and Specificity of Serum Immunoglobulin G and Immunoglobulin G4 Levels in the Diagnosis of Autoimmune Chronic Pancreatitis: Korean Experience. Pancreas 2007;35 (2):156–61.
6. Kwon S, Kim M, Choi E. The diagnostic criteria for autoimmune chronic pancreatitis. Pancreas 2007;34:279–286
7. Okazaki K. Autoimmune pancreatitis is increasing in Japan. Gastroenterology 2003;125 (5):1557–8.

8. Kim KP, Kim MH, Lee SS, Seo DW, Lee SK. Autoimmune pancreatitis: it may be a worldwide entity. Gastroenterology 2004;126 (4):1214.

9. Sutton R. Autoimmune pancreatitis – also a Western disease. Gut 2005;54 (5):581–3.

10. Members of the Criteria Committe for Autoimmune Pancreatitis of the Japan Pancreas Society. Diagnostic criteria for autoimmune pancreatitis by the Japan Pancreas Society. J Jpn Pancreas Soc 2002;17:585–7.

11. Kim KP, Kim MH, Kim JC, Lee SS, Seo DW, Lee SK. Diagnostic Criteria for autoimune chronic pancreatitis revisited. World J Gastroenterol 2006;12 (16):2487–96.

12. Chari ST, Smyrk TC, Levy MJ, et al. Diagnosis of autoimmune pancreatitis: The Mayo Clinic experience. Clin Gastroenterol Hepatol 2006;4 (8):1010–16; quiz 934.

13. Hamano H, Kawa S, Horiuchi A, et al. High serum IgG4 concentrations in patients with sclerosing pancreatitis. N Engl J Med 2001;344 (10):732–8.

14. Ghazale A, Chari ST, Smyrk TC, et al. Value of Serum IgG4 in the Diagnosis of Autoimmune Pancreatitis and in Distinguishing it From Pancreatic Cancer. Am J Gastroenterol 2007 (electronic version).

15. Suda K, Takase M, Fukumura Y, et al. Histopathologic characteristics of autoimmune pancreatitis based on comparison with chronic pancreatitis. Pancreas 2005;30 (4):355–8.

16. Ito T, Nishimori I, Inoue N, et al. Treatment for autoimmune pancreatitis: consensus on the treatment for patients with autoimmune pancreatitis in Japan. J Gastroenterol 2007;42 Suppl. 18:50–8.

17. Kamisawa T, Egawa N, Inokuma S, et al. Pancreatic endocrine and exocrine function and salivary gland function in autoimmune pancreatitis before and after steroid therapy. Pancreas 2003;27 (3):235–8.

18. Epstein O, Chapman RW, Lake-Bakaar G, Foo AY, Rosalki SB, Sherlock S. The pancreas in primary biliary cirrhosis and primary sclerosing cholangitis. Gastroenterology 1982;83 (6):1177–82.

19. Uchida K, Okazaki K, Asada M, et al. Case of chronic pancreatitis involving an autoimmune mechanism that extended to retroperitoneal fibrosis. Pancreas 2003;26 (1):92–4.

20. Aparisi L, Farre A, Gomez-Cambronero L, et al. Antibodies to carbonic anhydrase and IgG4 levels in idiopathic chronic pancreatitis: relevance for diagnosis of autoimmune pancreatitis. Gut 2005;54 (5):703–9.

Part VII
Gastrointestinal Autoimmune Diseases

59
Autoimmune Gastritis

Ban-Hock Toh, Senga Whittingham and Frank Alderuccio

Abstract   Autoimmune gastritis is a chronic gastritis that may remain asymptomatic for many years before progression to gastric atrophy, depletion of stocks of vitamin B_{12} with clinical manifestations of pernicious anemia. Autoantibodies to gastric parietal cells, the molecular target of which is the gastric H/K ATPase, is the simplest screening test for autoimmune gastritis. Intrinsic factor autoantibodies, the second autoantibody test, typically segregate with the development of pernicious anemia; these antibodies have two actions – inhibition of vitamin B_{12} binding with intrinsic factor in the stomach and prevention of its transport into the body via the terminal ileum. Autoantibodies to gastric parietal cells and to intrinsic factor are present in 90 and 70%, respectively, of patients with pernicious anemia. As the gastritis evolves, the histology of the stomach shows increasing infiltration by lymphocytes accompanied by increasing destruction of parietal cells and zymogenic cells until the loss of mature cells is complete, the mucosa is atrophic, and there is intestinal metaplasia. This histologic evolution is accompanied by biochemical changes: loss of acid, depletion of pepsinogen I, and increased secretion of gastrin by the gastric antrum. Finally, when the stocks of vitamin B_{12} are exhausted, clinical and hematologic signs of megaloblastic anemia and its complications become evident. Although immunosuppressive drugs will check the autoimmune reaction allowing maturation of gastric parietal cells, the preferred treatment is vitamin B_{12} replacement.

Keywords   Autoimmune gastritis · parietal cell · gastric H/K ATPase · intrinsic factor

Pernicious anemia is the most common cause of vitamin B_{12} (cobalamin) deficiency that affects about 2% of persons who are more than 60 years old (1, 2, 3). It is the end-stage of autoimmune gastritis characterized by the loss of gastric parietal cells and zymogenic cells from the gastric mucosa. The loss of intrinsic factor-secreting parietal cells and the associated inhibitory antibodies to intrinsic factor in the gastric juice leads to vitamin B_{12} malabsorption and megaloblastic anemia. Whereas earlier studies suggested that the disease is restricted to Northern Europeans, later studies reported the disease in black and Latin-American subjects, and more recently in Chinese subjects (4). Although silent for 20–30 years until the end stage, the underlying gastritis can be predicted many years before anemia develops by the presence of circulating autoantibodies to gastric parietal cells.

History

Thomas Addison first described the clinical features of pernicious anemia (1849), whereas Austin Flint later linked the anemia to disease of the stomach (1860). An "extrinsic factor" (later identified as vitamin B_{12}) was implicated by Castle (1953) following the earlier observation by Minot and Murphy (1926) that feeding with cooked liver cured the anemia. The discovery of autoantibody markers of the disease (circulating parietal cell and intrinsic factor antibodies) laid the groundwork for the underlying pathogenesis of autoimmune gastritis.

Pathogenesis

The gastric H/K ATPase ("proton pump") is the molecular target of the humoral and cellular immune response in autoimmune gastritis (Figure 59.1). Autoantibodies to the gastric parietal cells bind to the 100-kD catalytic (α) subunit and the 60- to 90-kD glycoprotein (β) subunit of the H/K–ATPase. Studies of human autoimmune gastritis and of mouse models (5) have led to our current understanding of the destructive role of gastric H/K ATPase-specific Th1 CD4 T cells in the genesis of the gastritis and of the protective role of Foxp3-expressing CD4 CD25 regulatory T cells. The accompanying loss of zymogenic cells has been

From: Y. Shoenfeld et al. (eds.): *Diagnostic Criteria in Autoimmune Diseases*, DOI: 10.1007/978-1-60327-285-8_59,

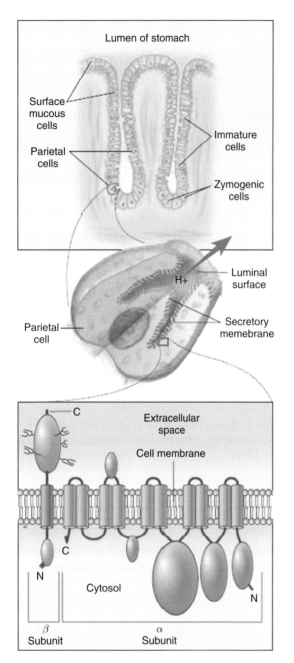

FIGURE 59.1. Gastric parietal cell H/K ATPase as the molecular target in autoimmune gastritis associated with pernicious anemia. The top panel represents a gastric gland, showing the location of parietal cells in relation to zymogenic cells, immature cells, and surface mucous cells. The middle panel represents a stimulated gastric parietal cell, showing the lining membrane of the secretory canaliculus on which gastric H+/K+ ATPase is located. The bottom panel represents the catalytic α and glycoprotein β subunits of gastric H+/K+ ATPase, showing their orientation in the lining membrane of the secretory canaliculus of the parietal cell. "N" denotes the N-terminal of protein and "C" the C-terminal of protein [Reprinted with permission from Toh et al. (1)].

attributed to arrested maturation of a mucosa that is attempting to regenerate following a Fas-dependent autoimmune attack on parietal cells. How tolerance to the gastric H/K ATPase and to gastric intrinsic factor is lost remains enigmatic. The gastric mucosal pathogen *Helicobacter pylori* induces autoantibodies directed against gastric H/K-ATPase in 20–30% of infected patients (6). The presence of these autoantibodies is associated with the severity of gastritis, increased atrophy, and apoptosis in the corpus mucosa, and patients with these autoantibodies who are infected with *H. pylori* display histopathological and clinical features that are similar to those of autoimmune gastritis. T-cell cross-reactivity between H/K ATPase and *H. pylori* has also been demonstrated with T-cell epitopes on the H/K ATPase in a mouse model overlapping corresponding epitopes identified in humans. HLA-DR molecules of an infected individual have been implicated in this cross-reactive recognition (7). The observation that mRNA expression levels of H/K-ATPase in the gastric mucosa increased 250-fold after *H. pylori* eradication (8) raises the prospect of an increased antigenic load that could favor either tolerance or autoimmunity. However, a role for *H. pylori*, invoking molecular mimicry to the gastric H/K ATPase, in the genesis of human autoimmune gastritis that leads to end-stage pernicious anemia requires long-term longitudinal studies of progression from asymptomatic autoimmune gastritis to overt pernicious anemia for substantiation. It seems likely that *H. pylori* is infrequently found in pernicious anemia because the development of atrophic body gastritis destroys its niche in the gastric antrum.

Clinical Manifestations

The median age at diagnosis is 60 years with slightly more women affected than men. The main clinical features at presentation are listed in Table 59.1. The usual presentation is with symptoms of anemia. Vitamin B_{12} deficiency results in atrophic glossitis and megaloblastosis of small intestinal epithelial cells that result in malabsorption accompanied by diarrhea. Neurologic complications include peripheral neuropathy and lesions in the postero-lateral columns of the spinal cord (subacute combined degeneration) and in the cerebrum (megaloblastic madness) that progress from demyelination to axonal degeneration and neuronal death. These neurologic complications arise because of the fundamental role of vitamin B_{12} in central nervous system (CNS) function at all ages, especially the methionine-synthase-mediated conversion of homocysteine to methionine essential for nucleotide synthesis and for genomic and non-genomic methylation (9). Complications affecting the CNS are now seldom seen because they occur at the end stage of vitamin B_{12} deficiency. Intestinal metaplasia

TABLE 59.1. Symptoms and signs of pernicious anemia at presentation.

1. Pallor and fatigue due to anemia
2. Loss of appetite and a sore, smooth, and red tongue due to atrophic glossitis
3. Diarrhea due to malabsorption of vitamin B_{12} and intestinal changes
4. Peripheral numbness, muscle wasting, diminished tendon reflexes, loss of perception to light touch and vibration, and spastic ataxia due to peripheral neuropathy and subacute combined degeneration of the spinal cord

in the gastric mucosa is a risk factor for adenocarcinoma development. There is a 3-fold excess risk of gastric carcinoma and a 13-fold excess risk for gastric carcinoid tumors associated with the hypergastrinemia consequent to achlorhydria. The prevalence of gastric adenocarcinoma in patients with pernicious anemia is 1–3%, whereas 2% of patients with gastric adenocarcinoma have pernicious anemia. Gastric cancer also develops in the context of infection with *H. pylori*, which infects 50% of the world's population and is responsible for inducing chronic gastric inflammation that progresses to atrophy, metaplasia, dysplasia, and gastric cancer (10).

Predisposing Genetic Factors

A genetic predisposition to pernicious anemia is suggested by clustering of the disease and of gastric autoantibodies in families, and by its association with the autoimmune endocrinopathies. About 20% of the relatives of patients with pernicious anemia have the disease. These relatives, especially first-degree female relatives, also have a higher frequency of gastric autoantibodies than normal subjects. Disease concordance has been observed in 12 sets of monozygotic twins. Evidence of an association between pernicious anemia and particular molecules of the major histocompatibility complex is weak, but earlier studies distinguished between patients with pernicious anemia and those with pernicious anemia and other autoimmune endocrinopathies. A candidate gene *NALP* that encodes NACHT leucine-rich-repeat protein 1, a regulator of the innate immune system on chromosome 17p13, has been identified in vitiligo-associated multiple autoimmune diseases (11). The group includes various combinations of generalized vitiligo with organ-specific autoimmune diseases such thyroid disease, latent autoimmune diabetes in adults, pernicious anemia, and Addison's disease as well as systemic autoimmune diseases such as rheumatoid arthritis, systemic lupus erythematosus, and psoriasis. NALP1 is thought to activate the innate immune system in response to bacterial pathogen-associated molecular patterns. It is widely expressed at low levels but at high levels in immune cells, particularly T cells and recruits adapter proteins to a complex termed the *NALP1 inflammasome* that activates the proinflammatory cytokine interleukin-1β (11, 12). Pernicious anemia is a feature of autoimmune polyendocrinopathy syndrome type 1 arising from mutations of the autoimmune regulatory (AIRE) gene (13).

Association with other Autoimmune Diseases

Pernicious anemia may be associated with the autoimmune endocrinopathies including particularly autoimmune thyroiditis, type 1 diabetes mellitus, and more rarely primary Addison's disease, primary ovarian failure and primary hypoparathyroidism. Pernicious anemia is also associated with the antireceptor autoimmune diseases that include Graves' disease, myasthenia gravis, and the Lambert–Eaton syndrome.

Pathologic Features

Autoimmune gastritis is manifest pathologically as type A chronic atrophic gastritis that affects the parietal cell-containing fundus and body of the stomach with sparing of the gastric antrum. It is distinguished from type B chronic atrophic gastritis that typically starts in the antrum and is associated with *H pylori* infection and low concentrations of serum gastrin concentrations that follow destruction of the gastrin-producing cells associated with the antral gastritis. Autoimmune gastritis is characterized histologically by a mononuclear cellular infiltrate in the submucosa that extends into the lamina propria between the gastric glands accompanied by degeneration of mature parietal cells and zymogenic cells. In the established lesion, there is marked reduction in the number of gastric glands, and the parietal cells and zymogenic cells are lost from the gastric mucosa and replaced by mucus-containing cells (intestinal metaplasia). A long-term study over 6–7 years reported that atrophic gastritis and intestinal metaplasia of the fundus and body are lesions that persist due to ongoing autoimmunity irrespective of the presence or absence of *H.pylori* infection (14). Progression of the histological appearance of autoimmune gastritis is summarized in Table 59.2.

TABLE 59.2. Histologic stages of progression of autoimmune gastritis.

1. Lymphocytic infiltration of the gastric mucosa, arising in the submucosa and extending into the mucosa
2. Degeneration of mature gastric parietal and zymogenic cells
3. Gastric atrophy with loss of gastric parietal and zymogenic cells and their replacement by cells with an intestinal phenotype (intestinal metaplasia)

Serologic Features

Serum antibodies to gastric parietal cells and to intrinsic factor remain the mainstay for the serologic diagnosis of autoimmune gastritis and pernicious anemia. Parietal cell autoantibodies directed against the gastric H/K ATPase are diagnostic of asymptomatic autoimmune gastritis. Found in about 90% of patients with pernicious anemia and in about 30% of first-degree relatives of patients with pernicious anemia and in patients with autoimmune endocrinopathies, they reflect the underlying presence of autoimmune gastritis. In normal subjects there is an age-related increase in the prevalence of parietal-cell autoantibodies, from 2.5% in the third decade to 9.6% in the eighth decade. Two specificities of intrinsic factor antibodies have been identified; one reacts with the vitamin B_{12} binding site and the other impedes transport of vitamin B_{12} through the mucosa of the terminal ileum. Thus, these two specificities play a major role in the malabsorption of vitamin B_{12} and the development of pernicious anemia. They are detected in about 70% of patients with pernicious anemia. The serology together with the features of pernicious anemia is summarized in Table 59.3.

Hematologic Features

The hematologic features are those of low serum vitamin B_{12} levels and of megaloblastic anemia characterized by peripheral blood features of macrocytosis, hypersegmented polymorphonuclear leukocytes, anemia, leukopenia, thrombocytopenia, or pancytopenia. Bone marrow typically reveals megaloblasts and large myeloid precursors.

A Schilling test, now outmoded but an excellent diagnostic test, will confirm that the vitamin B_{12} deficiency is the result of intestinal malabsorption due to intrinsic-factor deficiency. The low urinary excretion of orally administered vitamin B_{12} is increased when vitamin B_{12} is administered with intrinsic factor.

Biochemical Features

Hypo- or achlorhydria is indicative of destruction of the acid-producing gastric parietal cells. Total (pentagastrin-resistant) achlorhydria is diagnostic of pernicious anemia because it is the only gastric lesion that results in achlorhydria. A magnesium hydrogen breath test to assess achlorhydria avoids the need for intubation (15). A low serum pepsinogen I concentration reflects the destruction of zymogenic cells. Hypergastrinemia is the result of sparing of the antrum from the autoimmune reaction and stimulation of the gastrin-producing G cells by the loss of acid-producing gastric parietal cells.

Gastric Biopsy

The presence of type A chronic atrophic gastritis can be confirmed by gastric biopsy.

Diagnostic Criteria

There are no internationally accepted criteria for the diagnosis of either autoimmune gastritis or pernicious anemia. For autoimmune gastritis in asymptomatic subjects, we suggest that the presence of parietal autoantibody is diagnostic of the underlying gastric pathology. For pernicious anemia, we suggest fulfilment of minimum criteria listed in Table 59.4.

Prognosis

The prognosis of asymptomatic subjects with parietal cell autoantibody-positive autoimmune gastritis is unknown. Given that the latent period is unusually long, sometimes 20–30 years or more between the onset of asymptomatic autoimmune gastritis and end-stage pernicious anemia, these patients should be subjected to regular review of their serologic and hematologic status.

TABLE 59.3. Hematology, biochemistry, serology, and pathology of pernicious anemia.

1. Hematology: Megaloblastic anemia characterized by macrocytes, poikylocytes, hypersegmented polymorphonuclear leukocytes, leukopenia, and thrombocytopenia in a peripheral blood film and megaloblasts in a bone marrow smear. Low serum levels of vitamin B_{12} with normal folic acid levels. Impaired urinary excretion of vitamin B_{12} due to its malabsorption measured by Schilling test
2. Biochemistry: Achlorhydria, low levels of serum pepsinogen I, and high levels of serum gastrin
3. Serology: Parietal cell antibody, intrinsic factor antibodies
4. Histopathology on gastric biopsy: Type A chronic atrophic gastritis affecting the fundus and body of the stomach with sparing of the antrum

TABLE 59.4. Minimum diagnostic criteria for pernicious anemia.

1. Parietal cell and/or intrinsic factor antibodies
2. Anemia, macrocytosis
3. Low serum levels of vitamin B_{12}
4. Hypergastrinemia and/or low serum pepsinogen I

In the case of pernicious anemia, provided the diagnosis is firmly established and vitamin B_{12} replacement therapy commenced before the onset of neurologic complications, the prognosis is good. However, patients and particularly young patients with autoimmune gastritis and pernicious anemia should be monitored by regular gastroscopy examination for development of gastric adenocarcinoma and gastric carcinoids even though the risk is small.

Prediction

As parietal cell antibodies are diagnostic of asymptomatic autoimmune gastritis, these antibodies may predict the subsequent development of pernicious anemia. However, it is not known whether the gastric pathology of asymptomatic subjects with parietal cell antibody will progress to the stage of total exhaustion of gastric parietal cells to lead to pernicious anemia in the lifetime of the patient. Whether or not the autoimmune process proceeds to this end-stage depends on a number of checks and balances including genetic predisposition to disease and regulation of the autoimmune response through the T-lymphocyte compartment of the immune system and possibly diet.

Although intrinsic factor antibodies typically segregate with overt pernicious anemia, they have also been reported in asymptomatic subjects together with parietal cell antibody.

Early abnormalities of gastric function identified as low acid secretion assessed by the magnesium hydrogen breath test, low serum pepsinogen I concentration, and hypergastrinemia (15) were reported in parietal cell antibody-positive first-degree relatives of patients with pernicious anemia with low serum levels of vitamin B_{12} (16).

Iron deficiency arising as a result of reduced iron absorption due to decreased acid secretion may precede the development of pernicious anemia (17, 18). This has been attributed to the requirement of gastric acid to reduce iron from its ferric to ferrous form for its absorption. Autoimmune gastritis, defined as hypergastrinemia with parietal cell antibody, was encountered in 20–27% of patients with obscure or refractory iron deficiency anemia and is four to six times more common than celiac disease causing unexplained iron deficiency. The unique clinical features of the iron deficiency anemia was first described by Faber and others over 100 years ago (19), including refractoriness to oral iron treatment, female predominance, relatively young age, increased prevalence of thyroid disease, and tendency to progress to pernicious anemia. Obscure iron deficiency in young women may therefore be a predictor of the development of pernicious anemia. Iron deficiency has also be reported to occur frequently in patients with pernicious anemia (20).

TABLE 59.5. Markers of progression from parietal cell-positive autoimmune gastritis to pernicious anemia.

1. Hypergastrinemia
2. Low serum pepsinogen I
3. Hypo- or achlorhydria

TABLE 59.6. Indications for screening for autoimmune gastritis and pernicious anemia.

1. First-degree relatives of patients with pernicious anemia
2. Autoimmune thyroid disease
3. Type 1 diabetes

In patients with type 1 diabetes, serum pepsinogen I and elevated levels of serum gastrin and parietal cell antibody were identified as early markers of pernicious anemia (21). The highest parietal cell antibody titers ($\geq$1:640) identified patients with significantly higher levels of plasma gastrin and lower levels of pepsinogen I. It has been estimated that among patients with type 1 diabetes mellitus about 25% are at risk of developing gastric autoimmunity (22).

In a study of patients with autoimmune thyroid disease, high serum gastrin levels in parietal cell antibody-positive patients with low vitamin B_{12} was identified in 31% of patients (23); atrophic gastritis was confirmed by biopsy in a subset of these patients. This study suggests that the occurrence of autoimmune thyroid disease may be a predictor of the associated disease of pernicious anemia. Similarly, in a study of children with autoimmune thyroid disease, 30% had detectable parietal cell antibody and hypergastrinemia was found in 45% of the parietal cell antibody-positive children showing that autoimmune gastritis is an early event in juvenile autoimmune thyroid disease and that elevated gastrin levels is a reliable marker of gastric atrophy (24).

Table 59.5 summarizes markers that may predict progression from asymptomatic autoimmune gastritis to pernicious anemia, and Table 59.6 summarizes indications for screening for autoimmune gastritis and pernicious anemia.

Therapy: Oral Versus Intramuscular Injection of Vitamin B_{12}

Although immunosuppressive drugs will check the autoimmune reaction allowing maturation of gastric parietal cells, the preferred treatment is vitamin B_{12} replacement. The standard treatment is monthly intramuscular injections of at least 100 μg of vitamin B_{12} to correct the vitamin deficiency and the complications particularly neurologic complications. There is recent interest in oral treatment with vitamin B_{12} on the grounds that about 1% of the vitamin is absorbed by mass action in the absence of intrinsic factor. The evidence derived from limited studies of randomized controlled trials comparing the effectiveness of oral versus intramuscular vitamin B_{12} to treat vitamin B_{12} deficiency suggests that 2000 µg doses of oral vitamin B_{12} daily and 1000 µg doses initially daily and thereafter weekly and then monthly may be as effective as intramuscular administration in obtaining short-term hematologic and neurologic responses in vitamin B_{12}-deficient patients (25). The survey supports the report of a previous study that showed that patients that received 1000 µg of oral vitamin B_{12} daily for up to 18 months maintained satisfactory serum B_{12} levels and showed normal hematology and neurology (26). These latter findings of response to oral vitamin B_{12} treatment are entirely consistent with the original report of a curative response following the feeding of patients with cooked liver (containing vitamin B_{12}) as reported by Minot and Murphy in 1926 (27), a discovery that led to the award of a Nobel prize shared with Whipple.

Acknowledgments. Supported by the National Health and Medical Research Council of Australia.

References

1. Toh BH, van Driel IR, Gleeson PA. Pernicious anemia. *N Engl J Med* 1997 November 13; 337(20): 1441–8. Review.
2. Toh BH, Alderuccio F. Pernicious anaemia. *Autoimmunity* 2004 June; 37(4): 357–61. Review.
3. Toh BH, Whittingham S, Alderuccio F. Gastritis and Pernicious anemia. In: *The Autoimmune Diseases* 4th Ed, Elsevier Academic Press, 2006, pp. 527–46.
4. Wun Chan JC, Yu Liu HS, Sang Kho BC, Yin Sim JP, Hang Lau TK, Luk YW, Chu RW, Fung Cheung FM, Tat Choi FP, Kwan Ma ES. Pernicious anemia in Chinese: A study of 181 patients in a Hong Kong hospital. *Medicine (Baltimore)* 2006 May; 85(3): 129–38.
5. Field J, Biondo MA, Murphy K, Alderuccio F, Toh BH. Experimental autoimmune gastritis: Mouse models of human organ-specific autoimmune disease. *Int Rev Immunol* 2005 January–April; 24(1–2): 93–110. Review.
6. Bergman MP, Vandenbroucke-Grauls CM, Appelmelk BJ, D'Elios MM, Amedei A, Azzurri A, Benagiano M, Del Prete G. The story so far: Helicobacter pylori and gastric autoimmunity. *Int Rev Immunol* 2005 January–April; 24(1–2): 63–91. Review.
7. Bergman M, Del Prete G, van Kooyk Y, Appelmelk B. Helicobacter pylori phase variation, immune modulation and gastric autoimmunity. *Nat Rev Microbiol* 2006 February; 4(2): 151–9. Review.
8. Osawa H, Kita H, Ohnishi H, Hoshino H, Mutoh H, Ishino Y, Watanabe E, Satoh K, Sugano K. Helicobacter pylori eradication induces marked increase in H+/K+-adenosine triphosphatase expression without altering parietal cell number in human gastricmucosa. *Gut* 2006 February; 55(2): 152–7. Epub 2005 May 4.

9. Reynolds E. Vitamin B12, folic acid, and the nervous system. *Lancet Neurol* 2006 November; 5(11): 949–60. Review.
10. Fox JG, Wang TC. Inflammation, atrophy, and gastric cancer. *J Clin Invest* 2007 January; 117(1): 60–9.
11. Jin Y, Mailloux CM, Gowen K, Riccardi SL, LaBerge G, Bennett DC, Fain PR, Spritz RA. NALP1 in vitiligo-associated multiple autoimmune disease. *N.Engl J Med* 2007 March 22; 356(12): 1216–25.
12. Taieb A. NALP1 and the inflammasomes: Challenging our perception of vitiligo and vitiligo-related autoimmune disorders. *Pigment Cell Res* 2007 August; 20(4): 260–2.
13. Eisenbarth GS, Gottlieb PA. Autoimmune polyendocrine syndromes. *N Engl J Med* 2004 May 13; 350(20): 2068–79. Review.
14. Lahner E, Bordi C, Cattaruzza MS, Iannoni C, Milione M, Delle Fave G, Annibale B. Long-term follow-up in atrophic body gastritis patients: Atrophy and intestinal metaplasia are persistent lesions irrespective of Helicobacter pylori infection. *Aliment Pharmacol Ther* 2005 September 1; 22(5): 471–81.
15. Humbert P, López de Soria P, Fernández-Bañares F, et al. Magnesium hydrogen breath test using end expiratory sample to assess achlorhydria in pernicious anemia patients. *Gut* 1994; 35: 1205–8.
16. Junca J, de Soria PL, Granada ML, Flores A, Marquez E. Detection of early abnormalities in gastric function in first-degree relatives of patients with pernicious anemia. *Eur J Haematol* 2006 December; 77(6): 518–22. Epub 2006 October 17.
17. Hershko C, Ronson A, Souroujon M, Maschler I, Heyd J, Patz J. Variable hematologic presentation of autoimmune gastritis: Age-related progression from iron deficiency to cobalamin depletion. *Blood* 2006 February 15; 107(4): 1673–9. Epub 2005 October 20.
18. Hershko C, et al. The anemia of achylia gastrica revisited. *Blood Cell Mol Dis* 2007 May 8; Epub ahead of print.
19. Faber K. Achylia gastrica mit Anämie. *Med Klin* 1909; 5: 1310–25.
20. Carmel R, Weiner JM, Johnson CS. Iron deficiency occurs frequently in patients with pernicious anemia. *JAMA* 1987; 257: 1081–3.
21. Alonso N, Granada ML, Salinas I, Lucas AM, Reverter JL, Junca J, Oriol A, Sanmarti A. Serum pepsinogen I: An early marker of pernicious anemia in patients with type 1 diabetes. *J Clin Endocrinol Metab* 2005 September; 90(9): 5254–8.
22. Lam-Tse WK, Batstra MR, Koeleman BP, Roep BO, Bruining MG, Aanstoot HJ, Drexhage HA. The association between autoimmune thyroiditis, autoimmune gastritis and type 1 diabetes. *Pediatr Endocrinol Rev* 2003 September; 1(1): 22–37. Review.
23. Ness-Abramof R, Nabriski DA, Braverman LE, Shilo L, Weiss E, Reshef T, Shapiro MS, Shenkman L. Prevalence and evaluation of B12 deficiency in patients with autoimmune thyroid disease. *Am J Med Sci* 2006 September; 332(3): 119–22.
24. Segni M, Borrelli O, Pucarelli I, Delle Fave G, Pasquino AM, Annibale B. Early manifestations of gastric autoimmunity in patients with juvenile autoimmune thyroid diseases. *J Clin Endocrinol Metab* 2004 October; 89(10): 4944–8.

25. Butler CC, Vidal-Alaball J, Cannings-John R, McCaddon A, Hood K, Papaioannou A, Mcdowell I, Goringe A. Oral vitamin B12 versus intramuscular vitamin B12 for vitamin B12 deficiency: A systematic review of randomized controlled trials. *Fam Pract* 2006 June; 23(3): 279–85. Review.

26. Nyholm E, Turpin P, Swain D, Cunningham B, Daly S, Nightingale P, Fegan C. Oral vitamin B12 can change our practice. *Postgrad Med J* 2003 April; 79(930): 218–20.

27. Minot GR, Murphy WP. Treatment of pernicious anemia by a special diet. 1926. *Yale J Biol Med* 2001 September–October; 74(5): 341–53.

60
Ulcerative Colitis

Karsten Conrad and Martin W. Laass

Abstract Ulcerative colitis (UC) is a chronic relapsing–remitting inflammatory bowel disease (IBD) characterized by mucosal ulceration, rectal bleeding, diarrhea, and abdominal pain. In contrast to Crohn's disease (CD), UC is restricted to the colon and the inflammation is limited to the mucosal layer. Classic UC begins in the rectum and affects the colon in a retrograde fashion. Dependent on the anatomic extent of involvement, patients can be classified as having proctitis, left-sided colitis, or pancolitis. Inflammatory arthropathies and primary sclerosing cholangitis (PSC) are the most common and clinically most important extraintestinal manifestations in UC patients. The etiopathogenesis of UC is incompletely understood, but immune-mediated mechanisms involving specific T-cell subsets are responsible in genetically predisposed individuals for dysregulated immune responses against intraluminal (bacterial) antigens. The diagnosis is based on history, clinical, endoscopical, and histological features (presence of architectural distortion, e.g., transmural or superficial patchy infiltration, and/or acute inflammatory cells). Autoantibodies [antineutrophil cytoplasmic antibodies (ANCAs) and goblet cell autoantibodies (GABs)] may be helpful in the early diagnosis of UC and in differentiating it from CD.

Keywords Ulcerative colitis · primary sclerosing cholangitis · ANCA

Ulcerative colitis (UC) is a chronic inflammatory bowel disease (IBD) of unknown etiology characterized by mucosal ulceration, rectal bleeding, diarrhea, and abdominal pain. In contrast to Crohn's disease (CD), UC is restricted to the colon and the inflammation is limited to the mucosal layer.

Epidemiology

The UC is a worldwide distributed disease with differences in its frequency in dependence on ethnical background and geographic localization. Prevalence rates for UC range from 90 to 220 per 100,000 population in Northern Europe and Northern America (1). UC is three to five times more prevalent in Jewish people. Among Caucasians, the annual incidence fluctuates between 3 and 15 per 100,000 population (2, 3). The disease is less common in Eastern and Southern Europe, and at least 10 times less common in Asian, African, and Oriental populations. Rising incidence and prevalence have also been shown for these ethnic groups, suggesting additional environmental and lifestyle effects on the pathogenesis of UC (4).

UC is slightly more common in men than in women. Any age group from infants to the elderly can be affected, but the peak age of onset is between 15 and 30 years with a second but smaller peak between 50 and 70 years (4). It is estimated that 20–30% of patients with UC and CD have the onset of their symptoms below the age of 18 years, although diagnosis is often delayed.

History

Descriptions of bloody diarrhea and dysentery date back to antiquity. The first report suggesting that patients were dying from UC was published in 1793 (Matthew Baillies's "Morbid Anatomy of Some of the Most Important Parts of the Human Body"). After the first case report of a "simple ulcerative colitis" in 1859 by Samuel Wilks from Guy's Hospital (London), the disease was described in greater detail in 1875 by S. Wilks and W. Moxon and in 1909 by H.P. Hawkins. In 1935, Hurst described the UC with its typical sigmoid endoscopical changes. He considered this disease as infectious dysenteria that secondary develops into chronic disease due to additional factors (5). An

From: Y. Shoenfeld et al. (eds.): *Diagnostic Criteria in Autoimmune Diseases*, DOI: 10.1007/978-1-60327-285-8_60,
© 2008 Humana Press, Totowa, NJ

involvement of immune mechanisms in the pathogenesis of UC was suggested since the 1960 s by clinical features, therapeutic efficacy of immunosuppressive drugs, histopathological findings, studies on animal models, and the detection of anticolon antibodies (5). Recently, UC is regarded as an inflammatory disease with increased responsiveness of the gut mucosal immune system involving T-cell subsets in genetically susceptible individuals. It belongs to the group of chronic IBD (see also Chapter "Crohn's Disease").

Pathogenesis

Although autoimmune reactions occur, UC does not fulfil the criteria for a classical autoimmune disease. UC can be considered as an immune-mediated disorder that develops in genetically predisposed individuals because of dysregulated immune responses against intraluminal (bacterial) antigens. The mechanisms of the development of those aberrant reactivities and of the dysregulated activation of immunologic effector pathways and the subsequent tissue injury as well as the triggering genetic and environmental factors are intensively studied (6, 7). Recently, UC has been defined as an atypical Th2 response mediated by CD1d-restricted NKT cells that produce high levels of IL-13 (8). Furthermore, studies on animal models of colitis suggest an important role of the Th17 pathway in chronic intestinal inflammation (7). The activation of T cells by bacterial superantigens might lead to a dysregulated, but intense immune activity causing the remission and flare-up cycle of mucosal inflammation in patients with UC (9). The elucidation of abnormal immune mechanisms in UC will facilitate the development of novel therapeutic options with greater efficacy.

Approximately 5–10% of all patients with IBD have a positive family history, which is considered the greatest risk factor for developing IBD. The concordance rate for UC in monozygotic twins is 10% and in dizygotic twins 3%, demonstrating genetic contribution to UC (10). For IBD nine susceptibility loci (designed IBD1–IBD9) have been described. Most of them are CD associated, but IBD2 on chromosome 12q14 and IBD3 encompassing the HLA region on chromosome 6p have been identified as susceptibility regions for UC (11). In contrast to CD, where smoking is a strong independent risk factor, smoking is associated with less severe course of UC.

Clinical Manifestations

UC is characterized by perianal bleeding, diarrhea with small voluminous mucous-bloody stool, abdominal cramps, and fatigue (12). UC always involves the rectum and extends proximally to involve a variable amount of the colon (Table 60.1). Although by definition UC is restricted to the

TABLE 60.1. Ulcerative colitis (UC) types according to the localization of the inflammation, and symptoms and signs of UC at presentation.

	Prevalence at presentation (%)
Type of UC	
Proctitis/proctosigmoiditis	40–50
Left-side colitis (up to flexura sinistra)	30–40
Pancolitis (in rare cases with additional backwash ileitis)	25–30
Symptoms and signs	
Diarrhea	70–90
Abdominal pain	30–70
Weight loss	35–45
Rectal bleeding	50–90
Growth impairment in children	5
Extraintestinal manifestation	2–15

colon, nonspecific mucosal inflammation in the terminal ileum ("backwash ileitis") may be found. The involvement of the upper gastrointestinal tract is a controversial issue especially in the pediatric population with UC. In contrast to adults, pancolitis in children with UC is more common with rates between 60 and 90%. The clinical picture mainly depends on the extent of bowel involvement, disease activity, and extraintestinal manifestations and complications (Tables 60.1 and 60.2). Inflammatory arthropathies and primary sclerosing cholangitis (PSC) are the most common and clinically most important extraintestinal manifestations in UC patients. PSC is diagnosed in about 2–10% of UC patients.

TABLE 60.2. Extraintestinal manifestations of ulcerative colitis (UC).

	Manifestation[a]
Musculoskeletal	• Peripheral arthropathy: colitic type of arthritis[b] (10%; 15–20% of *active UC*); symmetrical polyarthritis of small joints • Ankylosing spondylitis[c] (1–26%)/sacroiliitis (up to 24%), enthesopathy (4%)
Skin	• Erythema nodosum[b,c] (up to 19%) • Pyoderma gangrenosum (0.5–2%)
Ophthalmologic	• Episcleritis[b] (1.5–4%) • Uveitis
Hepatobiliary	• Primary sclerosing cholangitis (PSC) (2–10%) • Autoimmune hepatitis (AIH), rare (often PSC/AIH overlap)
Growth and development in children	• Delayed puberty • Delayed growth

[a] Manifestations that seem to be connected with UC because of clinical associations or pathological mechanisms. Not included: extraintestinal concomitant manifestations (nephrolithiasis, cholelithiasis) and non-disease specific complications (osteoporosis, thromboembolic manifestations).
[b] Associated with disease activity.
[c] May precede bowel symptoms.

Pathological Features

Pathological features are listed in Table 60.4. Histologically, UC is characterized by diffuse inflammatory cell infiltration of the mucosa and a reduction in mucus-secreting goblet cells. Furthermore, the regular arrangement of glandular crypts is disrupted.

Laboratory Features

Laboratory features are no disease-specific markers. They are determined to detect inflammatory processes or deficiencies due to malnutrition and may help to assess disease activity and course as well as complications. The main laboratory abnormalities observed in UC are summarized in Table 60.3.

Serological Features

Several autoantibody specificities have been described in sera of UC patients (Table 60.3). Currently, atypical antineutrophil cytoplasmic antibodies (ANCAs) and anti-intestinal goblet cell autoantibodies (GABs) are used as diagnostic parameters.

ANCAs

ANCAs (pANCA, xANCA, atypical ANCA) that are different from the vasculitis-associated ANCA can be found in 50–70% of UC patients. They are not UC-specific because they are also detectable in patients with various immune-mediated diseases including CD (5–25%), PSC (up to 88%), and autoimmune hepatitis (up to 81%). A positive ANCA and a negative test for antibodies against mannan of *Saccharomyces cerevisiae* (ASCA) or antigens of exocrine pancreas (PAB) indicate that UC is more likely than CD(13). Although several autoantibodies that are directed against granulocyte antigens such as lactoferrin, bactericidal permeability increasing protein (BPI), cathepsin G, lysozyme, β-glucuronidase, catalase, α-enolase, high-mobility group (HMG) nonhistone chromosomal proteins (HMG-1 and HMG-2), and nuclear envelope-associated proteins have been found in UC patients in varying frequencies (2–57%), the exact target antigen(s) of UC-associated ANCA are not known (14). Hence, indirect immunofluorescence (IIF) on human neutrophils is the only widely available detection method. The presence of ANCA detected by IIF or of individual target antigens detected by specific immunoassays does not correlate with activity, extent, or duration of the disease.

GABs

GABs are directed against a component of a mucin produced by intestinal goblet cells. They are detectable by IIF on intestinal tissues or cancer cells which were differentiated into goblet cells or by immunoassays (ELISA, Western blot) using purified mucin prepared from human intestinal tissue. GABs are strongly associated with the presence of IBD. In most studies, GAB is found to occur in 15–28% of patients with UC, whereas the occurrence of GAB is very rare in sera from patients with other intestinal diseases (including CD) as well as other organ specific or systemic diseases and healthy controls. GAB can also be found in rare cases of a variant form of autoimmune enteropathy with depletion of goblet cells. If the autoantigenic targets used for testing are properly chosen and prepared, GABs are highly specific (pathognomonic) for UC (15).

Besides ANCA and GAB other autoantibodies with probable clinical and/or pathogenic relevance have been described. The earliest indication of autoimmunity was the detection of antibodies against colonic epithelial cells. The human tropomyosin isotype 5 (hTM5) is likely to be an autoantigen of the anticolon reactivities because it is expressed on the surface of colonic but not small bowel enterocytes, and its expression is upregulated in the colon epithelium of patients with UC. Autoreactive B- and T-cell responses against hTM5 and a positive correlation of UC activity and anti-hT5 autoantibody responses have been detected. Furthermore, hTM5-specific IgG autoantibodies present in UC sera were able to destroy colonic cells by antibody and complement-mediated lysis suggesting a pathogenic role of these autoantibodies (16).

TABLE 60.3. Biochemical and serological features of ulcerative colitis (UC).

Biochemical feature	Changes
Erythrocyte sedimentation rate (ESR)	↑
Thrombocytes	↑
Mean red cell volume	↓↓↓
Albumin	↓
CRP	↑/↑↑
Fecal calprotectin	↑↑↑
Autoantibodies	**Frequencies and relevance**
Atypical ANCAs	50–70%
GABs	15–28%
	Diagnostic marker of UC (specificity up to 100%)
Tropomyosin isotype 5	64%
	Associated with disease activity
HMG-1/HMG-2	32–33%
	Seem to be associated with disease activity

ANCA, antineutrophil cytoplasmic antibody; CRP, C-reactive protein; GAB, goblet cell autoantibody; HMG, high-mobility group.
The semiquantitative (↑↑) system indicates the extent of the observed abnormalities.

Diagnostic Criteria

UC is primarily a clinical diagnosis, confirmed by pathomorphological, histological, and autoantibody findings. There are several definitions or criteria used to classify patients as having UC (17). The epidemiological diagnosis of UC relies on the presence of (a) bloody diarrhea with negative stool cultures and (b) endoscopic evidence of diffuse continuous mucosal inflammation involving the rectum and extending to a point more proximal in the colon. The presence of "backwash ileitis" does not exclude a diagnosis of UC. The most important diagnostic criteria are listed in Table 60.4. There are several UC activity indices (e.g., modified Truelove and Witts severity index or more recently the Mayo score) for classification and prognosis of UC, but none has been validated either in adults or in pediatric clinical trails. For clinical practice it is sufficient to describe disease activity as mild (up to four bloody stools per day), moderate (four to six bloody stools per day and minimal toxicity), or severe (more than six stools per day and signs of toxicity, such as fever, tachycardia). In fulminant colitis as the most severe form, there are more than 10 bloody stools per day with anemia requiring blood transfusion and colonic dilation on plain abdominal radiographs as a sign of toxic megacolon.

Prognosis

In general, life expectancy in UC patients seems to be normal (18). Ten years after diagnosis of UC, about one quarter of patients had undergone proctocolectomy. Most of the patients have an intermittent course with intermittent relapses. Patients with UC have an increased risk of developing malignancies especially colorectal cancer. Surveillance colonoscopy should be performed in UC patients yearly starting 10 years after diagnosis as cancer risk increases with duration of colitis. Patients with PSC have an additional predisposition for cholangiocarcinoma with prevalence ranges from 6 to 36% and an estimated annual incidence of 0.5–1%. The long-term use of aminosalicylates is lowering the risk of colorectal cancer.

Prediction

The strongest risk factor for UC is having a relative with the disease. The presence of ANCA, GAB, or hTM5 antibodies in unaffected family members could reflect a genetic and/or environmental factor predisposing to disease or could also be indicative of presymptomatic disease (14, 15, 16). In 25% of patients with UC, ANCAs were found to be positive before disease manifestation (19). Further studies are necessary to evaluate the exact predictive value of these UC-associated autoantibodies.

Therapy

Oral aminosalicylates, either mesalazine (5-aminosalicylic acid) or sulfasalazine (a combination of 5-aminosalicylate and sulfapyridine), are the principal therapeutic agents for induction of remission in mild to moderate disease and for maintenance therapy (20). Topical therapy with aminosalicylates is an alternative therapeutic approach for patients with left-sided disease or proctitis. Severe or moderate UC not responding to aminosalicylates requires treatment with prednisolone (or equivalent) oral or intravenous at a dose of 1–2 mg/kg weight, up to 60 mg per day. In patients with

TABLE 60.4. Diagnostic features of ulcerative colitis (UC).

	Feature
Clinical features (symptoms should be present for at least 2 weeks)	• Diarrhea • Gross or occult rectal bleeding • Abdominal pain with or around time of defecation • Exclusion of intestinal infection (appropriate enteric pathogens include *Salmonella, Shigella, Yersinia, Campylobacter, E coli 0157:H7, Clostridium difficile*)
Laboratory features	• Iron deficiency anemia • Thrombocytosis • Hypalbuminemia • Autoantibodies (GAB, atypical ANCA) • Elevated fecal calprotectin
Endoscopic features	• Diffuse, continuous involvement of the mucosa starting at the rectum and extending proximally to a variable extent • Loss of vascular pattern • Loss of haustra • Edematous, erythematous appearance of the mucosa • Minute surface erosions • Pseudopolyps with long-standing UC • Friability (contact hemorrhage–mucosa bleeds when touched by endoscope) • Mucopurulent exudates
Histological features	• Increased mononuclear inflammation in the lamina propria • Mucin depletion • Crypt distortion, branching, and atrophy • Villous transformation of mucosal surface • Crypt abscesses

chronic or steroid-dependent disease immunosuppressive treatment with azathioprine or 6-mercaptopurine should be started as maintenance therapy. In patients with steroid refractory or dependent disease and in patients not responding to standard therapy, infliximab or another anti-tumor necrosis factor α (anti-TNFα) antibody may be an option to induce and maintain remission. In fulminant colitis, not responding to steroids, intravenous cyclosporine has become an alternative therapy, avoiding urgent colectomy. Total proctocolectomy with ileal pouch-anal canal anastomosis may be required in patients with toxic megacolon, in cases of fulminant colitis or in the prevention of colon cancer.

References

(1) Ekbom A. The changing faces of Crohn's disease and ulcerative colitis. (2003) In: Targan, S.R., Shanahan, F., and Karp, L.C. (eds.), Inflammatory Bowel Disease: From Bench to Bedside. 2nd ed. Dordrecht/Boston/London: Kluwer Academic Publishers, pp. 5–20.

(2) Mendeloff, A.I., Calkins, B.M. (1988) The epidemiology of idiopathic inflammatory bowel disease. In: Kirsner, J.B., Hawkins, C.F. Inflammatory Bowel Disease, 3rd ed. Lea & Febiger, Philadelphia, p. 3.

(3) Calkins, B.M., Mendeloff, A.I. (1986) Epidemiology of inflammatory bowel disease. *Epid Rev* 8: 60–91.

(4) Hanauer, S.B. (2006) Inflammatory Bowel Disease: Epidemiology, Pathogenesis, and Therapeutic Opportunities. *Inflamm Bowel Dis* 12: S3–9.

(5) Kirsner, J.B. (2001) Historical origins of current IBD concepts. *World J Gastroenterol* 7: 175–84.

(6) Wen, Z., Fiocchi, C. (2004) Inflammatory bowel disease: autoimmune or immune-mediated pathogenesis? *Clin Dev Immunol* 11: 195–204.

(7) Bamias, G., Cominelli, F. (2007) Immunopathogenesis of inflammatory bowel disease: current concepts. *Curr Opin Gastroenterol* 23: 365–9.

(8) Fuss, I.J., Heller, F., Boirivant, M., Leon, F., Yoshida, M., Fichtner-Feigl S., Yang Z., Exley M., Kitani A., Blumberg, R.S., Mannon P., Strober, W. (2004) Nonclassical CD1d-restricted NK T cells that produce IL-13 characterize an atypical Th2 response in ulcerative colitis. *J Clin Invest* 113: 1490–77.

(9) Shiobara, N., Suzuki, Y., Aoki, H., Gotoh, A., Fujii, Y., Hamada, Y., Suzuki, S., Fukui, N., Kurane, I., Itoh, T., Suzuki, R. (2007) Bacterial superantigens and T cell receptor β-chain-bearing T cells in the immunopathogenesis of ulcerative colitis. *Clin Exp Immunol* 150: 13–21.

(10) Baumgart, D.C., Carding, S.R. (2007) Inflammatory bowel disease: Cause and immunobiology. *Lancet* 369: 1627–40.

(11) Newman, B., Siminovitch, K.A. (2005) Recent advances in the genetics of inflammatory bowel disease. *Curr Opin Gastroenterol* 21: 401–7.

(12) Podolsky, D.K. (2002) Inflammatory bowel disease. *N Engl J Med* 347: 417–29.

(13) Conrad, K., Schmechta, H., Klafki, A., Lobeck, G., Uhlig, H., Gerdi, S., Henker, J. (2002) Serological differentiation of inflammatory bowel diseases. *Eur J Gastroenterol Hepatol* 14: 1–7.

(14) Bossuyt, X. (2006) Serologic markers in inflammatory bowel disease. *Clin Chem* 52: 171–81.

(15) Conrad, K., Bachmann, M.,Stöcker, W. (2006) Anti-intestinal goblet cell antoantibodies. In: Shoenfeld, Y., Gershwin, M.E., Meroni, P.L. (eds.), *Autoantibodies*, 2nd ed. Elsevier, Amsterdam, pp. 417–22.

(16) Ebert, E.C., Geng, X., Lin, J., Das, K.M. (2006) Autoantibodies against human tropomyosin isoform 5 in ulcerative colitis destroys colonic epithelial cells through antibody and complement-mediated lysis. *Cell Immunol* 244: 43–9.

(17) North American Society for Pediatric Gastroenterology, Hepatology, and Nutrition: Colitis Foundation of America; Bousvaros, A., Antonioli, D.A., Collett, R.B., Dubinsky, M.C., Glickman, J.N., Gold, B.D., Griffith A.M., Jevon, G.P., Higuchi, L.M. Hyams, J.S., Kirschner, B.S., Kugathasan, S., Baldassano, R.N., Russo, P.A. (2007) Differentiating ulcerative colitis from Crohn disease in children and young adults: Report of a working group of the North American Society for Pediatric Gastroenterology, Hepatology, and Nutrition and the Crohn's and Colitis Foundation of America. *J Pediatr Gastroenterol Nutr* 44: 653–74.

(18) Winther, K.V., Jess, T., Langholz, E., Munkholm, P., Binder, V. (2003) Survival and cause-specific mortality in ulcerative colitis: follow-up of a population-based cohort in Copenhagen County. *Gastroenterology* 125: 1576–82.

(19) Israeli, E., Grotto, I., Gilburd, B., Balicer, R.D., Goldin. E., Wiik, A., Shoenfeld Y. (2005) Anti-Saccharomyces cerevisiae and autineutrophil cytoplasmic antibodies as predictors of inflammatory bowel disease. *Gut* 54: 1232–6.

(20) Sutherland, L., MacDonald, J.K. (2006) Oral 5-aminosalicylic acid for induction of remission in ulcerative colitis. The Cochrane Database of Systematic Reviews 2006, Issue 2. Art. No.: CD000543.pub2. DOI: 10.1002/14651858. CD000543.pub2.

61
Inflammatory Bowel Disease

Miquel Sans and Carolina Figueroa

Abstract Inflammatory bowel disease (IBD) includes two main entities, Crohn's disease (CD) and ulcerative colitis (UC), with increasing incidence in the developed world. These are chronic, inflammatory disorders of unknown aetiology, characterized by leucocyte infiltration of the bowel wall which results in intestinal ulceration, causing abdominal pain, diarrhoea, bloody faeces and weight loss, among many other symptoms. IBD pathophysiology is very complex, requiring a genetic predisposition, the influence of certain environmental factors and a dysregulated immune system, as effector element. Both IBD genetics and the role of the intestinal microbiota in the development of IBD are at present the focus of intense research activity. There are no pathognomonic signs or symptoms of IBD. Therefore, diagnosis of CD and UC has to be based on a convincing combination of symptoms, biochemical abnormalities, mucosal endoscopic appearance, histological examination of mucosal biopsies and radiographic findings. It also requires to rule out other entities, such as infectious colitis. Treatment of UC and CD is primarily based, at present, on a sequential use of aminosalicylates, antibiotics, steroids, immunosuppressants and infliximab. However, IBD therapy is far from satisfactory and a significant proportion of CD and UC patients still require surgical treatment.

Keywords Inflammatory bowel disease · Crohn's disease · ulcerative colitis · bowel inflammation · epidemiology · diagnosis · treatment

Introduction

Inflammatory bowel disease (IBD) includes two main entities, Crohn's disease (CD) and ulcerative colitis (UC). CD can involve any portion of the digestive tract, from the oral mucosa to the anus. Lesions have a characteristic discontinuous distribution and affect all the wall layers in depth. On the contrary, UC only affects the colon. In this case, lesions can involve a variable but continuous proportion of the colon length, always starting in the rectum, and only the mucosal layer is affected. Both CD and UC are chronic, inflammatory disorders of unknown aetiology, characterized by leucocyte infiltration of the bowel wall which results in intestinal ulceration, causing abdominal pain, diarrhoea, bloody faeces and weight loss, among many other symptoms. In spite of the recent advances, including the biological therapy, treatment of IBD must be considered at present far from satisfactory, as shown by the high surgical requirement, which still is 30% for UC and 70% for CD patients.

Epidemiology

The incidence and prevalence of IBD have markedly increased in the last decades in the developed world, resulting in a present estimation of 1.5 million IBD patients in Europe and a similar figure in the USA (1). Similarly to other chronic, immune-mediated conditions, striking geographical differences in IBD prevalence have been shown between rich (Europe and the USA) and less developed (Africa and Asia) areas. This observation has led to the "hygiene hypothesis," which suggests that a high rate of infections, and especially of parasite infestations, at early stages of life would result in a Th2-predominant training of the immune system, which would protect from the later development of IBD (2). The sharp increase in IBD incidence observed in the last decades in the Mediterranean area as well as in some South American countries, such as Chile or Argentina, closely paralleling their social and economic development, strongly supports the hygiene hypothesis. Both

From: Y. Shoenfeld et al. (eds.): *Diagnostic Criteria in Autoimmune Diseases*, DOI: 10.1007/978-1-60327-285-8_61,
© 2008 Humana Press, Totowa, NJ

CD and UC age of onset peaks around 20–40 years, with no gender differences.

Pathogenesis

Although the aetiology of CD and UC remains elusive, key progress has been done in our understanding of IBD pathogenesis. It is now widely accepted that IBD develops in genetically susceptible subjects due to the interaction with environmental factors, tobacco being the best known of them. The intestinal flora also plays a key role and recent work has clearly proven that defects in the recognition of microbial antigens and also in the host defence against microbes, in combination with a deregulated immune system, will finally result in IBD.

The volume of research undertaken on IBD genetics in recent years has been tremendous. Genome-wide linkage studies pointed towards more than 10 chromosomal regions and fine-mapping of these regions led to the identification of a number of genes, including *CARD15* (*NOD2*), *DLG5*, *OCTN1* and *2*, *TLR4* and *CARD4* (*NOD1*). With the recent completion of the human genome project, whole genome association studies have now become possible and have identified additional genes (*IL23R*, *IRGM*, *PTGER4*, *ATG16L1*) for CD and UC, that have subsequently been replicated. At present, the *CARD15* gene is still the most understood susceptibility gene, explaining around 30% of the genetic predisposition to CD (3).

The demonstration that the CARD15 genetic variants associated to CD impairs the recognition of the bacterial product muramyl dipeptide by its receptor, the NOD2 protein, has reinforced the concept that the intestinal flora play a key role on IBD pathogenesis. Previously, a body of evidence accumulated both in humans and animal models, demonstrating that the presence of intestinal flora is mandatory for the development of bowel inflammation. The similarities existing between IBD and infectious colitis, at both the clinical and the pathological levels, has led to the search of an infectious pathogen as the single, causative agent of IBD. However, none of the microorganisms studied, including several viruses, *E. coli* and *M. paratuberculosis*, seem to cause CD or UC. At present, the researcher's efforts are focusing on the specific properties of the gut microbiota in IBD patients. So far, an increased number of bacteria firmly adhered to the intestinal mucosa as well as a marked reduction in the microbiota diversity have been described in IBD patients (4).

Clinical Manifestations

Both CD and UC are very heterogeneous conditions, and in each patient, clinical manifestation will mainly depend on disease extension, flare severity, presence of extraintestinal manifestations and development of certain IBD-related complications, such as bowel strictures, perianal disease, internal fistulas and intraabdominal abscesses. The most frequent symptoms in CD patients are diarrhoea, abdominal pain and weight loss, whereas UC patients typically present with diarrhoea and presence of blood and mucus in the stools. Other symptoms frequently observed in CD and UC patients are listed in Table 61.1. The already mentioned heterogeneity of CD and UC has prompted in the last years the development of several clinical classifications of IBD. Among them, the Vienna classification of CD and, most recently, the Montreal classification of CD and UC are the most widely accepted (Table 61.2) (5, 6). In the case of CD patients, both classifications are based on three main characteristics, namely age at onset, disease location and clinical behaviour, which have proven to have a key impact on CD severity. In the case of UC patients, disease extension is the most relevant feature. Interestingly, disease phenotype is not a stable characteristic of CD patients. Thus, close to 90% of CD cases have an inflammatory phenotype at diagnosis, whereas most of them have developed a more complicated, either stenosing or penetrating, phenotype, after 10 years of follow-up (7).

TABLE 61.1. Most frequent symptoms of Crohn's disease and ulcerative colitis.

Crohn's disease	Ulcerative colitis
Diarrhoea	Haematochezia
Abdominal pain	Diarrhoea
Weight loss	Rectal tenesmus
Fever	Faecal urgency/incontinence
Delayed growth (children)	Abdominal pain
Perianal disease	Fever
Extraintestinal manifestations	Extraintestinal manifestations

TABLE 61.2. Montreal classification of Crohn's disease.

(1) Age at onset
    A1 – Diagnosed at the age of 16 years or before
    A2 – Diagnosed at the age of 17–40 years
    A3 – Diagnosed above 40 years of age
(2) Disease location
    L1 – Ileal
    L2 – Colonic
    L3 – Ileo-colonic
    + "L4" (if it exists, location proximal to terminal ileum)
(3) Disease behaviour
    B1 – Inflammatory (non-stenosing, non-penetrating)
    B2 – Stenosing
    B3 – Penetrating
    + "p" (if it exists, perianal disease)

TABLE 61.3. Key pathological features of Crohn's disease and ulcerative colitis.

Pathological findings	Crohn's disease	Ulcerative colitis
Crypt distortion	+	+++
Architecture alteration	+	+++
Lamina propria neutrophils	+	+
Mononuclear cell infiltrate	+++	+
Lymphoid aggregates	+++	No
Granuloma	+++	No
Giant multinuclear cells	+++	No

Pathological Features

The most characteristic pathological feature of both CD and UC is a dense, chronic inflammatory infiltrate that includes lymphocytes, macrophages and plasmatic cells, among other cell types. This inflammatory infiltrate affects all the bowel layers in CD and is limited to the mucosa, as well as the submucosa in severe flares, in UC patients. Another typical pathological feature of both diseases is the disruption of the normal architecture of the mucosa, which looses the regular disposition of the glands. Although none of the pathological changes observed in these patients is completely specific of IBD in general, or CD or UC in particular, the presence of granulomas strongly suggests the diagnosis of CD, once other granulomatous conditions, such as intestinal tuberculosis, are ruled out. The most relevant pathological features of IBD, and their relative frequency of presentation in both CD and UC patients, is described in Table 61.3 (8).

Biochemical Features

Similarly to the pathological findings, there are no specific biochemical markers in IBD and blood tests are often normal in inactive CD and UC patients. On the contrary, when IBD patients experience a flare, this is reflected by a marked increase in the serum levels of the C-reactive protein (CRP) and other acute-phase markers as well as by many other changes, not only at the blood level but also in faecal markers, such as calprotectin.

The most widely used biochemical parameter in IBD patients is the CRP. The synthesis of this acute-phase protein is markedly upregulated in the liver in response to a variety of stimuli, including infectious and inflammatory processes, which confers to this marker a low specificity and therefore a very limited usefulness for the initial diagnosis of IBD. However, the measurement of serum levels of CRP is a good indicator of inflammatory activity in both CD and UC patients. CRP has been included in several indexes of IBD activity and, of note, is the most frequently used

biochemical parameter in IBD clinical trials. In addition, and due to its short half-live, CRP is also very useful to monitor the early response to IBD therapies (9).

Among the many biochemical changes present in active CD and UC patients, the erythrocyte sedimentation rate (ESR) has been also frequently used. However, in addition to the inflammatory activity, this parameter is also influenced by other concomitant processes, such as anaemia or hypoalbuminemia, which are frequently found in IBD patients. Many IBD patients present leucocytosis and thrombocytosis. Again, these changes can also be caused by concomitant infections (the first) or iron deficiency (the second), being therefore very unspecific.

For many years a number of serological tests, including p-ANCA, ASCA, Omp-c, c-byr and many others, have been used to try to help physicians in either the initial diagnosis of IBD or to identify subgroups of CD or UC patients with a certain clinical course. Although they might be of some help, especially in cases of indeterminate colitis, they have not reached wide acceptance and use in clinical practice.

More recently, several studies have demonstrated the usefulness of calprotectin, a faecal marker, to both predict early relapse in inactive IBD patients and to monitor the response of active IBD patients to therapy (10).

Endoscopy

Endoscopy is a key tool for physicians treating IBD patients, because diagnosis of both CD and UC is primarily based on the endoscopic appearance or the intestinal mucosa and the histological analysis of the colonic or ileal biopsies, obtained at endoscopy. The main endoscopic features of CD and UC are displayed on Table 61.4.

In addition to the initial diagnosis, the conventional endoscopy is also useful for IBD patients in other settings, such as monitoring the response to IBD therapies

TABLE 61.4. Key endoscopic features of Crohn's disease and ulcerative colitis.

Endoscopic findings	Crohn's disease	Ulcerative colitis
Mucosal surface	Nodular or polypoid	Granular
Distribution of lesions	Segmentary	Diffuse/continuous
Aphthoid ulcers	Yes	No
Ulcer characteristics	Great variety in size and depth	Small and superficial (bigger in severe cases)
Pseudopolyps	Infrequent	Frequent
Rectal involvement	<50%	Almost 100%
Ileal involvement	Frequent	No

at the mucosal level. In that respect, achieving the mucosal healing has proven to have a key impact on the clinical outcome of CD and UC patients, as recently demonstrated (11).

The recent development of the chromoendoscopy and magnification endoscopy, as well as other more sophisticated endoscopic techniques, such as narrow band imaging, and endomicroscopy, will be very helpful in the screening of dysplasia and colorectal cancer in IBD patients, especially in those with a long-lasting pancolitis. Several studies have demonstrated that the use of chromoendoscopy/magnification endoscopy, which allows targeted biopsies, is clearly superior to the conventional strategy for the screening of dysplasia in IBD, which was based on the analysis of a high number of random colonic biopsies (12).

Radiological Study

With the exception of small bowel barium studies used to identify ileal or proximal involvement by CD, radiological techniques are usually of limited usefulness in the initial diagnosis of IBD. On the contrary, they have other frequent indications for IBD patients, in clinical practice. Both pelvic magnetic resonance imaging (MRI) and ultrasound endoscopy are the first choice examinations to fully characterize perianal disease as well as other penetrating complications of CD (13). Abdominal computerized tomography (CT) or MRI are routinely used to study abdominal abscesses. Leucocyte-labelled scintigraphy has been used for many years as an alternative technique to complete the study of extension in CD and UC patients. However, MRI might replace scintigraphy in this indication in the near future.

Diagnostic Criteria

As already mentioned, there are no symptoms, biochemical changes, pathological features or endoscopic findings that can be considered as completely specific or CD or UC. For that reason, diagnosis of these entities mainly relies on a combination of clinical suspicion with typical endoscopic and histologic findings, along with an active process of ruling out other conditions. The criteria of Lennard-Jones, published in 1989 to uniform the diagnosis of CD (Table 61.5) and UC (Table 61.6), have been widely accepted to date (14).

TABLE 61.5. Diagnostic criteria of Crohn's disease[a]

	Examination or endoscopy	Radiology	Biopsy	Surgical specimen
Distribution				
Proximal lesions	+	+	+	+
Anal lesions	+	+		+
Segmentary distribution	+	+	+	+
Transmural lesions				
Fissure		+		+
Abscess	+	+		+
Fistula	+	+		+
Stenosis	+	+		+
Pathology findings				
Ulcers			+	+
Lymphoid aggregates			+	+
Mucin retention			+	
Granulomas			+	+

[a] Adapted from Lennard-Jones JE (14).
Diagnosis of Crohn's disease is established if
(1) Granuloma is found at pathological examination + 1 other criteria;
(2) in the absence of granuloma at pathological examination 3 criteria.

TABLE 61.6. Diagnostic criteria of ulcerative colitis[a]

Inclusion criteria	Exclusion criteria
Diffuse mucosal involvement, without granuloma (at pathological examination)	Infectious colitis (microbiology)
Rectal involvement (at endoscopy)	Ischaemic colitis (risk factors, location, pathological findings)
Involvement, in continuity with the rectum, of a variable portion of the colon (at endoscopy of barium radiography)	Actinic proctitis/colitis (previous radiotherapy/pathological findings)
	Solitary rectal ulceration (location, pathological findings)
	Crohn's disease (small bowel involvement, pathological findings)
	Complex anal lesions (physical examination)
	Granuloma (pathological findings)

[a] Adapted from Lennard-Jones JE (14).

Therapy

Crohn's Disease

Treatment choice depends on disease location, severity and the presence of stenosing or penetrating complications (15). Oral or intravenous steroids have been for many years the most frequently used treatment for moderate to severe flares of CD. Oral mesalazine can be also used in mild to moderate cases, although its efficacy is less that that of delayed-release formulations of budesonide, which are at present the first choice of treatment for mild to moderate ileitis. In patients with moderate or severely active CD refractory to steroids, infliximab, a monoclonal antibody to TNF-α, is indicated (16). Failure to infliximab usually leads to surgical treatment. Patients with mild to moderate chronically active CD as well as CD patients developing steroid dependency are usually treated with immunosuppressants, such as azathioprine, mercaptopurine or methotrexate. In case of failure, infliximab has proven to be efficacious in this setting. As maintenance therapy, once disease remission is achieved, several drugs including azathioprine, mercaptopurine, methotrexate and infliximab, but not mesalazine, have proven to reduce the risk of relapse during follow-up. Stricturing CD in the absence of inflammatory activity requires bowel surgery. Perianal disease as well as internal penetrating CD cases are the most difficult to treat. These CD patients must benefit from a combined medical and surgical approach, including drainage of abscesses, placement of setons, the use of antibiotics and immunosuppressants and, in most cases, infliximab (17).

Ulcerative Colitis

Similarly to CD, both disease location and severity will lead the treatment choice in UC patients. In patients with distal colitis (especially in proctitis and proctosigmoiditis), rectal mesalazine has proven to be superior to both oral mesalazine and rectal steroids. In patients with extensive, mild to moderate UC, oral mesalazine is the treatment of choice. In cases not responding to oral mesalazine, oral steroids are the second line of therapy, whereas in patients with severely active UC intravenous steroids will be used. In cases of moderate to severely active UC, resistant to steroids, two options are at present available, cyclosporin A and infliximab (18, 19). In the absence of a face-to-face study, comparing the usefulness of both drugs, treatment must be individualized and selected according to each centre preference. Failure to these rescue therapies requires urgent surgical treatment, which will initially consist of procto-colectomy with derivative ileostomy, followed later on by proctectomy, ileo-anal pouch and reconstruction of the faecal transit. Recent evidence suggests that the addition of rectal treatment improves the results of conventional therapy in patients with extensive UC. Patients developing a mild to moderate, chronically active UC as well as UC patients developing steroid dependency are treated with immunosuppressants, such as azathioprine or mercaptopurine. In case of failure, infliximab has

proven to be efficacious in these patients. As a maintenance therapy, oral and/or topical mesalazine (according to disease extension) is the first option of treatment.

Prognosis

In highly heterogeneous diseases, such as CD and UC, the development of prognostic markers has been an unmet need and the subject of intense research for many years. Unfortunately, none of the clinical, biochemical, endoscopical, serological or genetic markers studied so far either has gained wide acceptance or has reached clinical practice. However, a recent report from the French GETAID group has suggested and validated a clinical prognostic index (20). More complex indexes, combining clinical, serological and genetic markers, are under development at present.

References

1. Lakatos PL. Recent trends in the epidemiology of inflammatory bowel diseases: Up or down? *World J Gastroenterol* 2006 October 14; 12(38): 6102–8.
2. Danese S, Sans M, Fiocchi C. Inflammatory bowel disease: The role of environmental factors. *Autoimmun Rev* 2004 July; 3(5): 394–400.
3. Vermeire S. Review article: genetic susceptibility and application of genetic testing in clinical management of inflammatory bowel disease. *Aliment Pharmacol Ther* 2006 October; 24(Suppl. 3): 2–10.
4. Swidsinski A, Ladhoff A, Pernthaler A, Swidsinski S, Loening-Baucke V, Ortner M, Weber J, Hoffmann U, Schreiber S, Dietel M, Lochs H. Mucosal flora in inflammatory bowel disease. *Gastroenterology* 2002 January; 122(1): 44–54.
5. Gasche C, Scholmerich J, Brynskov J, D'Haens G, Hanauer SB, Irvine EJ, Jewell DP, Rachmilewitz D, Sachar DB, Sandborn WJ, Sutherland LR. A simple classification of Crohn's disease: Report of the Working Party for the World Congresses of Gastroenterology, Vienna 1998. *Inflamm Bowel Dis* 2000 February; 6(1): 8–15.
6. Silverberg MS, Satsangi J, Ahmad T, Arnott ID, Bernstein CN, Brant SR, Caprilli R, Colombel JF, Gasche C, Geboes K, Jewell DP, Karban A, Loftus EV Jr, Peña AS, Riddell RH, Sachar DB, Schreiber S, Steinhart AH, Targan SR, Vermeire S, Warren BF. Toward an integrated clinical, molecular and serological classification of inflammatory bowel disease: Report of a Working Party of the 2005 Montreal World Congress of Gastroenterology. *Can J Gastroenterol* 2005 September; 19(Suppl. A): 5–36.
7. Louis E, Collard A, Oger AF, Degroote E, Aboul Nasr El, Yafi FA, Belaiche J. Behaviour of Crohn's disease according to the Vienna classification: Changing pattern over the course of the disease. *Gut* 2001 December; 49(6): 777–82.

8. Geboes K. Pathology of inflammatory bowel diseases (IBD): Variability with time and treatment. *Colorectal Dis* 2001 January; 3(1): 2–12.

9. Solem CA, Loftus EV Jr, Tremaine WJ, Harmsen WS, Zinsmeister AR, Sandborn WJ. Correlation of C-reactive protein with clinical, endoscopic, histologic, and radiographic activity in inflammatory bowel disease. *Inflamm Bowel Dis* 2005 August; 11(8): 707–12.

10. Konikoff MR, Denson LA. Role of fecal calprotectin as a biomarker of intestinal inflammation in inflammatory bowel disease. *Inflamm Bowel Dis* 2006 June; 12(6): 524–34.

11. Frøslie KF, Jahnsen J, Moum BA, Vatn MH; IBSEN Group. Mucosal healing in inflammatory bowel disease: Results from a Norwegian population-based cohort. *Gastroenterology* 2007 August; 133(2): 412–22. Epub 2007 June 2.

12. Kiesslich R, Fritsch J, Holtmann M, Koehler HH, Stolte M, Kanzler S, Nafe B, Jung M, Galle PR, Neurath MF. Methylene blue-aided chromoendoscopy for the detection of intraepithelial neoplasia and colon cancer in ulcerative colitis. *Gastroenterology* 2003 April; 124(4): 880–8.

13. Schwartz DA, Wiersema MJ, Dudiak KM, Fletcher JG, Clain JE, Tremaine WJ, Zinsmeister AR, Norton ID, Boardman LA, Devine RM, Wolff BG, Young-Fadok TM, Diehl NN, Pemberton JH, Sandborn WJ. A comparison of endoscopic ultrasound, magnetic resonance imaging, and exam under anesthesia for evaluation of Crohn's perianal fistulas. *Gastroenterology* 2001 November; 121(5): 1064–72.

14. Lennard-Jones JE. Classification of inflammatory bowel disease. *Scand J Gastroenterol Suppl* 1989; 170: 2–6; discussion 16–9.

15. Travis SP, Stange EF, Lémann M, Oresland T, Chowers Y, Forbes A, D'Haens G, Kitis G, Cortot A, Prantera C, Marteau P, Colombel JF, Gionchetti P, Bouhnik Y, Tiret E, Kroesen J, Starlinger M, Mortensen NJ; European Crohn's and Colitis Organisation. European evidence based consensus on the diagnosis and management of Crohn's disease: Current management. *Gut* 2006 March; 55(Suppl. 1): i16–35.

16. Baert FJ, D'Haens GR, Peeters M, Hiele MI, Schaible TF, Shealy D, Geboes K, Rutgeerts PJ. Tumor necrosis factor alpha antibody (infliximab) therapy profoundly down-regulates the inflammation in Crohn's ileocolitis. *Gastroenterology* 1999 January; 116(1): 22–8.

17. Present DH, Rutgeerts P, Targan S, Hanauer SB, Mayer L, van Hogezand RA, Podolsky DK, Sands BE, Braakman T, DeWoody KL, Schaible TF, van Deventer SJ. Infliximab for the treatment of fistulas in patients with Crohn's disease. *N Engl J Med* 1999 May 6; 340(18): 1398–405.

18. Lichtiger S, Present DH, Kornbluth A, Gelernt I, Bauer J, Galler G, Michelassi F, Hanauer S. Cyclosporine in severe ulcerative colitis refractory to steroid therapy. *N Engl J Med* 1994 June 30; 330(26): 1841–5.

19. Rutgeerts P, Sandborn WJ, Feagan BG, Reinisch W, Olson A, Johanns J, Travers S, Rachmilewitz D, Hanauer SB, Lichtenstein GR, de Villiers WJ, Present D, Sands BE, Colombel JF. Infliximab for induction and maintenance therapy for ulcerative colitis. *N Engl J Med* 2005 December 8; 353(23): 2462–76.

20. Consigny Y, Modigliani R, Colombel JF, Dupas JL, Lémann M, Mary JY; Groupe d'Etudes Thérapeutiques des Affections Inflammatoires Digestives (GETAID). A simple biological score for predicting low risk of short-term relapse in Crohn's disease. *Inflamm Bowel Dis* 2006 July; 12(7): 551–7.

62
Celiac Disease

Nicola Bizzaro and Elio Tonutti

Abstract   Celiac disease (CD) is a chronic small-bowel disorder of autoimmune origin, occurring both in children and adults, and is one of the most common disorders in Western countries, with an estimated frequency of 1:100–200 in the general population. This disease is genetically determined and has a strong HLA association with the DQ2 and DQ8 alleles. The serological markers of the disease are tissue transglutaminase, endomysial and gliadin antibodies. Histological demonstration of typical intestinal alterations, together with clinical improvement when patients are on a gluten-free diet, is the gold standard for a definite diagnosis.

Keywords   Celiac disease · transglutaminase antibodies · endomysial antibodies · gliadin antibodies · HLA

Celiac disease (CD) is a gluten-sensitive enteropathy of autoimmune origin, characterized by inflammation and villous atrophy of the small-bowel mucosa, that impairs nutrient absorption. The disease has a strong genetic background, affecting mainly susceptible individuals bearing the antigens codified by HLA class II DQ2/DQ8 alleles. The classical presentation in children includes severe gastrointestinal symptoms such as abdominal distension, diarrhea, abdominal pain and weight loss, whereas iron-deficient anemia is the most common symptom in adult CD. The serological markers of the disease are tissue transglutaminase, endomysial and gliadin antibodies. Histological demonstration of typical intestinal alterations, together with clinical improvement when patients are on a gluten-free diet, is the gold standard for a definite diagnosis.

Epidemiology

In contrast to what was believed until a few years ago, CD is a relatively common disorder. The false conviction that it was a rare disease was due to the fact that most patients are asymptomatic or have only mild gastrointestinal symptoms that may go unrecognized (1, 2). The development of highly sensitive immunological methods for identifying diagnostic antibodies has enabled an increasing number of patients with CD, with vague or asymptomatic clinical presentations, to be identified. Population-based studies indicate now that approximately 0.5–1% of the

Western European and Northern American populations suffer from CD (3, 4).

History

Samuel Gee (5) in 1888 provided the first thorough description of the clinical features of childhood CD. In 1953, Dicke (6), a Dutch pediatrician, observed that the ingestion of certain cereal grains were harmful to children with this disease, and Paulley (7) in 1954 provided the first description of the histopathological findings of the intestinal lesions.

The presence of antibodies directed against gluten proteins in the serum of patients suffering from CD was reported in the late 1950s. For many years, the determination of antigliadin antibodies (AGAs), the alcohol-soluble fraction of gluten, was the only serological test to identify CD patients. The discovery of anti-endomysial autoantibodies (EMAs), and later of antitransglutaminase antibodies (anti-tTG), in the 1990s has changed the serological approach to the diagnosis of CD.

Pathogenesis

CD is initiated by the ingestion of gliadin, which is present in foods containing wheat, barley and rye. It seems that in CD patients, the integrity of the tight junction system of

From: Y. Shoenfeld et al. (eds.): *Diagnostic Criteria in Autoimmune Diseases*, DOI: 10.1007/978-1-60327-285-8_62,
© 2008 Humana Press, Totowa, NJ

the intestinal epithelium cells is compromised enabling the passage of macromolecules such as the gluten in the submucosa. Gliadin peptides are then modified by the enzyme tTG located in the extracellular space of the intestinal mucosa. Conversion of glutamine residues into glutamic acid by tTG facilitates the binding of gliadin peptides to HLA antigens of class II DQ2 or DQ8 expressed on antigen-presenting cells. In individuals with this genetic make-up, an immune response leading to the synthesis of cytokines and specific anti-tTG and AGA antibodies can be triggered. However, the fact that approximately 25–30% of the population in the Western hemisphere express HLA-DQ2 or HLA-DQ8 and are exposed to large amounts of gluten daily, but only a minority develop CD, indicates that other currently unknown factors are involved in the development of the disease.

Clinical Manifestations

CD is characterized by multiform clinical expressions (8). Signs and symptoms at presentation are shown in Table 62.1.

The classical form of CD in children consists of gastrointestinal symptoms starting between 6 and 24 months of age, after the introduction of gluten in the diet. Children with CD frequently have gastrointestinal symptoms such as diarrhea, vomiting, abdominal pain or abdominal distension, and growth retardation. However, most CD patients, especially adults, do not present gastrointestinal disorders but manifest signs resulting from malabsorption (hypochromic iron-deficient anemia, osteopenia, tooth enamel defects, etc.) or other symptoms whose trigger mechanism is unclear (hypertransaminasaemia, headache or joint pains). Gluten intolerance may also manifest as a skin disorder (dermatitis herpetiformis); patients with skin lesions typical of this disease present serological positivity for anti-tTG IgA, and the histological alterations of the intestinal mucosa typical of CD.

Patients suffering from some disorders (especially Hashimoto's thyroiditis, type I diabetes, IgA deficiency and Down's syndrome) have a higher risk (3–5 times) of developing CD than the normal population. In patients belonging to those at-risk groups, it is advisable to perform serological tests for CD even in the absence of symptoms.

Pathological Features

CD is characterized by varying degrees of atrophy of the intestinal mucosa, with a reduction in the height, or disappearance, of the villi.

The degree of intestinal lesion is defined on the basis of the widely used Marsh-Oberhuber classification (9), which describes the degree of architectural changes in the mucosa and outlines three categories of lesions associated with CD:

1. *Type 1—infiltrative*: architecturally normal small-bowel mucosa and intraepithelial lymphocytosis (>40 intraepithelial lymphocytes (IELs) per 100 epithelial cells); these features are suggestive but not diagnostic of CD.
2. *Type 2—infiltrative-hyperplastic*: normal villous architecture, intraepithelial lymphocytosis (>40 IELs per 100 epithelial cells), crypt hyperplasia (regenerative aspect shown by elongation of the crypts, reduction in muciferous activity and increase in number of mitoses). These histopathological features are non-specific and clinical correlation is indicated.
3. *Type 3—atrophic*: villous atrophy of different degree, associated with intraepithelial lymphocytosis (>40 IELs per 100 epithelial cells) and crypt hyperplasia.

TABLE 62.1. Signs and symptoms of CD.

Typical symptoms	Atypical symptoms secondary to malasorbption	Atypical symptoms independent of malasorbption	Associated conditions
Chronic diarrhea	Sideropenic anemia	Dental enamel defects	Type 1 diabetes
Failure to thrive	Short stature	Aphtous stomatitis	Dermatitis herpetiformis
Abdominal distension and pain	Osteopenia	Glossitis	Primary biliary cirrhosis
Vomiting	Osteoporosis	Ataxia	Autoimmune thyroiditis
Weight loss	Fatigue	Epilepsy	Sjögren's syndrome
	Apatia	Polyneuropathy	Addison's disease
	Delayed puberty	Alopecia	Down's syndrome
	Gaseousness and flatulence	Pericarditis	Turner's syndrome
	Hemorrhage	Dilatative cardiomyopathy	IgA deficiency
	Bruising	Arthritis	
	Steatorrhea	Myopathy	
	Constipation	Recurrent abortion	
	Dispepsia	Infertility	
	Nausea	Hypertransaminasaemia	
		Vitiligo	

4. Type 3 lesions are further subcategorized based on villous height in:

(a) type 3a—mild villous atrophy.
(b) type 3b—moderated villous atrophy.
(c) type 3c—total villous atrophy (flat mucosa and no visible villi).

Serological Features

The serological diagnosis of CD is based on the detection of class IgA AGA, EMA and anti-tTG antibodies. In patients with an IgA deficiency, AGA, EMA or anti-tTG tests of the IgG class are used. The diagnostic accuracy (sensitivity and specificity) of the serological markers in adult and pediatric patients and in subjects with IgA deficiency, is shown in Table 62.2.

As tTG has been identified as the main antigen recognized by antiendomysium antibodies (10), ELISA tests have been developed to identify both IgG and IgA anti-tTG antibodies, and this test may now be considered the best tool for the serological identification of CD (11).

Anti-tTG testing can also be used to monitor CD patients following a diet in which the autoantibodies gradually decline, until they disappear.

With the discovery of anti-tTG antibodies, the use of AGA IgA and AGA IgG tests is no longer recommended for detecting CD (12). However, the recent identification of the immunodominant antigen sites of gliadin and the resulting development of specific tests for these epitopes refocused the attention on AGA and the possibility of their use in certain clinical situations, such as the diagnosis of CD at pediatric age, as anti-tTG and EMA autoantibodies may appear after the age of 2–5 years (13).

Diagnostic Criteria

Diagnostic criteria were proposed in 1990 by the European Society for Pediatric Gastroenterology, Hepatology and Nutrition (14) (Table 62.3). Recently, the North American

TABLE 62.3. Revised criteria for the diagnosis of CD proposed by the ESPGHAN (14).

1	History and clinical presentation compatible with CD
2	Serological screening compatible with CD
3	Histological findings compatible with CD
4	Obvious clinical and serological response to GFD
5	Subject >2 years old
6	Rule out other clinical conditions mimicking CD

Society for Pediatric Gastroenterology, Hepatology and Nutrition has developed clinical guidelines for the diagnosis and treatment of CD (12).

A possible diagnostic algorithm involves the use of anti-tTG IgA ELISA as a highly sensitive screening test, followed by a highly specific EMA confirmation test if the anti-tTG ELISA test result is positive. If the sample also tests positive for EMA IgA, the serological diagnosis of CD is practically certain, while if it tests negative for EMA IgA, determination of haplotype HLA DQ2/DQ8 is advisable (15). Confirmation of the serological diagnosis of CD requires an intestinal biopsy in all cases. Because the histological changes in CD may be patchy, it is recommended that multiple biopsy specimens be obtained.

Although a small-bowel biopsy is recommended to establish the diagnosis, the availability of accurate serologic tests has reduced the need for a second biopsy. A second biopsy can now be reserved for selected patients who have an unsatisfactory or equivocal clinical response to a strict gluten-free diet (GFD).

IgA anti-tTG assay cannot be used in patients with IgA deficiency and should be replaced by IgG-class antibody tests. Anti-tTG IgG antibody assay is considered a better test than AGA IgG for identifying individuals with selective IgA deficiency (12, 16, 17).

Prediction

Some individuals test positive for anti-tTG/EMA or AGA without any histologically detectable damage to the intestinal mucosa. These cases are classed as "latent celiac disease," and must be monitored on a long-term basis to evaluate the appearance of symptoms and/or intestinal damage, because it has been demonstrated that the detection of antibodies can precede the appearance of clinical symptoms by many years (18). In preserved serum samples, the predictive value of anti-tTG antibodies was 60% at 10 years (13).

Therapy

The keystone of CD treatment remains a GFD in which all foods containing the offending cereal grains are avoided. The response to gluten withdrawal is generally rapid;

TABLE 62.2. Diagnostic accuracy of serologic markers of CD in adults, children and in subjects with IgA deficiency.

	Sensitivity %	Specificity %
AGA IgA	52–100	47–94
AGA IgG	57–100	71–100
tTG IgA adults	91–99	97–100
tTG IgG adults	30–50	90–93
tTG IgA children	96	99
tTG IgG children	30–50	85–90
EMA IgA	93–96	99–100
tTG IgG in IgA def.	90	100

gastrointestinal symptoms usually improve within 2 to 3 weeks. When CD patients follow a GFD, the normal architecture of the intestinal villi is restored and, in patients with dermatitis herpetiformis, the skin lesions heal. Lack of improvement within 6 to 8 weeks after the institution of a GFD should prompt a search for inadvertent ingestion of gluten by the patient or for an associated disease.

After 6–12 months of a totally GFD, the anti-tTG IgA antibodies decrease, and eventually disappear. This characteristic of CD enables the anti-tTG IgA test to be used to monitor patients' compliance with their diet even if the disappearance of anti-tTG IgA does not correlate completely with a normal histological pattern.

It has been shown that the early recognition of silent CD and the subsequent introduction of a GFD can reduce the risk of developing some important complications such as osteoporosis and intestinal lymphoma.

References

1. Catassi, C., Ratsch, I., Fabiani, E., Ricci, S., Bordicchia, F., Pierdomenico, R., et al. (1995) High prevalence of undiagnosed coeliac disease in 5280 Italian students screened by antigliadin antibodies. *Acta Paediatr* **84**, 672–6.

2. Ivarsson, A., Persson, L.A., Juto, P., Peltonen, M., Suhr, O., and Hernell, O. (1999) High prevalence of undiagnosed coeliac disease in adults: a Swedish population-based study. *J Intern Med* **245**, 63–8.

3. Catassi, G., Rätsch, I.M., Fabiani, E., Rossini, M., Bordicchia, F., Candela, F., et al. (1994) Coeliac disease in the year 2000: Exploring the iceberg. *Lancet* **343**, 200–3.

4. Not, T., Horvath, K., Hill, I.D., Partanen, J., Hammed, A., Magazzù, G., et al. (1998) Celiac disease risk in the USA: high prevalence of antiendomysium antibodies in healthy blood donors. *Scand J Gastroenterol* **33**, 494–8.

5. Gee, S. (1888) On the coeliac affection. *St Barth Hosp Rep* **24**, 17–20.

6. Dicke, W.K., Weijers, H.A., van de Kamer, J.H. (1953) Coeliac disease. II. The presence in wheat of a factor having a deleterious effect in cases of coeliac disease. *Acta Paediatr Scand* **42**, 34–42.

7. Paulley, J.W. (1954) Observation on the aetiology of idiopathic steatorrhoea; jejunal and lymph-node biopsies. *BMJ* **490**, 1318–21.

8. Rostom, A., Catherine, D., Cranney, A., Saloojee, N., Sy, R., Garritty, C., et al. (2005) The diagnostic accuracy of serological tests for celiac disease: a systematic review. *Gastroenterology* **128**, S38–46.

9. Oberhuber, G., Granditsch, G., and Vogelsang, H. (1999) The histopathology of coeliac disease: time for a standardized report scheme for pathologists. *Eur J Gastroenterol Hepatol* **11**, 1185–94.

10. Dieterich, W., Ehnis, T., Bauer, M., Donner, P., Volta, U., Riecken, E.O., et al. (1997) Identification of tissue transglutaminase as the autoantigen of celiac disease. *Nat Med* **3**, 797–801.

11. National Institutes of Health. (2005) National Institutes of Health consensus development conference statement on celiac disease. June 28–30, 2004. *Gastroenterology* **128**, S1–9.

12. Hill, I.D., Dirks, M.H., Liptak, G.S., Colletti, R.B., Fasano, A., Guandalini, S., et al. (2005) Guideline for the diagnosis and treatment of celiac disease in children: Recommendations of the North American Society for Pediatric Gastroenterology, Hepatology and Nutrition. *J Ped Gastroenterol Nutr* **40**, 1–19.

13. Simell, S., Kupila, A., Hoppu, S., Hekkala, A., Simell, T., Stahlberg, M.R., et al. (2005) Natural history of transglutaminase autoantibodies and mucosal changes in children carrying HLA-conferred celiac disease susceptibility. *Scand J Gastroenterol* **40**, 1182–91.

14. Walker-Smith, J.A., Guandalini, S., Schmitz, J., Shmerling, D.H., and Visakorpi, J.K. (1990) Revised criteria for diagnosis of celiac disease. *Arch Dis Child* **65**, 909–11.

15. Tonutti, E., Bizzaro, N. (2006).Anti-tissue transglutaminase and anti-endomysial antibodies. In: Shoenfeld, Y., Gershwin, M.E., Meroni, P.L. (eds). *Autoantibodies*, 2 nd edition. Amsterdam: Elsevier, pp. 443–50.

16. Dahlbom, I., Olsson, M., Forooz, N.K., Sjöholom, A.G., Truedsson, L., and Hansson, T. (2005) Immunoglobulin G (IgG) anti-tissue transglutaminase antibodies used as markers for IgA deficient celiac disease patients. *Clin Diag Lab Immunol* **12**, 254–8.

17. Lenhardt, A., Plebani, A., Marchetti, F., Gerarduzzi, T., Not, T., Meini, A., et al. (2004) Role of human-tissue transglutaminase IgG and anti-gliadin IgG antibodies in the diagnosis of coeliac disease in patients with selective immunoglobulin A deficiency. *Dig Liv Dis* **36**, 730–4.

18. Paparo, F., Petrone, E., Tosco, A., Maglio, M., Borrelli, M., Salvati, V.M., et al. (2005) Clinical, HLA, and small bowel immunohistochemical features of children with positive serum antiendomysium antibodies and architecturally normal small intestine mucosa. *Am J Gastroenterol* **100**, 2294–8.

Part VIII
Cutaneous Autoimmune Diseases

63
Cutaneous Lupus Erythematosus

Annegret Kuhn, Vincent Ruland and Gisela Bonsmann

Abstract Cutaneous lupus erythematosus (CLE) is a chronic inflammatory autoimmune disorder, comprising a broad spectrum of clinical manifestations. Various environmental factors influence the clinical expression of CLE and a striking relationship has emerged between sunlight exposure and the various subtypes of this disease. However, the diverse pathophysiological mechanisms in CLE are currently under investigation. A detailed patient's history, evaluation of the activity and damage, histological analysis of skin biopsy specimens, phototesting, and serological investigations support the diagnosis of CLE, and also provide important information on the appropriate therapeutic strategy. Until now, antimalarial agents remain the treatment of choice for CLE.

Keywords Autoimmune disorder · CLASI · photosensitivity · skin manifestations · treatment

Lupus erythematosus (LE) is a chronic inflammatory autoimmune disease with a heterogeneous clinical presentation. In contrast to the multi-organ disease of systemic LE (SLE), patients with cutaneous LE (CLE) present with manifestations primarily confined to the skin.

Epidemiology

The incidence of SLE in the general population varies according to the characteristics of the population studied, such as predominant age, sex, race, ethnicity, and national origin. In Europe, the annual incidence of SLE ranges from 3.3 to 4.8 cases per 100,000 persons per year, and in the United States, the annual incidence of SLE has been reported to range from 2.0 to 7.6 cases per 100,000 persons per year (1). Cutaneous manifestations appear in 72–85% of patients with SLE and can occur at any stage of the disease; however, most studies focus on SLE, and a systematic epidemiological analysis of the various CLE subtypes has not been performed. The incidence of CLE has been estimated to be 2–3 fold higher than that of SLE. Recently, a study from Stockholm County, Sweden, suggested that Ro/SSA-positive SCLE patients have an estimated incidence of 0.7 per 100,000 persons per year as compared with an incidence of SLE in Sweden of 4.8 per 100,000 persons per year (2).

History

In 1845, Hebra described a "butterfly erythema" which he named "seborrhoea congestive"; however, the term *lupus érythémateaux* was not used until 1851 by Cazénave, who distinguished non-infectious skin lesions from cutaneous tuberculosis (lupus vulgaris), referring to an earlier report by Biett on this disease termed *erytheme centrifuge*. In the following years, Kaposi performed clinical and histological studies on the relation of cutaneous lesions and systemic organ manifestations of this disease. He recognized the presence of discoid skin lesions in SLE and extensively described the butterfly rash as a facial cutaneous sign of SLE. Therefore, Kaposi is nowadays recognized as the first describer of SLE and his continuous effort is reflected in several publications between 1869 and 1880. In addition, systemic organ manifestations in the context of LE were also mentioned in 1895 by Osler in his work titled "On the visceral complications of erythema exsudativum multiforme".

Pathogenesis

The complexity of CLE makes understanding of the underlying pathomechanisms difficult and, at the same time, implies multifactorial aspects of the pathogenic

From: Y. Shoenfeld et al. (eds.): *Diagnostic Criteria in Autoimmune Diseases*, DOI: 10.1007/978-1-60327-285-8_63,
© 2008 Humana Press, Totowa, NJ

course. Irritative stimuli, various drugs, and especially UV radiation can lead to the induction of skin lesions (3, 4). Furthermore, genetic factors also seem to be involved in the development of CLE subtypes. For example, a high association with HLA-A1,-B8, and -DR3 can be demonstrated in patients with SCLE (5). In addition, SCLE seems to be significantly associated with a single-nucleotide polymorphism in the TNF-alpha gene promoter (–308 A), which encodes for high TNF-alpha expression (6). Congenital homozygous deficiency of C1q is not only a risk factor for appearance of SLE, but has also been shown to be a predisposing factor for photosensitive CLE. More recently, the potential significance of apoptosis in the pathogenesis of CLE has been emphasized. A significant increase of apoptotic keratinocytes has been found in primary and UV-induced skin lesions of patients with different subtypes of CLE compared with healthy controls (7). Furthermore, in most patients with CLE, the number of apoptotic nuclei increased significantly between days 1 and 3 after UV exposure, suggesting that late apoptotic cells accumulate in the skin of patients with this disease. Detection of an increased number of apoptotic cells in the epidermis of CLE patients may reflect an increase in apoptosis; however, a deficient clearance of apoptotic debris could also lead to the increased number of apoptotic keratinocytes. The hypothesis that clearance of apoptotic cells in the skin of patients with CLE is either impaired or delayed is in analogy to the growing evidence that defects in the clearance of apoptotic cells may be important in triggering the immune response in SLE.

Classification

The clinical expression of CLE shows great variety and consequently, has led to the practice of identifying different subtypes of the disease. However, the development of a unifying concept for skin manifestations of the disease has proven difficult. In 1977, Gilliam proposed a classification system that divided the cutaneous lesions into LE-specific and LE-nonspecific manifestations by histological analysis of skin biopsy specimens (8). The LE-specific cutaneous findings encompass the various subtypes of CLE, which were subdivided into three different categories as defined by constellations of clinical features, histological changes, laboratory abnormalities, and average duration of skin lesions: acute CLE (ACLE), subacute CLE (SCLE), and chronic CLE (CCLE). In contrast, skin lesions, such as urticarial vasculitis and livedo reticularis, are some of the most common LE-nonspecific cutaneous lesions and are mostly associated with SLE, reflecting potentially serious complications. Since the initial formulation of the Gilliam nomenclature and classification system more than two decades ago, several attempts have been made to improve this system and to provide new

TABLE 63.1. Düsseldorf classification of cutaneous lupus erythematosus 2004[a].

| Acute cutaneous lupus erythematosus (ACLE) |
| Subacute cutaneous lupus erythematosus (SCLE) |
| Chronic cutaneous lupus erythematosus (CCLE) |
| Discoid lupus erythematosus (DLE) |
| Lupus erythematosus profundus (LEP) |
| Chilblain lupus erythematosus (CHLE) |
| Intermittent cutaneous lupus erythematosus (ICLE) |
| Lupus erythematosus tumidus (LET) |

[a] Modified after Kuhn and Ruzicka 2004 (8).

approaches to the problem of classification of the cutaneous manifestations of LE. In recent years, a further subtype with characteristic clinical, histological, and photobiological features, named LE tumidus (LET), has been analyzed and defined as a separate entity of CLE. The course and prognosis in these patients is generally more favorable than in those with other subtypes of CLE and therefore, a revised classification system, including LET as the intermittent subtype of CLE (ICLE), was suggested in 2004 (8) (Table 63.1).

Clinical Manifestations

ACLE usually occurs in association with systemic manifestations preceding the onset of a multisystem disease by weeks or months. Sun exposure is a common exogenous factor capable of precipitating ACLE, and some patients even report an exacerbation of their systemic symptoms after exposure to sunlight. Furthermore, infections, especially with subtle types of viruses, or certain drugs, such as hydralazine, isoniazide, and procainamide, have also been found to induce or aggravate this disease (4). Localized ACLE commonly presents as the classic "malar rash" or "butterfly rash" in the central portion of the face and may only affect the skin transiently preceding the onset of a multisystem disease. The skin lesions typically begin with symmetric, small, discrete erythematous macules and papules on the cheek and nose, occasionally associated with fine scales that gradually become confluent. Facial edema may be severe in some patients. Localized facial ACLE lesions have also been seen in 15% of patients with SCLE. Generalized ACLE is less common and its onset usually coincides with exacerbation of systemic organ manifestation and prolonged disease activity. It is characterized by a widespread, symmetrically distributed, maculopapular erythematous, sometimes puritic rash with accentuation of the UV-exposed areas. Hands and feet are often involved, whereas knuckles are typically spared. Skin lesions of generalized ACLE may mimic a drug eruption or even on rare occasions can simulate toxic epidermal necrolysis (TEN-like ACLE). Superficial ulceration of the oral or nasal mucosa is frequent in ACLE, the hard palate is most commonly affected but labial, gingival, buccal, and lingual mucosa may also be involved. ACLE skin lesions usually heal without scarring.

SCLE is a distinct entity with specific clinical and serological features, further associated with a distinctive immunogenetic background including the 8.1 ancestral haplotype, the common Caucasoid haplotype that is carried by most people who type for HLA-B8, -DR3. This subtype is characterized by the production of anti-Ro/SSA antibodies and can be triggered by UV light as well as a number of different drugs, such as thiazide diuretics, calcium channel blockers, ACE inhibitors, and allylamine antifungals (5). The characteristic skin lesions of SCLE appear in a symmetric distribution on sun-exposed areas (i.e. extensor sites of the upper extremities, V-area of the neck, shoulders, trunk, and less commonly, the face) and present initially as erythematous macules or papules that evolve into scaly, papulosquamous or annular/polycyclic plaques. Approximately 50% of patients show predominantly papulosquamous or psoriasiform lesions whereas the other half has the annular/polycyclic variant; few patients develop a mixed form with both types of lesions. Individual annular lesions expand and merge with polycyclic confluence and central hypopigmentation. As a "clue" of the disease, SCLE can subside with characteristic vitiligo-like hypopigmentation but never leads to scarring as in DLE. Vesicles can arise at the active margins of the lesions and TEN-like SCLE can develop as a severe manifestation of the disease. SCLE may exhibit mild systemic symptoms, such as arthralgia and myalgia but no more than 10%–15% experience complications of SLE over their lifetime.

Discoid LE (DLE) is the most common subtype of CCLE and can occur as localized DLE (80%) with lesions above the neck or as disseminated DLE (20%) with lesions above and below the neck. This disseminated form of DLE, especially when involving the trunk, is associated with an increased risk of progression to SLE (9). Antinuclear antibodies (ANAs) in low titer are detected in 30–40% of patients with DLE; however, less than 5% have the high ANA titer that is seen in SLE. Anti-Ro/SSA antibodies are found only occasionally in DLE patients. The first morphological sign of DLE is a well-defined, coin-shaped (discoid) erythematous patch of varying size followed by follicular hyperkeratosis, which is adherent to the skin. By removing the adherent scale, follicle-sized keratotic spikes similar to carpet tacks can be seen ("carpet tack sign"). The lesions slowly expand with active inflammation and hyperpigmentation at the periphery, leaving depressed central atrophy and scarring, teleangiectasia, and hypopigmentation. The central atrophic scarring is highly characteristic for this subtype. DLE lesions occur primarily in UV-exposed areas, such as the scalp, face, ears, neck, and arms, but may also be found palmo-plantar and in inguinal folds (4). At the scalp, DLE can progress to the point of total, irreversible scarring

alopecia. Mucous membrane involvement can be found in approximately 25% of patients with DLE, but does not necessarily reflect systemic manifestation or high disease activity (10). The buccal mucosa is most commonly involved, with discoid plaques showing erythema, radiating white striae, and teleangiectasia. Furthermore, DLE can follow any form of trauma to the skin (Koebner's phenomenon or isomorphic response).

Further subtypes of CCLE are LE profundus/panniculitis (LEP) and chilblain LE (CHLE). LEP is characterized by indurated nodules or plaques resulting in deep lipatrophy; CHLE is characterized by purple, painful plaques in cold-exposed acral areas, mostly on toes and fingers that may become hyperkeratotic and ulcerate.

LET has recently been defined as a distinct entity of CLE and this subtype is now included in the new classification as intermittent cutaneous LE (ICLE) (8). In several regards, LET differs from other variants of CLE; scarring, the hallmark of DLE, does not occur in LET, even in patients with recurrent skin lesions. Anti-Ro/SSA and anti-La/SSB antibodies have been found in not more than 10% of patients with LET and association with systemic disease seems to be very rare in patients with this subtype (11). Clinically, LET is characterized by succulent, urticaria-like, single or multiple plaques with a bright, reddish or violaceous smooth surface. The swollen appearance of the lesions and the absence of clinically visible epidermal involvement are the most important features of LET. The borders are sharply limited, and, in some cases, there is a tendency for the lesions to coalesce in the periphery, producing a gyrate configuration, or to swell in the periphery and flatten in the center. The skin lesions of patients with LET are primarily found on sun-exposed areas, such as face, upper back, V-area of the neck, and extensor aspects of the arms; phototesting confirmed that patients with LET are more photosensitive than those with other subtypes of CLE.

American College of Rheumatology (ACR) Criteria

The criteria established by the American College of Rheumatology (ACR) include 11 clinical and laboratory features that were originally intended only for the classification of SLE, providing some degree of uniformity to the patient populations of clinical studies (12). However, these criteria assign too much weight to the skin as one expression of a multi-organ disease; characteristic skin lesions for differentiating DLE from SCLE are not included in this list. In CLE patients with primarily cutaneous manifestations, application of the ACR criteria often results in overestimation of SLE (13). For example, while 48% of patients with SCLE have been described as fulfilling four or more of the

ACR criteria, none had serious CNS or renal disease (5). However, subsequent studies have revealed that only about 10–15% of patients with SCLE go on to develop severe clinical manifestations of SLE. Therefore, the ACR classification criteria are currently being re-evaluated, including dermatological control groups such as rosacea and amyopathic dermatomyositis.

Cutaneous Lupus Erythematosus Disease Area and Severity Index (CLASI)

Several disease activity scores (SLEDAI, ECLAM, BILAG) have been established for SLE to determine the disease activity of individual patients via scoring methods. Although the disease activity scores include dermatological criteria, such as butterfly rash, generalized erythema, and oral ulcer, they are not suitable for judging activity of CLE subtypes. For this reason, a new scoring system (CLASI = cutaneous lupus erythematosus disease area and severity index) has been developed for CLE patients, taking into account both anatomical region (e.g. face, chest, arms) and morphological aspects (e.g. erythema, scale/hypertrophy, dyspigmentation, scarring) of skin lesions (14). Furthermore, "activity" and "damage" of the disease can be judged separately and scoring from 0 to 3 points can be assigned to each lesion. Alopecia is analyzed with a separate scoring system, while differentiating between non-scarring (0 to 3 points) and scarring (0 to 6 points) forms. So far, the CLASI has been validated in 9 patients, and clinical responsiveness needs to be evaluated in a prospective clinical trial, which is ongoing.

Histology

To confirm the diagnosis of CLE, histological examination of skin biopsy specimens is recommended in correlation with clinical evaluation of the lesions. The different subtypes of CLE often show similar histological features with superficial and deep perivascular and periadnexal lymphocytic infiltrate as well as the so-called "interface-dermatitis", a lymphocytic infiltrate of the dermoepidermal junction. Characteristic are the vacuolar degeneration of the dermoepidermal junction and necrotic keratinocytes in the lower epidermal layers as well as the thickening of the basement membrane as a late consequence (15). Individual histological criteria may lead toward the diagnosis of clinical variants of CLE, i.e. in ACLE, histological findings are usually less prominent relative to the impressive clinical picture. In fully developed DLE lesions, there is prominent ortho- and parahyperkeratosis, follicular plugging, and epidermal atrophy. SCLE lesions generally have less hyperkeratosis and follicular plugging compared with DLE. The periappendageal inflammation that is characteristic of DLE is less prominent in SCLE and ACLE. Lobular lymphocytic panniculitis is characteristic for LEP; however, the absence of the characteristic epidermal and dermal changes of CLE can make the histological diagnosis sometimes challenging when there is no overlying DLE. Abundant mucin deposition between collagen bundles is characteristic for LET and, usually, there is no sign of epidermal involvement or vacuolar degeneration of the dermoepidermal junction.

As a non-invasive technique, reflectance confocal microscopy (RCM) has recently been evaluated in the context of DLE, by taking 4-mm punch biopsies from lesional skin (16). RCM was able to identify interface changes as well as dermal, epidermal, and adnexal inflammatory cell infiltration in a high percentage of cases. This non-invasive technique might be helpful in biopsy site selection; however, further studies are necessary.

Direct Immunofluorescence

Direct immunofluorescence (DIF) can be performed in skin biopsy specimens of patients with CLE, detecting deposits of the immunoglobulins IgG, IgM, and in rare cases, IgA, as well as of the complement component C3 at the dermoepidermal junction. However, uncommon manifestations of CLE, such as LEP and CHLE, have been infrequently investigated or have proved negative in DIF studies. Furthermore, the number of positive results varies greatly among different studies (4). This might be due to the controversies concerning terminology of DIF, which have clouded this field from the beginning. Some groups use the term "lupus band test" (LBT) to refer to lesional and non-lesional DIF findings in LE, whereas others reserve this designation for reference to immunofluorescence examination of non-lesional skin only. The strongest clinical association of positive DIF in non-lesional, sun-protected skin has been with SLE, and patients with DLE without clinical or laboratory evidence of extracutaneous disease have been uniformly negative. Furthermore, DIF findings at the dermoepidermal junction are not specific for LE, because similar deposits can also be found in normal or sun-damaged skin, especially in the face, and in other non-LE dermatological conditions.

Phototesting

More than hundred years ago, it was first suspected that sunlight was involved in the induction of LE, partly due to the fact that this disease seemed to accumulate in spring and summer. Subsequently, "photosensitivity" was listed as one of the ACR criteria for the classification of SLE, although it is poorly defined as "a result of an unusual reaction to sunlight by patient's history or physician's observation" (12). A detailed clinical history is important for the diagnosis and assessment of photosensitivity in patients with LE including several key components, such as the morphology of the rash, duration, distribution, and the relationship to sun exposure and specific symptoms (e.g., pain, pruritus, burning, blistering, and swelling). However, a negative history of photosensitivity does not necessarily exclude sensitivity to sunlight (3). This might be due to the fact that the development of UV-induced skin lesions in patients with CLE is characterized by a latency period of up to several weeks. For this reason, a relationship between sun exposure and exacerbation of CLE does not seem obvious to the patient and therefore, it might be difficult for some patients to link sun exposure to their disease.

Owing to the clinical evidence demonstrating the clear relationship between sunlight exposure and skin manifestations of CLE, experimental light testing with different wavelengths has been developed to better define UV sensitivity in patients with a photosensitive form of the disease. Phototesting can be carried out by irradiating defined test areas with single doses of 60–100 J/cm^2 UVA and/or 1.5 MED UVB daily for three consecutive days using a standardized protocol (3) (Table 63.2). Interestingly, there are substantial differences in the clinical subtypes of CLE with regard to responses to the different UV wavelength. Patients with LET have been found to be the most photosensitive subtype of CLE, because phototesting revealed characteristic skin lesions in 72% of these patients. In contrast, pathological skin reactions were induced by UV irradiation in 63% of patients with SCLE, in 60% of patients

with ACLE, and in 45% of patients with DLE. However, it is still unclear why sometimes skin lesions cannot be reproduced under the same conditions several months after the initial phototesting and why UV irradiation does not show positive results in all patients tested, providing indirect evidence for various factors in the pathophysiology of CLE.

Biochemical Features

Laboratory tests can be divided into primary screening tests to confirm the diagnosis of CLE and secondary tests aimed toward ruling out systemic organ manifestations (Table 63.4).

Serological Features

High titers of antinuclear antibodies (ANAs) and detection of anti-dsDNA antibodies should raise suspicion of SLE and can also be a marker for transition from CLE to SLE. In various immunofluorescence studies using HEp-2 cells, ANAs ranged from 10–21% in DLE, from 69 to 72% in SCLE, and from 90–98% in SLE patients (17). These results were compared to examination with enzyme-linked

TABLE 63.2. Protocol of phototesting in patients with cutaneous lupus erythematosus[a].

Test site	Non-UV exposed, unaffected areas of the upper back or extensor aspects of the arm
Size of test field	Defined test areas that should be sufficiently large to provide reactions (e.g. 4 × 5 cm)
Dosage	60–100 J/cm^2 UVA and/or 1.5 MED UVB on three consecutive days
Light sources	UVA: UVASUN 3000 (330–460 nm), Waldmann; or UVA1 Sellamed 2000 (340–440 nm), (Sellas Medizinische Geräte, Gavelsberg, Germany) UVB: UV-800 with flourescent bulbs, Philipps TL 20 W/12 (285–350 nm), (Waldmann, Villingen/Schwenningen, Germany)
Evaluation	24, 48 and 72 h up to 4 weeks after irradiation
Criteria for positive photoprovocation	- Induced skin lesions clinically resemble LE - Skin lesions develop slowly over several days or weeks - Skin lesions persist up to several months - Histopathological analysis confirms clinical diagnosis

[a] Modified after Kuhn et al. 2006 (21).

TABLE 63.3. Diagnostic parameters of different subtypes of cutaneous lupus erythematosus[b].

CLE Subtype	ACLE	SCLE	DLE	LET
Clinical presentation				
Edema/induration	+	(+)	++	+++
Desquamation	+	++	++	0
Hypopigmentation	0	+++	++	0
Hyperpigmentation	0	0	++	0
Follicular hyperkeratosis	0	0	+++	0
Scarring	0	0	+++	0
Photosensitivity	++	+++	+	+++
Histopathology				
Orthohyperkeratosis	0	(+)	++	0
Interface dermatitis	+	++	++	0
Thickened basement membrane	+	++	+++	0
Lymphocytic infiltrate	+	++	+++	+++
Interstitial mucin deposition	+	++(+)	++	+++
Direct immunofluorescence (DIF)				
Lesional skin	+++	++	+++	+
Non-lesional, sun-protected skin	++(+)	(+)	0	n.d.
Serology (autoantibodies)				
ANA (HEp-2 cells)	+++	++	+	+
Anti-dsDNA	+++	0	0	0
Anti-Sm	++	0	0	0
Anti-Ro/SSA	+	+++	0	+
Anti-La/SSB	+	++(+)	0	+
Prognosis/Risk SLE	+++	+	(+)	0–(+)

[b] Modified after Kuhn et al. 2006 (22).

In this table, specific characteristics have been simplified and graded, because percentages given for DIF and antibody serology vary greatly in literature owing to small patient groups.

TABLE 63.4. Diagnostic procedure in cutaneous lupus erythematosus[a].

Screening when suspecting CLE
Patient's history
Clinical evaluation
Histopathology (and DIF) from skin biopsy
Phototesting
Laboratory analysis ESR, differential white cell count, creatinine, AST,
                  ASL, AP, LDH
                  Urine analysis
                  ANA titer and pattern (HEp-2 cells)
Laboratory procedure after histological confirmation of CLE
CRP, CPK, protein electrophoresis, PTT, TSH basal
24-hr urine analysis: creatinine clearance, protein
IgG, IgM, IgA
C3, C4 (CH50, C1q if indicated)
RF, circulating immunocomplexes
ANA differentiation (ENA)
Anti-dsDNA antibodies (ELISA, RIA, and/or CLIFT)
Anti-phospholipid antibodies (anti-cardiolipin antibodies, lupus
    anticoagulans, VDRL)
Antithyroid antibodies
Cryoglobulins, cold agglutinins (in cases of suspicion)

[a] Modified after Kuhn et al. 2006 (21)

immunosorbent assay (ELISA), leading to detection of slightly higher percentages in CLE: 30% in DLE and 79% in SCLE. Anti-Ro/SSA antibodies have been detected in 70–90% and anti-La/SSB antibodies in 30–50% of patients with SCLE and are highly characteristic for this subtype (5). The incidence of anti-Sm, anti-RNP, and anti-phospholipid antibodies in CLE is low and usually associated with systemic organ manifestation. The laboratory features can be complemented by further serological examinations (Table 63.4). In SCLE, association of rheumatoid factor with anti-Ro/SSA antibodies has been described in more than 30%. Furthermore, complement factors such as C2 and C4 are usually within normal range in CLE—if there is no genetic complement deficiency—separating the disease from SLE with complement consumption. The determination of hemolytic complement activity (CH50) should be restricted to individual cases of CLE with high suspicion of systemic disease or in associated hypocomplementemic urticarial vasculitis. In these cases, C1q and anti-C1q antibodies should also be measured.

Prognosis

Prognosis of CLE depends heavily on the clinical subtype of the disease and its severity. In general, CLE prognosis is regarded as more benign than that of SLE. Approximately 5% of DLE patients experience transition to SLE and 50% of SCLE patients fulfill four or more ACR criteria, but less (10–15%) may develop systemic organ manifestations. Several risk factors exist that can influence the prognosis of CLE. For example, familial aggregation and twin studies in SLE have suggested that genetic factors play an important role in the predisposition of the disease. Inherited complement deficiencies also influence disease susceptibility. Patients with homozygous deficiences of the early complement components of C2 and C4 are at risk of developing not only SLE but also CLE. Recently, familial CHLE was described as a monogenic form of CLE, mapping to chromosome 3p21 by investigation of a large German family with 18 affected members, suggesting a highly penetrant trait with autosomal dominant inheritance (18). The gender of patients also seems to be important, since studies have shown that male patients with SLE develop skin manifestations more often.

Prediction

The prognosis of CLE depends on the severity and extent of visceral involvement; however, it is still difficult to predict which cases will develop systemic organ involvement and transition to SLE. Some signs of systemic manifestations, such as minimal proteinuria and arthralgia, are often registered in CLE and 14–27% of patients with DLE, and 67–70% of patients with SCLE have been shown to have mild extracutaneous involvement. Several risk factors may influence the course and prognosis of CLE: genetic predisposition, race and sex, clinical presentation, age at disease onset, and triggering factors such as exposure to UV light and drugs. In a prospective multicenter study, 296 patients with SLE or CLE (DLE and SCLE) were examined and variables most relevant for disease protection were collected. Data identified mild signs of nephropathy as the variable with strongest impact for distinction between SLE and CLE. High ANA titers (>1:320) and appearance of arthralgia also have a strong impact for distinction, while low ANA titers and anti-dsDNA antibodies seem to have little or no impact (9).

Therapy and Prevention

In patients with CLE, it is very important to provide instructions for protection from sunlight and artificial sources of UV irradiation as well as avoidance of potentially photosensitizing drugs (19). Topical corticosteroids show efficacy in the treatment of patients with all different subtypes of localized CLE; however, they are of limited value in the treatment of widespread skin lesions due to the well-known side-effects, such as atrophy, dyspigmentation, and teleangiectasia. Recently, different groups have found administration of calcineurin inhibitors to be useful in CLE, especially in ACLE, SCLE, and LET. In addition, physical therapy, such as cryotherapy or lasers, and dermatosurgical methods, may also be useful adjuncts.

TABLE 63.5. Antimalarial agents in cutaneous lupus erythematosus.

Adults:	Hydroxychloroquine:	≤6.5 mg/kg ideal body weight/day
	Chloroquine:	≤4.0 mg/kg ideal body weight/day
	Quinacrine:	100 to max. 200 mg/day
	(Cessation of smoking!)	
Children:	Hydroxychloroquine:	6.0 mg/kg ideal body weight/day for 1 month, afterward ≤5.0 mg/kg ideal body weight/day
	Chloroquine:	≤3.5 mg/kg ideal body weight/day

The mainstay of treatment for widespread or localized disfiguring skin manifestations in patients with CLE, irrespective of the subtype of the disease, are antimalarial agents (Table 63.5). Our understanding of the use of combinations of antimalarial agents (hydroxychloroquine or chloroquine in addition to quinacrine) in therapy-refractory cases of CLE and proper dosing according to the ideal body weight limits problems with toxicity (20). Meanwhile, it is well known that smoking reduces the efficacy of treatment with antimalarial agents and can also induce and aggravate CLE. Further treatment options, such as methotrexate, dapsone, retinoids, clofazimine, and thalidomide, are helpful for patients with resistant disease; however, side-effects need to be taken into consideration (21). Recent advances in biotechnology resulted in the development of several novel systemic agents for the treatment of autoimmune diseases. However, further controlled clinical trials are necessary for their approval and new therapeutic strategies are currently developed.

References

1. Jiménez S, Cervera R, Ingelmo M, Font J. The Epidemiology of Lupus Erythematosus. In: Kuhn A, Lehmann P, Ruzicka T (eds), Cutaneous Lupus Erythematosus. Berlin, Heidelberg, New York: Springer, 2004;33–44.
2. Popovic K, Nyberg F, Wahren-Herlenius M et al. A serology-based approach combined with clinical examination of 125 Ro/SSA-positive patients to define incidence and prevalence of subacute cutaneous lupus erythematosus. Arthritis Rheum 2007;56:255–64.
3. Kuhn A, Beissert S. Photosensitivity in lupus erythematosus. Autoimmunity 2005;38:519–29.
4. Costner MI, Sontheimer RD, Provost TT. Lupus erythematosus. In: Cutaneous Manifestations of Rheumatic Diseases Sontheimer RD, Provost TT (eds), Williams & Wilkins, Philadelphia, 2003;15–64.
5. Sontheimer RD. Subacute cutaneous lupus erythematosus: 25-year evolution of a prototypic subset (subphenotype) of lupus erythematosus defined by characteristic cutaneous, pathological, immunological, and genetic findings. Autoimmun Rev 2005;4:253–63.
6. Werth VP, Zhang W, Dortzbach K, Sullivan K. Association of a promoter polymorphism of tumor necrosis factor-alpha with subacute cutaneous lupus erythematosus and distinct photoregulation of transcription. J Invest Dermatol 2000;115:726–30.
7. Kuhn A, Herrmann M, Kleber S et al. Accumulation of apoptotic cells in the epidermis of patients with cutaneous lupus erythematosus after ultraviolet irradiation. Arthritis Rheum 2006;54:939–50.
8. Kuhn A, Ruzicka T. Classification of cutaneous lupus eyrthematosus. In: Kuhn A, Lehmann P, Ruzicka T (eds), Cutaneous Lupus Erythematosus. Berlin, Heidelberg, New York: Springer, 2004:53–8.
9. Tebbe B, Mansmann U, Wollina U et al. Markers in cutaneous lupus erythematosus indicating systemic involvement. A multicenter study on 296 patients. Acta Derm Venereol 1997;77:305–8.
10. Loureno SV, Nacagami Sotto M, Constantino Vilela MA et al. Lupus erythematosus: Clinical and histopathological study of oral manifestations and immunohistochemical profile of epithelial maturation. J Cutan Pathol 2006;33:657–62.
11. Kuhn A, Richter-Hintz D, Oslislo C et al. Lupus erythematosus tumidus: A neglected subset of cutaneous lupus erythematosus. Arch Dermatol 2000;136:1033–41.
12. Tan EM, Cohen AS, Fries JF et al. The 1982 revised criteria for the classification of systemic lupus erythematosus. Arthritis Rheum 1982; 25:1271–7.
13. Albrecht J, Berlin JA, Braverman IM. Dermatology position paper on the revision of the 1982 ACR criteria for systemic lupus erythematosus. Lupus 2004;13:839–49.
14. Albrecht J, Taylor L, Berlin JA et al. The CLASI (Cutaneous Lupus Erythematosus Disease Area and Severity Index): an outcome instrument for cutaneous lupus erythematosus. J Invest Dermatol 2005;125:889–94.
15. Ackerman AB (ed.). Lupus erythematosus. In: Histologic Diagnosis of Inflammatory Skin Diseases. 2nd edn, Baltimore, Williams & Wilkins; 1997:525–46.
16. Ardigò M, Maliszewski I, Cota C et al. Preliminary evaluation of in vivo reflectance confocal microscopy features of Discoid lupus erythematosus. Br J Dermatol 2007;156:1196-203.
17. Wenzel J, Bauer R, Bieber T, Bohm I. Autoantibodies in patients with lupus erythematosus: spectrum and frequencies. Dermatology 2000;201:282–3.
18. Lee-Kirsch MA, Gong M, Schulz H et al. Familial chilblain lupus, a monogenic form of cutaneous lupus erythematosus, maps to chromosome 3p. Am J Hum Gen 2006;79:731–7.
19. Ting WW, Sontheimer RD. Local therapy for cutaneous and systemic lupus erythematosus: Practical and theoretical considerations. Lupus 2001;10:171–84.
20. Ochsendorf FR. Antimalarials. In: Kuhn A, Lehmann P, Ruzicka T (eds): Cutaneous Lupus Erythematosus. Berlin, Heidelberg, New York: Springer, 2004;347–72.
21. Kuhn A, Gensch K, Stander S, Bonsmann G. Cutaneous lupus erythematosus: Part 2: Diagnostics and therapy. Hautarzt 2006;57:345–60.
22. Kuhn A, Haust M, Bonsmann G. Kutaner Lupus erythematodes: Aktuelle klinische, diagnostische und therapeutische Aspekte. CME Dermatologie 2006;2:24-38.

64
Pemphigus and Bullous Pemphigoid

Daniel Mimouni and Michael David

Abstract   Pemphigus and bullous pemphigoid are organ-specific autoimmune disorders with an established immuno-logical basis but unknown etiology. Pemphigus has three variants categorized by the presence/absence of intraepithelial blisters and erosions of the skin and variable involvement of the mucous membranes. The diagnosis of pemphigus and bullous pemphigoid is based on the clinical picture and confirmed by specific immunopathological findings. In general, the natural history of pemphigus is characterized by constant progression with a high mortality risk; the prognosis of bullous pemphigoid is more favorable. There are no prognostic indexes for the different variations of the diseases. Treatment consists of systemic corticosteroids, corticosteroid-sparing agents, and specific immunobiologic agents. Bullous pemphigoid tends to be more responsive to treatment and may also respond to topical agents as well as anti-inflammatory drugs.

Keywords   Autoimmune bullous diseases · pemphigus · pemphigoid · desmogleins

Definition

Pemphigus and bullous pemphigoid are autoimmune blistering diseases with an established immunological basis but unknown etiology. Pemphigus is characterized by loss of cell–cell adhesion (acantholysis) mediated by auto-antibodies to epidermal cell-surface proteins (1). It has three major variants, pemphigus vulgaris, pemphigus foliaceus, and paraneoplastic pemphigus, differentiated by the presence/absence of intraepithelial blisters and erosions of the skin and variable involvement of the mucous membranes. Bullous pemphigoid is characterized by sub-epidermal bullae and in vivo deposition of autoantibodies and complement components and significant polymorpho-nuclear cell infiltrates along the epidermal basement membrane zone (2).

Epidemiology

Pemphigus vulgaris is the most common form of pemphigus in North America and Europe. Mean age of onset is 50–60 years, with an equal sex distribution. Its prevalence in the general population is 1–10 per million. Although the disease affects members of all races, epidemiologic data suggest a wide geographic variability, with higher rates in Jews of northern European origin (3). Bullous pemphigoid is the most common of the autoimmune blistering skin diseases. It occurs mainly in older patients (4).

Pathogenesis

There is solid evidence that pemphigus autoantibodies are not just surrogate markers for the disease, but pathogenic (5). The autoantibodies are invariably found in serum and bound in lesional epithelia; the severity of the disease correlates with the serum autoantibody titer. Transpla-cental transfer of pemphigus antibodies may induce a short-term blistering eruption in neonates, and passive transfer of human pemphigus antibodies to mice pro-duces acantholysis and intraepidermal detachment, reproducing the human disease with precision (5). Two desmosomal proteins have been identified as the target antigens in pemphigus: desmoglein 1 in pemphigus folia-ceus (molecular weight 165 kDa) and desmoglein 3 in pemphigus vulgaris (molecular weight 130 kDa). The

From: Y. Shoenfeld et al. (eds.): *Diagnostic Criteria in Autoimmune Diseases*, DOI: 10.1007/978-1-60327-285-8_64,

desmogleins are part of the family of molecules called cadherins, which are known to play a major role in cell–cell adhesion.

The pathogenesis of bullous pemphigoid involves circulating autoantibodies to two protein antigens: BP antigen 1 (230 kD) and BP antigen 2 (180 kD), also known as type XVII collagen. These antigens are key components of the epidermal hemidesmosomes, which are adhesion structures that anchor the epidermal basal cells to the underlying basement membrane.

Clinical Manifestations

The lesions of pemphigus vulgaris typically occur first in the oropharyngeal mucosa and subsequently in the skin. Other mucosa such as the genitalia and conjunctiva may be involved as well. The primary skin lesion consists of flaccid bullae that break to form a large painful erosion, which usually fails to heal without specific intervention. The most common sites are the scalp, face, and trunk, although all parts of the body may be affected.

The clinical manifestations of bullous pemphigoid differ from those of pemphigus vulgaris. Oral lesions are rare, and the skin lesions are typically polymorphic and cause significant itching. They may present as erythematous urticarial papules or plaques of the trunk and flexor parts of the extremities. Subsequently, tense blisters arise, sometimes producing an extensive bullous eruption.

Pathologic Features

Histologic study of pemphigus vulgaris lesions typically reveals suprabasal acantholysis. Histologic skin sections from patients with bullous pemphigoid typically show separation of the basal epidermis from the adjacent dermis (subepidermal plane) with eosinophils in the dermis.

Immunofluorescence and Serologic Features

Direct immunofluorescence study of skin tissue from patients with pemphigus vulgaris shows IgG and C3 deposition on the epithelial cell surface. The immunoserologic hallmark of the disease is the presence of serum anti-desmogleins 1 and 3. By contrast, on immunofluorescence study of tissue from patients with bullous pemphigoid, IgG and C3 are deposited along the basement membrane; the immunoserologic hallmark is the presence of serum anti-BP antigens 1 and 2. The finding of these typical patterns on indirect immunofluorescence study of serum samples using monkey esophagus as the substrate is diagnostically helpful. Other, nonroutine, serologic tests that can detect anti-desmoglein and anti-BP antibodies with more accuracy include ELISA and immunoblotting (6).

Diagnostic Criteria

At present, there are no universally recognized diagnostic criteria for pemphigus vulgaris or bullous pemphigoid. Table 64.1 summarizes the methods accepted at present. For a definitive diagnosis, we suggest positive findings on direct immunofluorescence combined with two of the major criteria or one of the major and one of the minor criteria identified in the table.

Prognosis

Pemphigus vulgaris has a chronic course, with remissions and flares. Left untreated, it progresses steadily, and is associated with a very high risk of mortality within 2 years. The introduction of corticosteroids has rendered the disease treatable, but not curable. The course and prognosis of bullous pemphigoid is more favorable. There are also remissions (sometimes spontaneous) and flares, but symptoms frequently disappear after a few months to a few years. There are at present no prognostic indices for the variations of the diseases.

TABLE 64.1. Diagnostic criteria for pemphigus vulgaris and bullous pemphigoid[a].

Criteria	Pemphigus vulgaris	Bullous pemphigoid
Major		
Clinical picture	Flaccid blisters and erosions in mucosa, skin, or both	Polymorphic eruption with tense blisters and erosions in skin (rarely mucosa)
Histopathology	Intraepidermal blisters with acantholysis	Subepidermal blistering with eosinophils
DIF	Deposition of IgG and C3 on epithelial cell surface	Deposition of IgG and C3 along the basement membrane
Minor		
IF	Deposition of IgG and C3 on epithelial cell surface	Deposition of IgG and C3 along the basement membrane
ELISA	Desmogleins 1 or 3	BP antigens 1 or 2
Immunoblot	Bands at 130 or 160 kDa	Bands at 180 or 230 kDa

[a] Obligatory conditions for definitive diagnosis: three major criteria or two major (one of which is positive DIF) and one minor criteria.
DIF: direct immunofluorescence; IF: indirect immunofluorescence.

Therapy

If pemphigus vulgaris is not treated definitively and promptly, the process "hardens," leading to epitope spreading (7, 8), which makes the disease more difficult to control. Even if the initial presentation is limited, the disease will generalize without systemic treatment. Initially, patients are administered systemic corticosteroids, either alone or in conjunction with other immunosuppressive agents. The most effective and often-used immunosuppressive agents are azathioprine, mycophenolate mofetil, and cyclophosphamide. More recent studies reported high efficacy for plasmapheresis, intravenous immunoglobulins (IVIG), and anti-CD20 (rituximab) (9, 10). Treatment with rituximab has yielded promising results in terms of long-standing remissions.

Bullous pemphigoid is more responsive to treatment than pemphigus. The therapeutic regimen is also based on corticosteroids (topical or systemic), alone or in conjunction with other immunosuppressive drugs, as well as anti-inflammatory agents (for cytokine inhibition).

References

1. Nousari HC, Anhalt GJ. Pemphigus and bullous pemphigoid. *Lancet* 1999; 354: 667–72.
2. Mimouni D, Nousari CH. Bullous pemphigoid. *Dermatol Ther* 2002; 15: 369–73.
3. Heymann AD, Chodick G, Kramer E, Green M, Shalev V. Pemphigus variant associated with penicillin use: A case-cohort study of 363 patients from Israel. *Arch Dermatol* 2007; 143: 704–7.
4. Joly P, Roujeau JC, Benichou J, et al. A comparison of oral and topical corticosteroids in patients with bullous pemphigoid. *N Engl J Med* 2002; 346: 321–7.
5. Anhalt GJ, Labib RS, Voorhees JJ, Beals TF, Diaz LA. Induction of pemphigus in neonatal mice by passive transfer of IgG from patients with the disease. *N Engl J Med* 1982; 306: 1189–96.
6. Bhol K, Tyagi S, Natarajan K, Nagarwalla N, Ahmed AR. Use of recombinant pemphigus vulgaris antigen in development of ELISA and IB assays to detect pemphigus vulgaris autoantibodies. *J Eur Acad Dermatol Venereol* 1998; 10: 28–35.
7. Seidenbaum M, David M, Sandbank S. The course and prognosis of pemphigus. A review of 115 patients. *Int J Dermatol* 1988; 27: 580–4.
8. Tuohy VK, Kinkel RP. Epitope spreading: a mechanism for progression of autoimmune disease. *Arch Immunol Ther Exp (Warsz)* 2000; 48: 347–51.
9. Ahmed AR Spigelman Z, Cavacini LA, Posner MR. Treatment of pemphigus vulgaris with rituximab and intravenous immune globulin. *N Engl J Med* 2007; 355: 1772–9.
10. Joly P, Mouquet H, Roujeau JC, D'Incan M, Gilbert D, Jacquot S, Gougeon ML, Bedane C, Muller R, Dreno B, Doutre MS, Delaporte E, Pauwels C, Franck N, Caux F, Picard C, Tancrede-Bohin E, Bernard P, Tron F, Hertl M, Musette P. A single cycle of rituximab for the treatment of severe pemphigus. *N Engl J Med* 2007; 357: 605–7.

65
Vitiligo

Sharon Baum, Aviv Barzilai and Henri Trau

Abstract   Vitiligo is a skin-depigmenting disorder that may be associated with other organ-specific autoimmune diseases. Vitiligo patients develop, with various frequencies, organ-specific autoantibodies, such as parietal, adrenal, and thyroid-related antibodies, but the meaning of these antibodies in vitiligo patients is unclear. Theories concerning the pathogenesis of vitiligo have concentrated on four different mechanisms: autoimmune, autocytotoxic, genetic, and neural. The autoimmune hypothesis focuses on the association of vitiligo with other autoimmune diseases. The autocytotoxic theory postulates that cytotoxic precursors to melanin synthesis accumulate occur in melanocytes causing cell death. The genetic hypothesis focuses on genetic data, and the neural hypothesis links segmental vitiligo with neurons that juxtapose melanocytes. Diagnosis is based mainly on clinical picture. Vitiligo can be treated in many ways. These include steroids, phototherapy, and topical immunomodulators. Multiple surgical modalities have offered patients significant benefits. For patients with generalized vitiligo, depigmentation of the remaining pigmented epidermis is sometimes the only alternative.

Keywords   Vitiligo · melanocytes · autoantibodies · steroids · phototherapy

Vitiligo is an acquired, sometimes progressive disorder in which some or all of the melanocytes in the interfollicular epidermis, and occasionally those in the hair follicles, are selectively destroyed. Vitiligo may be associated with other organ-specific autoimmune diseases, such as thyroid disease (Hashimoto's thyroiditis and Graves' disease), Addison's disease, pernicious anemia, insulin-dependent diabetes mellitus, and alopecia areata (1). Autoantibodies directed against these and other organ systems can also be present without clinical correlation. Pigmented cells in the eye and ear are sometimes affected (2, 3).

Epidemiology

The disease itself is not inherited, but the predisposition for vitiligo is inherited. Vitiligo is relatively frequent, with a rate of 1–2%. No sex-related difference in prevalence is reported. Vitiligo may appear at any time from birth to senescence, though the onset is most commonly observed in childhood or young adulthood. Approximately one half of those with vitiligo acquire the disease before the age of 20 years, and the incidence decreases with increasing age (4). Epidemiologic studies have shown that one-fourth to

one-third of patients with vitiligo have family members with the disease. Larger studies involving patients with vitiligo and their families conclude that the disease is neither transmitted as an autosomal recessive nor as a dominant trait. The finding that multiple unlinked autosomal loci on red blood cells (such as RH on chromosome 1, ACP1 on chromosome 2, and MN on chromosome 4) are associated with the disease suggests a multifactorial genetic pattern. These studies also demonstrate that close biologic relatives have a 4.5-fold increased risk of the development of vitiligo compared with controls (5).

Pathogenesis

The concept of vitiligo as an autoimmune disease was introduced following reports of autoantibodies found in serum from patients with active disease. This phenomenon has been studied in great detail, and antibodies directed against melanocytes are clearly more prevalent in patients with active vitiligo (6). These antibodies are generally reactive with intracellular antigens, but humoral immunity to pigment cells may constitute an epiphenomenon that occurs in response to cell damage. Evidence supporting a

From: Y. Shoenfeld et al (eds.): *Diagnostic Criteria in Autoimmune Diseases*, DOI: 10.1007/978-1-60327-285-8_65,

role for antibodies is provided by demonstrating that adoptive transfer of vitiligo serum can induce depigmentation of xenografted human skin in SCID mice and by demonstrating antibody-dependent cellular cytotoxicity in vitro (7). Recently, it was found that there is an inflammatory infiltrate surrounding expanding vitiligo lesions. Infiltrates consist of macrophages, as well as dendritic cell and T cells. No B cells are found in vitiligo skin (8).

Four pathogenic theories have been discussed, as follows:

- Autoimmune Hypothesis: The frequent association of vitiligo with autoimmune diseases, together with studies demonstrating that vitiligo patients can have autoantibodies and autoreactive T lymphocytes against pigmented cells, supports the theory that there is an autoimmune involvement in the etiology of the disease. Although the pathogenic mechanisms of T cells have recently been well studied in vitiligo, the role of autoantibodies in the disease remains obscure (Figure 65.1).

- Vitiligo may develop in patients with melanoma. The same process, autoimmune destruction of melanocytes, is thought to be responsible for both melanoma-associated vitiliginous depigmentation and common vitiligo. They appear identical histologically (9). As immune system effectors circulate freely in the plasma, the sites of depigmentation do not necessarily have to be near the actual melanoma and, in fact, can be quite distant from it. The major difference is their distribution: vitiligo usually begins centrally and spreads to the periphery whereas generalized vitiliginous lesions usually begin distally.

- Neural Hypothesis: The neural theory was based on the following: (a) case reports of patients afflicted with a nerve injury and vitiligo with decreased or absent skin

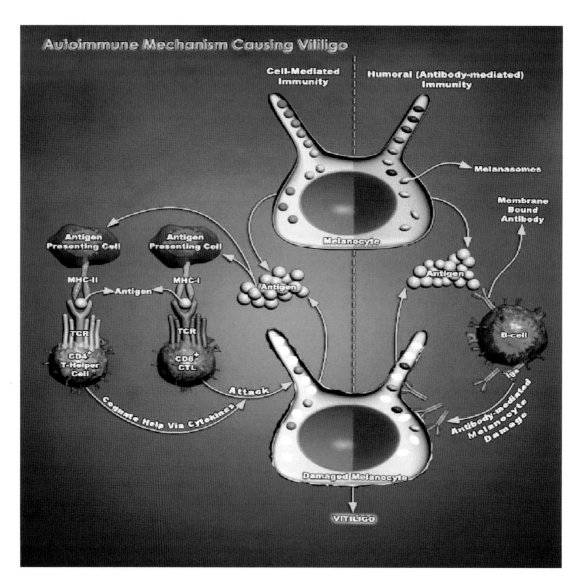

FIGURE 65.1. Schematic figure showing the autoimmune mechanism causing vitiligo.

findings in the denervated areas, (b) clinical evidence of segmental, dermatomal vitiligo, (c) increased sweating and vasoconstriction in vitiliginous areas implying increased adrenergic activity, and (d) depigmentation in animal models with disconnected nerve fibers (10). Keratinocytes and melanocytes from involved skin have also been shown to have increased monoamine oxidase A activity, with the former cells synthesizing 4-fold more norepinephrine and 6.5-fold less epinephrine than control keratinocytes. Increased urinary excretion of a dopamine metabolite, and norepinephrine and epinephrine metabolite, has been documented in vitiligo patients with active disease (11).

- Autocytotoxicity Theory: The autocytotoxic theory stems from the belief that increased melanocyte activity leads to its own demise. Electron micrograph examinations of vitiliginous interface and normal skin in patients with vitiligo demonstrated accumulation of extracellular granular material and basilar vacuolization of pigmented skin in patients with rapidly progressing disease. This theory has been supported by studies that have demonstrated an increased melanocyte susceptibility to precursor molecules (such as dopachrome) with exposure to melanotropin (also known as melanocyte-stimulating hormone). A second mechanism by which autocytotoxicity may occur is through inhibition of thioredoxin reductase, a free-radical scavenger located on the membrane of melanocytes. This enzyme is inhibited by calcium, which has been shown to be membrane bound in higher concentrations on vitiliginous keratinocytes relative to controls. Higher extracellular calcium levels cause increased superoxide radicals that lead to inhibition of tyrosinase by upsetting the equilibrium of oxidized and reduced thioredoxin in the epidermis, later causing vacuolization and eventually cell death (12).
- Genetic Hypothesis: Melanocytes have an inherent abnormality that impedes their growth and differentiation in conditions that support normal melanocytes. The premise that vitiligo, or a susceptibility to the disease, is inherited is based on the fact that familial aggregation is often seen. Epidemiologic studies have suggested a multifactorial genetic pattern. Attempts to associate specific HLA haplotypes have lead to variable results, limited by the small number of patients in each study.

It is believed that Vitiligo is a polygenic trait and that a convergence theory, combining elements of different theories across a spectrum of expression, is the most accurate etiology.

Clinical Manifestations

Vitiligo appears as sharply circumscribed, cosmetically disturbing, white spots that stand out. The appearance is particularly noticeable when the unaffected skin is tanned.

The disease is categorized according to the extent of involvement and the distribution of depigmentation. Generalized vitiligo is the most common presentation with bilateral, symmetric depigmentation of the face (especially periorificial areas); neck; torso; extensor surfaces; or bony prominences of the hands, wrists, legs, axillae, or orifices. Involvement of the mucus membrane is frequently observed in the setting of generalized vitiligo. Vitiligo often occurs around body orifices such as the lips, genitals, gingiva, areolas, and nipples (Figures 65.2 and 65.3). Segmental vitiligo occurs in a dermatomal, asymmetric distribution; because of its earlier onset, recalcitrant course, and decreased association with autoimmune disease, it is considered a special type of vitiligo (13). Universal vitiligo implies loss of pigment over the entire body surface area. Most patients initially experience depigmentation in a sun-exposed site. Depigmentation of body hair in vitiliginous macules may be present. Although the color of the irides do not change in patients with even extensive vitiligo, depigmented areas in the pigment epithelium and choroid occur in up to 40% of patients. Moreover, the incidence of uveitis in patients with vitiligo is elevated, and the incidence of vitiligo in patients with uveitis is also higher than expected (2). The membranous labyrinth of the inner ear contains melanocytes. Because vitiligo affects all active melanocytes, auditory problems can result in patients with vitiligo. In a study of patients with vitiligo who were younger than 40 years of age, 16% had

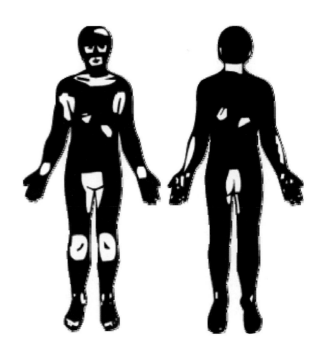

FIGURE 65.2. Schematic figure of the most common clinical presentation of vitiligo. It is bilateral, symmetric on the face (especially periorificial areas), neck, torso, extensor surfaces, or bony prominences of the hands, wrists, and legs.

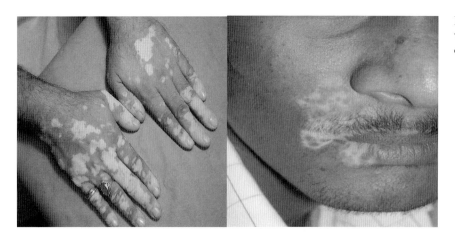

FIGURE 65.3. Typical clinical picture of vitiligo patient with depigmented lesions on dorsum of hand and around the lips.

hypoacusis in the 2–8 kHz range, which was of minimal disturbance to those affected (3).

Pathological Features

Histologically, in vitiliginous skin melanocytes are uniformly absent, supported by dopa and silver nitrate-negative staining and by monoclonal and polyclonal antibodies directed against melanocytes. Rarely, usually in early lesion, perivascular or lichenoid lymphocytic infiltrate and melanophages with only slight decrease in the number of melanocytes may be seen (Figure 65.4).

Diagnostic Criteria

The diagnosis of vitiligo is usually based on clinical examination of a patient with acquired, milk-white spots in typical sites. Wood's lamp test is helpful to differentiate different types of depigmentation. Only in a small number of particularly difficult cases, a skin biopsy may be required to differentiate vitiligo from other conditions. Occasionally the following specific tests are required to rule out the

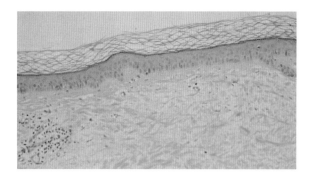

FIGURE 65.4. Histological picture of vitiligo presenting decreased number of melanocytes along the basal layer with mild superficial perivascular lymphocytic infiltration.

association with other autoimmune diseases: thyroid profile, blood sugar, complete blood count, Vit B12 levels, etc.

Although the pathogenic mechanisms of T cells have recently been well studied in vitiligo, the role of autoantibodies in the disease remains obscure. However, even if antibodies to melanocytes are not an agent of the disease, identifying their target antigens could provide for the development of diagnostic tests that are not yet available for vitiligo and could serve as markers for important T-cell responses in patients with the disease.

Prognosis

The course of the disease is unpredictable but is often progressive with phases of stabilised depigmentation. An extending vitiligo with enlarging macules or the development of new lesions is classified as the active form of the disease.

Therapy

Vitiligo can be treated in many ways (14). Two of the most common modalities, systemic and topical PUVA, use 8-methoxypsoralen and UV radiation in the 320–400 nm range. Corticosteroids have also been used to treat vitiligo. Multiple surgical modalities have offered patients significant benefits. For those patients with generalized vitiligo, depigmentation of the remaining pigmented epidermis is sometimes the only alternative.

Cosmetic Modalities

Visible depigmented macules and patches can be concealed with make-up or topical dyes. Cost, ease of application for focal vitiligo, and lack of side effects are specific advantages of topical cover-ups. However, patients unaccustomed to wearing make-up or involved in vigorous physical activity or patients with extensive disease may find topical cosmesis difficult.

Psoralen–UVA

The first modern use of light therapy in combination with purified topical and/or oral psoralens was by El Mofty in 1948. Meladinine, a derivative of coumarin consisting of 8-methoxypsoralen and 8-isoamyleneoxypsoralen, was found to be an effective oral and topical treatment. As late as 1967, sunlight was considered the most useful source of energy to repigment the skin of patients with vitiligo, with the use of oral and topical psoralens. With the realization that 8-methoxypsoralen optimally sensitized vitiliginous skin at 360 nm, the fluorescent blacklight became a useful light source, and the UVA light box was born. How PUVA therapy stimulates these inactive melanocytes is still unknown, but data have accrued to suggest possible mechanisms. Psoralens interact with double-stranded and supercoiled DNA, but with exposure to UV light, they covalently bind and inhibit DNA by forming photoadducts with thymine bases and cross-links between opposite pyrimidine base pairs. Consequently, RNA and protein synthesis are indirectly decreased. PUVA increases the size but not the number of melanosomes in keratinocytes. Kao and Yu determined that normal, cultured melanocytes exposed to PUVA experienced stimulation of tyrosinase activity, inhibition of DNA and protein synthesis, and depletion of epidermal growth factor expression (15). Serum from patients with vitiligo that previously demonstrated a positive indirect immunofluorescence with cultured melanocytes failed to react after PUVA treatment at 124 mJ/cm^2, therefore depleting vitiligo-associated melanocyte antigens. Decreasing the antigenic potential of antibodies directed against melanocytes and the density of Langerhans cells in treated skin, PUVA may, in part, immunologically mediate the repigmentation process. Melanotic melanocytes in the bulb and infundibulum of the hair follicle are destroyed in vitiliginous skin, although inactive cells in the middle and lower parts of the follicle and the outer root sheath are spared. Inactive melanocytes contain early structural, melanosomal proteins but do not contain enzymes required for melanogenesis (16). These cells in the outer root sheath activate (and thereby acquire structural and enzymatic proteins), proliferate, and mature as they migrate up the hair follicle into the epidermis and spread centrifugally. These active melanocytes are large, with elongated dendrites and intense DOPA oxidase activity. Research on mechanisms by which melanocytes migrate from the lower hair follicle to the epidermis has focused on cytokine release by keratinocytes. It has been postulated that basic fibroblast growth factor, which is released by cultured keratinocytes after UVB irradiation, is the mitogen for melanocytes. Oral PUVA therapy is used in patients with extensive vitiligo. Vitiligo on the trunk, proximal extremities, and face respond well to PUVA therapy, although distal extremities and periorificial or dermatomal depigmentation do not. In the past few years, there have been new therapeutic advances for vitiligo. These include narrowband ultraviolet B (NB-UVB) phototherapy, targeted phototherapy, topical immunomodulators such as calcineurine inhibitors, and vitamin D analogues in combination with ultraviolet light. NB-UVB phototherapy appears to be more effective and better tolerated than PUVA in vitiligo treatment in both children and adults, and it is currently considered the treatment of choice for patients with moderate to severe vitiligo. Major advantages of NB-UVB treatment include ease of treatment, no need for post-treatment ocular protection, and absence of systemic side effects. Targeted phototherapy with 308-nm excimer laser may be more effective attributable to the sparing of uninvolved skin, lower cumulative dosage, and shorter treatment times that may reduce the incidence of long-term side effects of phototherapy (17).

Topical and Systemic Steroids

About 32–58% of patients experience full repigmentation of the vitiliginous areas, and an additional 16–40% patients experience partial repigmentation with the use of steroids. High-potency steroids are used for localized, depigmented areas for 1–2 months, at which time therapy is slowly tapered to a lower-strength preparation. Because of potentially severe side effects, systemic corticosteroid treatment is not warranted in the treatment of vitiligo. Long-term follow-up of patients treated with topical steroids has been limited; therefore, it is difficult to ascertain its efficacy (18). Since 2002, some studies and case reports have discussed the application of topical immunomodulators in the treatment of vitiligo alone or in combination with other treatments. In a randomized, double-blind, right–left comparison study by Lepe et al., 20 children with active vitiligo were treated with 0.1% tacrolimus or 0.05% clobetasol twice a day for 2 months. The results have shown that tacrolimus was almost as effective as clobetasol (19).

Surgical Treatment

If topical steroids or PUVA treatments fail to repigment, surgical alternatives exist. These treatments regimens are most often limited to segmental or localized vitiligo, although they can be successful in generalized disease. Surgical modalities may be considered in inactive, nonprogressive disease only; moreover, areas such as the dorsal fingers, ankles, forehead, and hairline tend not to repigment well. The treatments include epidermal grafting, autologous minigrafting, transplantation of in vitro cultured epidermis, and transplantation of noncultured melanocytes (20).

References

1. Amerio P, Tracanna M, De Remigis P, et al., Vitiligo associated with other autoimmune diseases: Polyglandular autoimmune syndrome types 3B + C and 4. *Clin Exp Dermatol* 2006 September; 31(5): 746–9.

2. Cowan C, Halder R, Grimes P, et al., Ocular disturbances in vitiligo. *J Am Acad Dermatol* 1986; 15: 17–24.

3. Tosti A, Bardazzi F, Tosti G, et al., Audiologic abnormalities in cases of vitiligo. *J Am Acad Dermatol* 1987; 17: 230–3.

4. Spritz RA. The genetics of generalized vitiligo and associated autoimmune diseases. *Pigment Cell Res* 2007 August; 20(4): 271–8.

5. Nath SK, Majumder PP, Nordlund JJ. Genetic epidemiology of vitiligo: Multilocus recessivity crossvalidated, *Am J Hum Genet* 1994; 55: 981–90.

6. Kemp EH, Waterman EA, Weetman AP. Autoimmune aspects of vitiligo. *Autoimmunity* 2001; 34: 65–77.

7. Norris DA, Kissinger RM, Naughton GK, Bystryn JC. Evidence for immunologic mechanisms in human vitiligo: patients' sera induce damage to human melanocyes in vitro by complement-mediated damage and antibody-dependent cellular cytotoxicity. *J Invest Dermatol* 1988; 90: 783–9.

8. Le Poole IC, van den Wijngaard RM, Westerhof W, Das PK. Presence of T cells and macrophages in inflammatory vitiligo skin parallels melanocyte disappearance. *Am J Pathol* 1996 April; 148(4): 1219–28.

9. Merimsky O, Shoenfeld Y, Baharav F et al. Melanoma-associated hypopigmentation: Where are the antibodies? *Am J Clin Oncol* 1996; 19: 613–618.

10. Kovacs SO. Vitiligo. *J Am Acad Dermatol.* 1998 May; 38(5 Pt 1): 647–66.

11. Schallreuter KU, Wood JM, Pittelkow MR, et al. Increased monoamine oxidase A activity in the epidermis of patients with vitiligo. *Arch Dermatol Res* 1996; 288: 14–18.

12. Al-Fouzan A, Al-Arbash M, Fouad F et al. Study of HLA class I/II and T lymphocyte subsets in Kuwaiti vitiligo patients. *Eur J Immunogenet* 1995; 22: 209–13.

13. Freedberg IM, Eisen AZ, Wolff K et al. Vitiligo in Fitzpatrick's dermatology in general medicine. Sixth edition, 2003, McGraw-Hill, New York.

14. Grimes P. Vitiligo. An overview of therapeutic approaches, Dermatol Clin 1993; 11: 325–38.

15. Kao C, Yu H. Comparison of the effect of 8-methoxy-psoralen (8-MOP) plus UVA (PUVA) on human melanocytes in vitiligo vulgaris and in vitro. *J Invest Dermatol* 1992; 98: 734–40.

16. Horikawa T, Norris D, Johnson TW, et al., DOPA-negative melanocytes in the outer root sheath of human hair follicles express premelanosomal antigens but not a melanosomal antigen or the melanosome-associated glycoproteins tyrosinase, TRP-1, and TRP-2, *J Invest Dermatol* 1996; 106: 28–35.

17. Casacci M, Thomas P, Pacifico A, Bonnevalle A, Paro Vidolin A, Leone G. Comparison between 308-nm monochromatic excimer light and narrowband UVB phototherapy (311–313 nm) in the treatment of vitiligo – a multicentre controlled study. *J Eur Acad Dermatol Venereol* 2007 August; 21(7): 956–63.

18. Forschner T, Buchholtz S, Stockfleth E. Current state of vitiligo therapy – Evidence-based analysis of the literature. *J Dtsch Dermatol Ges* 2007 June; 5(6): 467–75.

19. Lepe V, Moncada B, Castanedo-Cazares JP, Torres-Alvarez MB, Ortiz CA, Torres-Rubalcava AB. A double-blind randomized trial of 0.1% tacrolimus vs 0.05% clobetasol for the treatment of childhood vitiligo. *Arch Dermatol* 2003; 139: 581–5.

20. Boersma BR, Westerhof W, Bos JD. Repigmentation in vitiligo vulgaris by autologous minigrafting: Results in nineteen patients. *J Am Acad Dermatol* 1995; 33: 990–5.

66
Psoriatic Arthropathy

Gleb Slobodin and Elias Toubi

Abstract Psoriatic arthritis (PsA) is a common inflammatory psoriatic arthropathy that characteristically occurs in individuals with psoriasis. Varied presentations of PsA may delay the timely diagnosis and treatment in some patients. Recently accepted 'CASPAR' classification criteria are highly specific and allow the diagnosis of PsA even in the absence of skin psoriasis (PsA sine psoriasis) or in the presence of positive rheumatoid factor. New treatment modalities, particularly biological medicines, allow better control of varied manifestations of PsA.

Keywords Psoriasis · arthritis · autoimmunity

Introduction

Psoriatic arthritis (PsA) is a common inflammatory psoriatic arthropathy that characteristically occurs in individuals with psoriasis. PsA was classified as a distinct entity for the first time in 1964, but the antiquity of this disease dates back to many centuries [1]. The many facets of PsA have historically complicated the timely diagnosis on the one hand, while its aggressive and destructive behavior has been recently recognized in up to 20% of affected persons on the other [2]. As such, PsA attracted much attention lately, which resulted in great progress in the understanding, classification, and treatment of the disease in the past years. This chapter will summarize the current experience in PsA in light of the recent developments in the field.

A Clinical Spectrum

Traditionally classified in the group of the spondyloarthritidies (SpA), PsA may manifest clinically in the whole gamut of patterns, which were first recognized by Moll and Wright (1973) [3]. Since then, many additional large series of patients with PsA have been published and much new data accumulated. We recognize today that PsA may not only be an oligoarticular or polyarticular disease, or affect peripheral or axial joints, or spine, but it may also evolve from one pattern to another with time [4]. These patterns may also overlap, particularly in patients with longstanding disease.

In most patients, PsA coexists with skin psoriasis, which may be extensive, limited, or even hidden with a patient unaware of its existence. On the contrary, in as many as 7–30% of patients, arthritis may precede the appearance of psoriatic skin lesions, called 'PsA *sine* psoriasis' [2]. In these patients, where a main prompt to the causation is absent, the right diagnosis of PsA will depend solely on the recognition of the specific features of the articular disease. Nevertheless, no single clinical, radiological, or laboratory sign, pathognomonic for PsA has been reported, thus raising the expert physician diagnosis to the traditional gold standard in the diagnosis of PsA [5].

Of five main patterns of PsA, both *oligoarticular* and *spinal* variants may be difficult to distinguish from the other members of the SpA group [6]. By clinical presentation and radiological features, these patterns of PsA are particularly similar to reactive arthritis, while a wide spectrum of skin rashes and lesions in the course of the latter may merely complicate the differential diagnosis. *Enthesopathy*, which is a characteristic feature of the whole group of SpA, may be particularly prominent in PsA, affecting frequently plantar fascia or Achilles tendons. Bone marrow edema adjacent to the entheseal insertion sites is characteristic in PsA and thought to be a manifestation of underlying osteitis. The involvement of the entheses at the very earliest stage of PsA has been demonstrated by magnetic resonance imaging (MRI) and led recently to an enthesis-based biomechanical hypothesis of disease pathogenesis [7]. *Dactylitis*, an inflammation affecting both the joints and the tendons of the whole digit may be seen in

From: Y. Shoenfeld et al. (eds.): *Diagnostic Criteria in Autoimmune Diseases*, DOI: 10.1007/978-1-60327-285-8_66,
© 2008 Humana Press, Totowa, NJ

16–48% of patients with PsA, being usually less common in other SpA. PsA is also featured by the relative asymmetry of sacroiliac/spinal involvement and more extensive paramarginal syndesmosmophytes and/or periosteal reaction compared to ankylosing spondylitis or SpA related to inflammatory bowel disease.

The evidence of features of SpA (inflammatory enthesopathy, dactylitis, spinal involvement, periosteal proliferation) in any further discussed pattern of PsA is of primary importance and may serve as a clue to the right diagnosis in many patients.

A distal pattern affecting the distal interphalangeal (DIP) joints must be mainly differentiated from osteoarthritis (OA), particularly inflammatory erosive OA. The joint involvement in these two disorders may be very similar both clinically and radiologically. A clue to the right diagnosis lies in the concomitant *psoriatic nail involvement* in most patients with PsA. Pitting is the most common psoriatic nail lesion, while onycholysis, nail-bed discoloration, subungual hyperkeratosis, transverse grooves, or longitudinal ridging may be seen as well [8]. Of interest, nail changes were reported to occur in about 90% of patients with PsA (all patterns), compared with 45% of psoriatic patients without arthritis. Recent MRI studies demonstrated that an involvement of the distal phalanges in the inflammatory process accompanies both the DIP joints involvement and psoriatic nail lesions in patients with PsA, being a potential connective link between the two phenomena [9].

Laboratory parameters of inflammation (erythrocyte sedimentation rate and C-reactive protein) are frequently normal or minimally elevated in PsA, not contributing much to the differential diagnosis in this setting. However, the fine interpretation of X-rays may help to differentiate between PsA and OA in some patients. The lack of apposition of adjacent bony margins would be characteristic for PsA, while in OA undulating osseous surfaces are usually closely applied. Pencil-in-cup appearance of the joints, irregular periosteal bone proliferation, or resorption of the distal tuft, if exist, may be diagnostic for PsA.

A polyarticular pattern must be distinguished from rheumatoid arthritis (RA). In this setting, PsA may be recognized by its tendency to asymmetry and involvement of the joints in the 'ray' pattern rather than in 'raw' pattern, typical for RA. The presence of erythema over the inflamed joint is unusual in RA, but may be seen frequently in PsA, probably reflecting the characteristic for psoriatic disease exaggerated angiogenesis. Concomitant involvement of DIPs, spine, or psoriatic nail lesions in PsA patients should not be unnoticed. Positive serology (both RF and anti-cyclic citrullinated peptide [anti-CCP] antibodies) may sometimes deceive, occurring in PsA (mainly polyarticular) in up to 10%–15%. Intriguingly, an association of a positive test for anti-CCP antibodies and HLA-DRB1-shared epitope in patients with PsA was reported

[10]. Radiologically, both PsA and RA are characterized by osseous erosions; however, irregular excrescences of bony proliferation and the lack of juxtaarticular osteoporosis would strongly favor the diagnosis of PsA.

Arthritis mutilans is the most destructive form of PsA, which may lead to an extensive and irreversible joint damage with appearance of the "telescoping" phenomenon and shortening of the digits in a short period of time. All aforementioned clinical and radiological features of PsA may contribute to the diagnosis, which necessitates an aggressive therapeutic approach.

Classification Criteria

At least six different criteria sets have been proposed since the first diagnostic criteria of Moll and Wright that included three main points: the existence of an inflammatory arthritis, the presence of psoriasis, and the seronegativity [3,11]. The many patterns of PsA necessitated, however, more specific classification criteria to distinguish PsA from other members of the SpA group, OA, RA, or gout, which may be frequent in patients with psoriasis. A case is even more complicated owing to high prevalence of both psoriasis and aforementioned rheumatic diseases leading to statistically sensible noncausal association of skin psoriasis and arthropathies.

Recently, an international group of experts in PsA, the **ClAS**sification of **P**soriatic **AR**thritis (CASPAR) study group, worked out a new, simple and highly specific classification criteria [3]. These criteria permit classification of an inflammatory articular disease as PsA when at least 3 of the following (current psoriasis gains 2 points, each other criterion gains 1 point) are met:

- current psoriasis (2 points) or personal or family history of psoriasis;
- typical psoriatic nail dystrophy;
- dactylitis;
- negative test for rheumatoid factor;
- juxtaarticular new bone formation (excluding osteophytes) on plain radiographs of the hand or foot.

The CASPAR criteria, which were developed on the basis of data analysis of 588 patients with PsA and 534 patients with other arthropathies, have a specificity of almost 99% and a sensitivity of 91.4%. In addition to their very high specificity, the CASPAR criteria are also progressive by permitting the diagnosis of PsA in the absence of psoriasis (PsA sine psoriasis) as well as in RF-positive patients. On the contrary, relatively low sensitivity, particularly in the early disease, may be the main limiting factor of these criteria.

Detailed comparison of the historical and current diagnostic and classification criteria for PsA may be found in [5,11].

PsA Mechanisms

Both cellular interactions and molecular pathways of inflammation in PsA have not been elucidated sufficiently. In general, synovial histopathology of PsA, whether oligo- or polyarticular, is closer to that of other SpA rather to RA. Particularly, the *increased synovial vascularity*, triggered by vascular growth factors, and massive *neutrophil infiltration* are characterisctic for PsA [12]. Of interest, both increased angiogenesis and abundance of neutrophils are seen also in psoriatic skin lesions.

Intracellular citrullinated peptides, frequently recognized in RA synovium, are not seen in PsA [12]. The synovial infiltrate in PsA, besides neutrophiles, is formed mainly by T lymphocytes, with also cells of B-lineage, macrophages, and dendritic cells present. Both CD4 and CD8 T cells, with the latter predominating in the joint effusions in PsA, may show oligoclonal expansions, suggesting an antigen-driven response [13]. However, the T-cell-activating antigens have not been identified so far. Of relevance, CD40L was recently reported overexpressed on stimulated T cells from patients with psoriatic arthritis when compared with RA patients and healthy volunteers [14]. Th17 lymphocytes, a recently reported lineage of proinflammatory T helper cells essential in both psoriasis and RA, are still uninvestigated in PsA.

The general pattern of T-cell-derived cytokines, including IL2, IL4, IL10, TNFβ, IFNγ in the synovial fluid in PsA has been found similar to that of RA, but in lower concentrations [15]. Of other inflammatory cytokines, *TNF-α* is abundant in PsA synovium, and likewise in both psoriatic skin lesions and inflammatory arthropathies. *Macrophages*, which usually serve as a main source of TNF-α, may differ in the inflamed synovium of PsA from that in RA by their numbers and subtypes, with more CD163+ macrophages found in PsA [12]. B-cells, presenting in the PsA synovium, participate in building of lymphoid aggregates there, which may point to antigen-driven B-cell development [16]. However, the precise organization and function of B-cells in PsA is not clear.

Dendritic cells (DCs) attracted much attention recently as a potential key player in psoriasis. Plasmacytoid CD123+ DCs serve there as a major interferon-α producer, while myeloid CD11c+ DCs produce a variety of cytokines and chemokines, being abundant in psoriatic skin lesions (reviewed in [17]). DCs, while recognized in the synovium and joint fluid in PsA [12], have not been studied yet enough in this disease.

Disturbed bone remodeling, as expressed by both extensive bone erosions and exaggerated bone formation in the same patients, is another characteristic and poorly understood feature of PsA. The receptor activator of nuclear factor-kappa B ligand (RANKL), TNFα, and IL-7 have been recently suggested as critical molecules involved in the activation of osteoclasts and subsequent bone resorption in PsA [18]. A reduction in the number of osteoclast precursors in the peripheral blood after anti-TNF treatment in patients with PsA was also reported. On the contrary, the mechanisms of increased bone formation and its potential relation to characteristic for PsA osteitis are not studied yet.

Progress and Problems in PsA Treatment

Better understanding of disease mechanisms allowed introducing new, highly specific and effective therapies in the arsenal of medicines for treatment of PsA in the past decade. Some of these therapies were translated to the field of PsA from the experience with RA and AS patients, while others were first used in patients with psoriasis. This new generation of "biologics" differs from those traditionally used in PsA such as methotrexate, sulfasalasine, cyclosporine, and other disease-modifying anti-rheumatic drugs (DMARDs) by their targeted action on a specific structure, leading to the neutralization of this structure (*i.e.* anti-TNF treatments) or interruption of immunological signal transduction and modulation of T-lymphocyte function (*i.e.* alefacept) [19].

While the efficacy of biologicals in PsA has been repeatedly appreciated in clinical trials and confirmed by evidence-based studies (reviewed in [19]), the precise effect of these therapies on the disease course is unknown, primarily because of the absence of accepted outcome measures in PsA. The used in the majority of clinical trials American College of Rheumatology (ACR) or Disease Activity Score (DAS) response criteria, developed for RA, as well as Psoriatic Arthritis Response Criteria (PsARC), are based mainly on the affected joints count, and as such may be acceptable in the polyarticular PsA, which shares some clinical similarities with RA. The widely agreed measures of improvement in oligoarticular, spinal, or predominant DIP patterns of PsA, as well as measures of enthesitis and dactylitis in PsA are still unavailable [20]. This lag between the appearance of new effective treatment modalities and the difficulties in assessment of some variants of PsA may lead to the underestimation of the severity of PsA and inappropriately chosen treatment in some patients. It has to be particularly mentioned that the blind translation of RA therapies (both traditional DMARDs and biologicals) for patients with PsA may be unwise, regarding the potential differences in the efficacy and toxicity of medicines in two different conditions. In addition, coordinated therapy, directed at both psoriatic skin lesions and affected joints, may be preferred in PsA patients. Finally, combination therapy of two or more nonbiologic DMARDs or biologic and nonbiologic DMARD (methotrexate being most frequently used) has repeatedly been shown superior to monotherapy in PsA.

Table 66.1 Available literature data on the efficacy of disease-modifying and biological medicines in psoriatic arthritis and psoriasis. [17, 19].

Treatment	Target	Peripheral PsA	Axial PsA or AS	Enthesitis	Dactylitis	Skin psoriasis
SSZ	?	Y	N	N	N	Y
MTX	Adenosine receptor ?	Y	N	N/A	N/A	Y
LEF	Pyrimidine	Y	N	N/A	N	Y
CS	Calcineurin	Y	N/A	N/A	N/A	Y
AZA	Inosinic acid	Y	N	N/A	N/A	N/A
Infliximab	TNFα	Y	Y	Y	Y	Y
Etanercept	TNFα	Y	Y	Y	N/A	Y
Adalimumab	TNFα	Y	Y	N/A	N/A	Y
Alefacept	CD2	Y	N/A	N/A	N/A	Y
Efalizumab	LFA-1	N	N/A	N/A	N/A	Y
Abatacept	CD80/86	N/A	N/A	N/A	N/A	Y
Pamidronate	osteoclasts	N/A	Y	N/A	N/A	N/A

SSZ = Sulfasalazine, MTX = Methotrexate, LEF = Leflunomide, CS = cyclosporine, AZA = azathioprine. Efficacy: Y = efficient; N = non-efficient; N/A = data are unavailable.

Take Home Messages

1. PsA is a distinct inflammatory arthropathy manifesting by synovitis, enthesitis, and osteitis.
2. No single clinical, radiological, or laboratory sign, pathognomonic for PsA has been reported, thus raising the expert physician diagnosis to the traditional gold standard in the diagnosis of PsA.
3. CASPAR classification criteria are simple and highly specific for PsA.
4. Increased vascularity, abundance of TNFα, and disturbed bone remodeling feature the histopathology of PsA; precise cellular interactions and molecular pathways of inflammation have not been elucidated yet.
5. The arsenal of medicines for PsA has been significantly expanded during the past decade, permitting highly effective mono- and combination therapy with traditional DMARDs and new biological medicines.

References

1. Pasero G, Marson P. The antiquity of psoriatic arthritis. Clin Exp Rheumatol 2006; 24:351–3.
2. Gladman DD, Antoni C, Mease P, Clegg DO, Nash P. Psoriatic arthritis: epidemiology, clinical features, course, and outcome. Ann Rheum Dis 2005; 64(Suppl II):ii14–7.
3. Moll JMH, Wright V. Psoriatic arthritis. Semin Arthritis Rheum 1973; 3:55–78.
4. Kane D, Stafford L, Bresnihan B, FitzGerald O. A prospective, clinical and radiological study of early psoriatic arthritis: an early synovitis clinic experience. Rheumatology 2003; 42:1460–8.
5. Taylor W, Gladman D, Helliwell P, MarchesoniA, Mease P, Mielants H, and the CASPAR study group. Classification criteria for psoriatic arthritis. Development of new criteria from a large international study. Arthritis Rheum 2006; 54:2665–73.
6. Gladman DD. Clinical, radiological, and functional assessment in psoriatic arthritis: is it different from other inflammatory joint diseases? Ann Rheum Dis 2006;65:(Suppl III):iii22–4.
7. McGonagle D, Lories RJU, Tan AL, Benjamin M. The concept of a "synovio-entheseal complex" and its implications for understanding joint inflammation and damage in psoriatic arthritis and beyond. Arthritis Rheum 2007; 56:2482–91.
8. Jiaravuthisan MM. Sasseville D, Vender RB, Murphy F, Muhn CY. Psoriasis of the nail: anatomy, pathology, clinical presentation, and a review of the literature on therapy. J Am Acad Dermatol 2007; 57:1–27.
9. Tan AL, Grainer AJ, Tanner SF, Emery P, McGonagle D. A high-resolution magnetic resonance imaging study of distal interphalangeal joint arthropathy in psoriatic arthritis and osteoarthritis: are they the same? Arthritis Rheum 2006; 54:1328–33.
10. Korendowych E, Owen P, Ravindran J, Carmichael C, McHugh N. The clinical and genetic associations of anti-cyclic citrullinated peptide antibodies in psoriatic arthritis. Rheumatol 2005; 44:1056–60.
11. Helliwell PS, Taylor WJ. Classification and diagnostic criteria for psoriatic arthritis. Ann Rheum Dis 2005; 64(Suppl II):ii3–8.
12. Kruithof E, Baeten D, De Rycke L, Vandooren B, Foell D, Roth J, Canete JD, Boots AM, Veys EM, De Keyser F. Synovial histopathology of psoriatic arthritis, both oligo- and polyarticular, resembles spondyloarthropathy more than it does rheumatoid arthritis. Arthritis Res Ther 2005; 7:R569–80.
13. Costello PJ, Winchester RJ, Curran SA, Peterson KS, Kane DJ, Bresnihan B, FitzGerald OM. Psoriatic arthritis joint fluids are characterized by CD8 and CD4 T cell clonal expansions that appear antigen driven. J Immunol 2001; 166:2878–86.
14. Daoussis D, Antonopoulos I, Andonopoulos AP, Liossis SNC. Increased expresion of CD154 (CD40L) on stimulated T cells from patients with psoriatic arthritis. Rheumatology 2007; 46:227–31.

15. Partsch G, Wagner E, Leeb BF, Broll H, Dunkey A, Smolen JS. T cell derived cytokines in psoriatic arthritis synovial fluids. Ann Rheum Dis 1998; 57:691–3.

16. Canete JD, Santiago B, Cantaert T, Sanmarti R, Palacin A, Celis R, GraellE, Gil-Torregrosa B, Baeten D, Pablos JL. Ectopic lymphoid neogenesis in psoriatic arthritis. Ann Rheum Dis 2007; 66:720–6.

17. Lowes MA, Bowcock AM, Krueger JG. Pathogenesis and therapy of psoriasis. Nature 2007; 445:866–73.

18. Colucci S, Brunetti G, Cantatore FP, Oranger A, Mori G, Quarta L, Cirulli N, Mancini L, Corrado A, Grassi FR, Grano M. Lymphocytes and synovial fluid fibroblasts support osteoclastogenesis through RANKL, TNF, and IL-7 in an in vitro model derived from human psoriatic arthritis. J Pathol 2007; 212:47–55.

19. Turkiewicz AM, Moreland LW. Psoriatic arthritis. Current concepts on pathogenesis-oriented therapeutic options. Arthritis Rheum 2007; 56:1051–66.

20. Gladman DD, Mease PJ, Krueger G, van der Heidje DMFM, Antoni C, Helliwell PS, Kavanaugh AF, Nash P, Ritchlin CT, Strand CV, Taylor W. Outcome measures in psoriatic arthritis. J Rheumatol 2005; 32:11.

Part IX
Cardiovascular and Pulmonary Autoimmune Diseases

67
Autoimmune Dilated Cardiomyopathy

Udi Nussinovitch and Yehuda Shoenfeld

Abstract   Dilated cardiomyopathy (DCM) is characterized by dilatation and contractile dysfunction of the myocardium. It may be secondary to various clinical conditions or idiopathic. Inhere we propose a new criteria system for diagnosis of an autoimmune DCM. The proposed criteria are based on the accumulating evidence stating that autoimmunity has a key role in some patients and, presumably, a different clinical entity. Diagnosis requires establishing the autoimmune basis of the disease following an echocardiographic diagnosis. This new proposed entity has a possible therapeutic significance, because we assume that patients with established autoimmune DCM will gain the greatest beneficial effect of immunosuppressive and immunomodulating treatment.

Keywords   Dilated cardiomyopathy (DCM) · autoantibodies · left ventricular end diastolic volume (LVEDV) · anti-α myosin heavy chain · anti β-1 adrenergic receptor

Dilated cardiomyopathy (DCM) is characterized by dilatation and contractile dysfunction of the myocardium. It may be generalized, or affect solely the left ventricle. Additionally, other abnormal preload and afterload anomalies should not coexist by definition (1, 2). In some patients, myocarditis and DCM can be referred to as acute and chronic phases of an inflammatory process (3). Idiopathic DCM is diagnosed after excluding secondary causes such as genetic factors and familial presentation, infections (usually viral agents), toxins or chemotherapeutic drugs, metabolic abnormalities, nutritional deficiencies, neuromuscular diseases, and inflammatory conditions (2, 4). Several predisposing conditions may coexist, along with immune abnormalities and autoantibodies that play a key role in the pathogenesis (5, 6). Autoimmunity may be triggered by various exogenous factors in predisposed individuals (6). DCM may also emerge in autoimmune rheumatic disorders such as systemic sclerosis, systemic lupus erythematosus, dermatomyositis and Churg–Strauss syndrome (2, 4). The pathogenesis of DCM is yet unclear, but antibodies to adenosine-diphosphate (ADP) and ATP mitochondrial translocator protein have been shown to cause cell lysis in rats (6). Anti-cardiac myosin is also assumed to be an important mediator in progression to DCM (6). It is assumed that compliment activation following antibodies deposition causes myocardial damage, and also that a local increase in TNFα, nitric oxide, mitogen-activated protein kinases (MAPKs) and cytokines amplify that damage (6). Cell mediated autoimmune response is another mechanism of myocardial damage caused in DCM (6).

Epidemiology

The reported prevalence of idiopathic DCM in the USA is 36 cases per 100,000 persons, and an annual incidence of 5–8 new cases for the same population size (4, 7). In the USA, annually 9000 deaths are attributed to DCM (8).

Pathogenesis

Clinical Manifestations

Familial presentation usually of dominant trait, with more then two affected family members, may be found in up to 25% of patients (2). Preliminary signs and symptoms usually begin between ages 20–50 years, although people of all ages might be affected (4). The common manifestations are symptomatic heart failure (in up to 95% of cases), usually with severe cardiac dysfunction, palpitations, chest pain and dyspnea on exertion. Systemic and pulmonary embolism are less common, and asymptomatic

From: Y. Shoenfeld et al. (eds.): *Diagnostic Criteria in Autoimmune Diseases*, DOI: 10.1007/978-1-60327-285-8_67,

TABLE 67.1. Symptoms and signs in autoimmune dilated cardiomyopathy (4).

Left and right heart failure symptoms	
initial presentation	75–85%
Overall	95%
Dyspnea on exertion	86%
Palpitation	30%
Peripheral edema	29%
Asymptomatic cardiomegaly	4–13%
Chest pain on exertion	
initial presentation	8–20%
Overall	35%
Systemic and pulmonary embolism	1.5–4%

TABLE 67.2. Serological circulating autoantibodies in dilated cardiomyopathy and normal subjects (3).

Autoantibody	Prevalence in DCM (%)	Healthy (%)
Inhibiting anti-β1 receptor	30–31	4–12
Stimulating anti-β1 receptor	95	0
Anti-β myosin heavy chain	44	2.5
Anti-α myosin heavy chain	20	2
Anti-M7	31	0
Anti-M2 receptor	39	7.5
Adenine-nucleotide translocator	57	0
BCKD-E2	60	0
Anti-sarcolemmal antibody	10	25
Anti-myolemmal antibody	9	12
Anti-fibrillary antibody	24	6
Anti-interfibrillary	41	3

BCKD-E2 = branched chain α-ketoacid dehydrogenase dihydrolipoyl transacylase.

cardiomegaly may also occur (Table 67.1) (4). Both supra-ventricular and ventricular tachyarrhythmia may arise but it is uncommon for syncope or sudden deaths to be the initial presenting symptom (4). Mortality rate is as high as 15–50% in 5 years, mostly because of ventricular arrhythmias and heart failure (7).

Laboratory Findings

Electrocardiography

The ECG recording might be normal, or present T-wave changes, Q waves – in cases of extensive fibrosis, atrioventricular conduction delay and bundle branch block. Tachyarrythmias, particularly atrial fibrillation, are common (2).

Pathological Features

Histologically, cellular hypertrophy, myocyte degeneration, interstitial fibrosis, and small clusters of lymphocytes may be present (4, 8). The heart muscle stains positive for complement membrane attack complex C5b-9, indicating that the complement system has a role in pathogenesis (9). Loss of intracellular cardiac myofilaments is associated with mortality (4).

Serological Features

Heart-specific autoantibodies may be found in about a third of patients including anti-α myosin heavy chain, anti-β-1 adrenergic receptor, anti-mitochondrial antigens such as adenine nucleotide, translocator, branched-chain ketoacid dehydrogenase, M7 adenosine diphosphate-adenosine triphosphate carrier protein, and many more (Table 67.2) (3, 4). Some of the autoantibodies mentioned in the table are absent or not as commonly found in healthy subjects, but may be disease and organ nonspecific (3).

Diagnostic Criteria

The most practical diagnostic procedure is echocardiography, although radionuclide scanning or angiography might be used as well in attempt to confirm diagnosis (7). Left ventricular dilatation, segmental or global hypokinesis, and reduced ejection fraction are present (4). Fulfilment of echocardiographic diagnostic criteria (Table 67.3a) requires an ejection fraction smaller than 45% and/or fractional shortening smaller than 25%. Also, it requires left ventricular end-diastolic dimension that exceeds 112% than expected according to age and body surface area. A cutoff of 117% was proposed in order to increase sensitivity in family members (2, 5). Affected first-degree relatives can be diagnosed in the presence of cardiac dilatation without systolic dysfunction if one minor criterion is present. The presence of three minor criteria without fulfiling the major criteria can also establish the diagnosis in suspected familial presentation (Table 67.3b) (7). Diagnosis requires excluding other causes of systolic dysfunction, hypertension greater than 160/100 mmHg, coronary artery disease (with >50% obstruction in a major artery), chronic alcohol abuse, sustained supraventricular tachycardia, systemic disease, pericardial or congenital heart disease, and cor pulmonale (7).

Endomyocardial biopsy may be required in order to exclude myocarditis, although it has a limited therapeutic effect (4).

DCM cannot be solely attributed to autoimmunity, and no criteria are currently available to define pure autoimmune cardiomyopathy. We propose a new criteria system for diagnosis of an autoimmune DCM (Table 67.4). The new criteria are based on establishing the autoimmune basis of the disease (10) following an echocardiographic diagnosis. Hence, establishing diagnosis of autoimmune-mediated

TABLE 67.3a. Echocardiographic criteria of dilated cardiomyopathy (2, 7).

Fulfilment of both criteria:
1. Ejection Fraction <45% and/or fractional shortening <25%
2. Left ventricular end diastolic dimention (LVEDD) >112% than expected according to age and body surface area. Cutoff of LVEDD >117% is preferred in familial presentation

Exclusion criteria:
1. Blood pressure >160/100 mmHg
2. Intravascular obstruction of main coronary artery lumen exceeds 50%
3. Alcohol intake >80 g/day for males, or >40 g/day for females
4. Persistent supraventricular tachyarrythmias
5. Systemic disease
6. Pericardial disease
7. Congenital heart disease
8. Cor pulmonale

DCM requires fulfilment of two major echocardiographic criteria and at least one minor criterion. The proponed minor criteria are (a) Proven mononuclear cell infiltrate with abnormal human leukocyte antigen (HLA) presentation; (b) Circulating anti-heart autoantibodies or autoreactive lymphocytes in patients and in unaffected family members; (c) In situ evidence of autoreactive lymphocytes and/or autoantibodies in cardiac tissue; (d) Disease induction in animal following transfusion of the patient's serum, antibodies, or lymphocytes; and (e) Proven clinical or echocardiographic improvement following immunoadsorption or immunosuppressive therapy.

This new proposed entity has a possible therapeutic significance, because we assume that patients with established

TABLE 67.3b. Echocardiographic criteria of familial dilated cardiomyopathy (7).

Major criteria
1. Defined criteria for dilated cardiomyopathy (as stated above)

Minor criteria
1. Unexplained supraventricular (atrial fibrillation or sustained arryhthmias) or ventricular arryhthmias, frequent > 100/24 h or repetitive (three or more beats with > 120 beats/min before the age of 50 years.
2. Left ventricular dilatation > 112% of the predicted value [29]
3. Left ventricular dysfunction: ejection fraction <50% or fractional shortening <28%;
4. Unexplained conduction disease: II or III atrioventricular conduction defects, complete left-ventricular bundle branch block, sinus nodal dysfunction;
5. Unexplained sudden death or stroke before 50 years of age;
6. Segmental wall motion abnormalities (<1 segmen or 1 if not previously present) in the absence of intraventricular conduction defect or ischaemic heart disease.

1. Affected
presence of the major criteria (left ventriculat dilatation and systolic dysfunction)
• or left ventricular dilatation (> 117%) + one minor criterion
• or three minor criteria

2. Unknown
• presence of one or two minor criteria

TABLE 67.4. Proposed diagnosis criteria of autoimmune mediated dilated cardiomyopathy.

Major
1. Fulfilment of echocardiographic criteria of dilated cardiomyopathy
2. Excluding secondary cardiac injury because of infections, alcohols, toxins or chemotherapeutic drugs, metabolic abnormalities, nutritional deficiencies, neuromuscular diseases, or collagen vascular disorders

Minor
1. Proven mononuclear cell infiltrate with abnormal human leukocyte antigen (HLA) presentation
2. Circulating anti-heart autoantibodies or autoreactive lymphocytes in patients and in unaffected family members
3. In situ evidence of autoreactive lymphocytes and/or autoantibodies in cardiac tissue
4. Disease induction in animal following transfusion of the patient's serum, antibodies, or lymphocytes
5. Proven clinical or echocardiographic improvement following immunoadsorption or immunosuppressive therapy

Supporting evidence but not considered criteria
1. Clinical course of exacerbation and remissions
2. Positive HLA DR4
3. Familial clustering of autoimmune diseases and/or family history of dilated cardiomyopathy (two or more affected individuals, or sudden cardiac death in a first-degree relative younger than 35 years)

Diagnosis requires two major and at least one minor criteria.

autoimmune DCM will gain the greatest beneficial effect of immunosuppressive and immunomodulating treatment. The proposed criteria are based on the accumulating evidence stating that autoimmunity has a key role in some patients and, presumably, a different clinical entity. Known autoimmune association includes mononuclear and T-lymphocyte infiltrating and HLA class II upregulation on cardiac endothelium, circulating and in situ autoantibodies, known autoantigens, familial aggregation and existence of other familial autoimmune diseases, weak HLA DR4 association, and a possible clinical course with exacerbation and remissions (2, 9, 11, 12). Additional indirect proof of autoimmunity is found by disease induction following transmitting of anti-myosin CD4 T cells from mice with myocarditis to SCID mice (9). Induction of experimental disease and autoimmune response in animals after immunization with cardiac-type α-myosin has been proven as well (3, 9, 13).

Criticism on Dignostic Criteria

Diagnosis of autoimmune DCM is based on establishing its autoimmune basis. Yet, there is partial *direct* evidence of the autoimmunity in DCM because it has never been attempted to induce the disease by direct transfer of autoantibodies in humans. Moreover, review of the relevant medical literature revealed that there is no report of transplacental transmission of immunoglobulins and secondary disease induction in newborns. Nevertheless, many other acknowledged autoimmune diseases have partial or no direct proof of its autoimmune basis (10).

The greatest pitfall of the proposed criteria is the limited practical use of some minor diagnostic criteria, mainly because of the need of invasive biopsy, or the required complex special laboratory exams.

Prediction of Onset

DCM commonly appears in familial clusters, and mild dilatation without systolic dysfunction may be found in 9–21% of asymptomatic relatives. This may represent early disease manifestation (3). Cardiac-specific autoantibodies increase the risk of future DCM (3). The use of echocardiography and anti-heart antibody screening in asymptomatic relatives can identify high-risk patients. The positive predictive value (PPV) of echocardiographic screening is 10%, that of anti-heart antibody screening is 7%, and combined PPV rises to 18% (5). Negative anti-heart antibodies have a negative predictive value of 98% over a 5-year follow-up period (5).

Prognosis

Prognosis is poor for symptomatic patients, and most of deaths are caused by progression of heart failure (4). Spontaneous partial remission may be found in 20–45% of patients, usually shortly after initial symptoms. Severe cardiac dilatation and dysfunction usually means worse prognosis. Other indications for poor prognosis include right ventricular dilatation and failure, global ventricular dysfunction, a spherical shape of the left ventricle, syncope, S3 heart sound, systemic hypotension, and pulmonary hypertension (4).

Therapy and Prevention

Lifestyle changes, including weight loss and refraining from smoking or consumption of alcohol, should be advised to all patients. Moderate physical activity is beneficial, and dietary recommendations are the same as in other causes of heart failure (4). Symptomatic patients should be treated with diuretics, vasodilators such as ACE inhibitors, hydralazine and nitrates, aldactone antagonists, digitalis, and beta-blockers (4, 6). Nevertheless, diuretics should not be considered as mono-therapy because of potential contribution to disease progression (2). Beta-blockers possibly eliminate the effect of stimulatory anti-β1 receptor antibodies (3). Patients with severe

left ventricular dysfunction, atrial fibrillation, past history of thromboembolism, and evidence of intracardiac thrombus should be treated with warfarin (2, 4). Despite this medical therapy, prognosis remains poor, and definite therapy often requires heart transplantation (6). Although the high risk of sudden cardiac death, class I antiarrythmic agents have paradoxically caused increased mortality. Amoidarone usage has shown conflicting results (2).

Automatic cardioverter-defibrillator may be beneficial for selected patients (4).

Although autoimmunity plays a role in pathogenesis, prednisone has shown disappointing therapeutic effects (4). Treatment with prednisone and azathioprine in selected patients has shown echocardiographic and clinical improvement, even though there was no change in the number of hospital admissions and death rates (14). The use of immunoadsorption has eliminated circulating autoantibodies such as anti-β1 adrenergic receptor. Moreover, further application of IgG substitution has increased contractile indexes (6) and decreased HLA class II expression and lymphocyte infiltration in the myocardium (1).

Intravenous immunoglobulin therapy has failed to improve cardiac function in controlled trials (6, 15).

The only definite therapy of advanced heart failure is cardiac transplantation but because of high demand, an alternative surgical procedure such as Batista procedure (partial left ventriculectomy) can be offered to selected patients. Left ventricular assisted devices can be used as a bridge to transplantation (2).

References

1. Felix SB, Staudt A. Non-specific immunoadsorption in patients with dilated cardiomyopathy: Mechanisms and clinical effects. *Int J Cardiol* 2006; 112: 30–3.
2. Elliott P. Cardiomyopathy. Diagnosis and management of dilated cardiomyopathy. *Heart* 2000; 84: 106–12.
3. Caforio AL, Mahon NJ, Tona F, McKenna WJ. Circulating cardiac autoantibodies in dilated cardiomyopathy and myocarditis: Pathogenetic and clinical significance. *Eur J Heart Fail* 2002; 4: 411–7.
4. Dec GW, Fuster V. Idiopathic dilated cardiomyopathy. *N Engl J Med* 1994; 331: 1564–75.
5. Caforio AL, Mahon NG, Baig MK, et al. Prospective familial assessment in dilated cardiomyopathy: Cardiac autoantibodies predict disease development in asymptomatic relatives. *Circulation* 2007; 115: 76–83.
6. Mobini R, Maschke H, Waagstein F. New insights into the pathogenesis of dilated cardiomyopathy: Possible underlying autoimmune mechanisms and therapy. *Autoimmun Rev* 2004; 3: 277–84.
7. Mestroni L, Maisch B, McKenna WJ, et al. Guidelines for the study of familial dilated cardiomyopathies. Collaborative Research Group of the European Human and Capital Mobility Project on Familial Dilated Cardiomyopathy. *Eur Heart J* 1999; 20: 93–102.

8. Rakar S, Sinagra G, Di Lenarda A, et al. Epidemiology of dilated cardiomyopathy. A prospective post-mortem study of 5252 necropsies. The Heart Muscle Disease Study Group. *Eur Heart J* 1997; 18: 117–23.

9. Eriksson U, Penninger JM. Autoimmune heart failure: new understandings of pathogenesis. *Int J Biochem Cell Biol* 2005; 37: 27–32.

10. Rose NR, Bona C. Defining criteria for autoimmune diseases (Witebsky's postulates revisited). *Immunol Today* 1993; 14: 426–30.

11. Limas CJ, Iakovis P, Anyfantakis A, Kroupis C, Cokkinos DV. Familial clustering of autoimmune diseases in patients with dilated cardiomyopathy. *Am J Cardiol* 2004; 93: 1189–91.

12. Caforio AL, Daliento L, Angelini A, et al. Autoimmune myocarditis and dilated cardiomyopathy: Focus on cardiac autoantibodies. *Lupus* 2005; 14: 652–5.

13. Jahns R, Boivin V, Lohse MJ. Beta 1-adrenergic receptor-directed autoimmunity as a cause of dilated cardiomyopathy in rats. *Int J Cardiol* 2006; 112: 7–14.

14. Wojnicz R, Nowalany-Kozielska E, Wojciechowska C, et al. Randomized, placebo-controlled study for immuno-suppressive treatment of inflammatory dilated cardiomyo-pathy: Two-year follow-up results. *Circulation* 2001; 104: 39–45.

15. McNamara DM, Holubkov R, Starling RC, et al. Controlled trial of intravenous immune globulin in recent-onset dilated cardiomyopathy. *Circulation* 2001; 103: 2254–9.

68

Are Autoimmune Manifestations in Human Dilated Cardiomyopathy Primary or Secondary Events?

Lara Elizabeth Pereira and Aftab Ahmed Ansari

Abstract Myocarditis is generally defined as inflammation of the myocardium that can result in dilated cardiomyopathy (DCM), which is characterized by dilation and impaired contraction of the left and/or right ventricles. In addition to the characteristic myocardial dysfunction associated with this disease, some patients develop an autoimmune response characterized by heart-specific autoantibodies and autoreactive T cells that exacerbate cardiac injury. Furthermore, DCM encompasses a heterogeneous group of clinical conditions that include collagen vascular disorders, hypersensitivity myocarditis, sarcoidosis, and peripartum cardiomyopathy (PPCM), and although the cause(s) for some cases may be defined, the etiology(ies) of the inflammation and particularly autoimmunity in many patients remain unclear and are therefore classified as idiopathic (IDCM). The purpose of this review is to highlight the pathogenic mechanisms thought to contribute to the onset and progression of the autoimmune response associated with IDCM with a focus on current and potential diagnostic techniques.

Keywords Idopathic dilated cardiomyopathy · cardiac-specific autoantibodies

Introduction

Heart-related diseases can be broadly categorized into three distinct but overlapping disease processes. These include those associated with coronary artery disease and inflammatory myocarditis and those termed cardiomyopathies. The cardiomyopathies, which are considered advanced myocardial disorders of unknown origin, are classified as dilated, restrictive, and hypertrophic on the basis of clinical, physiological, and morphological criteria established by the World Health Organization (1). Some DCM cases are associated with a specific cause such as alcohol- and doxorubicin-induced cardiomyopathy, etc., whereas the rest of the cases are simply referred to as IDCM (2). In addition to the characteristic myocardial abnormalities such as depressed contractility and an increase in ventricular chamber size in the absence of atherosclerotic coronary artery disease, valvular abnormalities, or pericardial disease, a cardiac-specific autoimmune response also develops in several cases (2,3,4,5,6). There is one school of thought that considers acute myocarditis as a precursor for IDCM in a select group of patients and both stages of disease exhibit autoimmunity with a more pronounced effect apparent during the acute myocarditis phase. It is presently unclear as to whether this autoimmunity is a cause or secondary effect of another etiology of IDCM, but evidence strongly suggests at least a contributing role for this mechanism in disease pathogenesis. Although several treatment strategies have been implemented, many have proven to be inconclusive and/or ineffective particularly in patients with severe and rapidly progressive myocarditis. Thus, cardiac transplantation still represents the only option for such cases. The following is a review of pathogenic mechanisms proposed to be responsible for the development of cardiac autoimmunity in IDCM and a summary of current/potential methods of diagnosis.

Prevalence

Given that myocarditis itself is generally asymptomatic, produces a broad range of symptoms and/or exhibits a sometimes rapid and fatal onset, the true incidence of IDCM is difficult to ascertain and is usually derived from post-mortem analyses (4, 5). Studies to date collectively implicate autoimmunity as a significant underlying condition in IDCM with ~25–75% of patients exhibiting

From: Y. Shoenfeld et al. (eds.): *Diagnostic Criteria in Autoimmune Diseases*, DOI: 10.1007/978-1-60327-285-8_68,
© 2008 Humana Press, Totowa, NJ

detectable levels of serum cardiac-specific autoantibodies (5). Greater than 50% of peripartum cardiomyopathy (PPCM) patients for instance test positive for circulating cardiac-specific antibodies (7). This heart condition afflicts certain women between the last month of pregnancy and 5 months post-partum, and although the disorder is associated with pregnancy, the true etiology of PPCM and the cardiac autoimmunity associated with it remains unknown.

Clinical Manifestations

The clinical presentation of IDCM, which is detailed in Table 68.1, is considerably varied ranging from acute heart failure symptoms to generalized signs of malaise that are typically not deemed to be cardiac related. Characteristics that allow for reasonable suspicion of IDCM include electrocardiographic abnormalities such as ventricular arrythmias, ventricular dilatation, elevated serum cardiac markers, and signs such as chest pain and recent flu-like symptoms (2, 4, 5). Particular attention is paid to younger patients who present with such clinical features especially if their patient history reveals few cardiac risk factors such as drug intake and/or alcohol abuse and absence of other cardiac diseases. The autoimmune aspect of this disease does not manifest as any distinct clinical symptom and can therefore only be confirmed following serological analyses to detect cardiac-specific autoantibodies.

Serological and Cellular Features

Autoimmune myocarditis is characterized by the presence of a number of circulating autoantibodies that target cardiac-specific antigens including the intracellular myocyte structural proteins such as cardiac myosin

TABLE 68.1. Typical clinical presentation of (autoimmune) myocarditis/IDCM.

Type of clinical feature	Description
Physical signs/symptoms	Chest pain, dyspnea, increased heart rate, flu-like syndrome including fever, arthralgias, fatigue.
Biochemical/serological markers	Leukocytosis, elevated sedimentation rate, eosinophilia, elevation in serum levels of cardiac-related enzymes including creatine kinase, troponin T and troponin I, elevation in cardiac-specific autoantibodies
Electrocardiographic/ echocardiogram markers	Ventricular arrhythmias, heart block, left and/or right ventricular dysfunction with/without cardiac dilatation, enlarged left ventricle, reduced left ventricular ejection fraction

TABLE 68.2. Serological markers of cardiac autoimmunity.

Intracellular		Cell-surface
Structural	Non-structural	
Myosin	ANT	Beta-1-adrenoreceptor
Actin	BCKD	M2-cholinergic receptor
Laminin	HSP60	
Vimentin	Transaldolase	
Desmin	Hyaluronidase	
Carnitin	Dnase B	
Tubulin	Stryptosyme sarcoplasmic ATPase	

(α and β), actin, troponin, vimentin, laminin and desmin, non-structural intracellular proteins such as the adenine nucleotide translocator (ANT), mitochondrial proteins such as the branched chain ketoacid dehydrogenase (BCKD) and finally cardiac-specific cell-surface receptor molecules such as beta-1-adrenergic and M2 cholinergic receptors (Table 68.2) (2, 3, 6). PPCM patients also exhibit similar autoantibody profiles but recent studies by us reveal a distinct set of antibodies present in high titers that are specific for as yet unidentified 25 and 33 kDa cardiac proteins (8). In addition to autoantibody production, a weak but significant association with HLA-DR4 and abnormal expression of HLA class II on cardiac endothelium has been described (9, 10). Increased levels of circulating cytokines in correlation with cardiac autoantibodies have also been reported, but this is yet to be confirmed by additional studies (3, 11).

Etiology, Pathology, and Pathogenic Mechanisms

IDCM can have a broad range of causes that are of infectious (viral, bacterial, fungal, and protozoal) and non-infectious (drugs, toxins) origins (2, 4, 5). The most common infectious agents include enteroviruses such as the coxsackie viruses, adenoviruses, cytomegalovirus and HIV, bacteria such as *Mycobacterium tuberculosis* and chlamydial species, and particularly the protozoan *Trypanosoma cruzi*. The myocyte necrosis associated with cardiac injury results from a combination of factors. Direct cytolytic effects of the infectious agents in addition to lymphocyte infiltrates and the production of proinflammatory/pro-apoptotic cytokines in response to the infection lead to tissue injury. Other characteristic abnormalities include interstitial fibrosis, myofilament loss, ultrastructural mitochondrial abnormalities, T-tubular dilation, and presence of intracellular lipid droplets. Drugs that are pharmacotoxic and/or induce allergic immune reactions are also thought to contribute to myocyte damage.

TABLE 68.3. Proposed etiologies of cardiac autoimmunity.

Proposed etiology	Pathogenic mechanism	Reference
Molecular mimicry	Cardiac proteins released as a result of myocardial injury share epitopes with infectious agents and therefore become targets for immune response that is already aggravated by infection	(2, 3, 5, 6, 12)
Genetics	Polymorphisms in chemokines/cytokines, difference in TCR repertoire, isoforms of autoantigens	(2, 3, 15)
Immune abnormalities	Dysfunction in regulatory T cells and/or cellular expression of PD-1 or its cognate ligand	(2, 4, 14)
Fetal microchimerism (PPCM cases)	Circulating fetal stem cells in pregnant women develop into APCs and present maternal cardiac antigens to maternal immune system in a semi-allogeneic MHC context	(7, 13)
Deficiency in pregnancy-related hormones (PPCM cases)	Contributes to defective cardiac remodeling required during pregnancy resulting in myocardial injury and exposure of unique self-antigens	(7, 13)

The cause of the autoimmune response that develops in some cases of IDCM is still unclear, but a number of pathogenic mechanisms have been proposed and are highlighted in Table 68.3. The release of otherwise cryptic cardiac antigens because of mycocyte necrosis caused either by infectious agents, particularly enteroviruses, and/or drugs/toxins become targets for an immune response already primed by the causative agent. Molecular mimicry has been implicated because microbial agents share epitopes with host cardiac cell self-proteins and recognition of such host proteins by the immune response is thought to initiate autoimmune disease (3, 12). In the case of PPCM patients with autoimmune myocarditis, a possible role for fetal microchimerism has been proposed where fetal stem cells found to be present in pregnant women may develop into Antigen presenting cells (APCs) that present maternal cardiac antigens to maternal T and B cells in a different semi-allogeneic MHC context resulting in a break in self-tolerance (13). A paucity of vasoactive hormones important for cardiac remodeling to accommodate the hemodynamic stress associated with pregnancy has also been noted in PPCM patients (13). This hormonal deficiency may contribute to cardiac damage resulting in the exposure of additional autoantigens. Studies from animal models of autoimmune myocarditis have also implicated dysfunction in certain components of the immune system as potential causes of the autoimmune response. The PD-1

knockout mouse, which lacks the T-cell surface PD-1 receptor required for mediating inhibitory signals, develops fatal DCM and cardiac-specific autoantibodies (14). In addition, the use of rapamycin in experimental models of autoimmune myocarditis significantly relieves disease symptoms (4), suggesting that regulatory T cells (Tregs) may also play a role as rapamycin has been shown to generate this cell subset and the lack thereof may contribute to autoimmunity. These findings therefore highlight that in all diagnosed cases of autoimmune myocarditis, factors described above in addition to other influences such as host genetics, which in itself has various levels of complexities because of polymorphisms, as well as nutritional deficiencies may also play a role and this autoimmune response is likely to be a consequence of a number of etiological factors. It is also necessary to stress that it is still unclear as to whether this autoimmunity initiates the disease process or if it is a secondary manifestation of pathology induced by other agents causing IDCM. However, evidence from several studies continues to support at least a contributing role for autoimmunity in the pathogenesis of this disease. This is especially highlighted by studies utilizing animal models of experimental autoimmune myocarditis where immunization with the cardiac antigen myosin alone is sufficient to induce cardiac disease (15). Animal model studies have further demonstrated the direct pathogenic effect of certain cardiac autoantibodies such as anti-ANT and anti-β1-adrenoreceptor (3).

Diagnostic Criteria and Detection Techniques

The diagnosis of IDCM in general involves a combination of factors given the ambiguous nature of this disease and preliminary steps involve careful examination of patient history and exclusion of predisposing factors such as drug/alcohol abuse and/or other heart diseases such as coronary artery disease. Patients, particularly those under 45 years of age, who exhibit electrocardiogram abnormalities such as ventricular arrhythmias or heart block and elevation in serum cardiac markers such as creatine kinase, troponin T, and/or troponin I are considered for further testing. The drawback of electrocardiogram methods is that readings often fail to distinguish between myocarditis and acute myocardial infarction or pericarditis but contrast enhanced cardiac magnetic resonance imaging enables differentiation between these. Endomyocardial biopsy (EMB) remains the gold standard for diagnosis of myocarditis (4, 5) but given its invasive nature and its association with complications during surgery, deciding which patient should undergo the procedure is often an arduous task. Patients with severe left ventricular dysfunction and those who fail to respond to conventional treatment for congestive heart failure are typically considered for EMB.

Standards set by the Dallas criteria require that the EMB test result be positive for both inflammatory infiltrates and myocyte damage. This procedure is however not without its shortcomings because errors in sampling and considerable variation in the interpretation of specimen results contribute to serious inconsistencies in diagnosis. The EMB technique that involves simple H8E staining and examination by light microscopy also lacks sensitivity such that specimens with low-infiltrate frequency and/or little myocyte damage are overlooked, which is a serious oversight given that even apparently mild cardiac tissue injury has been reported to result in heart failure (2). EMB also provides no information about viral infection and/or autoimmunity associated with IDCM, which is crucial for determining an appropriate treatment regimen. Thus, sensitive molecular techniques including polymerase chain reaction (PCR), real-time PCR, and reverse transcriptase PCR have become routine for detection of viral genomes in EMB samples (2, 4, 5). The autoimmune feature of IDCM is typically confirmed by the presence of circulating cardiac-specific autoantibodies. A number of techniques are utilized to determine the level of serum autoantibodies, which include indirect immunofluorescence (IFL), ELISA, and immunoblots (3). IFL typically results in the identification of a broad range of autoantibodies, with ELISA and immunoblot assays targeting a specific autoantigen highlighting that these techniques cannot be used interchangeably as antibody-screening tools. In addition, for a given detection technique, IDCM patients exhibit a variation in both the specificity and the spectrum of autoantibodies although myosin and the beta-1-adrenoreceptor appear to be the most consistent cardiac autoantigens identified. These differences in autoantibody repertoire make it difficult to develop a single assay or to set a standard autoantigen panel as diagnostic criteria for autoimmune myocarditis. Another level of complexity is added by the observation that low but significant titers of autoantibodies are detected even in healthy controls who exhibit no other clinical markers of myocarditis (2, 3). It is possible that these controls may prove to be future candidates of IDCM and should perhaps be monitored closely for the development of IDCM. The level of autoantibodies also changes over the course of infection with higher titers being detected during the acute phase than the chronic IDCM stage and thus the stage at which sampling occurs will also influence test results. It is unclear whether lower autoantibody titers in the chronic stage indicate that autoimmunity is no longer involved in pathogenesis or simply if cell-mediated autoimmune mechanisms are now predominant. Indeed, cardiac-specific autoreactive T cells have been reported in myocarditis cases with one such study describing a significant interferon (IFN)-γ response by T cells isolated from acute myocarditis patients to a flavoprotein predominant in cardiomyocyte mitochondria (16), suggesting that assays based on the reactivity of patient lymphocytes to cardiac autoantigens may also be potential diagnostic tools of myocardial autoimmunity. The cell-mediated autoimmune response has however been mostly studied in animal models of autoimmune myocarditis (17, 18), and so, routine diagnostic tests to detect cardiac-specific autoreactive T cells in patients have not been established. Attempts have been made to utilize inflammatory cytokines as markers of T-cell activation in autoimmune myocarditis, but these studies remain controversial given that no distinct correlation has been noted between these cytokines and cardiac autoantibodies. Correlations between autoimmune myocarditis and other factors such as HLA-typing and HLA-class II expression have however been observed, with a weak but significant association with HLA-DR4 and aberrant expression of HLA class II on cardiac tissue being reported. The potential use of these observations as diagnostic and/or prognostic markers of autoimmune myocarditis are reviewed in Table 68.4.

TABLE 68.4. Review of current and potential diagnostic criteria and techniques for autoimmune myocarditis.

Study reference	Diagnostic criteria	Diagnostic technique	Pros	Cons
(3)	Circulating autoantibodies	Indirect immunoflourescence, ELISA, Immunoblot	Can be specific (ELISA/immunoblots) or detect broad spectrum of Ab (IFL), most consistent diagnosis obtained with these techniques, potential predictive tool	Methods cannot be used interchangeably given different specificities, results influenced by stage of disease
(11)	Inflammatory cytokines	ELISA	Useful if combined with autoantibody detection and/or low/negligible levels of autoantibodies are detected	No consensus has been reached on cytokines associated with cardiac autoimmunity
(16)	Autoreactive T-cells	Proliferation & cytokine response to cardiac antigen	Useful if combined with autoantibody detection and/or low/negligible levels of autoantibodies are detected	Results may be influenced by isoform of antigen utilized in assay and/or stage of disease, fresh lymphocytes required for assay
(9)	HLA-typing	Serological method	Results not influenced by course of disease, may serve as prognostic/predictive marker	Serological method not as specific as molecular-based method
(10)	HLA class II expression on cardiac tissue	Conventional immunoflourescence on EMB samples	Useful if combined with Dallas criteria and/or level of lymphocyte infiltration is too low for detection by standard light microscopy	EMB sample required

Evidence for Cardiac-Specific Autoantibodies as Predictors of IDCM in Asymptomatic Individuals

Studies have documented a higher frequency of incidence of cardiac autoantibodies in asymptomatic relatives (~30%) of IDCM patients than non-familial individuals (~7%) (3). Relatives who tested positive for autoantibodies were younger and exhibited larger left-ventricular end-systolic dimension and reduced percentage of fractional shortening when compared with autoantibody-negative relatives, suggesting an association between early myocarditis disease symptoms and autoantibodies. Short-term follow-up studies of symptom-free relatives suggest that the presence of cardiac autoantibodies at baseline was more common among relatives who progressed to diagnosed myocarditis than those who did not, although continued monitoring of these groups is required to acquire definitive correlates. This finding lends support to the observation that higher antibody titers are detected in acute myocarditis patients than when they progress to IDCM. The development of new assays to detect other features of autoimmunity including cell-mediated and cytokine factors may contribute to the early detection and treatment of myocarditis, halting its progression to IDCM.

Treatment

Given that autoimmune mechanisms contribute to myocardial pathogenesis, studies have explored the potential beneficial effects of immunosuppressive drugs in IDCM patients and have noted improvements in left ventricular function with their use (2). Clinical trials involving immunoglobulin depletion (apheresis) from IDCM patients in an attempt to remove certain subclasses of pathogenic autoantibodies also produced encouraging results (2). However, in both cases, treatment did not significantly improve long-term survival of patients, therefore leaving heart transplantation as the only option. Other therapeutic options mainly include those that provide supportive care for clinical symptoms and include angiotensin-converting enzyme inhibitors, diuretics, beta-blockers, and ventricular assisted devices.

Thus, although several cardiac autoantigens have been identified in IDCM patients, the precise cause for the break in self-tolerance and whether there is a disease-initiating role for these autoantibodies is still undefined. Furthermore, IDCM is in itself a complex heterogeneous disease and is likely the result of a combination of host and external factors. Future studies aimed at identifying the antibodies and/or autoreactive T cells to major cardiac autoantigens are crucial for the development of immunotherapies aimed at treating the pathogenic autoimmune response associated with IDCM.

References

1. Richardson P, McKenna WJ, Bristow M. Report of the 1995 WHO/ISFC Task Force on the definition and classification of cardiomyopathies. *Circulation* 1996; 93: 841–2.
2. Ansari AA, Sundstrom JB, Forster O, Hilfiker-Kleiner D, Sliwa K. Myocardial autoantibodies and their clinical significance. In: Shoenfeld Y, Gershwin ME and Meroni PL, eds. *Autoantibodies*. 2 nd edn. Amsterdam, Netherlands: Elsevier Press, 2007: 355–65.
3. Caforio ALP, Mahon NJ, Tona F, McKenna WJ. Circulating cardiac autoantibodies in dilated cardiomyopathy and myocarditis: pathogenic and clinical significance. *Eur J Heart Fail* 2002; 4: 411–7.
4. Ellis CR, Salvo TD. Myocarditis: Basic and clinical aspects. *Cardiol Rev* 2007; 15: 170–7.
5. Feldman AM, McNamara DS. Myocarditis. *N Engl J Med* 2000; 343: 1388–98.
6. Kallwellis-Opara A, Dorner A, Poller WC, Noutsias M, Kuhl U, Schultheiss HP, Pauschinger M. Autoimmunological features in inflammatory cardiomyopathy. *Clin Res Cardiol* 2007; 96: 469–80.
7. Fett JD, Dowell DL, Carraway RD, Sundstrom JB, Ansari AA. One hundred cases of peripartum cacrdiomyopathy … and counting: What is going on? *Int J Cardiol* 2004; 97: 571–3.
8. Warraich RS, Sliwa K, Ansari AA, Sundstrom JB, Yacoub MH, Fett JD. Autoantibody profiles in patients with peripartum cardiomyopathy: A distinct entity to idiopathic dilated cardiomyopathy. *Eur Heart J* 2003; 24: 189.
9. Anderson JL, Carlquist JF, Lutz JR, DeWitt CW, Hammond EH. HLA A, B and DR Typing in idiopathic dilated cardiomyopathy: A search for immune response factors. *Am J Cardiol* 1984; 53: 1326–30.
10. Caforio ALP, Stewart JT, Bonifacio E, Burke M, Davies MJ, McKenna WJ, Bottazzo GF. Inappropriate major histocompatibility complex expression on cardiac tissue in dilated cardiomyopathy. Relevance for autoimmunity? *J Autoimmun* 1990; 3: 187–200.
11. Limas CJ, Goldenberg IF, Limas C. Soluble interleukin-2 receptor levels in patients with dilated cardiomyopathy. Correlation with disease severity and cardiac autoantibodies. *Circulation* 1995; 91: 631–4.
12. Li Y, Heuser JS, Cunningham LC, Kosanke SD, Cunningham MW. Mimicry and antibody-mediated cell signaling in autoimmune myocarditis. *J Immunol* 2006; 177: 8234–40.
13. Sundstrom JB, Fett JD, Carraway RD, Ansari AA. Is peripartum cardiomyopathy an organ-specific autoimmune disease? *Autoimmun Rev* 2002; 1: 73–7.
14. Nishimura H, Okazaki T, Tanaka Y, Nakatani K, Hara M, Matsumori A, Sasayama S, Mizoguchi A, Hiai H, Minato N, Honjo T. Autoimmune dilated cardiomyopathy in PD-1 receptor deficient mice. *Science* 2001; 291: 319–22.
15. Huber SA. Animal models of human disease. Autoimmunity in Myocarditis: Relevance of animal models. *Clin Immunol Immunopathol* 1997; 83: 93–102.

16. Cicek G, Shiltz E, Staiger J, Neumann F-J, Melcher I, Brandsch R. Specific stimulation of peripheral blood mononuclear cells from patients with acute myocarditis by peptide-bound flavin adenine dinucleotide (FAD), a naturally occurring autologous hapten. *Clin Exp Immunol* 2003; 132: 366–70.

17. Jane-Wit D, Tuohy VK. Autoimmune cardiac-specific T cell responses in dilated cardiomyopathy. *Int J Cardiol* 2006; 112: 2–6.

18. Smith SC, Allen PM. The role of T cells in myosin-induced autoimmune myocarditis. *Clin Immunol Immunopathol* 1993; 68: 100–6.

69
Rheumatic Fever

Yaniv Sherer and Yehuda Shoenfeld

Abstract   Rheumatic fever (RF) is an inflammatory condition involving the heart, joints, skin and brain that emerges following group-A streptococcal infection. Use of appropriate diagnostic criteria for RF is crucial in order not to under-diagnose this frequent condition that carries the risk of significant long-term morbidity. The most frequent and severe manifestation of RF is carditis. Echocardiography detects subclinical carditis in many patients lacking any clinical manifestation, up to 10 times more than cases having clinical evidence of disease, yet it is not part of the Jones criteria used for RF diagnosis. We suggest adding echocardiography (either as a screening method or for use in suspected RF cases) to the diagnostic criteria of RF in order not to miss any subclinical carditis associated with RF and to enable administration of early antibiotic therapy.

Keywords   Rheumatic fever · echocardiography · carditis · Jones criteria

Rheumatic fever (RF) is a systemic inflammatory condition affecting the peri-arteriolar connective tissue which occurs following a group-A streptococcal infection (1). Molecular mimicry between streptococcal and human proteins is considered as the triggering factor leading to autoimmunity in RF and rheumatic heart disease (RHD). Several HLA class II alleles are associated with the disease, mainly HLA-DR7. Cardiac myosin is one of the major autoantigens involved in rheumatic heart lesions, and several peptides from the light meromyosin region were recognized by peripheral and intralesional T-cell clones from RF and RHD patients (1). RF is believed to be caused by antibody cross-reactivity, i.e., molecular mimicry. Infection with group-A Streptococcus is estimated to cause over 500,000 deaths per year, the majority of which are related to RF and RHD (2).

The anti-phagocytic bacterial surface M protein is a major candidate antigen in the development of RF but also in the development of a vaccine to prevent RHD. Major obstacles in the development of an M-protein-based vaccine is the widespread diversity of circulating streptococcal strains and M protein types, and the possibility of inducing autoimmunity following vaccination as a result of molecular mimicry between the M protein and host tissue proteins (2). A recent study also links RF to the antiphospholipid syndrome (3). Antibodies to β2-glycoprotein-I were found in 24.4% of 90 RF patients, and the immunoglobulin G sera from RF

patients possessed significant anti-β-glycoprotein-I activity, whereas sera from antiphospholipid syndrome patients contained a considerable anti-streptococcal M protein. Furthermore, affinity-purified anti-β2-glycoprotein-I and anti-β2-glycoprotein-I-related peptide antibodies from antiphospholipid syndrome patients cross-reacted with streptococcal M protein and M5 peptide (3).

RF as a worldwide disease has very well-known diagnostic criteria. The updated Jones criteria that are currently used for the diagnosis of acute RF (ARF) are detailed in Table 69.1 (4). As RF is a condition carrying possible long-term morbidity and necessitating long-term therapy, these diagnostic criteria should be judged whether they over-diagnose or alternatively and more importantly under-diagnose RF. Jones criteria underwent several modifications over the years, and going over the four revisions made after the original Jones criteria, it seemed that modifications of these criteria were primarily corrective and perfective (5). Disease characteristics originally characterized as major manifestations were subsequently categorized as minor manifestations, and vice versa. In addition, 20 years after the original publication, a requirement for antecedent streptococcal infection was added (5).

Description of the clinical and demographic characteristics of RF episodes in Brazil disclosed that there was a predominance of females, in only one-third of the cases was the disease diagnosed at the first episode of RF, and

From: Y. Shoenfeld et al. (eds.): *Diagnostic Criteria in Autoimmune Diseases*, DOI: 10.1007/978-1-60327-285-8_69,

TABLE 69.1. Revised Jones criteria for acute rheumatic fever.

Major Criteria
1. Carditis: All layers of cardiac tissue are affected (pericardium, epicardium, myocardium, and endocardium). The patient may have a new or changing murmur, with mitral regurgitation being the most common followed by aortic insufficiency.
2. Polyarthritis: This is a migrating arthritis that typically affects the knees, ankles, elbows, and wrists. The joints are very painful and symptoms are very responsive to anti-inflammatory medicines.
3. Chorea: This is also known as Sydenham's chorea, or "St. Vitus' dance." There are abrupt, purposeless movements. This may be the only manifestation of ARF and its presence is diagnostic. May also include emotional disturbances and inappropriate behavior.
4. Erythema marginatum: This is a non-pruritic rash that commonly affects the trunk and proximal extremities, but spares the face. The rash typically migrates from central areas to periphery and has well-defined borders.
5. Subcutaneous nodules: Usually located over bones or tendons, these nodules are painless and firm.

Minor Criteria
1. Fever
2. Arthralgia
3. Previous rheumatic fever or rheumatic heart disease
4. Acute phase reactants: leukocytosis, elevated erythrocyte sedimentation rate (ESR), and C-reactive protein (CRP)
5. Prolonged P-R interval on electrocardiogram (ECG)

Evidence of preceding streptococcal infection: Any one of the following is considered adequate evidence of infection.
1. Increased antistreptolysin O or other streptococcal antibodies
2. Positive throat culture for group A β-hemolytic streptococci
3. Positive rapid direct group A streptococcus carbohydrate antigen test
4. Recent scarlet fever

A firm diagnosis requires that two major or one major and two minor criteria are satisfied, in addition to evidence of recent streptococcal infection (4).

the most frequent clinical manifestations were carditis (69.7%), arthritis (21.4%), and chorea (6.1%) (6). Mitral regurgitation was the most frequent lesion followed by a combination of mitral regurgitations and aortic regurgitation. Stewart et al. (7) tested whether Jones criteria are being used appropriately for the diagnosis of ARF. The medical records of patients discharged with a diagnosis of ARF were evaluated, and 32% did not fulfill the Jones criteria. It seemed that the criteria were used appropriately to diagnose initial episodes of ARF but less successfully in recurrent episodes (7). In another study, 35 patients with suspected ARF were prospectively studied (8). Half of them had a discharge diagnosis of definite ARF, whereas 31% posed diagnostic difficulties due to mild symptoms that failed to fulfill Jones criteria. Of note is that at least 29% of patients without prior recognized ARF or RHD had echo-cardiographic evidence of established RHD suggesting that previous episodes were missed (8). The authors suggested that "probable" and "possible" ARF should be considered in cases not fulfilling Jones criteria in order to enable these patients acquire prophylactic therapy at least until further follow-up in order not to miss ARF cases.

Another recent study aimed to elucidate whether Jones criteria for diagnosis of ARF are useful enough. Data from 81 cases of ARF were retrospectively collected, showing that cardiovascular and joint involvement were the most frequent manifestations (80.2 and 77.8% of the cases, respectively), girls had significantly more chorea, arthritis was more frequent than arthralgia, and fever was noted in half of the patients (9). Surprisingly, only 29.6% of the patients fulfilled Jones criteria for ARF requiring an evidence of previous group-A streptococcal infection, and when this mandatory requirement was disregarded, the percentage rose to 87.7% (9). It seems that strict adherence to Jones criteria might lead to under-diagnosis of ARF. A considerable variability with respect to diagnosis in cases of reactive arthritis has also been reported (10). Physicians were most likely to prescribe antibiotic prophylaxis in the presence of clear cardiac risk in ARF. This reflects the lack of universally accepted criteria for the diagnosis of post-streptococcal reactive arthritis and insufficient long-term data regarding carditis risk in this population (10).

Echocardiography is still not included in the Jones criteria, yet it is a very important diagnostic tool as many of the ARF-induced carditis cases are clinically inapparent (11). Karaaslan et al. (12) determined the prevalence and prognosis of subclinical valvulitis by analyzing 104 ARF patients. Of 53 patients who had no cardiac murmur, 23 (43.4%) had subclinical valvulitis. Isolated mitral regurgitation was the most frequent finding found in 82.6% of the patients, followed by combined mitral and aortic regurgitation and isolated aortic regurgitation (12). Subclinical valvulitis has been suggested as a finding that should be accepted as an evidence of carditis, which is a major diagnostic criteria for ARF (13). A recent review of the existing literature on the prevalence and outcome of subclinical carditis in ARF reported that its prevalence ranged from 0% in one study only to 53% in 23 articles (14). The weighted pooled prevalence of subclinical carditis in ARF was 16.8%. In addition, the prevalence of persistence or deterioration of subclinical carditis 3–23 months after ARF diagnosis was 44.7% (14).

A large study confirms these previous observations: the prevalence of RHD as detected by echocardiographic screening is approximately 10 times higher as compared with clinical screening (15). Whereas clinical examination detected RHD that was confirmed by echocardiography in 8 of 3677 children in Cambodia and 5 of 2170 children in Mozambique, echocardiographic screening detected RHD in 79 and 66 cases in these countries, respectively. The mitral valve was involved in 87.3–98.4% of the cases (15). It is not surprising therefore that suggestion for new guidelines have previously emerged. New Australian guidelines formulated in 2005 for the diagnostic criteria of ARF in high-risk populations include echocardiographic evidence of subclinical valvular disease, and polyarthralgia or aseptic monoarthritis as major manifestations (16).

As carditis is probably the most frequent manifestation of RF, and it is also the clinical manifestation of RHD which carries the long-term morbidity associated with this disease, any new diagnostic criteria of RF should include greater efforts to detect carditis even at its preclinical stages. Referring to the revised Jones criteria (Table 69.1), we believe that there is no doubt that echocardiography should be added to the major criterion named "Carditis" as it can detect RHD up to 10 times higher as compared with clinical screening. The decision of screening policy is subject to regional differences in RF prevalence among different populations, yet in case screening is undertaken, echocardiography should be a major part of it. In the absence of a screening system to detect RHD, the intention to use echocardiography as a diagnostic tool for subclinical carditis should be very high. In other words, every patient having any of the other four major criteria or alternatively two of the minor criteria should undergo an echocardiography in order to reveal the most frequent and devastating manifestation of RHD – carditis. The requirement of proof of preceding streptococcal infection is important for classification and RHD-related studies, yet in the case of established carditis suspected to be due to RF, proof for antecedent streptococcal infection should not halt any further preventive therapy for a given RF patient.

References

1. Guilherme, L., Ramasawmy, R., Kalil, J. (2007) Rheumatic fever and rheumatic heart disease: Genetics and pathogenesis. *Scand J Immunol* **66**, 199–207.
2. Olive, C. (2007) Progress in M-protein-based subunit vaccines to prevent rheumatic fever and rheumatic heart disease. *Curr Opin Mol Ther* **9**, 25–34.
3. Blank, M., Krause, I., Magrini, L., et al. (2006) Overlapping humoral autoimmunity links rheumatic fever and the antiphospholipid syndrome. *Rheumatology* **45**, 833–41.
4. Special Writing Group of the Committee on Rheumatic Fever, Endocarditis, and Kawasaki Disease of the Council on Cardiovascular Disease in the Young of the American Heart Association (1992) Guidelines for the diagnosis of rheumatic fever. Jones Criteria, 1992 update. *JAMA* **268**, 2069–73.
5. Shiffman, R.N. (1995) Guideline maintenance and revision. 50 years of the Jones criteria for diagnosis of rheumatic fever. *Arch Pediatr Adolesc Med* **149**, 727–32.
6. Borges, F., Barbosa, M.L., Borges, R.B., et al. (2005) Clinical and demographic characteristics of 99 episodes of rheumatic fever in Acre, the Brazilian Amazon. *Arq Bras Cardiol* **84**, 111–4.
7. Stewart, T., McDonald, R., Currie, B. (2005) Use of the Jones Criteria in the diagnosis of acute rheumatic fever in an Australian rural setting. *Aust N Z J Public Health* **29**, 526–9.
8. Ralph, A., Jacups, S., McGough, K., et al. (2006) The challenge of acute rheumatic fever diagnosis in a high-incidence population: A prospective study and proposed guidelines for diagnosis in Australia's Northern Territory. *Heart Lung Circ* **15**, 113–8.
9. Pereira, B.A., da Silva, N.A., Andrade, L.E., et al. (2007) Jones criteria and underdiagnosis of rheumatic fever. *Indian J Pediatr* **74**, 117–21.
10. Birdi, N., Hsoking, M., Clulow, M.K., et al. (2001) Acute Rheumatic fever and poststreptococcal reactive arthritis: Diagnosing and treatment practices of pediatric subspecialties in Canada. *J Rheumatol* **28**, 1681–8.
11. Keitzer, R. (2005) Acute rheumatic fever (ARF) and post-streptococcal reactive arthritis (PSRA)- an update. *Z Rheumatol* **64**, 295–307.
12. Karaaslan, S., Demiroren, S., Oran, B., et al. (2003) Criteria for judging the improvement in subclinical rheumatic valvulitis. *Cardiol Young* **13**, 500–5.
13. Wilson, N.J., Neutze, J.M. (1995) Echocardiographic diagnosis of subclinical carditis in acute rheumatic fever. *Int J Cardiol* **50**, 1–6.
14. Tubridy-Clark, M., Carapetis, J.R. (2007) Subclinical carditis in rheumatic fever: A systematic review. *Int J Cardiol* **119**, 54–8.
15. Marijon, E., Ou, P., Celermajer, D.S., et al. (2007) Prevalence of rheumatic heart disease detected by echocardiographic screening. *N Engl J Med* **357**, 439–41.
16. Carapetis, J.R., Brown, A., Wilson, N.J., et al. (2007) An Australian guideline for rheumatic fever and rheumatic heart disease: An abridged outline. *Med J Aust* **186**, 581–6.

70
Accelerated Atherosclerosis in Autoimmune Diseases

Nicoletta Ronda and Pier Luigi Meroni

Abstract   Atherosclerosis (AS) is a chronic inflammatory disease of arterial vessels, leading to chronic and acute ischemic damage or hemorrhages in virtually any organ. Atherosclerotic plaque formation is the result of inflammatory processes that mediate lymphocyte and macrophage infiltration, lipid intra- and inter-cellular deposition and eventually smooth muscle cell migration/proliferation and fibrosis. Immune responses against exogenous as well as self-antigens cooperate in triggering such processes. The atherogenic processes may be magnified and accelerated in patients with autoimmune rheumatic diseases (AIRDs) because of the underlying immune abnormalities, the consequent systemic inflammation and the effects of the concomitant chronic therapies. As a matter of fact, accelerated AS (AAS) is responsible for increased mortality and morbidity in almost all the AIRDs nowadays. Diagnostic strategies to detect early atherosclerotic lesions and to apply preventive therapeutical approaches have been proposed in order to avoid complications related to AAS in AIRD.

Keywords   Atherosclerosis · rheumatoid arthritis · systemic lupus erythematosus · antiphospholipid syndrome

Background

Atherosclerosis (AS) is a chronic inflammatory disease of arterial vessels, characterized by the development of discrete lesions, the atherosclerotic plaques and diffuse endothelial dysfunction, leading to chronic and acute ischemic damage or hemorrhages in virtually any organ. However, the most frequent localization of atherosclerotic tissue damage, especially relevant for the patient's survival and quality of life, is that in heart, brain, gut, kidney and limbs. The detailed description of the wide spectrum of clinical pictures in this disease is largely available in clinical literature, and is not object of the present work, aimed at focusing on the association between accelerated AS (AAS) and auto-immune diseases and on the autoimmune mechanisms acting in AS.

Pathogenesis of the Atherosclerotic Lesions

Atherosclerotic plaque is the result of complex processes including subendothelial space infiltration by lymphocytes and monocytes, lipid deposition in the extracellular space in association with matrix macromolecules and accumulation of lipid-laden macrophages (foam cells). Local chemical modifications (especially oxidation) of lipids increase their pro-inflammatory and immunogenic potential accelerating plaque evolution. With time free lipids accumulate, calcium deposition occurs and smooth muscle cells proliferate, migrate and transdifferentiate, producing matrix components and collagen. Fibroblasts migrating from the adventitia contribute to the fibrotic process and together with other resident or infiltrating cells remodel interstitium composition through the impaired balance between metalloproteases and their inhibitors. At any stage, the changes in chemical properties of intimal surface facilitate platelet and leukocyte adhesion and eventually thrombosis. Increases in the plaque thickness may reduce vessel lumen, effect which is clinically particularly relevant in specific sites, such as medium size vessels (tissue dysfunction or macroscopic infarction) and terminal vessels (tissue ischemia or infarction). The acute swelling and rupture is typical of soft plaques, rich in free lipids and inflammatory cells, and with a limited fibrous component and through thrombosis causes acute ischemic events. In spite of the increasing data on the molecular mechanisms acting in

From: Y. Shoenfeld et al. (eds.): *Diagnostic Criteria in Autoimmune Diseases*, DOI: 10.1007/978-1-60327-285-8_70,
© 2008 Humana Press, Totowa, NJ

plaque formation, consensus on the chronology and cause–effect relationship of described events is far from being reached, different authors claiming as primum movens dyslipidemia, platelets activation, neurogenic dysfunction, infections, etc.

In the last decade clinical studies and animal models, together with in vitro works, have provided evidence that immune responses are involved in plaque formation, through immune cell migration in intima and local activation, and through the action of autoantibodies. These immune responses may be triggered by infectious agents and/or neoantigen exposition on endothelium activated by stressors including classical atherogenic factors [1]. The primary rather than secondary role of immunity in plaque formation is supported not only by the demonstration of activated immunocompetent T lymphocytes and dendritic cells in early lesions in young subjects but also by experiments in which defective immune responses were shown to be protective against the plaque formation [2].

The involvement of autoimmune responses is proven by the identification of autoantigens, the results of studies on animal models (active immunization and passive transfer) and by clinical evidence. β2-Glycoprotein I (β2 GPI), the main target antigen recognized by antiphospholipid antibodies (aPLs), can be found in human AS specimens from carotid endarterectomies, it is abundantly expressed within the subendothelial regions and the intimal–medial border of human AS plaques, and it colocalizes with CD4$^+$ lymphocytes [1]. Immunization of mice with β2 GPI resulted in pronounced cellular response to β2 GPI and high titers of anti-β2 GPI antibodies associated with larger AS lesions containing abundant CD4$^+$ cells [1]. T lymphocytes from β2 GPI-immunized low-density lipoprotein (LDL)-receptor-deficient mice induce increase in fatty streaks dimension when injected in into syngenic mice, compared with control lymphocytes [1]. Oxidized LDL (OxLDL) is the oxidized form of LDL, which is more likely to undergo uptake by macrophages/foam cells. Anti-oxLDL antibodies are present in the serum of patients with AS and healthy individuals [3]. In multivariate analyses anti-oxLDL auto-antibodies discriminated better between patients with peripheral vascular disease and control subjects than did any of the different lipoprotein analysis. There was also a tendency for higher autoantibody levels in patients with more extensive AS [4]. Heat shock proteins (HSPs) are a family of phylogenetically highly conserved stress proteins, of which human HSP60 has been recognized as an important autoantigen in AS. Both circulating levels of HSP60, released by activated/damaged cells, and anti-HSP60 antibody correlate with clinically evident AS and sonographically demonstrable AS lesions [2]. Anti-HSP antibodies provide a possible link between AS, inflammation and infections, because of the cross-reactivity with microbial HSP and of the correlation between antimycobacterial HSP65 and sonographically demonstrable AS carotid lesion

and mortality from cardiovascular disease (CVD). Factors such as smoke, shear stress, hyperglycemia, oxLDL, oxygen radicals and pro-inflammatory cytokines promote HSP exposition on EC, and facilitate in situ autoantibody pro-inflammatory action.

Endothelium is considered univocally in all pathogenic hypothesis as pivotal in AS plaque development given its ability to regulate vessel tone and interfere with inflammatory processes and coagulation. Moreover, activated endothelial cells (ECs) express class II major histocompatibility complex (MHC) molecules, thus functioning as non-professional antigen-presenting cells (APCs) [5]. Thus, they might cooperate with the professional APCs of the vascular-associated lymphoid tissue in mounting the adaptive immune responses to endogenous (oxLDL, HSP or β2 GPI) or exogenous (infectious antigens) molecules that have been proposed as playing a role in the early phases of the atherosclerotic process. Thus, ECs are not only target for immune and non-immune aggression but also active elements in inducing vascular damage.

Also in acute AS complications, due to plaque rupture and thrombosis, immune reactions may be involved in augmenting the quota of inflammatory infiltrate (and thus plaque instability), macrophage cholesterol uptake (in the case of anti-oxLDL) and EC activation/damage with changes in surface properties (e.g., tissue factor expression and impairment of the fibrinolytic system).

Accelerated Atherosclerosis in AIRD

The described atherogenic processes may be magnified and accelerated in patients with AIRD because of the underlying immune system dysfunction, the presence of systemic inflammation and endothelial activation, and the effects of chronic therapies. Humoral and cellular effectors of both innate and adaptive immune responses are involved [6]. Gathering information of the mechanisms of AAS in autoimmune patients may be useful not only to improve risk stratification, diagnosis and management of vasculopathy in these patients, but also to identify mechanisms and clinical or laboratory parameters that could became useful as AS risk markers also in general population.

The prognosis of AIRD changed dramatically in the last decade. Earlier diagnosis, new therapeutical approaches and the improved use of the immunosuppressive agents modified the natural course of these diseases affecting in a positive way both morbidity and mortality. However, among novel factors determining the prognosis of AIRD is the AAS recorded in almost all diseases of the group. For example, CVDs now represent the main cause of death and of significant clinical complications both in rheumatoid arthritis (RA) and in systemic lupus erythematosus (SLE) patients. Large evidence for the association between AAS and SLE, RA, Sjögren's syndrome, systemic sclerosis (SSc) and vasculitis is available (7).

Pathogenesis of AAS in AIRD

The levels of autoantibody to oxLDL are higher in patients with SSc, systemic vasculitides and SLE as compared with healthy population and correlate with AS vasculopathy (8). In SLE patients, hyperproduction of specific antibodies including anti-oxLDL seems to occur as suggested by the correlation between the total immunoglobulin serum concentration and the level of anti-oxLDL antibodies, together with the lack of such correlation between total immunoglobulin and antibodies to unrelated antigens (Epstein–Barr virus and purified protein derivative). Anti-β2GPI antibodies, included in the autoantibodies described as atherogenic, are frequently detected in AIRD, and particularly in SLE. The autoantigen was found to be expressed on ECs obtained from different anatomical localizations in in vitro and in vivo studies; the binding of the autoantibodies to expressed or adhered β2GPI has been suggested to induce a cell signaling that ends in the induction of an endothelial pro-inflammatory and procoagulant phenotype (9). Interestingly, such an effect was reported in in vivo experimental models also, suggesting that it might be one of the actual pathogenic mechanisms for the thrombophilic state associated with the persistent presence of aPLs. aPLs thus might contribute not only to the plaque formation but also to atherothrombosis (9).

Other pathogenic autoantibodies, reported as able to activate/damage ECs, are antiendothelial cell antibodies (AECAs), which react with yet unknown EC membrane constituents and have been described in sera from different AIRDs (9). In most cases, AECAs were shown to induce a pro-inflammatory and a procoagulant phenotype in EC monolayers in vitro (9). In accordance with the hypothesis of a role for AECA in AS is their demonstration also in primary AS and in patients displaying conditions at risk of AS (10, 11). Other autoantibodies frequently occurring in AIRD have been reported to react with ECs because of their ability to recognize their own antigens "planted" on EC membrane, as already discussed for anti-β2GPI antibodies. This is the case for the anti-dsDNA antibodies that can react with DNA–histone complexes adhering on EC membranes through electric charge interactions. Such binding has been shown to induce EC activation in vitro (9).

In line with the endothelium perturbation mediated by several circulating immune mediators is the demonstration of an impaired endothelium-dependent vasodilation in AIRD patients. Such impairment is related to the reduction in vasodilator bioavailability (mainly nitric oxide), and it has been associated with the propensity of an individual to develop atherosclerotic disease (12).

Complement (C') activation by circulating immune complexes or by other mechanisms might also contribute endothelial perturbation/damage. Activated products of the C' cascade or even the cell membrane insertion of the membrane attack complex (MAC) play a role. The latter phenomenon was reported to result in the release of an array of growth factors and cytokines that induces proliferation, inflammation and thrombus formation in the vascular walls. C' activation and elevated plasma levels of pro-inflammatory cytokines/chemokines are features common to several AIRDs, and C' deposition has been reported in the atherosclerotic lesions recently (13). Thus, C' may be responsible for chronic inflammatory state that represents a risk factor for plaque formation and a condition favoring its instability and rupture.

Diagnostic Criteria

The diagnosis of atherosclerotic disease relies mostly on clinical picture (signs and laboratory parameters demonstrating tissue or organ damage) and on instrumental studies (echography, angiography). However, AS starts early in life and develops insidiously, and usually signs and symptoms show when the disease is in advanced stage. Moreover, acute organ damage or death may occur suddenly and do not allow for effective therapies. For these reasons, and for the major epidemiologic relevance of AS in developed countries, nowadays most of the scientific efforts are pointed to find sensitive and specific clinical conditions, laboratory parameters and instrumental data to assess and stratify AS risk and to suggest prevention strategies. Classical risk factors include non-modifiable factors (e.g., age, gender) and modifiable factors linked to lifestyle and diet (Table 70.1). The real risk assessment for each individual relies on score risk charts that take into account the great weight of association of risk factors (14). A

TABLE 70.1 Risk factors for atherosclerosis

Classic risk factors	Autoimmunity-related risk factors
HDL cholesterol (reverse relationship)	Autoimmune diseases
LDL cholesterol	Anti-oxLDL antibodies
ApoB/ApoAI[a]	Anti-HSP60/70 antibodies
Hyperomocysteinemia	Anti-B2GPI antibodies
Hyperuricemia[a]	
CRP[a]	
Fibrinogen[a]	
Age	
Male sex	
Genotypes	
Body weight	
Hypertension	
Diabetes	
Smoke	

[a] Emerging, but its clinical utility is still controversial.

consensus on the clinical use recommendation is established at present for some but not all the listed factors, because of difficulties in measures standardization or because of insufficient specificity. In addition to clinical and laboratory parameters, new imaging methods are being developed to detect asymptomatic arterial disease, especially those based on echography. So, besides the well-established significance of ankle–brachial index, which reflects the stenosis between aorta and distal leg arteries, the intima-media thickness evaluation is being increasedly used (15). Reduced flow-mediated vasodilation has been suggested to represent a useful and non-invasive method predictive for AAS in several conditions including AIRD; however, its standardization is still a matter of debate (16).

As discussed above, new factors have emerged as reliable markers correlating with chronic AS vascular lesion extension and acute complications (Table 70.1). In clinical practice, the diagnosis of an autoimmune disease should induce careful assessment of cardiovascular state in a given patient. Except for anti-β2GPI antibodies, the serum measurement of the listed autoantibodies is still unavailable in most laboratories for clinical use, but it could become used in the future.

Therapy

Current principles for prevention and therapy of AS are largely described in literature; in particular, more aggressive goals for risk factor reduction and strategies to reduce inflammation in AIRD have been suggested (17). However, current view does not yet include the idea that immunomodulation can affect AS and thus provide hope for the development of new strategies not only for autoimmune patients but also for the general population. Possible options have been summarized recently (18). Among them is the induction of oral tolerance to autoantigens associated with AS, manipulation of the cytokine network, gene therapy and the use of intravenous immunoglobulin (IVIg). IVIgs have many immunoregulatory and anti-inflammatory properties and have shown the ability to reduce plaque development in a model of murine AS. Looking at mechanisms specifically relevant in AS, it has been reported that IVIgs contain anti-idiotypic activity against anti-oxLDL antibodies, and they are able to reduce metalloproteinase-9 (MMP-9) activity; moreover, IVIgs include a subset of natural antiendothelial antibodies that, opposite to pathologic AECA, directly modulate endothelial function, reducing pro-inflammatory and pro-thrombotic properties of resting EC and inhibiting cytokine and metalloprotease secretion by EC activated with pro-inflammatory stimuli (19). Finally, IVIgs reduce cytokine secretion and the membrane expression of adhesion molecules on EC stimulated with TNF-α and oxLDL, and inhibit one of the pathways of internalization of oxLDL in EC (19).

Studies on autoimmune mechanisms involved in AS have shown that statins, besides their action on serum cholesterol levels, have anti-inflammatory and immunomodulatory effects by reducing monocyte adhesion to EC and endothelial secretion of cytokines and MHC class II expression (20).

Acknowledgments. Authors would like to thank Dr. Paola Panzeri for her assistance in revising the manuscript.

References

1. Shoenfeld, Y., Sherer, Y., and Haratz, D. (2001) Atherosclerosis as an infectious, inflammatory and autoimmune disease. *Trends Immunol* **22**, 293–5.
2. Wick, G., Knoflach, M., and Xu, Q. (2004) Autoimmune and inflammatory mechanisms in atherosclerosis. *Annu Rev Immunol* **22**, 361–403.
3. Wu, R. and Lefvert, A.K. (1995) Autoantibodies against oxidized low density lipoproteins (oxLDL): Characterization of antibody isotope, subclass, affinity and effect on the macrophage uptake of oxLDL. *Clin Exp Immunol* **102**, 174–80.
4. Bergmark, C., Wu, R., de Faire, U., Lefvert, A.K., and Swedenborg, J. (1995) Patients with early onset of peripheral vascular disease have high levels of autoantibodies against oxidized low density lipoproteins. *Arterioscler Thromb Vasc Biol* **15**, 441–5.
5. Rothermel, A.L., Wang, Y., Schechner, J., Mook-Kanamori, B., Aird, W.C., Pober, J.S., Tellides, G., and Johnson, D.R. (2004) Endothelial cells present antigens in vivo. *BMC Immunol* **16**, 5–24.
6. Doria, A., Sherer, Y., Meroni, P.L., and Shoenfeld, Y. (2005) Inflammation and accelerated atherosclerosis: basic mechanisms. *Rheum Dis Clin North Am* **31**, 355–62.
7. Shoenfeld, Y., Gerli, R., Doria, A., Matsuura, E., Cerinic, M.M., Ronda, N., Jara, L.J., Abu-Shakra, M., Meroni, P.L., and Sherer, Y. (2005) Accelerated atherosclerosis in autoimmune rheumatic diseases. *Circulation* **22**, 3337–47.
8. Matsuura, E., Kobayashi, K., Inoue, K., Lopez, L.R., and Shoenfeld, Y. (2005) Oxidized LDL/beta2-glycoprotein I complexes: New aspects in atherosclerosis. *Lupus* **14**, 736–41.
9. Meroni, P.L., Ronda, N., Raschi, E., and Borghi, M.O. (2005) Humoral autoimmunity against endothelium: Theory or reality? *Trends Immunol* **26**, 275–81.
10. George, J., Meroni, P.L., Gilburd, B., Raschi, E., Harats, D., and Shoenfeld, Y. (2000) Antiendothelial cell antibodies in patients with coronary atherosclerosis. *Immunol Lett* **73**, 23–7.
11. Faulk, W.F., Rose, M., Meroni P.L., Del Papa, N., Torry, R.J., Labarrere, C.A., Busing, K., Crisp, S. J., Dunn, M.J., and Nelson, D.R. (1999) Antibodies to human endothelial cells identify myocardial damage and predicts development of coronary artery disease in patients with transplanted hearts. *Hum Immunol* **60**, 826–32.

12. Bonetti, P.O., Lilach, O.L., and Lerman, A. (2003) Endothelial dysfunction. A marker of atherosclerotic risk. *Arterioscler Thromb Vasc Biol* **23**, 168–75.

13. Niculescu, F. and Rus, H. (2004) The complement activation in atherosclerosis. *Immunol Res* **30**, 73–80.

14. Fourth joint task force of the European Society of Cardiology and other Societies on Cardiovascular Disease prevention in clinical practise. (2007) European guidelines on cardioavascular disease prevention in clinical practise: Executive summary. *Eur Heart J* **28**, 2375–414.

15. Wong, N.D. (2007) Metabolic syndrome: Cardiovascular risk assessment and management. *Am J Cardiovasc Drugs* **7**, 259–72.

16. Roman, M.J., Naqvi, T.Z., Gardin, J.M., Gerhard-Herman, M., Jaff, M., and Mohler, E. (2006) American Society of Echocardiography; Society for Vascular Medicine and Biology. American society of echocardiography report. Clinical application of noninvasive vascular ultrasound in cardiovascular risk stratification: A report from the American Society of Echocardiography and the Society for Vascular Medicine and Biology. *Vasc Med* **11**, 201–11.

17. Salmon, J.E. and Roman, M.J. (2001) Accelerated atherosclerosis in systemic lupus erythematosus: implications for patient management. *Curr Opin Rheumatol* **13**, 341–4.

18. Sherer, Y. and Shoenfeld, Y. (2002) Immunomodulation for treatment and prevention of atherosclerosis. *Autoimmun Rev* **1**, 21–7.

19. Ronda, N., Bernini, N., Giacosa, R., Gatti, R., Baldini, N., Buzio, C., and Orlandini, G. (2003) Normal human IgG prevents endothelial cell activation induced by TNFα and oxidized low-density lipoprotein atherogenic stimuli. *Clin Exp Immunol* **133**, 219–26.

20. Riboldi, P., Gerosa, M., and Meroni, P.L. (2005) Statins and autoimmune diseases. *Lupus* **14**, 765–8.

71
Idiopathic Interstitial Pneumonias

Antoni Xaubet, Maria Molina-Molina and Anna Serrano-Mollar

Abstract   The idiopathic interstitial pneumonias are a group of diffuse parenchymal lung diseases of unknown etiology with varying degrees of inflammation and fibrosis. They are classified into seven clinicopathological entities: idiopathic pulmonary fibrosis, nonspecific interstitial pneumonia, desquamative interstitial pneumonia, respiratory bronchiolitis/interstitial lung disease, organizing pneumonia, acute interstitial pneumonia, and lymphoid interstitial pneumonia. The diagnosis of the interstitial idiopathic pneumonias is clinical-radiological-pathological and requires the presence of an appropriate histological pattern in pulmonary biopsy. In idiopathic pulmonary fibrosis, a set of criteria has been established to permit diagnosis with a sensitivity of more than 90% when lung biopsy samples are not available. The only established treatment is based on glucocorticoids and immunossupressants, while lung transplantation is required in later stages.

Keywords   Idiopathic interstitial pneumonias · interstitial lung diseases · idiopathic pulmonary fibrosis

Classification of Idiopathic Interstitial Pneumonias

The idiopathic interstitial pneumonias are a group of diffuse parenchymal lung diseases of unknown etiology with varying degrees of inflammation (alveolitis) and fibrosis. The histopathological classification of the idiopathic interstitial pneumonias has evolved over time, and was most recently codified in the American Thoracic Society/European Respiratory Society 2002 consensus classification statement (1). This classification separates the idiopathic interstitial pneumonias into seven clinicopathological entities (Table 71.1). Idiopathic pulmonary fibrosis is characterized by the presence of usual interstitial pneumonia in the histological examination of lung parenchyma. The usual interstitial pneumonia pattern is not synonymous with the diagnosis of idiopathic pulmonary fibrosis. This histological pattern can also be associated with collagen vascular diseases, drug-induced interstitial pulmonary disease, chronic hypersensitivity pneumonitis, and asbestosis. Nonspecific interstitial pneumonia may be associated with collagen vascular diseases, drug-induced interstitial pulmonary disease, hypersensitivity pneumonitis, and HIV infection. Desquamative interstitial pneumonia and respiratory bronchiolitis/interstitial lung disease are almost exclusively associated with cigarette smoking. Desquamtive interstitial pneumonia is

considered to represent a more advanced stage of respiratory bronchiolitis/interstitial lung disease because of its similar pathology. Organizing pneumonia can be idiopathic or associated with collagen vascular diseases, drug-induced interstitial pulmonary disease, radiotherapy, inhalation of toxic substances, pulmonary infections, or inflammatory bowel diseases. The term acute interstitial pneumonia is used exclusively for cases of idiopathic acute respiratory distress syndrome. Lymphoid interstitial pneumonia was previously considered to be a pulmonary lymphoproliferative disorder, a precursor of pulmonary lymphoma. However, it has now

TABLE 71.1. Classification of idiopathic interstitial pneumonias.

Clinical diagnosis	Pathological pattern
Idiopathic pulmonary fibrosis (IPF)	Usual interstitial pneumonia
Nonspecific interstitial pneumonia (NSIP)	Nonspecific interstitial pneumonia (NSIP)
Desquamative interstitial pneumonia (DIP)	Desquamative interstitial pneumonia (DIP)
Respiratory bronchiolitis interstitial lung disease (RBILD)	Respiratory bronchiolitis interstitial lung disease (RBILD)
Acute interstitial pneumonia (AIP)	Diffuse alveolar damage (DAD)
Organizing pneumonia (OP)	Organizing pneumonia (OP)
Lymphoid interstitial pneumonia (LIP)	Lymphoid interstitial pneumonia (LIP)

From: Y. Shoenfeld et al. (eds.): *Diagnostic Criteria in Autoimmune Diseases*, DOI: 10.1007/978-1-60327-285-8_71,
© 2008 Humana Press, Totowa, NJ

been demonstrated that this association is very rare. Lymphoid interstitial pneumonia is usually associated with other disorders, such as collagen vascular diseases, autoimmune diseases (Hashimoto's disease, myasthenia gravis, pernicious anemia, primary biliary cirrhosis), and immunodeficiencies (agammaglobulinemia) (1, 2, 3).

Clinical Manifestations

The most common symptoms are dyspnea on exertion and dry coughing. The onset of dyspnea is usually gradual but progressive. The onset of the disease may be insidious, subacute, or abrupt, depending on the type of idiopathic interstitial pneumonia. Some clinical entities can cause constitutional symptoms. The most useful information obtained from the physical examination is the presence of crackles and finger clubbing, although these signs are not present in all the diseases (3, 4, 5, 6, 7, 8, 9, 10). Table 71.2 summarizes the important clinical features.

Diagnostic Approach

Blood Tests

These are not useful for diagnosis, although they may reveal abnormalities in markers of inflammation (C-reactive-protein, erythrocyte sedimentation rate, gamma globulins). Positive anti-nuclear antibodies or rheumatoid factor occur in 10–20% of patients with idiopathic pulmonary fibrosis, although the titers are low.

Serological Markers

Several cytokines, growth factors, and other mediators have been analyzed in the serum of patients with idiopathic interstitial pneumonias. However, they are of no use for diagnostic purposes.

Radiology

Chest roentgenogram findings in patients with idiopathic interstitial pneumonias consist of interstitial patterns that affect both hemithoraces diffusely. They indicate the presence of an interstitial lung disease, but lack diagnostic specificity. The chest roentgenogram may be normal in 10% of cases at the time of diagnosis. High-resolution computed tomography is a more sensitive tool than chest roentgenogram in the evaluation of abnormalities of the pulmonary interstitium and it has become indispensable for diagnostic approach. The major imaging findings are ground glass opacities, consolidation, linear and reticular opacities, centrilobular nodules, traction bronchiectasis, and honeycombing. Their distribution is different in each disease and this narrows the differential diagnosis (Table 71.3). In idiopathic pulmonary fibrosis, high-resolution computed tomography findings are characteristic and are considered to be a diagnostic criterion. The specificity is 96%, but the sensitivity is low, as in 20–25% of patients the findings are atypical. In the other idiopathic pulmonary pneumonias, high-resolution computed tomography may be helpful in reaching a diagnosis, but not in making a specific diagnosis (11, 12).

Lung Function Testing

This reveals restrictive impairment, reduced diffusing capacity for carbon monoxide, and reduced hypoxemia exaggerated or elicited by exercise. In 15% of cases, lung function impairment is the first manifestation of the disease. Nevertheless, a normal lung function test does not exclude the diagnosis of idiopathic interstitial pneumonia. (1, 3, 4)

Bronchoalveolar Lavage

Cellular analysis of bronchoalveolar lavage (BAL) is useful in the diagnostic assessment of idiopathic interstitial pneumonias. In most cases, however, BAL serves as guide to diagnosis, by supporting a provisional diagnosis or suggesting an alternative. In idiopathic pulmonary fibrosis, BAL shows increased neutrophils and eosinophils. In

TABLE 71.2. Frequency and clinical characteristics of idiopathic interstitial pneumonias.

	IPF[a]	NSIP	DIP/RBILD	AIP	OP	LIP
Frequency	~47–64%	~14–36%	~10–17%	<2%	~4–12%	<2%
Onset	Insidious	Insidious/Subacute	Insidious/Subacute	Abrupt (1–2 weeks)	Subacute	Subacute
Finger clubbing	~20–50%	~10–30%	~50%	No	No	No
Crackles	~90%	~40%	~60%	No	~40%	No
Constitutional symptoms	No	Depends on etiology	No	Fever Arthralgias Asthenia Weight loss	Fever Weight loss	Fever Arthralgias Asthenia Weight loss

[a] For abbreviations, see Table 71.1.

TABLE 71.3. High-resolution computed tomography (HRCT) findings in idiopathic interstitial pneumonias.

Disease	Main HRCT findings	Distribution
IPF	Reticular opacities	Peripheral
	Honeycombing	Subpleural
	Traction bronchiectasis	Basal
	Architectural distortion	
	Only minimal focal ground glass	
NSIP	Ground glass opacities	Peripheral
	Reticular opacities	Subpleural
	Consolidation	Basal
	Traction bronchiestasis	
DIP	Ground glass opacities	Multifocal
	Reticular opacities	Peripheral
RBILD	Bronchial wall thickening	Multifocal
	Centrilobular nodules	Diffuse
	Ground glass opacities	
AIP	Consolidation	Diffuse
	Ground glass opacities	
OP	Consolidation	Subpleural
	Ground glass opacities	Peribronchiolar
LIP	Ground glass opacities	Diffuse
	Centrilobular nodules	
	Linear opacities	
	Thin-walled cysts	

For abbreviations, see Table 71.1

TABLE 71.4. Diagnostic criteria of idiopathic pulmonary fibrosis.

The following criteria must be fulfilled in the presence of a surgical biopsy showing usual interstitial pneumonia
- Exclusion of other known causes of interstitial lung diseases
- Abnormal pulmonary function studies: evidence of restriction and/ or impaired gas exchange
- Abnormalities characteristics of the disease on chest roentgenogram or HRCT

In the absence of surgical lung biopsy, the following four major criteria must be fulfilled, plus three of the minor criteria

Major criteria
- Exclusion of other known causes of interstitial lung diseases
- Abnormal pulmonary function studies: evidence of restriction and/ or impaired gas exchange
- Abnormal characteristics of the disease on HRCT
- Transbronchial lung biopsy or BAL showing no features to support an alternative diagnosis

Minor criteria
- Age >50 years
- Insidious onset of otherwise unexplained dyspnea on exertion
- Duration of illness >3 months
- Persistent, bibasilar, inspiratory crackles

HRCT: High-resolution computed tomography; BAL: bronchoalveolar lavage.

patients with increased lymphocytes, other possible alternative diagnoses should be excluded. In organizing pneumonia, BAL reveals marked lymphocytosis, often associated with moderate neutrophilia and/or eosinophilia, together with a decreased CD4+/CD8+ T-lymphocyte ratio. BAL does not shows findings useful for the diagnostic assessment in the other idiopathic interstitial pneumonias. (1, 3, 4)

Diagnostic Criteria

The diagnosis of the interstitial idiopathic pneumonias is clinical-radiological-pathological and requires the presence of an appropriate histological pattern in pulmonary biopsy. Transbronchial lung biopsy performed with a fiberoptic bronchoscope may only confirm the histological diagnosis of organizing pneumonia. The diagnosis of the other idiopathic interstitial pneumonias requires a surgical lung biopsy. In idiopathic pulmonary fibrosis, a set of criteria has been established that allows diagnosis to be made with a sensitivity of more than 90% when lung biopsy samples are not available (Table 71.4) (11, 13).

Therapy

The fundamental aims of treatment are to suppress the inflammatory (alveolitis) and fibrotic components of the disease. The suppression of alveolitis is the only useful treatment, because no antifibrotic drugs of proven efficacy are currently available. The drugs used are glucocorticoids, whether associated with immunosuppressants (azathioprine or cyclophosphamide) or otherwise. In idiopathic pulmonary fibrosis, the addition of N-acetylcistein to this therapeutic approach seems to stabilize the disease in some patients. The indications and duration of treatment vary according to the form of idiopathic interstitial pneumonia; the same is true of the clinical response. Lung transplant is the last therapeutic option for diseases that progress to fibrosis and cause respiratory failure. (14, 15, 16)

References

1. American Thoracic Society/European Respiratory Society international multidisciplinary consensus classification of idiopathic interstitial pneumonias: General principles and recommendations. Am J Respir Crit Care Med 2002; 165: 277–304
2. Kim DS, Collard HR, King TE. Classification and natural history of the idiopathic interstitial pneumonias. Proc Am Thorac Soc 2006; 3: 285–292
3. Xaubet A, Ancochea J, Blanquer R, Montero C, Morell F, Rodríguez Becerra E et al. Diagnosis and treatment of diffuse interstitial lung diseases. Arch Bronconeumol 2003; 39: 580–600
4. American Thoracic Society. Idiopathic pulmonary fibrosis: diagnosis and treatment; joint statement of the American Thoracic Society and the European Respiratory Society. Am. J. Respir. Crit. Care Med. 2000; 161: 646–664

5. Martinez FJ. Idiopathic interstitial pneumonias. Usual interstitial pneumonia versus nonspecific interstitial pneumonia. Proc Am Thorac Soc 2006; 3: 81–95

6. Portnoy J, Veraldi KL, Schwarz MI, Cool CD, Curran-Everett D, Cherniack RM et al. Respiratory bronchiolitis-interstitial lung disease. Chest 2007; 131: 664–671

7. Ryu JH, Myers JL, Capizzi SA, Douglas WW, Vassallo R, Decker PA. Desquamative interstitial pneumonia and respiratory bronquiolitis-associated interstitial lung disease. Chest 2005; 127: 178–84

8. Cordier JF. Cryptogenic organizing pneumonia. Eur Respir J 2006; 28: 422–446

9. Cha SI, Fressler MB, Cool CD, Schwarz MI, Brown KK, Lymphoid interstitial pneumonia: clinical features, associations and prognosis. Eur Respir J 2006; 28: 364–369

10. Bonaccorsi A, Cancellien A, Chilosi M, Trisolini R, Boaron M, Crimi N. Acute interstitial pneumonia: report of a series. Eur Respir J 2003; 21: 187–191

11. Hunninghake G.W., Zimmerman M.B., Schwartz D.A. Utility of a lung biopsy for the diagnosis of idiopathic pulmonary fibrosis. Am. J. Respir. Crit. Care Med. 2001; 164; 193–196

12. Gotway MB, Freemer MM, King TE. Challenges in pulmonary fibrosis. 1: Use of high resolution CT scanning of the lung for the evaluation of patients with idiopathic interstitial pneumonias. Thorax 2007; 62: 546–553

13. Raghu G, Mageta YN, Lockhart D, Schmidt RD, Wood DE, Godwin JD. The accuracy of the clinical diagnosis of new onset idiopathic pulmonary fibrosis and other interstitial lung diseases: a prospective study. Chest 1999; 116: 1168–1174

14. Wells AU. Antioxidant therapy in idiopathic pulmonary fibrosis: Hope is kindled. Eur Respir J 2006; 27: 664–666

15. Selman M, Navarro C, Gaxiola M. Idiopathic pulmonary fibrosis: In search of an effective treatment. Arch Bronconeumol 2005; 41 (Suppl. 5): 15–20

16. Walter N, Collard HR, King TE. Current perspectives on the treatment of idiopathic pulmonary fibrosis. Proc Am Thorac Soc 2006; 3: 330–338

72
Pulmonary Arterial Hypertension

Isabel Blanco and Joan Albert Barberà

Abstract Pulmonary arterial hypertension (PAH) is the most characteristic group of pulmonary hypertensive states. Among other conditions, PAH includes the idiopathic type and forms associated with connective tissue diseases (CTDs), particularly with systemic sclerosis, CREST syndrome, and mixed CTD. Pulmonary hypertension (PH) can be detected by transthoracic Doppler echocardiography. This procedure should be performed routinely once a year in patients with CTD with high risk to develop PAH. The diagnosis of PH needs to be confirmed by right heart catheterization. Recently developed drugs that modulate endothelial function have provided encouraging results in the treatment of PAH with improvement in symptoms, exercise tolerance, and survival.

Keywords Pulmonary hypertension · pulmonary circulation · endothelium · echocardiography · right heart catheterization · prostacyclin · endothelin-1 · phosphodiesterase-5

Concept and Classification

The pulmonary circulation is a low-resistance, high-compliance system that accommodates all the cardiac output, even in conditions where cardiac output is high, as it occurs during exercise. Pulmonary vascular resistance is about one-fifth of the systemic resistance and decreases when cardiac output increases because of the recruitment and distensibility of the pulmonary vessels.

Reference values of pulmonary haemodynamic measurements are summarized in Table 72.1. Pulmonary arterial hypertension (PAH) is defined by a mean pulmonary artery pressure (PAP) greater than 25 mmHg at rest or greater than 30 mmHg during exercise.

The most important clinical repercussion of PAH is the increase in the work load of the right ventricle. Usually, small increases in pulmonary pressure do not have significant haemodynamic repercussion. Nevertheless, when PAP increases markedly, especially if this occurs acutely, the right ventricle may fail and the patient may die because of cardiac failure.

The classification of pulmonary hypertension (PH) has changed over time. Currently, it is classified into five different classes or categories (Venice classification, 2003) (Table 72.2) (1):

TABLE 72.1. Pulmonary haemodynamics measurements in healthy subjects[a].

Variable	Reference value
CO (L/min)	4–8.3
CI (L/min/m^2)	2.6–4.5
PAP (mmHg)	8–20
PAOP (mmHg)	5–14
RAP (mmHg)	2–9
PVR (din·seg·cm^{-5})	40–240

[a] Adults, at rest and at sea level.
CO: cardiac output; CI: cardiac index; PAP: pulmonary artery pressure; PAOP: pulmonary artery occlusion pressure; PVR: pulmonary vascular resistance; RAP: right atrial pressure.

(a) PAH; (b) PH associated with left heart disease; (c) PH associated with respiratory diseases and/or hypoxaemia; (d) PH because of chronic thrombotic and/or embolic disease; and (e) miscellaneous.

Pathogenesis

Different processes may contribute to the pathogenesis of PAH, namely vasoconstriction, vascular remordelling and thrombosis. In PAH, there is an impairment of the

From: Y. Shoenfeld et al. (eds.): *Diagnostic Criteria in Autoimmune Diseases*, DOI: 10.1007/978-1-60327-285-8_72,
© 2008 Humana Press, Totowa, NJ

TABLE 72.2. Clinical classification of pulmonary hypertension[a].

1. Pulmonary arterial hypertension (PAH)
   Idiopathic
   Familial
   Associated with
      Connective tissue disease
      Congenital systemic to pulmonary shunts
      Portal hypertension
      HIV infection
      Drugs and toxins
      Other (thyroid disorders, glycogen storage disease, Gaucher's
         disease, hereditary hemorrhagic telangiectasia,
         haemoglobinopathies, myeloproliferative disorders,
         splenectomy)
   Associated with significant venous or capillary involvement
      pulmonary veno-occlusive disease
      pulmonary capillary haemangiomatosis
   Persistent pulmonary hypertension of the newborn
2. Pulmonary hypertension associated with left heart disease
   Left-sided atrial or ventricular heart disease
   Left-sided valvular heart disease
3. Pulmonary hypertension associated with lung diseases and/or chronic
   hypoxaemia
   Chronic obstructive pulmonary disease
   Interstitial lung disease
   Sleep-disordered breathing
   Alveolar hypoventilation disorders
   Chronic exposure to high altitude
   Developmental abnormalities
4. Pulmonary hypertension due to chronic thrombotic and/or embolic
   disease
   Thromboembolic obstruction of proximal pulmonary arteries
   Thromboembolic obstruction of distal pulmonary arteries
   Non-thrombotic pulmonary embolism (tumour, parasites, foreign
      material)
5. Miscellaneous
   Histiocytosis X
   Lymphangiomatosis
   Sarcoidosis
   Compression of pulmonary vessels (adenopathy, tumour,
      fibrosing mediastinitis)

[a] Adopted in the 3rd World Symposium on Pulmonary Arterial Hypertension.
Venice, 2003.

Idiopathic PAH

Clinical Presentation

Idiopathic PH (IPAH), formerly termed primary PH, is a rare disease of unknown aetiology. Its incidence ranges between 1 and 2 new cases per year per million adult inhabitants (3). After puberty, idiopathic PAH is more common in women than in men (women/men ratio: 1.7) and is more prevalent in persons 20–40 years old. IPAH is the most characteristic disease in the PAH category, and it is defined by the presence of PH, which is not produced by any other clinical condition.

PAH often presents with non-specific symptoms. The most common symptoms are exertional dyspnoea (72%), syncope or presyncope (40%) usually during exercise, chest pain (48%), fatigue (70%), and/or peripheral oedema (40%). Because of the low specificity of these symptoms and their progressive evolution, the diagnosis of PAH is usually delayed 2 or more years after symptoms appeared. Patients should be asked for the potential risk factors associated with PH, such as drugs (aminorex, fenfluramine) and associated conditions [HIV infection, connective tissue disease (CTD), liver disease or congenital heart disease].

At the physical inspection the most frequent signs are accentuated pulmonary component of the second heart sound, left parasternal lift, pansystolic murmur of tricuspid regurgitation, and diastolic murmur of pulmonary insufficiency. In presence of right ventricular dysfunction, there is an increased "v" wave in the jugular pulse, jugular vein distension, peripheral oedema, hepatomegaly and, sometimes, ascites.

It is important to asses to what extension the disease affects daily life activities using the modified New York Heart Association (NYHA) classification [World Health Organization (WHO) classification] (4).

endothelial function of pulmonary arteries that leads to an imbalance between endothelium-derived vasodilator and vasoconstrictive mediators. Vasoconstriction is promoted by an increased synthesis and release of vasoconstricting agents such as tromboxane-A2 and endothelin-1, and by a concomitant reduction in the expression of both prostacyclin and nitric oxide synthases (2). Endothelial dysfunction also promotes cell proliferation in the vessel wall (remodelling). Vascular remodelling affects small pulmonary arteries, which show medial hypertrophy, intimal proliferation, neointimal lesions, and necrotizing arteritis. In addition, plexiform lesions, focal proliferation of endothelial channels lined by myofibroblasts, and smooth muscle cells may be observed.

Diagnostic Evaluation

A high index of suspicion, detailed clinical history and careful physical examination are critical for the diagnosis of PH.

Suspicion of the disease might be raised by conventional examinations such as electrocardiography (ECG), usually showing right ventricular hypertrophy and right atrial dilatation; and chest X-ray that may show proximal pulmonary artery and/or right ventricular enlargement.

In the diagnostic process we distinguish several phases: suspicion, detection and characterization (Table 72.3) (4). The essential tool for the detection of PH is transthoracic Doppler echocardiography, which provides information on the morphology and function of the right ventricle, and allows the estimation of pulmonary artery systolic

72.3. Diagnostic process of pulmonary hypertension.

Phase	Examinations
Suspicion Chest X-ray, ECG	Symptoms, physical examination
Detection	Transthoracic echocardiogram (TTE)
Class and type identification	TTE (valvulopathy or left heart disease, congenital heart diseases)
	Pulmonary function tests: forced spirometry, static lung volumes, CO diffusing capacity and arterial blood gases
	Ventilation-perfusion (V-Q) scanning
	General analyses and evaluation of
	Thyroid function
	Hepatic function
	Autoimmune screening: anti-nuclear antibodies (ANA), anti-DNA, anti-centromer, anti-cardiolipin and anti-U1-RNP
	Serologies of HIV, B and C hepatitis
	Optional
	High resolution CT chest scan
	Angio CT chest scan
	Sleep study
	Pulmonary angiography if chronic thromboembolic pulmonary hypertension
	Transoesophagueal echocardiography
Evaluation and diagnosis	Haemodynamic diagnosis:
	Pulmonary haemodynamics (right heart catheterization)
	Acute vasodilator test
	Exercise capacity
	6-min walk test
	Cardiopulmonary exercise test (optional)

pressure from the measurement of the systolic regurgitant tricuspid flow velocity.

Other tests to be performed include pulmonary function tests, blood tests (including C and B hepatitis serology, HIV serology, liver function and antibodies associated with CTD), arterial blood gas measurements, high-resolution CT scan if interstitial lung disease is suspected, and ventilation-perfusion scan. Biopsy of the lung is contraindicated because of the high risk of the procedure.

It is mandatory to confirm the diagnosis of PH by right heart catheterization. During the procedure, it is important to perform an acute vasodilator test with inhaled nitric oxide or intravenous epoprostenol (5) to evaluate the possibility for vasodilator treatment. Measurements of PAP, cardiac output, right atrial pressure and pulmonary vascular resistance provide important prognostic information.

An additional step for disease characterization is the assessment of exercise tolerance. This is usually performed using the 6-min walk test (6 MWT). The distance covered during the test correlates with the functional class and the cardiac output, and it also has important prognostic significance.

Treatment

General Measures

Vigorous or intensive exercise should be avoided to prevent right heart failure and a low salt diet is recommended. Patients must avoid drugs that could worsen PAH (nasal decongestants, beta-blocking agents). Pregnancy should be avoided because it may worsen PAH and is associated with high mortality risk.

Pharmacological Treatment

Anticoagulation

The use of anticoagulants improves survival in PAH, although the scientific evidence for this recommendation is limited. Warfarin and acenocumarine are the most commonly employed agents. The target International Normalized Ratio (INR)) ranges between 1.5 and 2.5.

Calcium-Channel Blockers.

They are indicated in patients showing a significant response in the acute pulmonary vasodilator test (decrease in PAP >10 mmHg, final PAP <40 mmHg, with no change or increase in cardiac output) (6). Nevertheless, a positive response is observed only in 13% of cases (7). The most commonly used drugs are nifedipine, diltiazem and amlodipine. The use of verapamil is not recommended because of its poor vasodilating action and its negative inotropic effect. Adverse effects of calcium channel blockers include hypotension, ankle oedema and hypoxaemia.

Specific Therapy

Three major pathways are involved in the pathobiology of PAH: the NO-cGMP, the prostacyclin-cAMP and the endothelin-1 pathways. These pathways correspond to important therapeutic targets in this condition. Three classes of drugs are currently available that exert an effect in these pathways: prostanoids, endothelin-1 receptor antagonists and phosphodiesterase-5 inhibitors (Figure 72.1).

Prostanoids. Prostacyclin is a natural substance synthesized by the endothelium with vasodilator and antiproliferative properties. Available drugs include synthetic prostacyclin (epoprostenol) and prostacyclin analogues that can be administered by inhalation (iloprost) or subcutaneous infusion (treprostinil). Randomized clinical trials have shown that prostanoids improve pulmonary haemodynamics, increase exercise tolerance and improve symptoms in patients with PAH in functional class III–IV

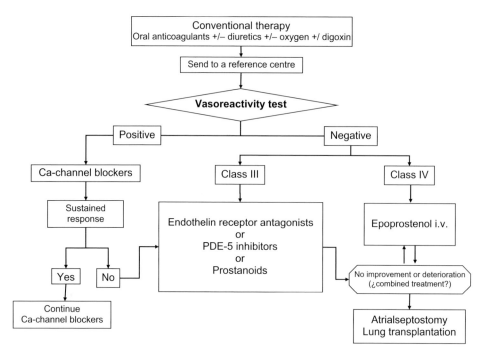

FIGURE 72.1. Treatment algorithm of pulmonary arterial hypertension in functional class III–IV. Adopted in the 3rd World Symposium on Pulmonary Arterial Hypertension (Venice 2003).

(8, 9). There is evidence that they also improve survival (8, 10). Epoprostenol must be administered by continuous intravenous infusion because its half life is very short (3–5 min). The drug is delivered by a continuous perfusion pump connected to a permanent central venous catheter. Main adverse effects are related to the administration method: dysfunction of the pump, catheter infections and venous thrombosis. The abrupt interruption of the perfusion may be life-threatening. The most common adverse effects of prostanoids are jaw pain, flushing, diarrhoea and headache. The development of tolerance is frequent, so it is usually necessary to increase doses progressively.

Iloprost has a more prolonged half life than epoprostenol and can be administered intravenously or by nebulization. Nebulized iloprost has the advantage of its selective deposition in the lung with less systemic side effects. Yet, it must be administered 6–9 times a day. The most important adverse effect is the potential to produce syncope (11). Treprostinil is administered continuously by a subcutaneous infusion. Its main adverse effects are erythema and pain at the insertion point (12). Both iloprost and treprostinil have shown beneficial effects in terms of symptoms, exercise tolerance and delay of clinical worsening (11, 12).

Endothelin-1 Receptor Antagonists. Endothelin-1 (ET-1) is a peptide produced by endothelial cells with vasoconstrictor and mitogenic actions. Bosentan is a dual, A and B, ET-1 receptor antagonist that is administered orally.

Controlled clinical trials have shown that it relieves symptoms, increases exercise tolerance and improves right ventricular function in patients with PAH in functional class II–IV (13). The most common adverse effect is the elevation of liver enzymes, which should be regularly monitored. Two selective inhibitors of ET-1 type A receptor have been recently approved for the treatment of PAH in patients in functional class III: sitaxsentan and ambrisentan.

Phosphodiesterase-5 Inhibitors. Phosphodiesterase-5 (PDE-5) inactivates intracellular cGMP. Therefore, PDE-5 inhibition increases the intracellular concentration of cGMP and produces vasodilatation. PDE-5 is extensively expressed in pulmonary vessels. Sildenafil is a selective inhibitor of PDE-5 that can be administered orally. Randomized controlled clinical trials have shown improvement in functional class, pulmonary haemodynamics and exercise tolerance in patients with PAH in functional class II–IV. The most frequent adverse effects are hypotension, migraine, dyspepsia and flushing. The currently approved dose in PAH is 20 mg/8 h (14). The efficacy of PDE-5 inhibitors such as tadalafil is currently being evaluated.

Combination therapy with more than one drug acting on different pathways is an appealing option in patients not responding to a single drug. Yet, scientific evidence supporting the use of combined therapy in PAH is still scarce. Furthermore, optimal combination regimes, potential interactions between drugs and adverse effects have not yet been established. For this reason, the initiation of combination therapy in patients clinically deteriorating with one drug is better handled in reference centres.

Supporting Treatments

Supporting treatments in PAH are addressed to treat complications associated with the disease, namely right heart failure and hypoxaemia.

Treatment of right heart failure includes low salt diet, diuretics and digital. Diuretics are indicated in patients presenting clinical signs of right ventricular insufficiency. They must be administered with caution because excessive depletion could lead to an inadequate filling of the right ventricle and worsen ventricular function.

The use of digoxin is restricted to patients who have atrial rhythm abnormalities and in patients receiving high doses of calcium-channel blockers to counteract their negative inotropic effect.

In patients with arterial hypoxaemia supplemental oxygen should be provided.

Invasive Treatments

Atrial septostomy is a procedure addressed to create a shunt in the interatrial septum. It permits decompression of the right heart, but it decreases arterial oxygenation. The procedure is associated with high risk and must be performed in experienced centres (15). Lung and heart-lung transplantation is indicated in patients not responding to specific therapy including intravenous epoprostenol (15). Postoperative mortality in PAH is higher than in other transplant indications. For this reason patients must be carefully selected.

The evidence for effective therapy improving survival and quality of life in patients with PAH is compelling. Treatment is likely to be most effective if applied earlier in the course of the disease and, given the complexity of these patients and of the treatments involved, this condition is best treated by experienced clinicians at centres with expertise in all aspects of diagnosis assessment and management.

Prognosis

The median life expectancy from the time of diagnosis in patients with IPAH, before the availability of specific therapy was 2.8 years (1616). Nowadays, survival has improved considerably and survival ratios >75% at 3 years are being reported with the use of new specific therapies (10).

PAH Associated with CTD

PH is a well-recognised complication of CTDs such as systemic sclerosis (SSc), especially in its limited form, mixed CTD (MCTD) and systemic lupus erythematosus (SLE). Occasionally it may also occur in association with interstitial lung disease. The prevalence of PH in CTDs has been reported to be up to 38%. In SSc, pulmonary complications, such as interstitial lung disease and PAH, are currently the leading causes of death. Patients with SSc and associated PAH have a particularly poor prognosis compared with those without PAH.

PAH associated with CTDs is the second most prevalent type of PAH after the idiopathic form. In patients with connective tissue disease associated PAH, systemic sclerosis is the underlying disease with the highest prevalence (75%), followed by MCTD (9%) and SLE (7%) (17).

Compared to idiopathic PAH, PH associated with connective tissue disorders is more prevalent in women (women/men ratio 4:1) and presents in older age (66 years old). In scleroderma, PAH is more frequent in its limited form (CREST) (3:1) and usually presents with concomitant disorders such as pulmonary fibrosis (diagnosed by CT scan) and left heart disease (systemic hypertension and cardiomiopathy).

Clinical presentation and lung pathology of PAH in CTD is indistinguishable from the idiopathic form. For these reason the diagnostic process and treatment are analogous (18) (Table 72.3, Figure 72.1).

Echocardiography is the main tool for detecting PAH. Accordingly, it should be performed routinely once a year in all patients with high risk to develop PH (SSc, CREST and MCTD).

Pulmonary function testing is useful in distinguishing vasculopathic from fibrotic alterations in patients with SSc who may associate both disorders. In patients with pulmonary fibrosis, forced vital capacity (FVC) and CO diffusing capacity (DL_{CO}) decrease concurrently, being the ratio FVC (%predicted)/DLco (%predicted) <1.4. If pulmonary vasculopathy is the most significant alteration, DL_{CO} decreases out of order compared to FVC, FVC(%)/DL_{CO}(%) ratio >1.8. In mixed fibrotic-vasculopathic pulmonary alteration the FVC(%)/DL_{CO}(%) ratio ranges between 1.4 and 1.8.

Treatment of PAH associated with CTDs (4, 19) follows the general algorithm proposed for PAH (Figure 72.1).

Immunosuppressive therapy might be effective in a minority of patients, mainly in those suffering from conditions other than SSc. The combination of ciclofosfamide and prednisone as been effective in improving pulmonary haemodynamics and exercise tolerance in patients with functional class I/II (20).

Acknowledgements. This work has been supported by a research fellowship grant from the Spanish Society of Respiratory Medicine (SEPAR) to I. Blanco and a research grant from the Fondo de Investigación Sanitaria (IP05/0244).

References

1. Simonneau G, Galie N, Rubin LJ, et al. Clinical classification of pulmonary hypertension. *J Am Coll Cardiol* 2004; 43: 5S–12S.

2. Humbert M, Morrell NW, Archer SL, et al. Cellular and molecular pathobiology of pulmonary arterial hypertension. *J Am Coll Cardiol* 2004; 43: 13S–24S.

3. Humbert M, Sitbon O, Chaouat A, et al. Pulmonary arterial hypertension in France: Results from a national registry. *Am J Respir Crit Care Med* 2006; 173: 1023–30.

4. Galie N, Torbicki A, Barst R, et al. Guidelines on diagnosis and treatment of pulmonary arterial hypertension. The Task Force on Diagnosis and Treatment of Pulmonary Arterial Hypertension of the European Society of Cardiology. *Eur Heart J* 2004; 25: 2243–78.

5. Morales-Blanhir J, Santos S, de JL, et al. Clinical value of vasodilator test with inhaled nitric oxide for predicting long-term response to oral vasodilators in pulmonary hypertension. *Respir Med* 2004; 98:225–34.

6. Rich S, Kaufmann E, Levy PS. The effect of high doses of calcium-channel blockers on survival in primary pulmonary hypertension. *N Engl J Med* 1992; 327: 76–81.

7. Sitbon O, Humbert M, Jais X, et al. Long-term response to calcium channel blockers in idiopathic pulmonary arterial hypertension. *Circulation* 2005; 111: 3105–11.

8. Barst RJ, Rubin LJ, Long WA, et al. A comparison of continuous intravenous epoprostenol (prostacyclin) with conventional therapy for primary pulmonary hypertension. The Primary Pulmonary Hypertension Study Group. *N Engl J Med* 1996; 334: 296–302.

9. Galie N, Seeger W, Naeije R, Simonneau G, Rubin LJ. Comparative analysis of clinical trials and evidence-based treatment algorithm in pulmonary arterial hypertension. *J Am Coll Cardiol* 2004; 43: 81S–88S.

10. Sitbon O, Humbert M, Nunes H, et al. Long-term intravenous epoprostenol infusion in primary pulmonary hypertension: Prognostic factors and survival. *J Am Coll Cardiol* 2002; 40: 780–8.

11. Olschewski H, Simonneau G, Galie N, et al. Inhaled iloprost for severe pulmonary hypertension. *N Engl J Med* 2002; 347: 322–9.

12. Simonneau G, Barst RJ, Galie N, et al. Continuous subcutaneous infusion of treprostinil, a prostacyclin analogue, in patients with pulmonary arterial hypertension: a double-blind, randomized, placebo-controlled trial. *Am J Respir Crit Care Med* 2002; 165: 800–4.

13. Rubin LJ, Badesch DB, Barst RJ, et al. Bosentan therapy for pulmonary arterial hypertension. *N Engl J Med* 2002; 346: 896–903.

14. Galie N, Ghofrani HA, Torbicki A, et al. Sildenafil citrate therapy for pulmonary arterial hypertension. *N Engl J Med* 2005; 353: 2148–57.

15. Klepetko W, Mayer E, Sandoval J, et al. Interventional and surgical modalities of treatment for pulmonary arterial hypertension. *J Am Coll Cardiol* 2004; 43: 73S–80S.

16. D'Alonzo GE, Barst RJ, Ayres SM, et al. Survival in patients with primary pulmonary hypertension. Results from a national prospective registry. *Ann Intern Med* 1991; 115: 343–9.

17. Coghlan JG, Handler C. Connective tissue associated pulmonary arterial hypertension. *Lupus* 2006; 15: 138–42.

18. Galie N, Manes A, Farahani KV, et al. Pulmonary arterial hypertension associated to connective tissue diseases. *Lupus* 2005; 14: 713–7.

19. Badesch DB, Tapson VF, McGoon MD, et al. Continuous intravenous epoprostenol for pulmonary hypertension due to the scleroderma spectrum of disease. A randomized, controlled trial. *Ann Intern Med* 2000; 132: 425–34.

20. Sanchez O, Sitbon O, Jais X, Simonneau G, Humbert M. Immunosuppressive therapy in connective tissue diseases-associated pulmonary arterial hypertension. *Chest* 2006; 130: 182–9.

Part X
Neurological Autoimmune Diseases

73
Multiple Sclerosis

Ron Milo and Ariel Miller

Abstract   Multiple sclerosis (MS) is a chronic inflammatory disease of the central nervous system (CNS) of immune-mediated pathogenesis. It is characterized pathologically by perivascular infiltrates of mononuclear inflammatory cells, demyelination and axonal loss, with the formation of multiple plaques in the brain and spinal cord, and clinically by a variety of neurological signs and symptoms disseminated in time and space. The clinical course, presentation and the pathology are highly variable among patients, making it a very heterogenous disease. The diagnosis of MS is based on clinical measures, supported by paraclinical evidence [predominantly magnetic resonance imaging (MRI)], together with the exclusion of other similar diseases. The currently used McDonald criteria for the diagnosis of MS incorporate MRI measures into the clinical ones, thus allowing early diagnosis of definite MS, even in patients after the first demyelinating episode or clinically isolated syndrome (CIS). Based on these criteria, current and future effective disease-modifying therapies that may slow down disease activity and reduce future disability can be delivered earlier, aiming at prevention of irreversable neurological damage, while tailored to the individual patient.

Keywords   Demyelination · magnetic resonance imaging · McDonald criteria

Multiple sclerosis (MS) is a chronic inflammatory disease of the central nervous system (CNS) of immune-mediated (probably autoimmune) pathogenesis. It is characterized pathologically by perivascular infiltrates of mononuclear inflammatory cells, demyelination and axonal loss, with the formation of multiple plaques in the brain and spinal cord, and clinically by a variety of neurological signs and symptoms disseminated in time and space.

History

It is Jean Martin Charcot of la Salpétrière hospital in Paris to be credited for the first clear and detailed description of the disease as a separate and defined entity. In a series of original articles published in 1868 on "La sclerose en plaques," and later in his published lectures and clinical presentations (1), he made definite links between the diverse symptomatology of the disease and its pathological changes, recognizing inflammatory cells, loss of myelin, proliferation of glial fibers and nuclei and axonal damage, alongside clinical features, including cognitive decine. His observations led also to the development of the first diagnostic criteria for MS, namely the Charcot triad (nystagmus, ataxia and disarthria). Although not being the first to recognize the disease, Charcot's great contribution was in defining and framing MS in a clear and organized manner, using modern medical approach. In 1884, Pierre Marie, Charcot's greatest pupil and successor as Chair of Neurology at the Salpêtrière hospital, suggested the infectious etiology for MS, which is still considered most likely.

The ability to induce an MS-like autoimmune disease in mammals by immunization with myelin or myelin antigens from the CNS [experimental autoimmune encephalomyelitis (EAE)] (acute disseminated encephalomyelitis, EAE), first described in 1933, the detection of increased proportion of gamma globulins in the cerebrospinal fluid of MS patients using electrophoresis in 1940, and several later large epidemiological and twin studies, led to the hypothesis that MS involves an autoimmune response to a self-antigen in genetically susceptible individuals, induced by a hitherto unknown environmental-infectious agent. The successful introduction of ACTH corticosteroids for the treatment of MS relapses in the 1960s, and the start of long-term treatment with immunosuppressive drugs in the 1970s added support to the theory of the immune-mediated nature of MS.

The application of MRI during the last 25 years dramatically improved our ability to visualize MS lesions in the

From: Y. Shoenfeld et al. (eds.): *Diagnostic Criteria in Autoimmune Diseases*, DOI: 10.1007/978-1-60327-285-8_73,

TABLE 73.1. Heterogeneity of MS pathology (2).

	Pattern I (12%)	Pattern II (53%)	Pattern III (30%)	Pattern IV (4%)
	CTL + macrophage-mediated demyelination	Antibody-mediated demyelination	Distal oligodendrogliopathy and apoptosis	Primary oligodendroglia degeneration
Possible mediators	TNF-α, ROI, proteinases	Anti-MOG; anti-Glc (anti-Glycan); anti-aquaporin; others?	Ischemia/toxic virus-induced	Metaboloc defect

brain and spinal cord, and the continuous introduction of non-conventional MRI techniques may now allow for more accurate measurements of axonal loss, atrophy or the so-called "normal-appearing" brain tissue.

Interferon-β-1b, the first effective preventive treatment for MS, has been introduced in 1993, signaling the way to many current and future promising disease-modifying agents.

Pathological Features

Histologically, the MS plaques, which are scattered in the white matter of the CNS, show perivenular infiltration of mononuclear inflammatory cells (T lymphocytes, monocytes/macrophages, B cells and plasma cells), demyelination, reduced number of oligodendrocytes, transected axons and astrocyte proliferation with resultant gliosis. Four categories of the disease have been recently defined based on the location and extension of plaques, immunopathological mechanisms, complement activation and the patterns of oligodendrocytes' destruction (2) (Table 73.1)

Pathogenesis

MS is believed to be mediated mainly (but not exclusively) by autoreactive Th1 cells recognizing auto-antigen(s) that are activated in the periphery by mechanism(s) yet to be unveiled (options include molecular mimicry with an infectious environmental factor peptide; superantigens; breakdown of immunological tolerance by other mechanisms, etc.). These activated T cells proliferate, express a variety of receptors and adhesion molecules, secrete proinflammatory mediators and metalloproteinases, activate the blood–brain barrier (BBB) and interact with it to enter into the brain, where they undergo reactivation by the local autoantigen(s) presented by MHC class II molecules expressed on activated microglia, astrocytes and macrophages. This initiates a loop of local inflammatory reaction in which cytokines, chemokines and other mediators secreted by the activated cells attract and activate other components of the immune system (macrophages, cytotoxic T cells, B cells, astrocytes and complement) and perpetuate a concerted attack on myelin, axons and glia, mediated by cytotoxic cells and cytokines, phagocytosis, proteases, antimyelin antibodies, complement, glutamate,

NO and other reactive oxygen intermediates. The resultant edema, demyelination, axonal transection, loss of oligodendrocytes and activation of astrocytes contribute to neurological dysfunction, to the formation of the acute plaques followed later by gliotic scars and to loss of brain volume. Other processes such as apoptosis, Th1 to Th2 shift, release of growth factors and cytokines by activated glia, and changes in the cytokine milieu follow, which contribute to downregulation and resolution of the local inflammatory response. This enables the release of conduction block, reorganization of functional pathways at the cellular and the system level, remyelination and some regenerative activity, and signals functional recovery. These restorative mechanisms are only partially and temporarily effective, as accumulation of irreversible axonal loss over time is significant, astrocyte reactivity seals the lesion, and gliosis causes a physical barrier to further remyelination, reducing the capacity to accommodate cumulative deficits, and marking transition to the stage of persistent deficit. Loss of trophic support from glia to axons may contribute to the chronic axonal degeneration and the increased clinical deficit that is characteristic of the progressive phase of the disease (3).

Clinical Manifestations

MS affects mainly young people with onset usually at the age of 20–40 years and is two to three times more common in females. At its onset it can run either a relapsing–remitting (RR-MS, 85%) or primary progressive (PP-MS, 15%) course (Figure 73.1). Symptoms of relapses (attacks) usually develop within hours to days, persist for several days to weeks and then gradually subside. The typical clinical presentation of PP-MS is usually of a slowly progressive myelopathy, seen more in males aged >40 years. Common symptoms at disease onset are summarized in Table 73.2 (4). Over time, more and more RR-MS patients (about 50% after 10 years) convert to the secondary-progressive phase of the disease (SP-MS), where relapses either stop or diminish in number, and disability gradually accumulates even between relapses. A subgroup of patients (5–7%) runs a progressive-relapsing course, which is characterized by a chronic-progressive course from onset, with superimposed relapses (5). The severity of symptoms, relapse rate and progression of disability vary considerably among patients, and some 15–20% of

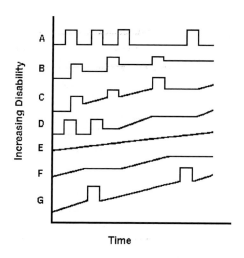

FIGURE 73.1. Main clinical courses seen in multiple sclerosis (MS) patients: relapsing–remitting (A, B), secondary-progressive (C, D), primary-progressive (E, F), progressive-relapsing (G).

TABLE 73.2. Initial symptoms of multiple sclerosis (MS) (4).

	Prevalence (%)
Sensory symptoms	35–40
Weakness in one or more limbs	25–40
Visual loss	17–29
Diplopia	12
Altered balance and gait	18
Vertigo	5
Bladder and bowel symptoms	5

the patients have "benign MS" [determined retrospectively as having no or low level of disability and retaining full function in all systems 15 years after disease onset].

A variety of chronic symptoms may affect MS patients during their chronic ongoing disease, which impact on social, family, occupational and personal life. These include visual disturbances (due to optic neuritis or diplopia), fatigue (in up to 90% of the patients), spasticity and/or ataxia with related gait problems, tremor, paroxysmal symptoms (seizures, tonic spasms, trigeminal neuralgia, paresthesia/dysesthesia), cognitive decline (in 50–75%, mainly in the domains of retrieval memory, attention, concentration, speed of information processing, executive functions and visuo-spatial orientation), depression and other affective disorders, bladder and bowel dysfunction, sexual dysfunction, heat sensitivity, dysphagia, dysarthria, sleep disorders and pain.

Diagnosis/Laboratory Data

There is no single laboratory test diagnostic for MS; however, several tests may support the clinical diagnosis of the disease. Cerebrospinal fluid analysis demonstrates oligoclonal IgG bands, which indicate intrathecal synthesis of immunoglobulins and inflammatory pathology in more than 90% of the patients. Delayed latencies of the visual, somatosensory and auditory evoked potentials on electrophysiological studies of these central sensory pathways, as well as prolonged central motor conduction times, are characteristic of demyelination, and may point to clinically silent lesions. Blood tests are usually used to rule out other diseases that may mimic MS.

Imaging

Magnetic resonance imaging (MRI) is the most sensitive test to detect and demonstrate the MS lesions. It is used to support the diagnosis, estimate lesion load and disease activity, measure brain atrophy and axonal loss, follow disease progression, provide prognosis, serve as a surrogate marker and provide outcome measures in clinical trials. MS lesions are hyperintense on T2-weighted, proton density or FLAIR imaging, and hypointense or isointense on T1-weighted imaging (Figure 73.2). They are typically ovoid in shape, of small size (3–8 mm on average, although giant plaques may occur) and located mainly in the periventricular white matter. They tend to be perpendicular to the ventricles, involve the corpus callosum and U-fibers and may enhance with gadolinium, especially during active inflammation, due to disruption of the BBB (6). Some MRI techniques used in MS, their pathological correlates and applications are summarized in Table 73.3 (6,7).

Diagnostic Criteria

Several sets of criteria have been developed before the MRI era for the clinical diagnosis of MS, based on the principle of objective evidence for CNS white matter lesion dissemination in time and space (Allison & millar, 1954; McAlpine, 1965; Schumacher, 1965; Rose, 1976; McDonald & Halliday, 1979; Poser, 1983). The availability of new treatments for MS which can modify the disease course and slow disease progression, and the recognition that significant damage to the CNS may occur early in the course of the disease, made it necessary to diagnose MS as soon as possible. The recent Mcdonald criteria and their 2005 revision (8) (Table 73.4) allow earlier definite diagnosis of MS, even after the first CIS suggestive of the disease, using MRI criteria to establish a second episode, thus helping earlier decision on therapy. The Barkhof MRI criteria help in confirming appropriate dissemination in space (Table 73.4a), whereas dissenination in time may be determined by another MRI performed at least 30 or 90 days following the first CIS (Table 73.4b), and preferably should be conducted at least 30 days from termination of steroid treatment.

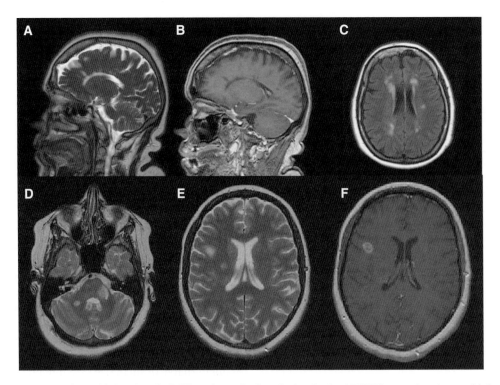

FIGURE 73.2. MRI imaging in multiple sclerosis (MS) patients. Patient 1: A – Sagittal T2W image showing multiple oval high signal (hyperintene) lesions perpendicular to the corpus callosum; B – Sagittal T1W image showing the same lesions as hypointense "black holes"; C – Axial FLAIR image showing multiple periventricular, partially confluent, white matter hyperintense lesions. Patient 2: D, E – Axial T2W showing multiple infratentorial and supratentorial white matter hyperintense lesions of different size; F – Post-gadolinium T1W image showing enhancement of a subcortical lesion seen in E.

When the original McDonald criteria applied at 1 year were compared to the "gold standard" of the previous Poser criteria for the diagnosis of clinically definite MS at 3 years in patients with CIS, high sensitivity (83%),

TABLE 73.3. Magnetic resonance imaging in multiple sclerosis (MS) (7, 8).

Imaging technique	Pathology	Application
T1W (unhenhanced)	Axonal loss; "Black holes"	Correlation with disability
T1W (enhanced)	BBB disruption	Disease activity
T2W	Nonspecific: inflammation, demyelination, edema, gliosis	Burden of disease
FLAIR	Comparable to T2W	Increased resolution
MR Spectroscopy	Axonal loss	Research; biochemical imaging
Magnetization transfer	Demyelinated areas	Research; structural integrity; normal-appearing white matter
Diffusion tensor MRI	Demyelination; axonal loss	Abnormalities in the normal appearing white and gray matters
Functional MRI		Research; cerebral function and reorganization; prognosis

specificity (83%), positive predictive value (75%), negative predictive value (89%) and accuracy (83%) were achieved (6). The recent MRI criteria modifications result in maintaining the high specificity (>90%) of the original McDonald criteria, and achieving higher sensitivity and accuracy (86%) in the definite diagnosis of MS after the first CIS (10). The McDonald criteria identifies earlier and more than three times as many patients with clinially definite MS, compared with the previous Poser criteria. Some limitations of these criteria are the following:

1. Limited access in some parts of the world to advanced technologyies such as MRI; thus, the diagnosis of possible MS should be made, until a second clinical episode.
2. The paraclinical tests incorporated into the criteria should be of high quality and sensitivity and should be used reliably and uniformly in order to achieve the expected high accuracy of the criteria.
3. Criteria may be too stringent for dissemination in space.
4. MS is a highly heterogenous disease, and these criteria that approach the most typical clinical presentation may be less sensitive in atypical cases (pediatric or elderly populations, PP-MS, non-western-european ethnic origin, or atypical clinical presentations).
5. Although MRI is highly sensitive for MS lesions, it is not specific. Similar white matter lesions can be seen in a

TABLE 73.4. The Revised McDonald Diagnostic Criteria for MS (9).

Clinical presentation	Additional data needed for MS diagnosis
≥2 attacks; objective clinical evidence of ≥2 lesions	None
≥2 attacks; objective clinical evidence of 1 lesion	Dissemination in space, demonstrated by: •MRI OR • ≥2 MRI-detected lesions consistent with MS plus positive CSF OR • Await further clinical attack implicating a different site
1 attack; objective clinical evidence of ≥2 lesions	Dissemination in time, demonstrated by: • MRI OR • Second clinical attack
1 attack; objective clinical evidence of 1 lesion (monosymptomatic presentation; clinically isolated syndrome)	Dissemination in space, demonstrated by: •MRI OR • ≥2 MRI-detected lesions consistent with MS plus positive CSF AND Dissemination in time, demonstrated by: • MRI OR • Second clinical attack
Insidious neurologic progression suggestive of MS	• One year of disease progression (retrospectively or prospectively determined) AND • 2 out of 3 of the following: a. Positive brain MRI (9 T2 lesions or ≥ 4 T2 lesions with positive visual evoked potentials; b. Positive spinal cord MRI (≥2 focal T2 lesions); c. Positive CSF

variety of other diseases; many of them share some clinical features with MS. Relying too heavily on MRI may result in overdiagnosis of MS and unnecessary treatments.

TABLE 73.4a. MRI criteria for dissemination in space (9).

Three of the following:
• ≥1 gadolinium-enhancing lesion(s) or 9 T2 hyperintense lesions
• ≥1 infratentorial lesion(s)
• ≥1 juxtacortical lesion(s)
• ≥3 periventricular lesions
(a spinal cord lesion is equivalent to a brain infratentorial lesion; an enhancing spinal cord lesion is equivalent to an enhancing brain lesion, and individual spinal cord lesions can contribute together with individual brain lesions to reach the required number of T2 lesions).

TABLE 73.4b. MRI criteria for dissemination in time (9).

1. Detection of gadolinium enhancement ≥3 months after the onset of the initial clinical event if not at the site of the initial event.
OR
2. Detection of a new T2 lesion if it appears any time compared with a reference scan done at least 30 days after the onset of the initial clinical event.

Overall, these criteria still emphasize the clinical nature of the diagnosis, the need to demonstrate dissemination in time and space, the use of supportive and confirmatory paraclinical examination to speed the process and to help eliminate false-negative and false-positive diagnoses, focus on specificity rather than sensitivity and call for the need to eliminate better explanations for the diagnosis.

Management

The last 15 years have seen major progress in the management of MS. Advances in the understanding of the immunology and pathology of MS resulted in the development of new therapies. Several disease-modifying agents that favorably affect disease activity and progression have been approved for use, and pipelines are loaded with many other promising immunomodulatory agents and other methods, in various stages of clinical evaluation (11,12).

1. For acute relapse, the standard treatment is a short course of high-dose corticosteroids (usualy intravenous methylprednisolone 500–1000 mg/day for 3–5 days, followed, in most cases, by tapering down of oral prednisone for additional 1–2 weeks). Severe attacks of CNS demyelination not adequately responding to corticosteroida may be treated with plasma exchange (13).
2. Prevention of disease activity: Six disease-modifying drugs [three types of interferon-β (Betaferon/Betaseron, Avonex and Rebif), glatiramer acetate (GA, Copaxone, mitoxantrone (Novantrone) and natalizumab (Tysabri)] have been approved so far for the prevention of disease activity in MS, after showing efficacy in reducing relapse rate and severity, slowing down accumulation of disablity and positively affecting MRI markers of disease activity and progression (13, 14) (Table 73.5). The three interferons also delay the development of definite MS after the first CIS (13).
3. Symptomatic treatment in MS is best delivered by a multidisciplinary approach that integrates physiotherapy, social and psychological interventions and medical treatments aimed at each of the individual symptoms (15).

Extensive basic and clinical research throughout the world continues to explore new therapies for MS. Strategies

TABLE 73.5. Approved disease-modifying drugs fo MS (13, 14).

Medication	Trade name	Dose, route of administration	Indications
Interferon β-1b	Betaferon/ Betaseron	SC 250 µg every other day	RR-MS SP-MS
Interferon β-1a	Avonex	IM 30 µg × 1/w	RR-MS
Interferon β-1a	Rebif	SC 22/44 µg × 3/w	RR-MS
Glatiramer acetate	Copaxone	SC 20 mg/day	RR-MS
Mitoxantrone	Novantrone	IV 12 mg/m^2 every 3 months (max. 140 mg/m^2)	Aggressive relapsing MS
Natalizumab	Tysabri	IV 300 mg every 4 weeks	RR-MS

include antigen-specific therapy, therapies that target specific regulatory molecules of the immune system, trapping lymphocytes in the lymph nodes, using other immunomodulatory, immunosuppressive and neuroprotective agents, transplantation of pluripotential stem cell and more (11,12). Current and probably next generation of MS drugs seem to be only partially and not equally effective for different patients. Two strategies may approach these limitations: combination therapies (16) and pharmacogenetics, which studies genetic variations between individuals that may account for differential responsiveness to given therapies (17, 18). This may shift the focus from treating the disease to treating the patient (*Personalized Medicine*), where treatment is tailored to the individual patient, combining immunomudulatory, neuroprotective and repair-promoting strategies, individually selected according to the patient's genetic makeup, disease subtype and activity.

References

1. Charcot JM. Histologie de la sclerose en plaques. *Gaz Hop, Paris*, 1868; 41: 554–5, 557–8, 566.
2. Lucchinetti C, Bruck W, Parisi J, et al. Heterogeneity of multiple sclerosis lesions: Implications for the pathogenesis of demyelination. *Ann Neurol* 2000; 47: 707–17.
3. Compston A, Coles A. Multiple sclerosis. *Lancet* 2002; 359: 1221–31.
4. Matthews B. Symptoms and signs of multiple sclerosis. In: Compston A (ed.), *McAlpine's Multiple Sclerosis*. Churchill Livingstone, London; 1998.
5. Lublin FD, Reingold SC. Defining the clinical course of multiple sclerosis: Results of an international survey. National Multiple Sclerosis Society (USA) Advisory Committee on Clinical Trials of New Agents in Multiple Sclerosis. *Neurology* 1996; 46(4): 907–11.
6. Bakshi R, Hutton GJ, Miller JR, Radue EW. The use of magnetic resonance imaging in the diagnosis and long-term management of multiple sclerosis. *Neurology* 2004; 63: S3–11.
7. Filippi M, Bakshi R, Rovaris M, Comi G. MRI and Multiple Sclerosis: What happened in the last 10 years? *J Neuroimaging* 2007; 17: S1–2.
8. Polman CH, Reingold SC, Edan C, et al. Diagnostic criteria for multiple sclerosis: 2005 revisions to the "McDonald criteria." *Ann Neurol* 2005; 56: 840–6.
9. Dalton CM, Brex PA, Miszkiel KA, Hickman SJ, MacManus DG, Plant GT, Thompson AJ et al. Application of the new McDonald criteria to patients with clinically isolated syndromes suggestive of multiple sclerosis. *Ann Neurol* 2002; 52: 47–53.
10. Swanton JK, Fernando K, Dalton CM, Miszkiel KA, Thompson AJ, Plant GT, Miller DH. Modification of MRI criteria for multiple sclerosis in patients with clinically isolated syndromes. *J Neurol Neurosurg Psychiatr* 2006; 77: 830–3.
11. Fontoura P, Steinman L, Miller A. Emerging therapeutic targets in multiple sclerosis. *Curr Opin Neurol* 2006; 19: 260–6.
12. Blevins G, Martin R. Future immunotherapies in multiple sclerosis. *Semin Neurol* 2003; 23: 147–58.
13. Kieseier BC, Hartung HP, Current disease-modifying therapies in multiple sclerosis. *Semin Neurol* 2003; 23: 133–46.
14. Polman CH, O'Connor PW, Havrdova E, et al. A randomized, placebo-controlled trial of natalizumab for relapsing multiple sclerosis. *N Engl J Med* 2006; 354: 899–910.
15. Kesselring J, Beer S. Symptomatic therapy and neurorehabilitation in multiple sclerosis. *Lancet Neurol* 2005; 4: 643–52.
16. Costello F, Stuve O, Weber MS, Zamvil SS, Frohman E. Combination therapies for multiple sclerosis: Scientific rationale, clinical trials, and clinical practice. *Curr Opin Neurol* 2007 June; 20(3): 281–5.
17. Kirstein-Grossman I, Beckmann JS, Lancet D, Miller A. Pharmacogenetic development of personalized medicine: Multiple sclerosis treatment as a model. *Drugs News Perspectives* 2002; 15: 558–67.
18. Grossman I, Avidan N, Singer C, Goldstaub D, Hayardeny L, Eyal E, Ben-Asher E, et al. Pharmacogenetics of Glatiramer Acetate therapy for Multiple Sclerosis reveals drug-response markers. *Pharmacogenet Genomics* 2007; 17: 657–66.

74
Myasthenia Gravis

Alexander Gorshtein and Yair Levy

Abstract   Myasthenia gravis (MG) is a chronic autoimmune disease of neuromuscular junction characterized by painless weakness of skeletal muscles, which appears or becomes more pronounced upon physical exertion. MG is a highly heterogeneous disease which may be difficult to suspect and diagnose. Currently there are no diagnostic criteria for MG. In this article we review the epidemiology, the pathogenesis, the clinical characteristics, the diagnostic tests available for the diagnosis of the disease, and propose diagnostic criteria for the disease, based on the clinical assessment and auxiliary serologic, pharmacologic and electrodiagnostic tests.

Keywords   Myasthenia gravis · autoantibodies to acetylcholine receptor · diagnostic criteria · autoantibodies to muscle-specific kinase · clinical manifestations · epidemiology

Myasthenia gravis (MG) is a chronic autoimmune disease affecting neuromuscular transmission. MG is characterized by painless muscular weakness, which develops or becomes more pronounced upon physical exertion.

History

In 1672, Willis reported the first case of the disease in the medical literature. In 1879, Erb recognized the disease as a separate entity, when he had reported three cases of "a new probably bulbar symptom complex." Jolly described the fading response of muscle contractions to prolonged electrical stimulation, and named the disease "myasthenia gravis pseudoparalytica" in 1895. In 1934, Walker had shown that injection of physostigmine leads to increase of strength in a patient with MG. In 1960 Simpson had postulated the autoimmune nature of MG (1). In 1970s, the pathogenicity of acetylcholine antibodies was demonstrated by passive transfer experiments, and plasma exchange and immunosuppressive therapies were introduced.

Epidemiology

The annual incidence of MG had increased during the last decades from 0.25 to 0.5 per 100,000 to 1–2 per 100,000 in the general population (2). This change is primarily related to the increase in the incidence of MG in male and female patients older than 65 years. The incidence of the disease peaks in the third decade in female patients, whereas there is a bimodal distribution of MG in males, with peaks in third and sixth decades (3). The reported prevalence of the disease ranges from 20 to 40 people per 100,000 (2). MG occurs in 40% of patients in whom thymoma is diagnosed.

The onset of MG associated with thymoma peaks in fourth and fifth decades (4). There is female predominance among thymoma patients with MG. Similarly to some other autoimmune diseases, MG with autoantibodies to AChR is strongly correlated to HLA antigens B8 and DR3 (5).

Pathogenesis

MG is the best understood autoimmune neurologic disease. Activated $CD4^+$ T-helper cells drive the autoimmune response in MG (6). The disease is primarily mediated by autoantibodies against AChR. The impairment in neuro-muscular transmission and muscular weakness inflicted by these autoantibodies is explained by several mechanisms, which include functional blockade of AChR, increased degradation of AChR, and the complement-mediated destruction of the postsynaptic folds (6). Passive transfer of purified antibodies against AChR to laboratory animals induces experimental MG. Similarly, passive vertical

From: Y. Shoenfeld et al. (eds.): *Diagnostic Criteria in Autoimmune Diseases*, DOI: 10.1007/978-1-60327-285-8_74,

transfer of the autoantibodies to neonate leads to the expression of the disease. Elimination of the autoantibodies by plasma exchange ameliorates the manifestations of MG. Hereby MG fulfils the Koch postulates for the autoantibody-mediated autoimmune disease. The thymus is thought to be involved in the pathogenesis of MG, because it is pathologically abnormal in the majority of MG patients (7).

Clinical Manifestations

MG characteristically presents as painless weakness of skeletal muscles, which appears or becomes more pronounced upon physical exertion, and improves with rest. Sensorium, tendon reflexes, and cerebellar functions are not affected by the disease. Symptoms at the presentation of the disease are listed in Table 74.1(8). Ptosis and diplopia appear early in the course of the disease in the majority of patients. Facial and bulbar muscle involvement manifests by difficulty in speech and facial expressions, chewing, and dysphagia. Limb weakness is usually proximal, although small hand muscles can be involved. Life-threatening weakness of respiratory muscles is termed myasthenic crisis. It usually occurs in the first years of the disease and is frequently provoked by an intercurrent infection. The clinical severity of MG is usually graded by a modification of a scale developed by Osserman (Table 74.2)(9, 10). The clinical course of MG is quite variable: in some patients, the weakness remains confined to a single group of muscles for many years (usually extraocular and eyelid muscles), whereas in about 85% it eventually progresses to a generalized weakness. Fluctuations in the severity of MG may occur during the first years after the onset of the disease.

Pathological Features

Thymus is histopathologically abnormal in 80–90% of patients with MG (7). The usual finding in about two-thirds of patients, more so in younger ones, is thymic hyperplasia, characterized by lymphoid follicles with active germinal centers. Thymomas are diagnosed in 10–15% of patients.

TABLE 74.1. Presenting symptoms at the onset of MG.

	Prevalence
Ocular only	40%
Ocular and bulbar	11%
Ocular and generalized	17%
Bulbar only	17%
Total bulbar	43%
Extremities	17%
Generalized	14%
Respiratory dysfunction	0.7%

TABLE 74.2. Modification of Osserman's clinical classification of MG.

I: Ocular signs and symptoms only
II: Generalized myasthenia:
  IIa: Mild disease
  IIb: Moderate disease
III: Severe generalized disease
IV: Myasthenic crisis

Electron microscopy of neuromuscular junctions from patients with MG demonstrates significantly diminished number of AChR, simplification of postsynaptic folds, and deposits of IgG and complement (11).

Serological Features

Autoantibodies against acetylcholine receptor (AChR) can be detected in up to 90% of patients with generalized MG, and in about 50% of patients with ocular disease (12). The presence of these antibodies is not correlated to the severity of disease. MG, in which autoantibodies against AChR are undetectable, is termed seronegative disease. Autoantibodies to muscle-specific kinase (MuSK) are specific for seronegative MG (13, 14, 15). The prevalence of these antibodies in seronegative MG is highly variable in different geographic regions; it ranges from 4% in Chinese patients to 22% in Netherland patients and up to 40–70% in North American and other European cohorts of patients (13, 14, 15). These antibodies are usually detected in young female patients with predominantly facial and bulbar involvement, and their presence is correlated to the severity of disease (14, 15). Another group of antibodies detected in MG are striational antibodies, which target sarcomeric proteins of striated muscle – titin, ryanodine receptor, myosin, actin, and other proteins (16). The association of these antibodies with thymoma was discovered in 1960 (17). Striational antibodies can be detected in about 80% of MG patients with thymoma. Testing these antibodies has similar test accuracy in predicting thymomas as computed tomography scan (16). Striational antibodies are more prevalent in older patients and in MG patients with more severe disease (16). These features make these antibodies important prognostic markers in MG patients. The pathogenic role of striational antibodies in MG has not been proven.

Diagnostic Criteria

Currently, there are no diagnostic criteria for MG. MG is a highly heterogenous disease, sometimes termed a great imitator of neurology because of a puzzling fluctuating weakness. The differential diagnosis of MG includes drug-induced myasthenia, Lambert–Eaton myasthenic syndrome, botulism, intracranial mass lesions, progressive external ophthalmoplegia, and other disorders (12). Intracranial and orbital lesions should be excluded by appropriate imaging. The association of MG with autoimmune diseases of the thyroid gland may pose an additional diagnostic challenge, particularly in cases of thyroid ophthalmopathy. Table 74.3 presents advantages and disadvantages of the tests currently used for the diagnosis of MG, their sensitivity and specificity in the diagnosis of the disease, and the clinical correlations of autoantibodies detected in MG patients (12, 13, 14, 15, 16). No test is accurate enough to be solely relied on for the diagnosis of MG. Edrophonium (Tensilon) test is especially useful for ocular MG, but it is not specific for MG, and the drug may cause cholinergic side effects. Electrodiagnostic tests (repetitive nerve stimulation and single fiber electromyography) are sensitive, but non-specific, and they are operator dependent. The sensitivity of serologic tests is low in patients with ocular myasthenia. The finding of a mass in the anterior mediastinum suggestive of thymoma may support the diagnosis of MG. Table 74.4 presents our proposed diagnostic criteria for MG in patients older than 2 years. Clinical weakness and the response to an anticholinergic drug should be measured by an objective instrument, such as quantitative MG score for disease severity, implemented for the group of muscles tested (10). Because autoantibodies to MuSK are specific for seronegative MG, they should be tested only in patients negative for autoantibodies to AChR. Striational antibodies were not included because of their low sensitivity and specificity for the

TABLE 74.3. Diagnostic tests in MG.

Test	Advantages for serologic tests – disease correlations	Disadvantages	Sensitivity	Specificity
Edrophonium (Tensilon)	Immediate results, valuable for oMG	CI: acute glaucoma, known sensitivity to medication, and mechanic urinary and intestinal obstruction. Cholinergic side effects	85% in oMG	Duration of action is short for evaluation of several groups of muscles (neostigmine may be preferred)
			60% in gMG	False positive results in ALS, intracranial tumors, supranuclear palsy
Autoantibodies to AChR	No correlation with disease activity	Insensitive for oMG	40–60% in oMG	Specific for MG
			80–90% in gMG	Negative result does not exclude MG.
Autoantibodies to MuSK	Marked female predominance, young onset, predominantly bulbar weakness, wasting of bulbar muscles Correlate with disease activity	Large geographic variability in the prevalence	4–70% of patients with seronegative MG	Highly specific for seronegative MG
Striational antibodies	More prevalent in older patients, correlate with disease severity, associate with thymoma.	Pathogenic role has not been proven	10–30% in gMG	Non-specific for MG
			60–85% in MG with thymoma	Valuable for prediction of thymoma and as prognostic determinants
Repetitive nerve stimulation	May be combined with edrophonium test	Unpleasant to patients	50–60% in oMG	Not specific- reduction in CMAP may occur in motor neuron, neuromuscular junction, and muscle diseases
		Operator dependent	70–80% in gMG, up to 90% in proximal muscle testing	
Single fiber electromyography	Highly sensitive	Time consuming	90–99% for oMG and gMG	Not specific – abnormal jitter may occur in motor neuron, neuromuscular junction, and muscle diseases
		Dependent on patient cooperation and operator skill		

ALS: amyotrophic lateral sclerosis; CI: contraindications; CMAP: compound muscle action potential; LEMS: Lambert–Eatom myasthenic syndrome; gMG: generalized MG; oMG: ocular MG.

TABLE 74.4. Proposed diagnostic criteria for myasthenia gravis (MG). Definite diagnosis of MG requires a positive clinical criterion and a serologic criterion, or a clinical criterion and both pharmacologic and electrophysiologic criteria. Probable MG is diagnosed when a positive clinical criterion and either pharmacologic or electrophysiologic criteria are fulfilled. See text for clarifications.

1. Clinical criterion – fluctuating muscular weakness and fatiguability without impairment in sensorium, reflexes, and cerebellar functions
2. Pharmacologic criterion – improvement in muscular weakness upon administration of an anticholinergic medication
3. Serologic criterion – presence of autoantibodies to AChR or MuSK
4. Electrophysiologic criterion – evidence of a defect in neuromuscular transmission (a decrement of >10% in the amplitude of the compound muscle action potential on repetitive nerve stimulation and/or an increase in jitter on single fiber studies)

diagnosis of MG. A positive clinical criterion and a serologic criterion, or a clinical criterion and both pharmacologic and electrophysiologic criteria provide the definite diagnosis of MG, whereas probable MG is diagnosed when a positive clinical criterion and either pharmacologic or electrophysiologic criteria are fulfilled. It should be stressed that these diagnostic criteria reflect our personal opinion and that they should be further refined and tested before their implementation in the diagnosis of MG.

Therapy

The therapies currently used for the treatment of MG can be divided into several groups, which include modulators of neuromuscular transmission, immunosuppressive, and immunomodulatory therapies. Anticholinesterase drugs ameliorate myasthenic weakness by temporary improvement of neuromuscular transmission in most patients with MG, but they rarely lead to the complete resolution of symptoms (12). Overdosage of these drugs may cause increasing weakness and muscarinic side effects. Immunosuppressive drugs used in MG include corticosteroids, azathioprine, mycophenolate mofetil, cyclophosphamide, cyclosporine, and tacrolimus. Rituximab – a monoclonal antibody to B-lymphocyte surface antigen CD20 – has been effective in several cases of refractory MuSK-positive MG. Thymectomy is a frequently implemented immunomodulatory treatment for the patients younger than 60 years (12), and even for older patients, but its benefit in non-thymomatous MG has not been established in prospective studies (18). In patients with non-thymomatous MG, thymectomy can only be considered an option to increase the probability of remission or improvement (18). A Cochrane review had evaluated the role of

intravenous immunoglobulin (IVIG) in the treatment of MG (19). The authors have not found enough data to recommend IVIG for the treatment of chronic MG. However, a more recent study had proven the effectiveness of IVIG in patients with worsening weakness because of MG (20). In severe exacerbations of MG, no difference was found between IVIG and plasma exchange, but an easier way of employment and a better safety profile make IVIG a preferred treatment for this indication. Some corticosteroid-dependent MG patients may benefit from etanercept – a soluble recombinant dimeric fusion protein based on TNF-alpha receptor, which binds to TNF-alpha and blocks its biologic activity.

References

1. Simpson JA. Myasthenia gravis, a new hypothesis. *Scot Med J* 1960; 5: 419.
2. Flachenecker P. Epidemiology of neuroimmunological diseases. *J Neurol* 2006; 253(Suppl. 5): V/2–V/8.
3. Mantegazza R, Baggi F, Antozzi C, et al. Myasthenia Gravis (MG): Epidemiological data and prognostic factors. *Ann N Y Acad Sci* 2003; 998: 413–23.
4. Potagas C, Dellatolas S, Tavernarakis A, et al. Myasthenia gravis: Changes observed in a 30-years retrospective clinical study of a hospital-based population. *J Neurol* 2004; 251: 116–7.
5. Matej H, Noakowska B, Kalamarz M, et al. HLA antigens and susceptibility to myasthenia gravis. *Arch Immunol Ther Exp (Warsz)* 1987; 35: 795–801.
6. Conti-Fine BM, Milani M, Kaminski HJ. Myasthenia gravis: past, present, and future. *J Clin Invest* 2006; 116: 2843–54.
7. Hohlfeld R, Wekerle H. The thymus in myasthenia gravis. *Neurol Clin* 1994; 12: 331–42.
8. Oosterhuis HJGH. Myasthenia gravis. A survey. *Clin Neurol Neurosurg* 1981; 83: 105–35.
9. Osserman KE. *Myasthenia Gravis*. New York: Grune and Stratton; 1958: 79–86.
10. Jaretzki A III, Barohn RJ, Ernstoff RM, et al. Myasthenia gravis: Recommendations for clinical research standards. Task Force of the Medical Scientific Advisory Board of the Myasthenia Gravis Foundation of America. *Ann Thorac Surg* 2000; 70: 327–34.
11. Engel AG, Tsujihata M, Lindstrom JM, Lennon VA. The motor end plate in myasthenia gravis and in experimental autoimmune myasthenia gravis. A quantitative ultrastructural study. *Ann N Y Acad Sci* 1976; 274: 60–79.
12. Drachman DB. Myasthenia gravis. *N Eng J Med* 1994; 330: 1797–810.
13. Hoch W, McConville J, Helms S, Newsom-Davis J, Melms A, Vincent A. Auto-antibodies to the receptor tyrosine kinase MuSK in patients with myasthenia gravis without acetylcholine receptor antibodies. *Nat Med* 2001 March; 7(3): 365–8.

14. Evoli A, Tonali PA, Padua L, et al. Clinical correlates with anti-MuSK antibodies in generalized seronegative myasthenia gravis. *Brain* 2003; 126: 2304–11.

15. Lavrnic D, Losen M, Vujic A, et al. The features of myasthenia gravis with autoantibodies to MuSK. *J Neurol Neurosurg Psychiatr* 2005; 76: 1099–102.

16. Romi F, Skeie GO, Gilhus NE, Aarli JA. Striational antibodies in myasthenia gravis: Reactivity and possible clinical significance. *Arch Neurol* 2005; 62: 442–6.

17. Strauss AJL, Seegal BC, Hsu KC, Burkholder PM, Nastuk WL, Osserman KE. Immunofluorescence demonstration of a muscle binding, complement-fixing serum globulin fraction in myasthenia gravis. *Proc Soc Exp Biol Med* 1960; 105: 184–91.

18. Skeie GO, Apostolski S, Evoli A, et al. Guidelines for the treatment of autoimmune neuromuscular transmission disorders. *Eur J Neurol* 2006; 13: 691–9.

19. Gajdos P, Chevret S, Toyka K. Intravenous immunoglobulin for myasthenia gravis. *Cochrane Database Syst Rev* 2006; 2: CD002277.

20. Zinman L, Ng E, Bril V. IV immunoglobulin in patients with myasthenia gravis: a randomized controlled trial. *Neurology* 2007; 68: 837–41.

75
Lambert-Eaton Myasthenic Syndrome

Bethan Lang

Abstract   The Lambert-Eaton myasthenic syndrome (LEMS) is an autoimmune disorder affecting the peripheral nervous system, characterised by proximal muscle weakness and autonomic dysfunction. Approximately 60% of patients have an associated small cell lung carcinoma (SCLC). LEMS is the most studied of the paraneoplastic neurological syndromes. Approximately 90% of patients have autoantibodies to voltage-gated calcium channels (VGCCs), transmembrane proteins found on the presynaptic nerve terminal, in the cerebellum and on the surface of the SCLC. It has been postulated that antibodies raised against determinants on the tumour may cross-react with the VGCC at the nerve terminal resulting in the neurological dysfunction.

Keywords   Lambert-Eaton myasthenic syndrome · voltage-gated calcium channel · VGCC · small cell carcinoma of the lung · SCLC · paraneoplastic disorder

The Lambert-Eaton Myasthenic Syndrome (LEMS)

The disorder was first characterised by Lambert and colleagues who described a patient who presented with a myasthenic-like illness and an associated bronchial carcinoma. Subsequent studies demonstrated electrophysiologically that the transmission defect was quite different to that of myasthenia gravis (1).

Lambert-Eaton myasthenic syndrome (LEMS) is an antibody-mediated disorder of the peripheral nervous system, characterised by proximal muscle weakness and autonomic dysfunction. In contrast to myasthenia gravis, there is little respiratory involvement and there is little ocular and bulbar muscle involvement. Approximately 60% of LEMS patients present with a SCLC, an aggressive lung carcinoma that almost invariably associates with smoking (2). SCLC represents 20–25% of all diagnosed cases of lung cancer and is a tumour of neuroendocrine origin that expresses functionally active voltage-gated calcium channels (VGCCs) on their surface (3). It has been hypothesised that autoantibodies raised initially against VGCCs expressed on the surface of the cancer cells may cross-react with VGCCs located on the presynaptic peripheral nerve terminal and thereby induce the neurological symptoms.

Epidemiology

The incidence of LEMS in the general population is around 1:100,000. However, the overall prevalence of LEMS in all SCLC patients is closer to 3% (4). The age of onset of LEMS can range between 17 and 79 years. A younger onset is found in patients without an associated neoplasm (2).

LEMS with Cancer Detected (CD-LEMS)

Fifty to sixty per cent of LEMS patients have an associated malignancy, most commonly SCLC, usually evident within 2 years of onset. Nearly 100% of these patients will have had a significant smoking history. Within this subgroup, males out number females 2:1 but this may simply reflect smoking habits in the population. Most CD-LEMS patients present with neurological problems months to years before the detection of the tumour and interestingly the survival time of these tumour-associated LEMS patients is significantly longer than patients with SCLC alone (5, 6).

From: Y. Shoenfeld et al. (eds.): *Diagnostic Criteria in Autoimmune Diseases*, DOI: 10.1007/978-1-60327-285-8_75,

413

LEMS with no Carcinoma Detected, Idiopathic LEMS, (NCD-LEMS)

The remaining 40% of patients never develop a tumour, even after prolonged follow-up. Epidemiologically, the onset of the disorder is earlier and the male to female distribution is more equal in this group than in those with CD-LEMS. There is also a higher incidence (30–40%) of other autoimmune diseases; many patients have a past or current history of other organ-specific auto-immune diseases such as thyroiditis, coeliac disease, myasthenia or vitiligo. HLA studies have shown an over-representation of HLA DR3-B8-A1, a haplotype known to associate with other autoimmune diseases including myasthenia gravis (7).

Pathogenicity

LEMS is an autoimmune disorder of the peripheral ner-vous system in which autoantibodies to specific subtypes of VGCCs have been described. The autoimmune aetiol-ogy has been established by a series of passive-transfer experiments in which the clinical and electrophysiologi-cal features have been transferred to mice by injection of serum or IgG derived from patients with LEMS (8). Additionally, freeze-fracture electron microscopy of the presynaptic nerve terminal, in both patients and in the passive-transfer mouse model, has shown a marked reduction in the number and paucity of the active zone particles, thought to be the morphological representa-tions of the VGCCs (9). It has been postulated, at least in the case of CD-LEMS, that antibodies raised against functionally active VGCCs on the SCLC surface can cross-react with VGCCs in the nervous system. The underlying aetiology in the NCD-LEMS cases is unknown yet.

Clinical Features

LEMS is a disorder of proximal muscle weakness and autonomic dysfunction, for example abnormal sweating, dry mouth, postural hypotension and impotence in males (2, 10) (see Table 75.1). Deep tendon reflexes are reduced or absent. Many patients find that the strength improves initially on exercise but the improvement will lessen as exercise is sustained.

Diagnostic Features

Diagnosis is usually through electrophysiological methods and serological investigation. As the disorder is strongly associated with an underlying tumour and since the

TABLE 75.1. Clinical features of LEMS.

	%
Weakness	
Proximal weakness is usual greater than distal. Patients are often aware of a fatiguable element to their weakness. Patients mostly improve with brief sustained exercise	100
Autonomic dysfunction	80
Dry mouth	
Male impotence	
Constipation	
Impaired sweating	
Cranial nerve involvement (often mild/transient)	25–50
Diplopia	
Ptosis	
Cerebellar features (predominantly in the CD-LEMS group)	9

For a full review, see O'Neill et al., 1988 (2).

neurological signs usually predate the detection of the tumour, CT and MRI of the thorax are recommended at diagnosis and that paraneoplastic aetiology is considered up to 5 years after, especially in patients with a smoking history.

Electrophysiological Studies

Clinical electrophysiological examination of patients usually shows low amplitude of compound muscle action potentials (CMAPs). A decline in CMAPs occurs during repetitive nerve stimulation at low frequency but marked facilitation occurs at higher rates (greater than 10 Hz) and after volun-tary contraction (1). In single fibre EMG, abnormal jitter and/or blocking is usually seen. The underlying defect is a reduction in the amount of the neurotransmitter acetylcho-line released per nerve impulse, which results in the failure to generate action potentials. However, during repetitive nerve stimulation the release of acetylcholine initially increases, and transmission improves.

A recent study has shown that there is no obvious dif-ference in the clinical or electrophysiological features between seropositive or seronegative cases of LEMS (11).

Laboratory Studies

VGCC is a multimeric family of proteins, which can be divided into a number of functionally distinct subtypes according to their electrophysiological, pharmacological, and biochemical properties. Neurotransmitter release at the peripheral neuromuscular junction is primarily con-trolled by P-/Q-type VGCC, a channel that is also found in high density in the cerebellum and on the surface of SCLC.

Methods of Detection

Neurotoxins derived from the venom of the fish-eating cone snails bind with high affinity and specificity to the

P-/Q-type (ω-conotoxin MVIIC, ωCmTx) and the N-type (ω-conotoxin GVIA, ωCgTx) VGCCs. VGCCs solubilised from human neuroblastomas and SCLC cell lines have been used as a source of antigen; however, mammalian cerebellum has proved a much richer source of P-/Q-type VGCCs and low concentrations of ^{125}I-ωCmTx radiolabel this subtype only, avoiding any necessity for further purification. Similarly, ^{125}I-ωCgTx has been used to label N-type VGCCs found in high concentration in the cerebral cortex and both can be used in standard radioimmunoassay procedures (12, 13). Recently, a novel radioimmunoassay based on the binding of a spider venom peptide ^{125}I-ωPtxIIA to P-/Q- and N-type VGCCs has been described; however, this assay does not appear to offer any advantage over existing assays (14). Currently, there are no reliable ELISA-based assay systems for the detection of VGCC antibodies.

Serological Features

Antibodies to P-/Q-type VGCCs are found in 85–90% of patients; however, antibodies to N-type VGCCs are found in 40% of patients and about 25% of patients have antibodies to dihydropyridine-sensitive L-type VGCCs. Generally, N-type and L-type VGCC antibodies are only found in conjunction with P-/Q-type VGCCs and not in isolation, which means that 10–15% of patients are "seronegative" for any of the VGCC antibodies (Table 75.2). The P-/Q-type VGCC antibody titre does not appear to correlate with disease severity across a population, but within individual patients a good correlation is often observed. There do not appear any clinical differences between the seropositive and negative patients (10, 11). A few LEMS patients have been reported to have antibodies to the synaptic vesicle protein synaptotagmin, including some VGCC antibody-negative patients; however, the pathogenicity of these antibodies has not yet been established (15, 16).

In a number of large-scale studies of patients who presented initially to oncology clinics, 5–7% of patients with SCLC have been shown to have anti-VGCC antibodies, with only half having clinical features of LEMS.

TABLE 75.2. Autoantibodies detected in LEMS patients.

Antibodies detected	All LEMS (%)	CD-LEMS (%)	NCD-LEMS (%)	REF
All VGCC	85–90	90–100	76–91	12, 13
P-/Q-type VGCC	85–90	90–100	76–91	12, 13
N-type VGCC	40–50	40	22	12, 13
L-type VGCC	25	0	25	15
	All LEMS	VGCC Ab positive	VGCC Ab negative	
Synaptotagmin	25	17	8.5[a]	15, 16

[a] All patients were SCLC negative.

Antibodies to VGCCs have also been detected in the serum and CSF of a number of patients with paraneoplastic cerebellar degeneration; again only half of these patients demonstrated electrophysiological features of LEMS (17). Additionally, there are sporadic reports of patients with anti-VGCC antibody positive cerebellar ataxia in whom no tumour has been detected. Analysis of VGCC antibody titres in patients with other autoimmune or neurological disorders and healthy individuals has shown that false positives are extremely rare (12, 13).

Therapy

In LEMS, small randomised controlled trials have demonstrated that 3,4-diaminopyridine (3,4-DAP), which specifically blocks potassium channels at the nerve terminal and increases the duration of the nerve action potential, is effective. As with other autoimmune disorders of the peripheral nervous system, immunosuppressive therapies are used as adjuncts. A combination of prednisolone and azathioprine is often effective, with plasmapheresesis or intravenous immunoglobulins for severe disease, exacerbations or those intolerant of steroids (18).

In CD-LEMS, the treatment of the tumour, whether by chemotherapy or radiotherapy, is paramount. Chemotherapy is often the first choice, as it will have an additional immunosuppressive effect. Effective treatment of the tumour will frequently produce a marked improvement in strength.

Prognosis

The prognosis of patients with SCLC alone is particularly poor, with only 5–10% of patients surviving up to 5 years. There is now clear evidence that SCLC patients with VGCC antibodies and the clinical signs of LEMS have an increase in their median survival compared with antibody-negative patients (5, 6). It is not entirely clear whether this is due to the early detection of an underlying tumour or to a vigorous autoimmune attack on the tumour itself. In most patients with CD-LEMS, the tumour will be detectable within 2 years of diagnosis and LEMS patients who have shown neurological signs for longer than 5 years are at very low risk of developing a tumour. In non-CD-LEMS, adequate immunosuppressive therapy is usually effective and the patients can expect a normal life expectancy.

References

1. Elmqvist D, Lambert EH. (1968) Detailed analysis of neuromuscular transmission in a patient with the myasthenic syndrome sometimes associated with bronchogenic carcinoma. Mayo Clin Proc 43, 689–713.

2. O'Neill JH, Murray NM, Newsom-Davis J. (1988) The Lambert-Eaton myasthenic syndrome. A review of 50 cases. Brain 111, 577–596.

3. Oguro-Okano M, Griesmann G, Wieben E, et al. (1992) Molecular diversity of neuronal-type calcium channels identified in small cell lung carcinoma. Mayo Clin Proc 67, 1150–1159.

4. Elrington G, Murray NM, Spiro SG, Newsom-Davis J. (1991) Neurological paraneoplastic syndromes in patients with small cell lung cancer. A prospective survey of 150 patients. J Neurol Neurosurg Psychiatr 54, 764–767.

5. Maddison P, Newsom-Davis J, Mills KR, Souhamis RL. (1999) Favourable prognosis in Lambert-Eaton myasthenic syndrome and small cell lung carcinoma. Lancet 353, 117–118.

6. Wirtz P, Lang B, Graus F, et al. (2005) P/Q-type calcium channel antibodies, Lambert-Eaton myasthenic syndrome and survival in small cell lung carcinoma. J Neuroimmunol 164, 161–165.

7. Wirtz PW, Willcox N, van der Slik AR, Lang B, Maddison P, Koeleman BPC, Giphart MJ, Wintzen AR, Roep BO, Verscuuren JJGM. (2005) HLA and smoking in prediction and prognosis of small cell lung cancer in autoimmune Lambert-Eaton myasthenic syndrome. J Neuroimmunol 159, 230–237.

8. Lang, B, Newsom-Davis J, Prior C, Wray D. (1983) Antibodies to motor nerve terminals: an electrophysiological study of a human myasthenic syndrome transferred to mouse. J. Physiol (Lond) 344, 335–345.

9. Fugunaga H, Engel AG, Lang B, Newsom-Davis J, Vincent A. (1983) Passive transfer of Lambert-Eaton myasthenic syndrome with IgG from man to mouse depletes the presynaptic membrane active zones. Proc Natl Acad Sci USA 80, 7636–7640.

10. Nakao YK, Motomura M, Fukudome T, Fukuda T, Shiraishi H, Yoshimura T, Tsujihata M, Eguchi K. (2002) Seronegative Lambert-Eaton myasthenic syndrome Neurol 58, 1773–1775.

11. Oh SJ, Hatanaka Y, Claussen GC, Sher E. (2007) Electrophysiological differences in seropositive and seronegative Lambert-Eaton myasthenic syndrome. Muscle Nerve 35, 178–183.

12. Motomura M, Johnston I, Lang B, Palace J, Vincent A, Newsom-Davis J. (1997) An improved diagnostic assay for Lambert-Eaton myasthenic syndrome. J Neurosci 147, 35–42.

13. Lennon VA, Kryzer TJ, Griesmann GE, et al. (1995) Calcium channel antibodies in the Lambert-Eaton syndrome and other paraneoplastic syndromes. N Engl J Med 332, 1467–1474.

14. Martin-Moutot N, de Haro L, Dos Santos RG, Mori Y, Seagar M. (2006) Phoneutria nigriventer ω-Phonetoxin IIA: A new tool for anti-calcium channel autoantibody assays in Lambert-Eaton myasthenic syndrome. Neurobiol Dis 22, 57–63.

15. El Far O, Marqueze B, Leveque C, Martin-Moutot N, Lang B, Newsom-Davis J, Yoshida A, Takahashi M, Seagar MJ. (1995) Antigens associated with N and L type calcium channels in Lambert-Eaton myasthenic syndrome. J Neurochem 64, 1696–1702.

16. Takamori M, Hamada T, Komai K, Takahashi M, Yoshida A. (1994) Synaptotagmin can cause an immune-mediated model of Lambert-Eaton myasthenic syndrome in rats. Ann Neurol 35, 74–80.

17. Graus F, Lang B, Pozo-Rosich P, Saiz A, Casamitjana R, Vincent A. (2002) P/Q-type calcium channel antibodies in paraneoplastic cerebellar degeneration with lung cancer. Neurology 59, 764–766.

18. Skeie GO, Apostolski S, Evoli A, Gilhus NE, Hart IK, Harms L, Hilton-Jones D, Meilms A, Verschuuren J, Horge HW. (2006) Guidelines for the treatment of autoimmune neuromuscular transmission disorders E J Neurol 13, 691–699.

76
Amyotrophic Lateral Sclerosis

Bethan Lang

Abstract   Amyotrophic lateral sclerosis (ALS) is a rapidly progressive neurodegenerative disorder of the upper and lower neurones that is invariably fatal. Mutations in the superoxide dismutase gene are thought to be causative in some cases of familial ALS; however, in most sporadic cases the cause is unknown. Abnormalities in the immune system of some patients with ALS and the detection of immune components in the motor neurones of ALS patients have been reported. The reputed presence of autoantibodies to a range of different autoantigens, including voltage-gated calcium channels (VGCC), Fas antigen (Apo-1/CD95), gangliosides and glycolipids have been postulated as causative factors. However, as yet there is little evidence to support these hypotheses and so the detection of antibodies is not routinely used diagnostically in ALS.

Keywords   Amyotrophic lateral sclerosis · neurodegenerative disorder · motor neurones

Introduction

Amyotrophic lateral sclerosis (ALS) or motor neurone disease, also known as Lou Gehrig's disease, is a rapidly progressive, invariably fatal, neurodegenerative disease that affects the limbs, speech, swallowing and breathing. It is caused by degeneration of both the upper motor neurones located in the brain and lower motor neurones in the spinal cord resulting in the loss of voluntary movements. The dying back of the nerves results in the gradual weakening of the muscle and atrophy. Death usually occurs through respiratory failure (1).

Epidemiology

The incidence of ALS is approximately 1–2 per 100,000 with a prevalence of about 5 per 100,000, men being affected more commonly than women. The onset can occur at any age, but most commonly occurs in people between the age of 40 and 60 years. Approximately 10% of all cases are familial, in a fifth of these cases mutations in the copper-zinc superoxide dismutase gene (SOD1), an enzyme that protects the body from damage by free radicals, have been detected. The remaining 90% of cases are classified as sporadic and have no known hereditary component.

Diagnosis

There is no definitive diagnosis of ALS, although the presence of both upper and lower motor neurone signs is highly suggestive. If the disease is thought to be familial, the mutations in the SOD1 gene can be looked for. In the sporadic cases, the symptoms of ALS can initially be very similar to a variety of other more treatable disorders and a differential diagnosis of other motor disorders such as Guillain-Barré syndrome, multiple sclerosis, myasthenia gravis and stroke, need to be excluded (1).

Clinical Features

Typically, the onset of the clinical features of ALS is subtle and is often missed or ignored. The symptoms at presentation depend on which particular pathway is first involved. At presentation, about 65% of patients have mixed upper and lower motor neurone features, many will have a "bulbar" onset, the first symptoms experienced being difficulty in speaking and/or swallowing. Muscle weakness and atrophy alone at presentation may occur in some cases. Muscle cramps, parasthesias and pain are also often cited. Pain or sensory disturbance is not unknown, but is not a common feature of the disease; it is usually the absence of pain or sensory disturbance that helps to distinguish

From: Y. Shoenfeld et al. (eds.): *Diagnostic Criteria in Autoimmune Diseases*, DOI: 10.1007/978-1-60327-285-8_76,

ALS from radiculopathies. Progression usually occurs over 12–30 months with death usually occurring due to respiratory failure or pneumonia.

Electrophysiological Studies

Standard nerve conduction studies and electromyography on an ALS patient will show a typical pattern of severe chronic denervation with spontaneous fibrillation potentials, reduced number of spikes following exercise due to a reduced number of motor neurones and an increase in the amplitude and duration of the motor action potential of the surviving units. This effect reflects the increasing muscle fibre number in each motor unit as a result of a successful reinnervation by surviving units.

Aetiology

The cause of ALS is unknown; however, theories regarding the pathogenesis include glutamate excitotoxicity, free radical oxidative stress, viral infection, exposure to pesticides, neurotoxins, heavy metal poisoning and autoimmunity. In the context of this chapter, only autoimmunity will be discussed; for a general review, see (1).

General Autoimmunity

There are reports of an increased incidence of autoimmunity in ALS patients and in their close relatives, while serum antibodies have been reported in the serum of some ALS patients (2). Active immunisation with crude preparations of neuronal tissue has produced models of ALS-like disease. Engelhardt and colleagues induced a lower motor neuron-like disorder after immunisation with bovine motor neurones and a more acute disorder involving both lower and upper neurones, by inoculation with spinal cord homogenates in guinea pigs (2). There have also been a number of reports that immunoglobulins prepared from ALS sera cause neuromuscular dysfunction in passive transfer models and in neuronal cell cultures. ALS, but not control IgG, was subsequently detected in the microtubules and rough endoplasmic reticulum of lower motor neurones and spinal cord of mice receiving injections of ALS IgG (3). Culturing neuronal cells in ALS IgG has been said to cause increased intracellular calcium levels, cell shrinkage and membrane blebbing, which are morphological features of apoptotic cell death (4); however, the purity of the preparation has been questioned. Autoantibodies to a wide range of different autoantigens are now being reported in ALS sera.

Autoantibody Specificities

Antibodies to Voltage-Gated Calcium Channels (VGCCs)

The VGCCs are a family of ion channels that exhibit functional and regional specialisation. The L-type ($\alpha 1_s$) VGCC subtype is involved in mediating excitation and contraction coupling in skeletal muscle, while the P-/Q- and N-type VGCCs have been shown to mediate neurotransmitter release in peripheral and central nervous system. There have been a number of reports that ALS serum and Ig causes neuromuscular dysfunction in passive transfer models and alters calcium currents in neuronal cell cultures. Passive transfer of ALS immunoglobulin has been reported to be able to increase miniature end plate potential frequency but conversely decrease calcium currents at the neuromuscular junction of mice (2). The ability of ALS sera/Ig to bind to L-type VGCC specifically and to displace monoclonal antibodies against the alpha-1 VGCC subunit (5) has also been questioned and contamination of the ALS sera with proteases may account for some of the findings reported (6). Following the report by Lennon et al. (7), describing 23 of 78 ALS patients with low anti-P-/Q- or N-type VGCC antibodies, an anti-VGCC antibody radioimmunoassay was thought useful in the diagnosis of ALS. Since then, there have been a number of contradictory reports. Arsac and colleagues, using radioimmunoassay and ELISA, found only marginally positive titres to N-type VGCC in 2 of 25 ALS patients (8) and all ALS sera were negative when tested against L-type VGCCs derived from either brain or muscle; similar results have been found by others (see Figure 76.1) (9).

Antibodies to Fas

Fas (APO1 or CD95) is a member of the tumour necrosis factor receptor family that, following activation, can trigger apoptosis. Yi et al. (10) demonstrated that 26% of ALS patient sera, most of which were shown to contain anti-Fas antibodies, were able to induce apoptosis of a human neuroblastoma cell line, whereas sera from only 2 of 27 Alzheimer's patients without anti-Fas antibodies were not. Although the authors demonstrated that a monoclonal anti-Fas antibody with agonistic properties and soluble Fas-ligand were also able to induce apoptosis, they did not show that the effect elicited by the ALS sera was necessarily antibody-mediated. In a separate study (11), anti-Fas antibodies were detected in 25% of sporadic ALS patients, 22% of familial ALS patients and 50% of patients with Parkinson's disease. However, there was no correlation between the anti-Fas antibody titre and the length of the disease or its severity. The relevance of these findings

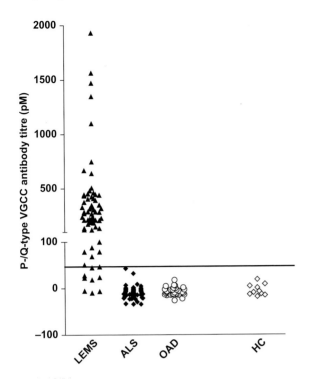

FIGURE 76.1. Serum antibodies to P-/Q-type VGCC in LEMS, ALS and controls. Antibody levels were measured by immuno-precipitation of human cerebellar VGCC labelled with ^{125}I-ω-conotoxin MVIIC (^{125}I-ω-CmTx). Antibody titres were considered positive if greater than 50 pmoles/litre of serum (pM); mean titre + 3 standard deviations above the mean of the healthy controls (HC, $n = 50$). Serum samples were available from 80 patients with Lambert-Eaton myasthenic syndrome (LEMS), 42 patients with amyotrophic lateral sclerosis (ALS), 30 patients with other autoimmune diseases (OAD), including myasthenia gravis, systemic lupus erythematosus or rheumatoid arthritis. (Modified from Ref. (9).

to ALS is in doubt as apoptosis-inducing anti-Fas antibodies have been detected in normal sera (12) and it has also been demonstrated that although cultured neuroblastomas express high levels of Fas, normal human neurones do not (13).

Antibodies to Gangliosides and Glycolipids

A few reports have described the presence of antibodies to specific gangliosides in the sera of patients with ALS. These include a report that 78% of ALS patients had IgM autoantibodies to GM1a or GD1a gangliosides, while these antibodies were present only in less than 10% of normal controls (14). Subsequent reports have failed to reproduce these results (15). Antibodies to sulphoglucuronyl paragloboside, a unique glycolipid present in both peripheral nerve and vascular endothelial cells, have also been reported in ALS; again the pathogenetic significance of these antibodies is unknown (16).

Treatment

Although autoimmunity has been postulated, immunotherapy has not been shown to be effective (17) and ALS remains largely untreatable. There are a number of symptoms that are amenable to treatment; however, most of these treatments are palliative and involved in maintaining the patients' quality of life.

Conclusions

Although there have been a number of different reports of antibodies in the sera of patients with ALS, results have been contradictory and there is no evidence that unequivocally proves their existence. The little evidence of pathogenicity has been challenged. The increased levels of autoantibodies in ALS may be related to a destructive immunological process in some patients. Therefore, testing for circulating antibodies has yet to be shown to have any clinical relevance.

References

1. Talbot K. (2002) Motor neurone disease. Postgrad Med J 78, 513–519.
2. Appel SH, Smith RG, Engelhardt JI, Stefani E. (1993) Evidence for autoimmunity in amyotrophic lateral sclerosis. J Neurol Sci 118, 169–174.
3. Engelhardt JI, Soos J, Obal I, Vigh L, Siklos L. (2005) Subcellular localisation of IgG from the sera of ALS patients in the nervous system. Acta Neurol Scand 112, 126–133.
4. Alexianu ME, Mohamed AH, Smith RG, Colom LV, Appel SH. (1994) Apoptotic cell death of a hybrid motoneuron cell line induced by immunoglobulins from patients with amyotrophic lateral sclerosis. J Neurochem 63, 2365–2368.
5. Kimura F, Smith GR, Delbono O et al. (1994) Amyotrophic lateral sclerosis patients antibodies label Ca2+ channel alpha-1 subunit. Ann Neurol 35, 164–171.
6. Nyormoi O. (1996) Proteolytic activity in amyotrophic lateral sclerosis IgG preparations. Ann Neurol 40, 701–706.
7. Lennon VA, Kryzer TJ, Griesmann GE, et al. (1995) Calcium channel antibodies in the Lambert-Eaton syndrome and other paraneoplastic syndromes. (1995) N Engl J Med 332, 1467–1474.
8. Arsac C, Raymond C, Martin-Moutot N, Dargent B, Couraud F, Pouget J, Seagar M. (1996) Immunoassays fail to detect antibodies against neuronal calcium channels in amyotrophic lateral sclerosis. Ann Neurol 40, 691–693.
9. Motomura M, Johnston I, Lang B, Palace J, Vincent A, Newsom Davis J. (1997) An improved diagnostic assay for Lambert Eaton myasthenic syndrome. J Neurosci 147, 35–42.
10. Yi FH, Lautrette C, Vermot-Desroches C, Bordessoule D, Couratier P, Wijdenes J, Preud'homme JL, Jauberteau MO. (2000) In vitro induction of neuronal apoptosis by anti-Fas antibody-containing sera from amyotrophic lateral sclerosis patients. J Neuroimmunol 109(2):211–20.
11. Sengun IS, Appel SH. (2003) Serum anti-Fas antibody levels in amyotrophic lateral sclerosis. J Neuroimmunol 142, 137–140.

12. Prasad NK, Papoff G, Zeuner A, Bonnin E, Kazatchkine MD, Ruberti G, Kaveri SV. (1998) Therapeutic preparations of normal polyspecific IgG (IVIg) induce apoptosis in human lymphocytes and monocytes: A novel mechanism of action of IVIg involving the Fas apoptotic pathway. J Immunol 161, 3781–3790.

13. Beecher B, D'Sousa SD, Troutt AB, Antel JP.(1998) Fas expression on human fetal astrocytes without susceptibility to fas-mediated cytotoxicity. Neuroscience 84(2), 627–634.

14. Pestronk A, Adams RN, Cornblath D, Kuncl RW, Drachmman DB, Clawson L. (1989) Patterns of serum IgM antibodies to GM1 and GD1a gangliosides in amyotrophic lateral sclerosis. Ann Neurol 25, 98–102.

15. Garcia Guijo C, Garcia-Merino A, Rubio G. (1995) Presence and isotype of anti-ganglioside antibodies in healthy persons, motor neuron disease, peripheral neuropathy, and other diseases of the nervous system. J Neuroimmunol 56, 27–33.

16. Ikeda J, Kohriyama T, Nakamura S. (2000) Elevation of serum soluble E-selectin and antisulfoglucuronyl paragloboside antibodies in amyotrophic lateral sclerosis. Eur J Neurol 7, 541–547.

17. Meucci N, Nobile-Orazio E, Scarlato G. (1996) Intravenous immunoglobulin therapy in amyotrophic lateral sclerosis. J Neurol 243, 117–120.

77
Paraneoplastic Neurological Syndromes

Tomeu Rossiñol and Francesc Graus

Abstract   Paraneoplastic Neurological Syndromes (PNS) are a group of neurological disorders affecting patients with cancer typically before any other clinical suspicion of an underlying oncological disease. PNS are admitted to have an autoimmune basis characterized by an immunological response against an antigen (onconeural antigen) expressed in both tumoral and neuronal cells. This view is supported by the presence of autoantibodies against onconeural antigens (antineuronal antibodies) associated to some subtypes of PNS. PNS are rare, affecting less than 1% of all patients with cancer, the most common being lung, breast and ovarian carcinoma, thymoma and Hodgkin's disease. Clinical manifestations are diverse according to the region of the nervous system affected (either central, peripheral or both) and the presence of clinical manifestations of theoretically unrelated areas of the nervous system is very suggestive of PNS. The major factor in the management of those patients is the prompt diagnosis and treatment of the underlying cancer, with immunosuppression as a complementary aid for treating the neurological manifestations. Recent diagnostic criteria and practical issues in management have been published in order to expand our knowledge and improve diagnosis and treatment of PNS.

Keywords   Paraneoplastic neurological syndromes · onconeural antigens · antineuronal antibodies

Paraneoplastic Neurological Syndromes (PNS) are a group of neurological disorders that may involve either the central or the peripheral nervous system and present exclusively or with high frequency in patients with cancer that usually is not diagnosed at the time the PNS appears (Table 77.1) (1). By definition, PNS are not explained by local, regional or metastatic infiltration, metabolic dysfunction, infection, secondary effects of the oncological therapy or cancer-related coagulopathy. Recent studies strongly support that most PNS are autoimmune disorders characterized by an immunological response against an antigen expressed in both tumor cells and neurons (2).

Epidemiology

PNS are rare disorders, affecting less than 1% of all patients with cancer. The most common tumors are lung, breast and ovarian carcinoma, thymoma and Hodgkin's disease. Median age at presentation ranges between 55 and 65 years, but, as expected, patients with PNS associated with Hodgkin's disease, ovarian teratoma and testicular tumors are younger. There is probably a global predominance in women (2–3:1), but some subtypes are characteristically in higher proportion in men.

History

An autoimmune explanation for PNS emerged in 1965 with the detection of antibodies reacting against neuronal cells. Further support to the autoimmune hypothesis was the description in 1985 of the anti-Hu antibody, found in patients with PNS associated with small-cell lung carcinoma (SCLC). Since then, more than 10 types of antibodies in serum and cerebrospinal fluid (CSF) have been described, associated with different PNS and tumors (Table 77.2) (2).

Pathogenesis

PNS are believed to be caused by the ectopic expression by tumor cells of an antigen, called onconeural antigen, which is identical to that present in the brain. An immune reaction mediated by antigen-specific cytotoxic

From: Y. Shoenfeld et al. (eds.): *Diagnostic Criteria in Autoimmune Diseases*, DOI: 10.1007/978-1-60327-285-8_77,

TABLE 77.1. Paraneoplastic neurological syndromes.

Syndromes of the central nervous system
   Encephalomyelitis
   LimbicEncephalitis
   BrainstemEncephalitis
   Subacute cerebellar degeneration
   Opsoclonus-myoclonus[b]
   Stiff-person syndrome
   Stiff-person syndrome
   Necrotizing myelopathy[a]
   Motor neuron diseases[a]

Syndromes of the peripheral nervous system
   Subacute sensory neuronopathy
   Sensorimotor neuropathies[b]
   Neuropathy with vasculitis[a]
   Autonomic neuropathies
   Chronic gastrointestinal pseudoobstruction
   Acute pandysautonomia[a]

Syndromes of the neuromuscular junction and muscle
   Myasthenia gravis
   Lambert-Eaton myasthenic syndrome[a]
   Acquired neuromyotonia[a]
   Dermatomyositis[a]
   Acute necrotizing myopathy[a]

Classical syndromes, defined as those almost always associated with cancer, are underlined.
[a] Neurological syndromes not associated with known onconeural antibodies.
[b] Associated with onconeural antibodies only with particular tumor types.

TABLE 77.2. Onconeural antibodies associated to PNS.

Antibody (sensitivity)	PNS	Associated cancer
Well-characterized antibodies		
Anti-Hu (ANNA-1) (> 80% except for subacute cerebellar degeneration and limbicencephalitis)	PEM, subacute sensory neuronopathy, subacute cerebellar degeneration, limbic Encephalitis, chronic gastrointestinal pseudoobstruction	SCLC
Anti-Yo (PCA-1) (>90%)	Subacute cerebellar degeneration	Ovarian, breast
Anti-Ri (ANNA-2) (low <5%)	BrainstemEncephalitis, opsoclonus-myoclonus	Breast, SCLC
Anti-CV2/CRMP5 (low, <20%)	PEM, chorea, subacute sensory neuronopathy, subacute cerebellar degeneration, limbicEncephalitis, chronic gastrointestinal pseudoobstruction	SCLC, thymoma
Anti-Ma2 (Probably >90%)	Limbic/Brainstem/Diencephalic encephalitis, subacute cerebellar degeneration	Testis, lung

TABLE 77.2. (CONTINUED)

Antibody (sensitivity)	PNS	Associated cancer
Anti-amphiphysin (low, except for stiff-person syndrome)	Stiff-person syndrome, others	Breast, SCLC
Partially characterized antibodies		
Anti-Tr (PCA-Tr) (probably high >80%)	Subacute cerebellar degeneration	Hodgkin's Lymphoma
Anti-NMDA[R] (probably high >80%)	Limbic encephalitis, hypoventilation	Ovaric teratoma
Anti-Zic4 (low, <5%)	Subacute cerebellar degeneration	SCLC
ANNA-3 (a few patients reported)	Various	SCLC
PCA-2 (a few patients reported)	Various	SCLC
Anti-mGluR1 (two patients reported)	Subacute cerebellar degeneration	Hodgkin's Lymphoma
Antibodies associated to PNS and to non-paraneoplastic neurological syndromes		
Anti-VGCC (40% in subacute cerebellar degeneration)	Lambert-Eaton myastenic syndrome, Subacute cerebellar degeneration	SCLC
Anti-Ach receptor (>90%)	Myasthenia gravis	Thymoma
Anti-VGKC (high in idiopathic cases)	LimbicEncephalitis, neuromyotonia	Thymoma, others
Anti-Ach nicotinic receptor (high?)	Subacute pandysautonomia	SCLC, others

ANNA-1: Antinuclear neuronal antibody type 1; PCA-1: Anti-Purkinje cell antibody type 1; ANNA-2: Antinuclear neuronal antibody type 2; CRMP5: Collapsing response mediator protein-5; PCA-Tr: Anti-Purkinje cell antibody-Tr; NMDA GluR: n-metil-D-aspartate type glutamate receptor; ANNA-3: Antinuclear neuronal antibody type 3: mGluR1: metabothropic glutamate receptor type 1; Ach: acetylcholine; VGCC: voltage-gated calcium channel; VGKC: voltage-gated potassium channel; SCLC: small-cell lung cancer.

T and B cells results in inflammatory infiltrates in the nervous system and tumoral tissue and the detection of antineuronal antibodies in the serum and CSF. The immune attack is initially directed against the tumor cells interfering with tumor growth (there are case reports of "spontaneous" remission of the tumor), and later misdirected against neuronal tissue that causes the clinical manifestations according to the region of the nervous system affected. Antineuronal antibodies probably are not pathogenic in most PNS because they recognize intracellular antigens and the PNS probably are mediated by T cells. However, with the exception of the Lambert-Eaton myasthenic syndrome (LEMS), no animal models have been developed to prove definitively that PNS are B- or T-cell mediated (2).

Clinical Manifestations

In PNS, the neurological manifestations appear before the diagnosis of the tumor. Patients usually develop a subacute clinical syndrome in weeks or a few months, that causes severe and irreversible neurological impairment in many instances. Clinicians should include PNS in differential diagnosis of subacute neurological disorders not explained by other conditions, particularly in patients older than 50 years. An important clinical clue is that PNS may present with a multifocal disease involving distant and apparently unrelated areas of the nervous system. The suspicion of PNS must be extreme in those syndromes that are defined as "classical" PNS because they are almost always associated with cancer (Table 77.1) (1, 3). In this chapter, we will describe in more detail some of these classical syndromes. The rest, including LEMS, myasthenia gravis and dermatomyositis, are described in other chapters of this book.

Serological Features

Several antibodies have been described associated to different clinical syndromes and specific tumors (Table 77.2). Specificity is very high for all these antibodies and only a few patients who are seropositive do not have cancer. Sensitivity varies depending on the antibodies (Table 77.2).

Diagnostic Criteria

According to recent criteria published in 2004 (4), the diagnosis of PNS should be based on the presence of cancer, the clinical syndrome (classical vs. non-classical), and the presence of well-characterized onconeural antibodies defined by laboratory tests that make an unambiguous identification of the antibody (Table 77.2). On the basis of these criteria, PNS are subdivided into "definite" or "possible" (Table 77.3). It is mandatory to exclude other possible causes for the neurological symptoms before the diagnosis of PNS is established. This classification does not rule out the possibility that "possible" PNS can include few clinical syndromes not directly related to cancer (i.e., coincidental associations) (4).

Management and Prognosis

The first step is to make an early diagnosis. This can be accomplished by knowledge of clinical clues to recognize PNS, serum or CSF antineuronal antibodies, good collaboration with radiologists to detect small tumors, and

TABLE 77.3. Diagnostic criteria for paraneoplastic neurological syndromes (PNS).

Definite PNS
1. A *classical* syndrome and cancer that develops within five years of the diagnosis of the neurological disorder.
2. A non-classical syndrome that resolves or significantly improves after cancer treatment without concomitant immunotherapy, provided the syndrome is not susceptible to spontaneous remission.
3. A non-classical syndrome with onconeural antibodies (well characterized or not) and cancer that develops within five years of the diagnosis of the neurological disorder.
4. A neurological syndrome (classical or not) with well-characterized onconeural antibodies (anti-Hu, Yo, CV2, Ri, Ma2, or amphiphysin), and no cancer.

Possible PNS
1. A *classical syndrome*, no onconeural antibodies, no cancer, but at high risk of having an underlying tumor.
2. A neurological syndrome (classical or not) with partially characterized onconeural antibodies and no cancer.
3. A non-classical syndrome, no onconeural antibodies, and cancer present within two years of diagnosis.

use of more sensitive imaging techniques, such as positron emission tomography (PET). However, even a negative PET does not rule out the presence of a microscopic tumor and serial examinations with PET or CT scan are indicated in patients with high risk of a PNS. Early tumor diagnosis is not only the best way to cure the tumor but also the best guarantee to improve or stabilize the PNS. The main objective in the management of a patient with a PNS is to cure the underlying cancer and to improve or stabilize (in those PNS associated with neuronal death) the neurological dysfunction.

The percentage of patients whose cancer is cured is far from optimal for two reasons: (a) the most frequent tumor associated with PNS, the SCLC, sometimes cannot be cured even when diagnosed in a limited disease stage and (b) the tumor of patients with PNS has usually invaded the regional lymph nodes when diagnosed. However, cure for the cancer is probably the best way to abrogate the immune response that is damaging the nervous system. The positive effect of tumor treatment has been observed in several PNS, such as paraneoplastic opsoclonus-myoclonus, LEMS, and anti-Hu-associated PNS (5).

Therapy

Several immunosuppressor therapies including corticosteroids, plasmapheresis and IVIG have been used in the treatment of PNS. The effect of these therapies is unclear because the number of patients treated is relatively low, patients also receive antineoplastic treatment, and randomized prospective studies are lacking. Although, theoretically, immunosuppression could exacerbate tumor growth, we did not find that these treatments were an adverse prognostic factor for survival. However, one must be cautious while using strong immunosuppressor therapies because a deleterious effect on the tumor growth could not be ruled out in isolated case reports (5).

The effect of immunotherapy in PNS has to be considered according to the type of PNS. In patients with LEMS and the opsoclonus-myoclonus syndrome, who have a functional, rather than an irreversible, neural damage, immunotherapy is effective. Paraneoplastic LEMS should be treated with corticosteroids but the response will depend on how effectively the tumor can be treated. Paraneoplastic opsoclonus-myoclonus syndrome may respond to IVIG treatment particularly when tumor therapy can induce a complete response. Unlike idiopathic cases, patients may remain with mild residual ataxia (5). In the other PNS, there is a variable degree of irreversible neuronal damage, so the objective of any immunotherapy should be stabilization rather than improvement of the neurological symptoms. However, the degree of neuronal damage probably is not the same among the different PNS. Improvement has been more frequently described in patients with limbicEncephalitis associated to testicular cancer and anti-Ma2 (Ta) antibodies. In contrast, patients with limbicEncephalitis and anti-Hu antibodies rarely improve. Patients with PCD and anti-Yo antibodies and those with PCD associated with SCLC almost never respond to any type of immunotherapy. Patients with anti-Tr antibodies and Hodgkin's disease usually follow the same pattern with the exception that around 15% improve. If the cause of the improvement is the tumor treatment or the immunotherapy is unclear, but there are a few case reports in which the improvement occurred before the onset of the treatment of the Hodgkin's disease. The poor response to immunotherapy in patients with PCD is emphasized by those patients who present PCD and LEMS at the same time. Immunotherapy improves the symptoms from LEMS but the cerebellar dysfunction remains stable or becomes worse (5).

Paraneoplastic Encephalomyelitis (PEM)

PEM is defined as the involvement of different areas of the nervous system over time, and is typically associated with anti-Hu, and less frequently with anti-CV2 or anti-amphiphysin antibodies. Multiple combinations of PNS syndromes are possible, with clinical predominance of one of them in 30% of cases at diagnosis and 60% during evolution. The most predominant PNS in patients with PEM is sensory neuronopathy, followed by limbicencephalitis, brainstem/cerebellar syndromes, and dysautonomia. SCLC is diagnosed in >80% of cases after a mean delay of 6.5 months after PEM appears. PEM has a dismal prognosis (median survival of 12 months) and causes an important disability (53% of patients are severely impaired for the activities of daily-living at the moment of diagnosis). Early diagnosis and treatment of the tumor (with or without immunotherapy) is the best current option to stabilize or improve PEM. Immunotherapy alone (mainly immunoglobulins, cyclophosphamide, methylprednisolone, plasmapheresis, or a combination of them) should be considered, especially when no tumor is found or when PEM appears after tumor diagnosis (6).

Paraneoplastic Limbic Encephalitis (PLE)

PLE is characterized by neurological manifestations attributable to limbic (medial temporal lobe) structures, manifested as short-term memory loss, seizures or psychiatric symptoms (depression, irritability and personality changes). Onset is over days or weeks in more than 80% of cases. Neurological manifestations occur before tumor diagnosis in 58% of cases, with a median interval of 3.5 months. Median age of patients is 55 years, with a slight predominance in men. Most PLE patients have at least two abnormal results in complementary exams (CSF, autoantibodies and MRI). CSF is abnormal in 60–80% of cases and MRI show abnormalities in one or both medial aspects of the temporal lobes in at least 50% of them (7). Antibody positivity is found in 60% of patients, conforming three main subtypes:

1. Anti-Hu-associated PLE: associated to SCLC in up to 90% of cases, this is the most frequent subtype of PLE, manifested as multifocal disease in 50% of cases as a part of the spectrum of PEM. PLE associated with SCLC may present other onconeural antibodies, mainly anti-CV2/CRMP5 or anti-amphiphysin or no antibodies. Prognosis is poor despite oncological and/or immunosuppressant therapy (6).
2. Anti-Ma2-associated PLE: limbic involvement occurs in 80% of cases, with brainstem (73%) and diencephalic involvement (38%). The presence of anti-Ma2 antibodies is associated with testicular cancer in 90% of cases. Improvement or stabilization occurs in up to 50% of the patients after oncological treatment, specially the cases with testicular tumor. Immunotherapy must be considered as an adjunctive therapy or when oncological treatment is not suitable (8).
3. Anti-NMDA-receptor PLE: presents in young patients (median age: 27 years) with psychiatric symptoms, generalized or partial complex seizures and decreased level of consciousness that requires prolonged mechanical ventilation. This subtype of PLE is associated with ovarian teratoma with particular good therapeutic response to tumoral resection and adjunctive immunotherapy in more than 90% of cases (9).

Opsoclonus-Myoclonus Syndrome (OMS)

OMS is defined by the presence of opsoclonus (involuntary and irregular saccadic eye movements in all directions), usually associated to arrhythmic action-myoclonus involving trunk, limbs and head. Symptoms of cerebellar dysfunction are frequent, such as ataxia and dysartria. Onset is usually subacute and, after excluding other etiologies, two subgroups must be taken into account: paraneoplastic and idiopathic, both of them with a presumed autoimmune basis. The most frequent neoplasms are neuroblastoma in children and breast or SCLC in adults, lacking specific antibodies in an important proportion of cases. Most frequently described antibodies are anti-Ri (associated with breast cancer) and anti-Hu or anti-amphipysin (both in SCLC, usually at low titers and with dubious significance). CSF is normal or discloses mild pleocytosis, and MRI usually has no alterations. Paraneoplastic opsoclonus-myoclonus syndrome may respond to IVIG treatment particularly when tumor therapy can induce a complete response. Unlike idiopathic cases, patients are more likely to remain with mild residual ataxia (10).

Paraneoplastic Cerebellar Degeneration (PCD)

PCD presents with a subacute history of weeks to months of truncal (wide-based gait) and appendicular ataxia (intention tremor) with or without dysatria, nystagmus, vertigo or diplopia. It usually stabilizes over 6 months but leaves the patient physically dependent in most cases. The pathological hallmark of PCD is the loss of Purkinje cells of the cerebellum (11). Several clinical–immunological associations have been identified:

1. Anti-Yo PCD accounts for up to 40% of cases of PCD and is one of the most homogeneous subgroup of PNS, affecting women with a median age of 60–65 years, 80% of them with gynecologic cancer (breast and ovary, usually localized and treatable). PCD appears before cancer in 61% of patients. Although PCD is not the main cause of death, most patients remain neurologically impaired, with almost null neurologic recovery after oncological or immunosuppressive therapy (12).
2. Anti-Hu PCD accounts for 32% of all PCD, affecting equally men and women after 65 years of age and initially manifested as a subacute picture (few weeks to 1 month) of cerebellar dysfunction that progresses to a multifocal disease, evolving to PEM. Prognosis is poor, with no neurological improvement to cancer therapy or immunosupression. The main cause of death is the PNS itself rather than the localized SCLC that is associated to the PCD in more than 85% of cases (6).

3. Anti-VGCC PCD occurs in patients with SCLC that present neurological involvement of the cerebellum and features of LEMS. This autoantibody is a useful marker of PCD linked to SCLC. In a series of patients with PCD and SCLC, 41% presented VGCC antibodies but only 16% had anti-Hu antibodies. VGCC antibodies may occur in cases of PCD and no clinical or electromyographic evidence of LEMS (13).
4. Anti-Tr PCD: represents 14% of all PCD. This type of PCD usually affects male patients with Hodgkin disease. The clinical symptoms are confined to the cerebellum without involvement of other areas of the nervous system. Tumor is found in 90% of cases (almost always a Hodgkin disease), with a mean time of 3.5 months, preceded by PCD in 80% of them. Anti-Tr autoantibodies may be present only in the CSF and usually disappear after successful treatment of the tumor. Unlike other PCD types, up to 15% of patients improve after treatment of the Hodgkin disease and immunotherapy (14). Infrequently, patients with PCD and Hodgkin disease may display other antibodies, such as anti-mGluR1. The cases described presented the PCD several years after successful treatment of the Hodgkin disease (2).

Subacute Sensory Neuronopathy (SSN)

The SSN is caused by damage to sensory neurons in the dorsal root ganglia. SSN is characterized by a subacute history (weeks) of pain and paresthesias with a multifocal and asymmetric pattern, invariably involving upper limbs during evolution. Lower limbs are also affected with variable intensity. Neurological examination shows abolition of the deep tendon reflexes and involvement of all modalities of sensation but with clear predominance of the joint position and vibratory senses. SSN appears as an isolated PNS in 24% of patients, being the predominant finding in 74% of anti-Hu PEM. SSN typically associates with clinical manifestations involving other areas of the nervous system. A relatively common involvement is the neurons in the myenteric plexuses that cause gastrointestinal pseudoobstruction (persistent vomiting, constipation and X-ray evidence of intestinal dilation). The typical SSN has a subacute onset and progresses rapidly to involve the four limbs and then may stabilize, although by the time its does so (6–9 months), the patient may be confined to bed or chair due to ataxia. In 10% of the patients, the neuropathy runs a mild, very slowly clinical evolution. These patients may remain ambulatory and with an independent life for years in absence of any antitumoral or immunosuppressive treatment. The CSF may show mild lymphocytic pleocytosis. EMG studies disclose abolished sensory nerve action potentials. Motor neurography is usually normal but may show evidence of mild denervation or slowed nerve conduction velocities (6).

SCLC underlies SSN in 70–80% of cases with anti-Hu antibodies (which have 99% specificity and 82% sensitivity), and is diagnosed after SSN appears in a median of 4.5 months. Other antibodies instead of anti-Hu can be detected, such as anti-CV2/CRMP5, and anti-amphiphysin. Oncological treatment is the mainstay therapy of SSN and the only independent predictor of stabilization or improvement. The role of immunotherapy is unclear (6).

References

1. Voltz R. Paraneoplastic neurological syndromes: an update on diagnosis, pathogenesis and therapy. Lancet Neurol 2002;1:294–305

2. Darnell RB, Posner JB. Paraneoplastic syndromes involving the nervous system. NEngl J Med 2003;349:1543–54.

3. Rudnicki SA, Dalmau J. Paraneoplastic syndromes of the spinal cord, nerve and muscle. Muscle Nerve 2000;23:1800–18.

4. Graus F, Delattre J-Y, Antoine JC, et al. Recommended diagnostic criteria for paraneoplastic neurological syndromes. J Neurol Neurosurg Psychiatry 2004;75:1135–40.

5. Vedeler CA, Antoine JC, Giometto B, et al. Management of paraneoplastic neurological syndromes: report of an EFNS Task Force. Eur J Neurol 2006;13:682–90.

6. Graus F, Keime-Guibert F, Reñe R, Benyahia B, Ribalta T, Acaso C, Escaramis G, Delattre JY. Anti-Hu-associated paraneoplasticEncephalomyelitis: analysis of 200 patients. Brain 2001;124:1138–48.

7. Humayun Gultekin S, Rosenfeld MR, Voltz R, Eichen J, Posner JB, Dalmau J. Paraneoplastic limbicEncephalitis: neurological symptoms, immunological findings and tumour association in 50 patients. Brain 2000;123:1481–94.

8. Dalmau J, Graus F, Villarejo A, Posner JB, Blumenthal D, Thiessen B, Saiz A, Meneses P, Rosenfeld MR. Clinical analysis of anti-Ma2-associatedEncephalitis. Brain 2004; 127:1831–44.

9. Dalmau J, Tüzüm E, Hai-yan W, et al. Paraneoplastic anti-N-methyl-D-aspartate receptorEncephalitis associated with ovarian teratoma. Ann Neurol 2007;61:25–36.

10. Bataller L, Graus F, Saiz A, Vilchez JJ, for the Spanish Opsoclonus-Myoclonus Study Group. Clinical outcome in adult-onset idiopathic or paraneoplastic opsoclonus-myoclonus. Brain 2001;124:437–43.

11. Shams'ili S, Grefkens J, de Leeuw B, et al. Paraneoplastic cerebellar degeneration associated with antineuronal antibodies: analysis of 50 patients. Brain 2003;126:1409–1418.

12. Peterson K, Rosenblum MK, Kotanides H, Posner JB. Paraneoplastic cerebellar degeneration. I. A clinical analysis of 55 anti-Yo antibody-positive patients. Neurology 1992;42:1931.

13. Mason WP, Graus F, Lang B, et al. Small-cell lung cancer, paraneoplastic cerebellar degeneration and the Lambert-Eaton myasthenic syndrome. Brain 1997;120:1279–1300

14. Bernal F, Shams'ili S, Rojas I, et al. Anti-Tr antibodies as markers of paraneoplastic cerebellar degeneration and Hodgkin's disease. Neurology 2003;60:230–4.

78

Guillain-Barré and Other Immune-Mediated Neuropathies

Avraham Unterman, Yehuda Shoenfeld and Joab Chapman

Abstract   Immune-mediated neuropathies are a heterogenic group of disorders caused by an autoimmune response and often associated with autoantibodies against various neuronal epitopes. Main pathophysiological mechanisms of nerve injury include immune-mediated demyelination, axonal damage, and vasculitic-induced nerve ischemia.

Diagnosis is based primarily on the clinical presentation and course, together with electrophysiological studies, testing for autoantibodies, and when needed, cerebrospinal fluid examination and nerve biopsy. Immune-mediated neuropathies frequently, though not universally, respond to immune therapies including corticosteroids, plasma exchange and intravenous immunoglobulins.

Keywords   Immune-mediated neuropathies · autoantibodies · Guillain-Barré syndrome · CIDP · multifocal motor neuropathy · vasculitic neuropathy

Immune-mediated neuropathies are a heterogenic group of disorders deemed to be caused by an autoimmune response directed against peripheral nerve antigens. They are often associated with autoantibodies against various neuronal epitopes, and frequently, though not universally, respond to immune therapies including corticosteroids, plasma exchange (PE) and intravenous immunoglobulins (IVIg) (1).

The major immune-mediated neuropathies and the associated autoantibodies, are listed in Table 78.1

Guillain-Barré Syndrome

Guillain-Barré syndrome (GBS) is an autoimmune acute peripheral neuropathy, causing limb weakness that progresses over a period of days and up to 4 weeks. The syndrome was described in 1916 by three French neurologists: Guillain, Barré, and Strohl, and is considered to be the most common cause of acute generalized paralysis. The four most common subtypes of GBS are acute inflammatory demyelinating polyneuropathy (AIDP), acute motor axonal neuropathy (AMAN), acute motor sensory axonal neuropathy (AMSAN) and the Miller Fisher's syndrome (MFS). The four types differ in their pathophysiology and immunological profiles, as well as in their worldwide incidence. In Western countries AIDP accounts for about

90% of all GBS cases, and AMAN accounts for most of the remaining 10% (2).

Epidemiology

GBS occurs throughout the world, affecting children and adults of all ages, with a median incidence of 1.3 cases/100,000 population (range, 0.4–4.0) (3). Men are affected approximately 1.5 times more than women (2). About two-thirds of GBS patients have an infection within a 6-week period prior to the diagnosis, generally either a flu-like episode or gastroenteritis (2, 3). The most frequent identifiable antecedent infectious organisms are Campylobacter jejuni (23–32%), cytomegalovirus (8–18%), Epstein-Barr virus (2–7%) and Mycoplasma pneumoniae (9%) (4).

Pathogenesis

There is considerable evidence supporting an immune mediated mechanism in GBS (5), though the pathophysiology is different in the various subtypes.

In AIDP the neuropathy is mainly demyelinating: macrophages invade the myelin sheaths and denude axons (2). Axonal damage can occur secondarily when the inflammation is severe. The histological appearance of AIDP resembles experimental autoimmune neuritis, which is caused predominantly by T cells directed against peptides from the myelin

From: Y. Shoenfeld et al. (eds.): *Diagnostic Criteria in Autoimmune Diseases*, DOI: 10.1007/978-1-60327-285-8_78,
© 2008 Humana Press, Totowa, NJ

TABLE 78.1. List of the major immune-mediated neuropathies (abbreviations in parentheses), and the main associated autoantibodies.

	Antibodies
Guillain-Barré syndrome (GBS)	
Acute inflammatory demyelinating polyneuropathy (AIDP)	Unknown
Acute motor axonal neuropathy (AMAN)	GM1,GM1b,GD1a,GalNac-GD1a
Acute motor sensory axonal neuropathy (AMSAN)	GM1, GM1b, GD1a
Miller Fisher's syndrome (MFS)	GQ1b, GT1a
Chronic inflammatory demyelinating polyneuropathy (CIDP)	Unknown
Multifocal motor neuropathy (MMN)	GM1
Paraneoplastic neuropathies	Hu, CV2
Vasculitic neuropathies	ANCA
Vasculitic neuropathy in primary vasculitis syndromes (e.g. PAN)	
Vasculitic neuropathy in connective tissue disorders (e.g. RA)	
"Nonsystemic" vasculitic neuropathy	
Neuropathies associated with monoclonal gammopathies	
Neuropathy in multiple myeloma	
Neuropathy in MGUS	
Neuropathy in other monoclonal gammopathies	

proteins P0, P2, and PMP22 (4). The exact role of T-cell-mediated immunity in AIDP remains unclear and there is also some evidence for the involvement of antibodies and complement (4).

In the axonal subtypes, AMAN and AMSAN, the main pathology is axonal injury rather than demyelinative one, and the pathophysiology is better understood. Strong evidence now exists that these axonal subtypes are caused by autoantibodies to gangliosides on the axolemma. An interesting observation is that the lipo-oligosaccharide from the Campylobacter jejuni bacterial wall contains ganglioside-like structures, thus promoting an immune response in some patients by the mechanism of molecular mimicry (2, 4). There is also evidence indicating a small increase in the risk of GBS following vaccination, especially with the influenza vaccine (6).

Serological Features

Several anti-ganglioside antibodies are associated both with AMAN (GM1, GM1b, GD1a and GalNac-GD1a in 64, 66, 45, and 33% of patients respectively) and with AMSAN (GM1, GM1b, GD1a) but not with AIDP (2, 4).

The Miller Fisher's syndrome, characterized by a triad of ophthalmoplegia, ataxia and areflexia, is associated with anti-GQ1b, a specific and sensitive anti-ganglioside antibody, present in more than 90% of the patients with MFS and absent in other forms of inflammatory neuropathy (4). Anti-GQ1b have been shown to damage the motor nerve terminal in vitro by a complement-mediated mechanism (4).

Clinical Course

Paresthesias and slight numbness in the toes and fingers are the earliest symptoms. The major clinical manifestation is weakness that evolves more or less symmetrically, and reaches its nadir 2–4 weeks after onset of symptoms.

The symptoms progress with an ascending pattern from the lower to the upper limbs in 56% of patients, involve the four limbs simultaneously in 32% of patients, and spread from the upper to the lower limbs in 12% of patients (2). The proximal as well as distal muscles of the limbs are involved. Involvement of the facial muscles is frequent, whereas the ocular motor muscles are usually spared, except with MFS. The weakness of the respiratory muscles may be severe enough to require assisted artificial ventilation in about 25% of the patients. More than half of the patients complain of pain and an aching discomfort in the muscles, mainly those of the hips, thighs and back. Autonomic involvement is common and may cause urine retention, ileus, sinus tachycardia, hypertension, cardiac arrhythmia, and postural hypotension.

After a variable plateau phase, recovery begins with return of proximal, followed by distal, strength over weeks or months. Between 4 and 15% of patients die, and up to 20% are disabled after a year despite modern treatment (4).

Diagnosis

Asbury and Cornblath's clinical criteria for the diagnosis of the Guillain-Barré syndrome (7) are widely accepted and are listed in Table 78.2.

The most important laboratory aids to the clinical diagnosis, are the electrophysiological studies and the CSF examination. The CSF is typically under normal pressure, contains an increased protein content, and is acellular or contains only a few lymphocytes (usually less than 10, rarely more than 50 mononuclear leukocytes/mm^3) (2). The protein content in the CSF may not be raised until 10 days after onset of disease and lumbar puncture may need to be repeated if the diagnosis remains doubtful (8).

Electrophysiological studies of both motor and sensory peripheral nerves play an important role in supporting the diagnosis, and help differentiate between the main

TABLE 78.2. Asbury and Cornblath's clinical criteria for Guillain-Barré syndrome diagnosis.

I. *Features Required for Diagnosis*
1. Progressive motor weakness of two or more limbs[a]
The degree ranges from minimal weakness of the legs, with or without mild ataxia, to total paralysis of the muscles of all four extremities and the trunk, bulbar and facial paralysis, and external ophthalmoplegia
2. Areflexia
Universal areflexia is the rule, though distal areflexia with definite hyporeflexia of the biceps and knee jerks will suffice if other features are consistent

II. *Clinical Features Strongly Supportive of the Diagnosis* (*in order of importance*)
1. Progression. Symptoms and signs of motor weakness develop rapidly but cease to progress by four weeks into the illness. Approximately 50% will reach the nadir by two weeks, 80% by three weeks, and more than 90% by four weeks
2. Relative symmetry
3. Mild sensory symptoms or signs
4. Cranial nerve involvement. Facial weakness occurs in approx. 50% and is frequently bilateral. Other cranial nerves may be involved (e.g., those innervating the tongue and muscles of deglutition, extraocular motor nerves). On occasion (less than 5%), the neuropathy may begin in the nerves to the extraocular muscles or other cranial nerves
5. Recovery. It usually begins 2–4 weeks after progression stops. May be delayed for months. Most patients recover functionally
6. Autonomic dysfunction. Tachycardia and other arrhythmias, postural hypotension, hypertension, and vasomotor symptoms, when present, support the diagnosis. These findings may fluctuate
7. Absence of fever at the onset of neuritic symptoms

III. *Features Casting Doubt on the Diagnosis*
1. Marked, persistent asymmetry of weakness
2. Persistent bladder or bowel dysfunction
3. Bladder or bowel dysfunction at onset
4. More than 50 mononuclear leukocytes/mm^3 in CSF
5. Presence of polymorphonuclear leukocytes in CSF
6. Sharp sensory level

IV. *Features That Rule Out the Diagnosis*
1. A current history of volatile solvents abuse. This includes huffing of paint lacquer vapors or addictive glue sniffing
2. Abnormal porphyrin metabolism indicating a diagnosis of acute intermittent porphyria
3. A history or finding of recent diphtheritic infection, either faucial or wound, with or without myocarditis
4. Features clinically consistent with lead neuropathy (upper limb weakness with prominent wrist drop; may be asymmetrical) and evidence of lead intoxication
5. The occurrence of a purely sensory syndrome
6. A definite diagnosis of a condition such as poliomyelitis, botulism, hysterical paralysis, or toxic neuropathy (e.g., from nitrofurantoin, dapsone, or organophosphates)

[a] Excluding Miller Fisher and other variant syndromes.

subtypes of GBS – i.e., between the demyelinating form (AIDP) and the axonal forms (AMAN and ASMAN). The particular electrophysiological abnormalities found in each subtype of GBS have been thoroughly described (4, 8). However, unlike the clinical diagnostic criteria, which have been agreed on, there is no consensus on electrophysiological criteria for classification. We direct readers to neurophysiological criteria proposed by Hughes and Cornblath for AIDP, AMAN, and AMSAN (4).

Treatment

IVIg (0.4 g/kg daily for 5 days) and plasma exchange have been shown to be similarly effective in accelerating the recovery, but do not significantly reduce mortality (1, 9, 10). IVIg has been found to be safer than PE, having a lower frequency of multiple complications (9). Thus, its efficacy, safety, and availability make IVIg the treatment of choice in many patients with GBS (9). A combination of plasma exchange and IVIg do not seem to produce significant extra benefit. Corticosteroids are not effective (10).

Chronic Inflammatory Demyelinating Polyneuropathy

Chronic inflammatory demyelinating polyneuropathy (CIDP) is a chronic acquired peripheral neuropathy, presumably of immunological origin. Both cell mediated and humoral processes have been suggested to play a role, but their extent and their target require further research and clarification (1).

Clinical Course

Typically, CIDP begins insidiously and evolves slowly, either in a steadily progressive or a relapsing-remitting manner, reaching its maximum severity after 8 weeks or more (compared to <4 weeks in AIDP) (11). The term subacute inflammatory demyelinating polyneuropathy has been used to describe an entity that progresses for 4–8 weeks (12). In three large series, symptoms at onset consisted of motor deficits (78–94% of patients), paresthesiae (64–79%), and pain (20–35%). At the chronic phase of the disorder motor deficits occur in 83–94%, sensory deficit in 72–89%, loss of tendon reflexes in 86–94%, and facial palsy in 4–15%, of patients. Dysautonomia is not a feature of CIDP (11).

Although a number of clinical similarities exist between the AIDP subtype of GBS and CIDP, there are also some important differences, such as the duration of disease progression and the response to treatment with corticosteroids. Table 78.3 compares some of the main clinical characteristics of AIDP and CIDP.

Diagnosis

The diagnosis of CIDP may be determined when a patient presents with a demyelinating polyneuropathy that progresses over more than 2 months, or evolves chronically over many months. The underlying demyelinating process is demonstrated by electrophysiological and, if needed, by pathological studies (e.g., sural nerve biopsy) (11). CSF examination may further support the diagnosis. As in AIDP, CSF is acellular or contains only a few mononuclear leukocytes (usually less than 10 cells/mm^3) and protein content is typically elevated. Yet, normal protein content is possible (found in up to 50% of patients, in some series) (11).

There are several proposed clinical and electrophysiological diagnostic criteria for CIDP. In 1991, an Ad Hoc Subcommittee of the American Academy of Neurology (AAN) proposed criteria for the diagnosis of CIDP that were to be used as a research tool. The AAN diagnostic criteria have been widely used in clinical practice and for inclusion in clinical trials. However, although the AAN electrodiagnostic criteria are highly specific, they are relatively insensitive and are fulfilled by only 50–60% of patients with typical clinical features of CIDP (11, 13). Since then, additional diagnostic criteria have been proposed. The newer INCAT (the Inflammatory Neuropathy Cause and Treatment group), Nicolas, and

Thaisetthawatkul criteria are as specific but more sensitive than the AAN criteria (13). Regardless of which criteria are chosen for use in clinical trials, patients who fall outside of these criteria (e.g., patients with normal electrophysiological studies) may still have CIDP and may benefit from immunomodulatory treatment (11, 13). Unfortunately, because of the lack of clarity with regard to the diagnostic criteria for CIDP, many patients remain untreated (13).

Treatment

Corticosteroids, intravenous immunoglobulins, plasma exchanges and immunosuppressive drugs are the main treatments used in this condition (1, 11, 14). The majority of patients will show an initial response to current treatments (11, 14). However, they fail to provide a durable clinical response (14). The relapsing form seems to carry a better prognosis than the progressive form (11).

Multifocal Motor Neuropathy

Multifocal motor neuropathy is a recently identified neuropathy characterized by slowly progressive, asymmetric limb weakness, usually affecting the upper limbs earlier (in about 70% of patients) and more severely than the lower limbs, with minimal or no sensory impairment (1, 15).

Epidemiology

The prevalence of MMN has been estimated to be approximately 1–2 per 100,000 (1, 16). Almost 80% of reported patients present their first symptoms between 20 and 50 years of age (1).

Pathogenesis

The pathogenesis of MMN is not completely known. Nevertheless the occurrence of serum antibodies, mostly IgM to the ganglioside GM1 in a proportion of patients ranging in different series from 25 to 80 % (15), and the frequent clinical improvement after immunological

TABLE 78.3. Comparison of the main clinical characteristics of AIDP and CIDP.

	AIDP	CIDP
Duration of disease progression	**<4 weeks**	**>8 weeks**
Wide spread polyneuropathy	present	present
High protein and absent or few cells in CSF	present	present
Demyelination	present	present
Secondary axonal damage	sometimes present	sometimes present
Antecedent infection	**2/3 of cases**	**16–32%**
Electrophysiological pattern	predominantly demyelinative	predominantly demyelinative
Association with auto-antibodies	not established	not established
Treatment with IVIg and PE	effective	effective
Treatment with corticosteroids	**ineffective**	effective

therapies suggest that the disease is immune mediated, even if the precise mechanism and the target antigens of this immune response are still unknown.

Diagnosis

A persistent, multifocal, partial motor conduction block (CB) is regarded as the neurophysiologic hallmark of MMN (1, 15). The American Association of Electrodiagnostic Medicine (AAEM) consensus criteria for definite CB (17) are: reduction of at least 50% in upper or 60% in lower limb proximal vs. distal compound muscle action potential (CMAP) amplitude with minimal temporal dispersion (no more than 30% increased CMAP duration).

However, applying these consensus criteria may result in under-diagnosis of the disorder in a subgroup of patients with MMN but without CB, who generally respond well to treatment (15, 16).

Treatment

Most patients with MMN respond to high-dose IVIg and some refractory patients have responded to cyclophosphamide. Glucocorticoids and PE are not effective (1).

Vasculitic Neuropathies

Peripheral neuropathy is a well-recognized consequence of systemic vasculitis, caused by vasculitic involvement of vasa nervorum resulting in nerve ischemia and Wallerian degeneration (18). Vasculitic neuropathies may be associated with primary vasculitis syndromes, such as polyarteritis nodosa, Churg-Strauss syndrome, and Wegener's granulomatosis, or with a vasculitis syndrome secondary to other systemic diseases, such as connective tissue disorders (e.g., rheumatoid arthritis and SLE) and malignancy (8, 18). In some cases (up to one third) of biopsy-proven vasculitic neuropathy, constitutional symptoms are absent and no underlying systemic disease can be detected (8), hence the name "nonsystemic" vasculitic neuropathy. However, clinically silent involvement of other organs is likely, and muscle biopsy often reveals vasculitic changes indicating that the underlying pathology is not confined to peripheral nerve (8).

Diagnosis

Recognition of vasculitis as the cause of peripheral neuropathy is important since the disorder is treatable. Systemic vasculitis should always be considered when mononeuropathy multiplex occurs in conjunction with constitutional symptoms, such as fever, anorexia, weight loss, malaise, and nonspecific pains. The diagnosis is straightforward in cases of known systemic vasculitis, but should also be considered in patients who otherwise seem healthy, since the neuropathy may be the first or only clinical manifestation of vasculitis (8).

Most patients have clinical features of mononeuropathy multiplex, with a subacute, progressive, generalized but asymmetric, painful, sensorimotor neuropathy (18). Laboratory tests often indicate features of systemic inflammation, such as an elevated sedimentation rate or positive anti-neutrophil cytoplasmic (ANCA) antibody, and electrophysiological studies shows multiple, asymmetric, axonal neuropathies. Nerve biopsy is necessary to establish the diagnosis in most cases, particularly in patients with "nonsystemic" vasculitic neuropathy (18).

Treatment

Long-term immunosuppressive therapy is required in most cases. High-dose prednisone combined with cyclophosphamide is standard initial therapy. In those with "nonsystemic" disease, cyclophosphamide should also be used if prednisone monotherapy is ineffective or the patient relapses with tapering (18). IVIg may be beneficial in cases of resistant vasculitic neuropathy (19).

Paraneoplastic Neuropathies

Paraneoplastic neuropathies are a heterogeneous group of autoimmune disorders, occuring in patients with cancer, most commonly small cell lung cancer, without a direct effect of the tumor mass or its metastases on the nervous system. They are associated in some patients with neuronal antibodies (mainly anti-Hu, less frequently anti-CV2). Paraneoplastic sensory neuronopathies are the most frequent, but there is often motor, autonomic, or central nervous system involvement as well. Neurologic symptoms often precede the detection of cancer. Therapy is directed at treating the cancer as well as suppressing the immune system response, but it is generally unsatisfactory.

References

1. Nobile-Orazio E. Treatment of dys-immune neuropathies. *J Neurol* 2005; 252: 385–95.
2. Cosi V, Versino M. Guillain-Barré syndrome. *Neurol Sci* 2006; 27(Suppl. 1): S47–51.
3. Hughes RA, Rees JH. Clinical and epidemiologic features of Guillain-Barré syndrome. *J Infect Dis* 1997; 176(Suppl. 2): S92–8.
4. Hughes RAC, Cornblath DR. Guillain-Barré syndrome. *Lancet* 2005; 366: 1653–66.
5. Shoenfeld Y, George J, Peter JB. Guillain-Barre as an autoimmune disease. *Int Arch Allergy Immunol* 1996; 109: 318–26.
6. Tishler M, Shoenfeld Y. Vaccination may be associated with autoimmune diseases. *Isr Med Assoc J* 2004; 6: 430–2.
7. Asbury AK, Cornblath DR. Assessment of current diagnostic criteria for Guillain-Barré syndrome. *Ann Neurol* 1990; 27: S21–4.

8. Crone C, Krarup C. Diagnosis of acute neuropathies. *J Neurol* 2007; 254: 1151–69.

9. Harel M, Shoenfeld Y. Intravenous immunoglobulin and Guillain-Barré Syndrome. *Clin Rev Allergy Immunol* 2005; 29: 281–7.

10. Hughes RA, Swan AV, Raphaël JC, Annane D, van Koningsveld R, van Doorn PA. Immunotherapy for Guillain-Barré syndrome: A systematic review. *Brain* 2007; 130: 2245–57.

11. Said G. Chronic inflammatory demyelinating polyneuropathy. *Neuromuscul Disord* 2006; 16: 293–303.

12. Oh SJ, Kurokawa K, de Almeida DF, Ryan HF Jr, Claussen GC. Subacute inflammatory demyelinating polyneuropathy. *Neurology* 2003; 61: 1507–12.

13. Sander HW, Latov N. Research criteria for defining patients with CIDP. *Neurology* 2003; 60: S8–15.

14. Ropper AH. Current treatments for CIDP. *Neurology* 2003; 60: S16–22.

15. Slee M, Selvan A, Donaghy M. Multifocal motor neuropathy: The diagnostic spectrum and response to treatment. *Neurology* 2007; 69: 1680–7.

16. Chaudhry V, Swash M. Multifocal motor neuropathy: Is conduction block essential? *Neurology* 2006; 67: 558–9.

17. Olney RK, Lewis RA, Putnam TD, Campellone JV Jr; American Association of Electrodiagnostic Medicine. Consensus criteria for the diagnosis of multifocal motor neuropathy. *Muscle Nerve* 2003; 27: 117–21.

18. Gorson KC. Vasculitic neuropathies: An update. *Neurologist* 2007; 13: 12–9.

19. Levy Y, Uziel Y, Zandman-Goddard G, Rotmen P, Amital H, Sherer Y, Langevitz P, Goldman B, Shoenfeld Y. Response of vasculitic peripheral neuropathy to intravenous immunoglobulin. *Ann N Y Acad Sci* 2005; 1051: 779–86.

79
Neuromylelitis Optica (Devic Syndrome)

Joab Chapman

Abstract Neuromyelitis optica (NMO), also known as Devic Syndrome, is defined clinically by severe inflammatory lesions in the optic nerves and spinal cord. Though it was lumped with multiple sclerosis for many years it is now a clearly defined disease entity by clinical, imaging and laboratory criteria. The main laboratory markers are high levels of antibodies to aquaporin 4 which is localized in the most affected areas. This disease may be the first of many to be separated out of the group of multiple sclerosis syndromes.

Keywords Neuromyelitis optica · Devic syndrome · aquaporin 4 · multiple sclerosis

The prototype of autoimmune disease which affects the white matter of the central nervous system is multiple sclerosis (MS). MS is defined by areas of inflammation in the white matter that are clinically associated with neurological deficits that relapse and remit over many years followed in many patients by progressive neuro-degeneration (1). Magnetic resonance imaging (MRI) allows visualization of the inflammatory lesions which are typically widely distributed in the periventicular and subcortical white matter and in the spinal cord. Though some laboratory findings such as oligoclonal IgG bands in the cerebrospinal fluid (CSF) and prolonged latencies of evoked potentials serve to confirm the diagnosis, there is no definitive laboratory test which can corroborate the clinical diagnosis. While it is believed that MS is an autoimmune disease, the lack of a definitive laboratory diagnosis of MS reflects the present lack of understanding of the cause of the disease and its exact pathogenesis. The current diagnostic criteria of MS have been recently re-defined (2, 11) (known as Mcdonald's criteria) but still depend almost exclusively on clinical and imaging findings and it is therefore more accurate to refer to MS as a syndrome than a disease. As a syndrome, our clinical definition of MS most likely includes a number of diseases with different causes and pathogenic mechanisms but have in common inflammatory damage to white matter tracts. Some of these diseases are probably genetic though a causative mutation for MS has not been found. An important step towards unraveling the different diseases making up the MS syndrome has been the definition of 4 clearly identifiable pathological pictures (3) each representing probably many separate disease entities.

One of syndromic variants of MS are a group of patients which have lesions confined to the optic nerve and spinal cord in a syndrome known as Devic and also named neuromyelitis optica (NMO) (4). This syndrome has raised much debate for many years, the key question being whether it represents a non-significant variation in the spectrum of MS or is a separate disease entity. The clinical data that supports NMO as a separate entity include the relatively specific involvement of the optic nerve and spinal cord by very severe clinical relapses which in many cases resolve only partially (4). This is also reflected in pathological studies which reveal areas of extensive necrosis which is unusual in MS. Imaging studies in NMO show extensive lesions of the spinal cord and relative sparing of the brain which also correlates with relative sparing of cortical function in these patients. Interestingly the major form of MS in Asia is more similar to NMO than western type MS.

The debate over NMO has been very much resolved over the past 5 years and it is now clear that it represents a well defined disease entity. The first major step forward was finding binding of NMO IgG to blood vessels in the brain and the development of a diagnostic test from this assay (5). This assay was found to correlate very well with the clinical manifestations of NMO which are clearly separate from MS. Further study of the NMO IgG found that it bound to a novel brain autoantigen, aquaporin-4 which is present at the astrocyte-endothelial junctions of the blood brain barrier (6) decrease in the levels of aquaporin-4 is also a very early and

From: Y. Shoenfeld et al. (eds.): *Diagnostic Criteria in Autoimmune Diseases*, DOI: 10.1007/978-1-60327-285-8_79,

TABLE 79.1. Diagnostic criteria for neuromyelitis optica NMO (9).

For definite (NMO) criteria require
1. optic neuritis,
2. myelitis, And at least two of three supportive criteria:
1. MRI evidence of a contiguous spinal cord lesion 3 or more segments, in length,
2. onset brain MRI nondiagnostic for multiple sclerosis
3. NMO-IgG seropositivity
CNS involvement beyond the optic nerves and spinal cord is compatible with NMO

significant stage in pathological NMO lesions which are clearly differentiated by this measure from MS lesions in histopathological studies (7). Oligoclonal IgG bands in the cerebrospinal fluid (CSF) are relatively uncommon in NMO relative to MS and may serve as an additional laboratory criteria for the disease (8). The currently accepted clinical criteria for NMO are detailed in the Table 79.1.

Myelitis is an anatomically defined autoimmune reaction occurring in the spinal cord. There are many causes of myelitis including an autoimmune reaction associated with viral infections, systemic autoimmune diseases such as systemic lupus erythematosus and sarcoid. The diagnosis is by clinical neurological and imaging evidence of damage to the spinal cord with a subacute course and associated with CSF pleocytosis and elevated protein. Many cases of myelitis are considered idiopathic and may be severe and recurrent. Since the clinical and laboratory diagnostic criteria for NMO have been re-defined (9), it has become apparent that some cases of severe recurrent longitudinally extensive myelitis fit the diagnosis of NMO (10).

The significant advances in diagnosing NMO and its variants offer a unique opportunity to develop specific and better therapies for this disease.

References

1. McDonald WI, Compston A, Edan G, et al. Recommended diagnostic criteria for multiple sclerosis: Guidelines from the International Panel on the diagnosis of multiple sclerosis. *Ann Neurol* 2001; 50(1): 121–7.
2. Polman CH, Reingold SC, Edan G, et al. Diagnostic criteria for multiple sclerosis: 2005 revisions to the "McDonald Criteria". *Ann Neurol* 2005; 58(6): 840–6.
3. Lucchinetti C, Bruck W, Parisi J, Scheithauer B, Rodriguez M, Lassmann H. Heterogeneity of multiple sclerosis lesions: Implications for the pathogenesis of demyelination. *Ann Neurol* 2000; 47(6): 707–17.
4. Mandler RN, Davis LE, Jeffery DR, Kornfeld M. Devic's neuromyelitis optica: A clinicopathological study of 8 patients. *Ann Neurol* 1993; 34(2): 162–8.
5. Lennon VA, Wingerchuk DM, Kryzer TJ, et al. A serum autoantibody marker of neuromyelitis optica: Distinction from multiple sclerosis. *Lancet* 2004; 364(9451): 2106–12.
6. Lennon VA, Kryzer TJ, Pittock SJ, Verkman AS, Hinson SR. IgG marker of optic-spinal multiple sclerosis binds to the aquaporin-4 water channel. *J Exp Med* 2005; 202(4): 473–7.
7. Roemer SF, Parisi JE, Lennon VA, et al. Pattern-specific loss of aquaporin-4 immunoreactivity distinguishes neuromyelitis optica from multiple sclerosis. *Brain* 2007; 130(Pt 5): 1194–205.
8. Bergamaschi R, Tonietti S, Franciotta D, et al. Oligoclonal bands in Devic's neuromyelitis optica and multiple sclerosis: Differences in repeated cerebrospinal fluid examinations. *Mult Scler* 2004; 10(1): 2–4.
9. Wingerchuk DM, Lennon VA, Pittock SJ, Lucchinetti CF, Weinshenker BG. Revised diagnostic criteria for neuromyelitis optica. *Neurology* 2006; 66(10): 1485–9.
10. Saiz A, Zuliani L, Blanco Y, Tavolato B, Giometto B, Graus F. Revised diagnostic criteria for neuromyelitis optica (NMO) : Application in a series of suspected patients. *J Neurol* 2007; 254(9): 1233–7.

80
Central Nervous System Vasculitis

Gisele Zandman-Goddard and Yehuda Shoenfeld

Abstract   Central nervous system (CNS) vasculitis refers to a spectrum of heterogeneous clinical disorders sharing the histopathology of blood vessel inflammation, leading to an array of neurological manifestations. We suggest a modified classification of CNS vasculitis: restricted to the CNS (Type I), associated with a systemic vasculitis as the predominant feature of an autoimmune disease (Type II), associated with other autoimmune diseases (Type III), associated with infectious diseases (Type IV), or associated with malignancies, drugs, and others (Type V). Type I CNS vasculitis is the most difficult to diagnose and is usually one of exclusion. We propose that magnetic resonance imaging (MRI)-guided biopsy should be the novel modification of the diagnostic criteria that includes clinical, laboratory, and imaging tests.

Keywords   CNS vasculitis · diagnostic criteria · classification · systemic vasculitis · autoimmune diseases · infections · malignancies · drugs

Introduction

Central nervous system (CNS) vasculitis refers to a spectrum of heterogeneous clinical disorders, sharing the histopathology of blood vessel inflammation and leading to an array of neurological manifestations related to ischemic injury to the brain involving the cortex, leptomeninges, and spinal cord. Immunopathogenic mechanisms incorporate leukocyte–endothelial interactions, immune complex injury, autoantibody damage, impairment of vascular tone, and alterations in coagulation. Whereas the systemic vasculitides are classically divided by the size of the blood vessels involved, CNS vasculitis has previously been dichotomized based on association with (secondary) or lack of (primary) other diseases. CNS vasculitis excludes a myriad of mimickers that are predominantly vasculopathies without evidence of inflammation. Because of the morbidity and mortality associated with the disease, and the potential utilization of immunosuppressive agents as the modality of therapy that harbor potential serious adverse events, it is imperative to assure a proper diagnosis (1, 2).

We suggest a modified classification of CNS vasculitis: restricted to the CNS (Type I), associated with a systemic vasculitis as the predominant feature of an autoimmune disease (Type II), associated with other autoimmune diseases (Type III), associated with infectious diseases (Type IV), or associated with malignancies, drugs, and others (Type V). In this chapter, we discuss the clinical and pathological manifestations of the different entities and the diagnostic criteria for this novel classification.

Classification of CNS Vasculitides (Table 80.1)

Type I (Primary, Isolated, Granulomatous)

Type I vasculitis presents equally in men and in women during the fourth to sixth decade. The classic presentation is progressive and cumulative with multifocal neurologic dysfunction. Headache and confusion are the most common presenting symptoms and the most common finding is hemiparesis. Ataxia of the limbs or gait and focal cortical dysfunction, including aphasia and seizures are also reported. To make the diagnosis even more difficult, every neurological symptom and sign has been reported in Type I CNS vasculitis. Nonspecific visual complaints occur in 15% of patients. Occasionally, patients present with multiple sclerosis-like disease or disease restricted to one portion of the nervous system. Perhaps, Type I vasculitis is a spectrum of disorders, which would explain the variability in clinical presentation and even response to therapy (3).

From: Y. Shoenfeld et al. (eds.): *Diagnostic Criteria in Autoimmune Diseases*, DOI: 10.1007/978-1-60327-285-8_80,
© 2008 Humana Press, Totowa, NJ

TABLE 80.1. Novel classification of CNS vasculitis.

Type	Other definition	Diseases
I	Isolated, primary, PACNS, granulomatous	None
II	Systemic vasculitis diseases as the predominant feature of autoimmune disease	PAN, MPA, CSS, WG, GCA, Takayasu's arteritis, Kawasaki disease
III	Other autoimmune diseases	SLE, SSc, RA, Sjögren's syndrome, MCTD, Behcet's, FMF, Cogan's syndrome, Susac syndrome
IV	Infectious diseases	Viral-VZV, HIV, CMV, HBV, HCV Bacterial-TB, Lyme, syphilis
V	Malignancies, drugs, and others	Malignancies – Hodgkin's and non-Hodgkin's lymphomas, hairy cell leukemia, neoplastic angioendotheliomatosis Drugs – Cocaine, opioids, amphetamines, and sympathomimetics including phenylpropanolamine, and methylphenidate.

CSS, Churg–Strauss syndrome; FMF, Familial Mediterannean Fever; GCA, giant cell arteritis; MPA, microscopic polyarteritis; PACNS, primary angiitis of the central nervous system; PAN, polyarteritis nodosa; WG, Wegener's granulomatosis.

The vascular inflammation is usually of a chronic granulomatous nature, with monocytes, histiocytes, lymphocytes, and plasma cells invading the walls of small arteries and veins, particularly in the leptomeninges. Larger vessels may be involved but are a minor portion of affected vessels. These pathological findings may distinguish Type I from Type II in that bifurcations are not affected and eosinophilia is not present, but fibrinoid necrosis may arise. The etiology and pathogenesis remains obscure.

Type II (Associated with Systemic Vasculitis as the Predominant Feature of an Autoimmune Disease)

The systemic vasculitides are a subset of autoimmune diseases characterized by a primary insult to the blood vessels resulting in inflammation and tissue ischemia of the various organs. The description of the various systemic vasculitides is beyond the scope of this chapter. CNS involvement in polyarteritis nodosa (PAN), occurs late in the progression of the disease, develops in up to 40% of patients, and is characterized by focal findings, (stroke and cerebral hemorrhage), diffuse manifestations such as seizures, and visual and oculomotor abnormalities (4, 5). In Churg–Strauss syndrome (CSS), a similar neuroclinical presentation to PAN is encountered, but less frequently, occurring in 25% of patients. In

Wegener's granulomatosis (WG), CNS involvement results from contiguous extension of the sinus granulomas, a small vessel vasculitis, or remote granulomas, and includes cranial neuropathies, cerebral hemorrhage, or thromboembolic events, but develops in 10% of patients (4, 5). Intracranial disease occurs infrequently in giant cell arteritis. Neuro-Behcet's syndrome occurs in up to 50% of patients, is more common in males, involves the small vessels with relapsing–remitting, disease sometimes progressive with focal or multifocal involvement (5). Headache (61.6%), upper motor neuron weakness (53.7%), brainstem, and cerebellar manifestations (49%) are most frequently reported (5). Patients with severe cases of hypersensitivity vasculitis (leukocytoclastic vasculitis) and occasionally patients with cryoglobulinemia types II and III develop seizures, encephalopathy, stroke, and cranial nerve involvement.

Type III (Associated with Other Autoimmune Diseases)

In the autoimmune diseases, the blood vessels are secondarily injured in the process of organ damage. Necrotizing and non-necrotizing vasculitides occur in systemic lupus erythematosus (SLE), systemic sclerosis (SSc), rheumatoid arthritis (RA), Sjögren's syndrome, and mixed connective tissue disease (MCTD). Among the autoimmune diseases, CNS involvement in SLE, occurring in 70% of patients, has been associated with 17 different focal or diffuse manifestations and 20 reported brain and systemic autoantibodies. Focal manifestations are more common in patients with secondary antiphospholipid syndrome (6).

Type IV (CNS Vasculitis Associated with Infections)

Viral, bacterial, fungal, and protozoan infections may cause vascular inflammation of the nervous system. Some of the infectious agents are associated with systemic vasculitis (hepatitis viruses); they may induce focal or diffuse neurological manifestations even in the absence of clinical systemic disease. Two worth noting are varicella zoster virus (VZV) and human immunodeficiency virus (HIV) infections. VZV can cause a large vessel vasculitis in immunocompetent patients leading to focal manifestations such as a stroke, following zoster of the contralateral trigeminal distribution, whereas small vessel vasculitis is encountered in immunocompromised patients as a progressive disease with fever, headache, seizures, and focal or multifocal deficits. The specific test for diagnosis is polymerase chain reaction (PCR) analysis and antibody testing of the cerebrospinal fluid (CSF) (4, 5).

HIV infection can cause a clinical picture of encephalitis or stroke. The neurological involvement can be the presenting feature of HIV infection, or AIDS. Complicating the issue, AIDS patients may develop a vasculitis as part of an opportunistic infection with VZV, cytomegalovirus (CMV), and toxoplasma. Furthermore, HIV patients may develop systemic vasculitis (7). The histopathology in these patients includes granulomatous, necrotizing, or eosinophilic vasculitis. Possibly, these reports incorporated patients with different types of vasculitis.

Type V (CNS Vasculitis Associated with Malignancies, Drugs, Others)

CNS vasculitis has been reported in individuals with lymphoma (Hodgkin's and non-Hodgkin's), hairy cell leukemia, neoplastic angioendotheliomatosis, and the pre-malignant lymphomatoid granulomatosis (1, 2). Cocaine, opioids, amphetamines, and sympathomimetics including phenylpropanolamine, and methylphenidate have been implicated in the development of CNS vasculitis. There are a number of causes for the CNS involvement among these individuals including histologically proven vasculitis and a higher incidence of co-infections with HIV, hepatitis B, and syphilis (1, 2, 5).

Diagnostic Procedures (Table 80.2)

There is a general consensus on the principles of the diagnosis of CNS vasculitis which is a potentially life-threatening disorder with increased morbidity due to irreversible

ischemia and infarction. Recognition of the neurological entities and excluding other diseases is of utmost importance because therapy will differ. Undiagnosed and untreated, the outcome of vasculitis is fatal. Absolute proof by tissue diagnosis is a prerequisite and without it empiric immunosuppressive therapy should not be instituted (3, 4, 5).

To establish the diagnosis of Type I CNS vasculitis, the guidelines are based on excluding the other types. This is successfully done by a systematic approach including the neurological, but also the non-neurological organ clinical assessment, appropriate hematological, chemistry, immunoserological and infectious disease serological laboratory tests, CSF analysis, neuroimaging, angiography, and magnetic resonance imaging (MRI)-guided biopsy.

Laboratory Tests

There is no specific laboratory test for the diagnosis of Type I CNS vasculitis. General laboratory tests are utilized for the purpose of excluding other types of CNS vasculitis and include complete blood count (CBC) and chemistry (SMAC). Coagulation screen, erythrocyte sedimentation rate (ESR), C reactive protein (CRP), complement levels, cryoglobulinemia, an autoantibody profile, angiotensin converting enzyme (ACE), and protein electrophoresis are useful for the diagnosis of Types II–III.

TABLE 80.2. Diagnostic procedures.

Description	Initial tests	Advanced procedure
General screening	CBC with differential, SMAC, ESR and CRP	Check for eosinophilia
Immunology serology	Appropriate immunoserological testing is recommended in the context of the clinical manifestations	HLA B5, pathergy test, EMG/NCV testing
		Peripheral nerve or organ involved biopsy (lung, kidney, temporal artery).
	ANA, anti-DNA Ab, ENA, anti-Scl 70, cANCA, pANCA, anti-MPO, anti-PR-3, HbsAg, anti-HCV	CSF analysis
CSF analysis	Cell count (pleocytosis of >5 cells/mm^3), protein elevation greater than 100 mg/dl, evidence of intrathecal synthesis of immunoglobulin and oligoclonal bands, acid-fast and immunoflorescence staining and culture, anti-Lyme Ab (ELISA, Western blot), VDRL, FTA-Abs, anti-varicella Ab, anti-HIV Ab (ELISA, Western blot), HbsAg, anti-HCV, cryoglobulins, culture and serology for protozoa and fungi, cytospin examination of the CSF for possible malignant cells.	Molecular genetic, immunoassay, and direct staining techniques to exclude spirochetal, fungal, mycobacterial, and viral infections, CSF PCR assay for *M. tuberculosis*, *Borrelia burgdorferi*, *T. pallidum*, VZV, HIV, HBV DNA, HCV RNA
Neuroimaging-MRI	The lesions are commonly bilateral and supratentorial; there may be involvement of the veins.	Enhancing of the perforating arteries and the meninges may be detected by MRI with injection of intravenous gadopentate dimeglumine
Angiography	Single or multiple areas of segmental narrowings and dilatations of the vessel, vascular occlusions, hazy vessel margins, and collateral formation.	
Brain biopsy	Segmental inflammation of small arteries and arterioles, intimal proliferation and fibrosis, with sparing of the media.	

ANA, antinuclear antibody (Ab); ANCA, -antineutrophil cytoplasmic Ab; CBC, complete blood count; CRP, C reactive protein; EMG, electromyography; ENA, extractable nuclear Ab; ESR, erythrocyte sedimentation rate; HBV, hepatitis B virus; HCV, hepatitis C virus; MPO, myeloperoxidase; NCV, nerve conduction study. SMAC, chemistry pannel.

PCR for infectious agents will aid in the diagnosis of Type IV CNS vasculitis. Hepatitis B and C screening will assist in the diagnosis of PAN (Type II).

CSF analysis is abnormal in 80–90% of patients. A mild lymphocytic pleocytosis and slightly elevated protein levels are most commonly detected, again being nonspecific. Furthermore, oligoclonal bands with an elevated IgG index, low glucose levels, and elevated leukocyte counts of several hundreds have all been reported. CSF analysis should include appropriate stains, cultures, serological tests, and cytology in order to establish the type of CNS vasculitis Some utilize serial CSF determination as a method for monitoring response to therapy (3, 5).

Neuroimaging

MRI is sensitive (50–100%) but not specific. Lesions suggestive of ischemia and inflammation will involve the cortex and white matter, some within known arterial territories. The lesions are commonly bilateral and supratentorial but have been described in the brainstem and cerebellar regions. There may be involvement of the veins (5, 8). Enhancing linear lesions corresponding to inflammation of the perforating arteries and enhancing of the meninges may be detected by MRI with injection of intravenous gadopentate dimeglumine (5, 8). An MRI should be performed to exclude multiple cerebral metastases, multicentric primary CNS tumors, hydrocephalus, and demyelinating diseases.

Analysis of CNS vasculitis with diffusion-weighted imaging and apparent diffusion coefficient mapping of the normal-appearing brain by conventional MRI has been reported to be advantageous in assessing CNS vasculitis, but cannot differentiate the type of vasculitis; hence further research is required (9, 10). Magnetic resonance angiography (MRA) currently remains an insufficient method to disclose fine vascular abnormalities frequently encountered in CNS vasculitis, and is not advantageous over conventional angiography. Functional imaging of the brain with single-photon-emission computerized tomography (SPECT) and positron-emission tomography (PET) may detect multifocal perfusion defects, have been widely investigated and utilized for the assessment of neuropsychiatric lupus, are usually evaluated in conjunction with MRI, but are not sensitive alone for the appropriate diagnosis, and are not specific for Type I CNS vasculitis. Electroencephalogram and brain computerized tomography are abnormal, nonspecific, and hence not recommended.

Angiography

The typical findings in cerebral angiography are single or multiple areas of segmental narrowings and dilatations along the course of the vessel, vascular occlusions, hazy vessel margins, and collateral formation. A prolonged circulation time can often be detected in the affected region (4). These findings are not specific for Type I CNS vasculitis and can be found in the other types and even in non-inflammatory vasculopathies. Complete reversal of abnormal angiographic findings is uncommon. The utilization of serial angiographies as follow-up in these patients is not established. The value of angiography is also not specific enough, and normal angiography results have been reported in many cases (3).

Brain Biopsy

Histological confirmation is the gold standard for the diagnosis of Type I and exclusion of the other types of CNS vasculitis. MRI-guided biopsy of enhancing lesions improves the sensitivity of the procedure substantially. In addition, biopsy that includes the leptomeninges, cortex, and subcortical tissue enhances the sensitivity of the diagnostic test. There is no significant difference between an open or sterotactic biopsy. There is a false-negative rate of 25% when the biopsy is blinded. False-positive findings are rare, but it is to be emphasized that the biopsy should be performed in the appropriate clinical, laboratory, and neuroimaging setting. Tissue sampling should be sent for culture and staining (11). MRI-guided brain biopsy including the leptomeninges is warranted. If a lesion is not visible, then a blinded biopsy from the non-dominant frontal or temporal pole including the leptomeninges is recommended (5).

The typical biopsy specimen reveals segmental inflammation of small arteries and arterioles, intimal proliferation, and fibrosis, with sparing of the media, and in some cases multinucleate giant Langerhans cells (12). The morbidity of brain biopsy is 2–3.3%, and hence the physician should not be deterred by this crucial procedure (5).

Diagnostic Criteria

Diagnostic criteria have been established by Calabrese in 1986 (13) and 1997 (3). They were modified by Moore (4) and recently by Svia (5) (Table 80.3). To properly diagnose CNS vasculitis, all of the criteria must be fulfilled. As in systemic vasculitis, the final diagnosis is based on histopathology. These criteria are based on the assessment of less than 200 patients that were reviewed in the literature over 20 years.

TABLE 80.3. Diagnostic criteria for CNS vasculitis (3, 4, 5).

Clinical	Features of a diffuse or focal CNS disease with a recurrent or progressive nature. Lasting at least 3 months.	Type I
	Evidence for an underlying systemic autoimmune disease	Types II–III
	Evidence for an underlying infection, malignancy, drug abuse, or other	Types IV–V
CSF	CNS inflammation	Type I
	CNS inflammation and infection	Type IV
	CNS inflammation and malignant cells	Type V
MRI		
Angiography	Segmental narrowing, ectasia, or beading	Type I
Brain biopsy	Vascular inflammation	Type I

Diagnostic Caveats

The utilization and interpretation of any one test whether it is physical exam, a blood test, neuroimaging, or tissue sampling are influenced by many factors and include the pre-test probability (11). The specificity and sensitivity of the diagnostic criteria for type I CNS vasculitis are shown in Table 80.4 (3, 5, 11). Type I CNS vasculitis is the most difficult to assess due to its rarity, the difficulty in obtaining adequate tissue sampling, and the necessity to exclude a multitude of other diseases. Calabrese et al. has evaluated this enigma extensively and reports in his seminal paper (3). The combination of normal MRI and normal CSF has a strong negative value and will exclude the possibility of CNS vasculitis in many patients (3).

The specificity and sensitivity of MRI-guided biopsy has not yet been reported but seems to increase the positive predictive value substantially. Hence, MRI-guided biopsy should be the novel modification of the diagnostic criteria. The importance of an added value of MRA and SPECT–PET has yet been to be established (14). As is shown in Table 80.4, only a combination of diagnostic modalities increases the sensitivity in establishing the proper diagnosis.

Therapy

The appropriate therapy for CNS vasculitis will be determined by the type of disease. The gold standard of therapy for Type I CNS vasculitis is high-dose steroids plus oral cyclophosphamide continued for 6–12 months after induction of remission. The limitation to evaluation of the beneficial potential of this modality of treatment is the rarity of disease, and possibly the difficulty of diagnosis. Upon establishing the underlying disease, appropriate therapy should be instituted for the systemic disorder. Thus, the treatment for Types II–III is based on the systemic autoimmune disease, and predominantly involves steroids and immunosuppressive agents. Intravenous immunoglobulin therapy has been beneficial in a few cases of patients with neuropsychiatric lupus (15). Antimicrobial agents should be utilized for type IV disease. Malignancies are treated by the chemotherapeutical protocol (3, 5).

TABLE 80.4. Sensitivity of diagnostic tests in Type I CNS vasculitis.

Test	Sensitivity (%)	Specificity (%)	PPV (%)	Comment
Abnormal CSF		40	37	
Abnormal CSF and biopsy	80–90			
Abnormal CSF and angiography	50–53	40		
MRI	77–100		43–72	Sensitivity may be increased with the FLAIR technique, enhancement of the leptomeninges, testing with SPECT or PET
MRI and biopsy	95–100			
MRI and angiography	75–80			
Angiography	100	26	37–50	Specificity may be increased if beading is found in multiple vessels in multiple vascular beds
Angiography and biopsy	60			
Blinded biopsy	74.4[a]	<100 (evaluate with the clinical picture)		
MRI guided biopsy	84		90–100	

[a] Reaching 87% if the biopsy includes the leptomeninges.
The combination of normal MRI and CSF test results has a strong negative predictive value and will exclude Type I CNS vasculitis, thus obviating the consideration for a brain biopsy (3).

References

1. Schmidley J.W. (2000) Central nervous system vasculitis. Chapter 57. Vascular disease of the nervous system. Bradley WG, Daroff RB, Fenichel GM, Marsden CD (eds.), *Neurology in Clinical Practice*. Boston, Butterworth Heinemann, pp. 1231–4.

2. Ropper A.H., Brown R.H. (2005) *Adam's and Victor's Principles of Neurology*, Eighth edition, New York, Mc-Graw-Hill Company, pp. 730–4.

3. Calabrese L.H., Duna G.F., Lie J.T. (1997) Vasculitis in the central nervous system. *Arthritis Rheum* 40: 1189–201.

4. Moore P.M., Richardson B. (1998) Neurology of the vasculitides and connective tissue diseases *J Neurol Neurosurg Psychiatr* 65: 10–22.

5. Siva A. (2001) Vasculitis of the nervous system. *J Neurol* 248: 451–68.

6. Zandman-Goddard G., Chapman J., Shoenfeld Y. (2007) Autoantibodies involved in neuropsychiatric SLE and antiphospholipid syndrome *Semin Arthritis Rheum* 36: 297–315.

7. Zandman-Goddard G., Shoenfeld Y. (2002) HIV and autoimmunity. *Autoimmun Rev* 1: 329–37.

8. Greenan T.J., Grossman R.I., Goldberg H.I. (1992) Cerebral vasculitis: MRI imaging and angiographic correlation *Radiology* 182: 65–72.

9. White M.L., Hadley W.L., Zhang Y. Dogar M.A. (2007) Analysis of central nervous system vasculitis with diffusion-weighted imaging and apparent diffusion coefficient mapping of the normal-appearing brain. *Am J Neuroradiol* 28: 933–7.

10. Hughes M., Sundgren P.C., Fan X., Foerster B., Nan B., Welsh R.C., et al. (2007) Diffusion tensor imaging in patients with acute onset of neuropsychiatric systemic lupus erythematosus: a prospective study of apparent diffusion coefficient, fractional anisotropy values, and eigen values in different regions of the brain. *Acta Radiol* 48: 213–22.

11. Calabrese L.H. (2002) Diagnostic strategies in vasculitis affecting the central nervous system. *Cleve Clin J Med* 69(Suppl. 2): SII105–8.

12. Lie J.T. (1997) Classification and histopathological spectrum of central nervous system vasculitis. *Neurol Clin* 15: 805–19.

13. Calabrese L.H., Mallek J.A. (1988) Primary angiitis of the central nervous system. *Medicine (Baltimore)* 67: 20–39.

14. Zhang, X., Zhu Z., Zhang F., Shu H., Li F., Dong Y. (2005) Diagnostic value of single-photon-emission computed tomography in severe central nervous system involvement of systemic lupus erythematosus: a case-control study. *Arthritis Rheum* 53: 845–9.

15. Zandman-Goddard G., Levy Y., Shoenfeld Y. (2005) Intravenous immunoglobulin therapy and systemic lupus erythematosus. *Clin Rev Allergy Immunol* 29: 219–228.

81
Autoimmune Epilepsy

Sarosh R. Irani and Bethan Lang

Abstract   Epilepsy is one of the most common neurological disorders; however, an underlying aetiology remains undetermined in the majority of cases. There is growing evidence of an autoimmune basis for a subset of epilepsies, and a number of antibodies have now been detected in the sera of patients with epilepsy. Many of these antibodies may not be pathogenic; however, those directed at ion channels or cell-surface receptors would be candidates in the direct causation of the disease. An example of such an antibody is the anti-voltage-gated potassium channel antibody. Other antibodies, such as those directed against glutamic acid decarboxylase, and neuronal gangliosides have a more uncertain role in aetiology but have been measured in many epileptics.

Keywords   Epilepsy · antibody · autoimmunity · voltage-gated potassium channel · glutamic acid decarboxylase

Introduction

Epilepsy affects around 0.5% of the population, making it one of the most common neurological diseases. Epilepsy can affect patients of all ages, with many cases proving significant therapeutic challenges. Although the clinical diagnosis of seizure episodes has been refined over many years, only the minority of patients can be given a specific underlying diagnosis to enable targeted treatment approaches. Such diagnoses are often based upon imaging technology, which allow the detection of underlying structural lesions such as vascular, malignant, traumatic and developmental insults. In addition, some of the remaining epilepsies are believed to have an underlying genetic aetiology. Such specific genes include those encoding potassium channels (benign familial neonatal convulsions) and nicotinic acetylcholine receptors (autosomal dominant nocturnal epilepsy). It is feasible to suggest that autoantibodies bind to and modulate the function of these and other ion channels, with a clinical phenotype similar to those produced by the genetic mutations. Hence, ion channels and surface receptors are now being implicated in the aetiology of autoimmune epilepsy.

Classification of Epileptic Syndromes

Many inconsistencies regarding the incidence of autoantibodies arise from the epilepsy literature and may be due to the technical and methodological differences used by the different laboratories to detect antibodies. Additionally, controversies in the systems used to classify the epilepsies may also account for some of the confusion encountered. Classification systems include those which are semiology based, dealing with the phenotype of seizures, or localisation-based, describing the cerebral anatomical origin of the seizure. In addition, some authors have suggested a treatment response classification for pragmatic management reasons. Utilisation of appropriate classification systems may allow for more accurate laboratory-based investigation of epilepsy and encourage some phenotype–antibody correlations to emerge.

Evidence for Autoimmunity in Epilepsy

Clinically, there is an increased incidence of epilepsy in many autoimmune diseases, including systemic lupus erythematosus, stiff-person syndrome (SPS) and type 1 diabetes (1). More specifically, a number of childhood epilepsies including Landau–Kleffner syndrome, West's syndrome and Lennox–Gastaut syndrome have been reported to respond well to intravenous immunoglobulin (IVIg), and sometimes steroid therapy. Furthermore, an HLA DR5 predisposition and increased serum immunoglobulin levels have been noted in Lennox–Gastaut syndrome.

From: Y. Shoenfeld et al. (eds.): *Diagnostic Criteria in Autoimmune Diseases*, DOI: 10.1007/978-1-60327-285-8_81,

TABLE 81.1. Autoantibodies in seizure disorders.

Antibody	Other associated diseases	Evidence for pathogenicity	Assay used to detect antibody
Anti-VGKC	Neuromyotonia, limbic encephalitis, Morvan's syndrome	Antibody titres fall in proportion to clinical improvements (2)	Radioimmunoassay using I^{125}-α-dendrotoxin (2)
Anti-GAD	Stiff-person syndrome, insulin-dependent diabetes mellitus, cerebellar ataxia	Sera from anti-GAD-positive patients down-regulates GABA currents (3)	Recombinant GAD65 used in an ELISA or iodinated in a radioimmunoassay (4)
Anti-NMDA	Limbic encephalitis, neuropsychiatric lupus	Nil	Transfected cell-based immunofluorescence (5).
Anti-GluR3	Rasmussen's encephalitis.	Active immunisation model (6).	ELISA using recombinant peptide (6). Radioimmunoassays have proved ineffectual in detecting GluR3 antibodies (7).

Below we discuss the main antibodies associated with epilepsy syndromes, their antigenic targets, methods for their detection and their likely relevance in disease pathogenesis (see Table 81.1).

Voltage-Gated Potassium Channel Antibodies

These antibodies were first described in the cramp fasciculation syndrome/neuromyotonia (NMT) spectrum of peripheral nervous system disease. Voltage-gated potassium channel antibodies (VGKCAbs) are seen in around 40% of these patients. Later, these antibodies were found in Morvan's syndrome, a rare combination of NMT with central nervous system (CNS) manifestations, which include cognitive impairment, hallucinations and autonomic disturbances.Most recently, VGKCAbs have been described in other CNS diseases: limbic encephalitis (LE) and epilepsy, using the same assay (2, 4). The highest titres of VGKCAbs are found in patients with acute or subacute onset of an encephalopathic disorder. Around 80% of these patients have seizures.

Autoantigen Definition

The Shaker family of VGKCs are composed of tetramers of Kv1 alpha subunits, each one associates with a beta subunit. In mammalian brain, the majority of Kv1 tetramers contain Kv1.1, Kv1.2, Kv1.4 and Kv1.6 and regulate the repolarisation properties of neuronal membranes. Kv1.1 may be the most important subunit in the CNS as Kv1.1 knockout mice develop spontaneous limbic seizures and show memory dysfunction, akin to patients with LE (8). Three of these subunits (Kv1.1, Kv1.2 and Kv1.6) bind alpha dendrotoxin (αDTX) with high specificity. αDTX is a neurotoxin derived from the venom from the green mamba (species *Dendroaspis*).

Autoantibody Definition

The Kv1 channels are responsible for membrane repolarisation following the depolarisation of the presynaptic terminal and subsequent release of neurotransmitter. Autoantibody binding to these Kv1 channels could cause channel dysfunction by pharmacological antagonism or by inducing channel down regulation. The lack of functional channels may result in prolonged depolarisation and neuronal hyperexcitability. In NMT, some groups have shown suppression of Kv1.6 currents with application of patient IgG (9). Furthermore, passive immunisation models have demonstrated transfer of IgG from NMT patients can electrophysiologically mimic the clinical syndrome of NMT (10). However, no such pathogenicity has yet been demonstrated with sera from patients with epilepsy.

Autoantibody Detection

VGKCs extracted from mammalian brain can be radiolabelled with I^{125}-αDTX and employed in a radioimmunoprecipitation assay. Briefly, serum, plasma or IgG is added to an aliquot of I^{125}-αDTX-labelled mammalian brain extract and, after a suitable incubation, precipitated by the addition of anti-human antisera and compared to the results obtained with healthy control serum. The results are usually reported in picomoles of I^{125}-toxin binding sites per litre of serum (pM). Values above 100 pM are reported as positive, with values above 400 pM being highly suggestive of CNS disease (2).

Clinical Utility

VGKCAbs can be associated with a spectrum of related CNS disorders, presenting with isolated seizures, cognitive impairment or a combination of the two. In a recent study of adult-onset epilepsy, 11% of patients had detectable VGKCAbs in their serum. Patients with higher titres were more commonly found to have a subacute, encephalopathic illness associated with their presentation, whilst those with lower titres tended to have less cognitive involvement (4). These low-titre VGKCAb-positive patients often suffered from "drug-resistant" temporal lobe epilepsy, a particularly difficult disease to manage. By analogy, patients presenting with LE show clinical hippocampal dysfunction, manifesting with amnesia and temporal lobe seizures, and concurrent MRI-proven mesial temporal lobe inflammation. The majority of these patients improve dramatically when promptly treated with corticosteroids. Seizures usually resolve before memory impairment, and clinical improvement is paralleled by a fall in VGKCAb tires (2). Thus, in the appropriate clinical setting, VGKCAbs may be considered a marker for the epileptic patients who are immunotherapy-responsive.

Glutamic Acid Decarboxylase Antibodies

Autoantigen Definition

Glutamic acid decarboxylase (GAD) is the rate-limiting enzyme in the synthesis of γ-aminobutyric acid (GABA) from glutamate. GABA is the major inhibitory neurotransmitter in the CNS. GAD exists in two isoforms: GAD 65 and 67. It is found predominantly in neurons but also in the β-cells of the pancreas. GAD is an intracellular protein, implying that antibodies against GAD would have to access the protein by traversing the intact cell membrane and are hence unlikely to have a pathogenic role.

Autoantibody Definition

Anti-GAD antibodies (anti-GAD Abs) were first described in around 40% of patients with insulin-dependent diabetes mellitus (IDDM) and in most patients with SPS. The antibody titres are much lower in IDDM than in SPS. Both of these conditions are associated with an increased risk of seizures, suggesting an association between anti-GAD Abs and epilepsy. Indeed, many more direct reports now exist. One early article described acute onset of drug refractory temporal lobe epilepsy in a young man. His seizures, refractory to multiple antiepileptic drugs, were eventually treated successfully with steroid therapy (11). In a survey of 100 patients with epilepsy, none of the patients with generalised epilepsy had anti-GAD Abs. However, from the patients with localisation-related epilepsy, 15% were anti-GAD Ab positive and 22% of these had very high titres, similar to SPS levels (12). By analogy with anti-VGKC Abs, these patients had temporal lobe epilepsy. This finding was confirmed in a larger study where high levels of anti-GAD Abs were also associated with drug-resistant temporal lobe epilepsy (4).

Autoantibody Detection

GAD reactivity in CNS disorders has traditionally been detected by immunohistochemical staining of GABA-rich regions of the brain, though this lacks specificity and quantification. ELISA methods using recombinant GAD protein as the immobilised antigen have been used, but now a commercially available radioimmunoassay using either I^{125}- or S^{32}-labelled recombinant GAD is available and provides a specific and quantitative assay.

Clinical Utility

Anti-GAD Abs appear in a number of diverse neurological syndromes from SPS and epilepsy to cerebellar ataxia and encephalomyelitis. Hence, they cannot be used without direct reference to the clinical syndrome. Occasional reports of low-level anti-GAD Abs in normal subjects, or those with a strong family history of diabetes, also cloud the utility of the assay alone. Despite these limitations, there are data suggestive of direct antibody pathogenicity. Cerebrospinal fluid (CSF) from a patient with high-level anti-GAD Abs was shown to suppress GABA-mediated transmission in cerebellar Purkinje cells (3). It was postulated that, in vivo, the GAD Abs would enter the cell via endocytosis and bind to the GAD in the cell cytoplasm, causing disruption of enzymatic activity.

Other Autoantibodies in Epilepsy

Anti-Ganglioside Antibodies

In an early report, anti-GM1 Abs have been detected, using ELISA techniques, in 4 of 64 of patients with epilepsy: again, all had partial seizures (13). Despite this finding not being replicated in a larger epileptic cohort (4), some older literature does suggest that intracerebral injection of anti-GM1 antiserum can produce seizures in rats which may be obviated by preadsorption against GM1 (14).

Anti-Glutamate Receptor Antibodies

Rasmussen's encephalitis (RE) is a chronic disease with refractory focal seizures, hemiparesis and encephalopathy. Early studies showed that rabbits immunised with glutamate receptor type 3 (GluR3), but not GluR1, 2, 5 or 6, fusion proteins developed encephalopathy, seizures and histopathological changes suggestive of RE (6). Since this finding, some groups have detected antibodies to GluR3 in sera from RE patients using ELISA. However, other groups were unable to confirm these findings using native protein expression techniques (7). More recent reports describe novel antigenic targets, including the alpha7 nicotinic subunit (15), suggesting possible heterogeneity in RE serology.

As with the anti-GluR3 Abs, antibodies directed against N-methyl D-aspartate (NMDA) receptors are excellent candidates to modulate CNS excitability. Indeed, a number of groups have detected antibodies against short peptide domains of NMDA subunits in patients with isolated epilepsy, using ELISA or western blotting (16). More recently, full-length NMDA heteromers have been expressed on the surface of mammalian cells shown to specifically bind antibodies from patients with seizures and paraneoplastic encephalitis (5). However, the pathogenic significance of such antibodies has not been fully investigated.

Others Autoantibodies

Antiphospholipid antibodies have been described at higher frequencies in epileptic populations, as have antibodies associated with coeliac disease, prompting successful treatment with a gluten-free diet (17). In addition, sera from epileptic patients have produced many as yet uncharacterised immunohistochemical staining patterns, using mammalian brain sections, suggesting other CNS Abs are pending characterisation.

Treatment and Prognosis

At the present time, only a few patients with pure autoimmune epilepsy have been treated with immunosuppressive therapies. However, drawing on paradigms from other antibody-associated CNS diseases, in particular non-paraneoplastic LE, there does seem to be benefit in the use of corticosteroids as first-line therapy. This can be supplemented with intravenous immunoglobulins (IVIg) or plasma exchange as required. As many of the antiepileptic "drug-resistant" epileptics are a particularly difficult group to manage, the novel use of immunosuppression in this population may impact favourably upon their prognosis.

Conclusions

Anti-neuronal antibodies are commonly detected in epileptic patients. Many such antibodies are directed against plausible epileptogenic targets including ion channels, such as voltage-gated potassium channels, and receptors, for example glutamate receptors. Although technical differences are likely to account for the discrepancies in findings between studies, a consistent emerging finding is the presence of anti-VGKC and anti-GAD antibodies in a significant proportion of the epileptic population. We await data to establish the pathogenicity of these antibodies.

References

1. Palace J, Lang B. (2000) Epilepsy: an autoimmune disease? *J Neurol Neurosurg Psychiatr* 69, 711–4.
2. Vincent A, Buckley C, Schott JM, Baker I, Dewar BK, Detert N, et al. (2004) Potassium channel antibody-associated encephalopathy: a potentially immunotherapy-responsive form of limbic encephalitis. *Brain* 127, 701–12.
3. Mitoma H, Song SY, Ishida K, Yamakuni T, Kobayashi T, Mizusawa H. (2000) Presynaptic impairment of cerebellar inhibitory synapses by an autoantibody to glutamate decarboxylase. *J Neurol Sci* 175, 40–4.
4. McKnight K, Jiang Y, Hart Y, Cavey A, Wroe S, Blank M, et al. (2005) Serum antibodies in epilepsy and seizure-associated disorders. *Neurology* 65, 1730–6.
5. Dalmau J, Tuzun E, Wu HY, Masjuan J, Rossi JE, Voloschin A, et al. (2007) Paraneoplastic anti-N-methyl-D-aspartate receptor encephalitis associated with ovarian teratoma. *Ann Neurol* 61, 25–36.
6. Rogers SW, Andrews PI, Gahring LC, Whisenand T, Cauley K, Crain B, et al.(1994) Autoantibodies to glutamate receptor GluR3 in Rasmussen's encephalitis. *Science* 265, 648–51.
7. Watson R, Jiang Y, Bermudez I, Houlihan L, Clover L, McKnight K, et al. (2004) Absence of antibodies to glutamate receptor type 3 (GluR3) in Rasmussen encephalitis. *Neurology* 63, 43–50.
8. Smart SL, Lopantsev V, Zhang CL, Robbins CA, Wang H, Chiu SY, et al. (1998) Deletion of the K(V)1.1 potassium channel causes epilepsy in mice. *Neuron* 20, 809–19.
9. Nagado T, Arimura K, Sonoda Y, Kurono A, Horikiri Y, Kameyama A, et al. (1999) Potassium current suppression in patients with peripheral nerve hyperexcitability. *Brain* 122, 2057–66.
10. Sinha S, Newsom-Davis J, Mills K, Byrne N, Lang B, Vincent A. (1991) Autoimmune aetiology for acquired neuromyotonia (Isaacs' syndrome). *Lancet* 338, 75–7.
11. Giometto B, Nicolao P, Macucci M, Tavolato B, Foxon R, Bottazzo GF. (1998) Temporal-lobe epilepsy associated with glutamic-acid-decarboxylase autoantibodies. *Lancet* 352, 457.
12. Peltola J, Kulmala P, Isojarvi J, Saiz A, Latvala K, Palmio J, et al. (2000) Autoantibodies to glutamic acid decarboxylase in patients with therapy-resistant epilepsy. *Neurology* 55, 46–50.
13. Bartolomei F, Boucraut J, Barrie M, Kok J, Dravet C, Viallat D, et al. (1996) Cryptogenic partial epilepsies with anti-GM1 antibodies: a new form of immune-mediated epilepsy? *Epilepsia* 37, 922–6.
14. Karpiak SE, Graf L, Rapport MM. (1976) Antiserum to brain gangliosides produces recurrent epileptiform activity. *Science* 194, 735–7.
15. Watson R, Jepson JE, Bermudez I, Alexander S, Hart Y, McKnight K, et al. (2005) Alpha7-acetylcholine receptor antibodies in two patients with Rasmussen encephalitis. *Neurology* 65, 1802–4.
16. Ganor Y, Goldberg-Stern H, Lerman-Sagie T, Teichberg VI, Levite M. (2005) Autoimmune epilepsy: distinct subpopulations of epilepsy patients harbor serum autoantibodies to either glutamate/AMPA receptor GluR3, glutamate/NMDA receptor subunit NR2A or double-stranded DNA. *Epilepsy Res* 65, 11–22.
17. Harper E, Moses H, Lagrange A. (2007) Occult celiac disease presenting as epilepsy and MRI changes that responded to gluten-free diet. *Neurology* 68, 533–4.

82
Autoimmune Chorea

Ziv Paz, Yehuda Shoenfeld and Joab Chapman

Abstract   Chorea is a movement disorder characterized by involuntary arrhythmic movement of a forcible, rapid, jerky type. The differential diagnosis of chorea is wide and finding the specific cause can be a challenging task. Autoimmune chorea can result from various immunological mechanisms. Sydenham chorea (SC) is a prototype of this group of diseases but other autoimmune conditions also present with chorea. This chapter reviews the autoimmune causes of chorea, defining diagnostic criteria based on clinical presentation and serological markers.

Keywords   Chorea · movement disorder · Sydenham chorea · Chorea gravidarum · antiphospholipid syndrome · SLE

Chorea is derived from the Greek word for dance. Chorea refers to involuntary arrhythmic movements of forcible, rapid, jerky type. The movements may be simple or quite complex. It is important to appreciate the difference between chorea and myoclonus, which present as a faster involuntary movement, involving single or several muscles or part of a single muscle.

Diseases characterized by chorea are listed in Table 82.1. Huntington chorea is a well-known disease presenting with chorea; the gene mutation was located to chromosome 4. However, the scope of this chapter is to discuss the acquired autoimmune etiologies for chorea.

Epidemiology

A review published by Piccolo and colleagues (1) describes the frequency of different causes of chorea. Of 23 cases admitted with chorea to two general hospitals, 5 were drug induced, 5 were AIDS related, and 6 were due to stroke. Sydenham chorea (SC) and arthritis were each found in one case. In four cases the etiology was not determined and only one patient had Huntington chorea.

Pathogenesis

The anatomic basis of chorea is inconsistent. In Huntington chorea, the involvement of the caudate nucleus and putamen is well established. Yet it is not uncommon to

TABLE 82.1. Diseases characterized by chorea.

Inherited disorders
Huntington disease
Benign hereditary chorea
Neuroacanthocytosis
Dentatorubropallidoluysian atrophy
Wilson disease
Rheumatic chorea
Sydenham chorea
Chorea gravidarum
Drug-induced chorea
Neuroleptic
Oral contraceptive
Phenytoin
L dopa and dopamine agonist
Cocaine
Chorea and systemic diseases
Systemic lupus erythematosus
Antiphospholipid syndrome
Thyrotoxicosis
AIDS
Paraneoplastic
Polycythemia vera
Stroke

observe lesions in these regions, such as old infarcts without chorea. Beyond a general dysfunction of the striatum, the precise localization of lesions in SC and other choreic diseases need to be determined.

From: Y. Shoenfeld et al. (eds.): *Diagnostic Criteria in Autoimmune Diseases*, DOI: 10.1007/978-1-60327-285-8_82,

Rheumatic Chorea

Two clinical entities are considered under this title: SC and chorea gravidarum.

Sydenham Chorea

SC is also known as St. Vitus dance, St. Johannis chorea, chorea minor, and rheumatic chorea. SC is a major manifestation of acute rheumatic fever and the most common cause of acquired chorea in childhood.

Epidemiology

The incidence of rheumatic fever and SC have declined significantly since the introduction of antibiotic treatment for streptococcal pharyngitis. However, SC is still common in developing countries and in untreated patients with rheumatic fever. In the United States, chorea complicates 18–36% of cases with rheumatic fever (2, 3). The average age at presentation is between 5 and 13 with female preponderance. Familial predisposition was described in the old literature (4).

Pathophysiology

SC is strongly associated with group A streptococcal infection. This condition is thought to be a result of autoantibodies directed originally against the pathogen antigenic component but eventually cross-react with the host antigen.

This phenomenon is called molecular mimicry. Antibodies against N-acetyl-β-D-glucosamine (NABG), a carbohydrate antigen of group A streptococci, are considered to be the mediators that lead to the different clinical manifestation of acute rheumatic fever. When these antibodies bind to lysoganglioside on the neuronal cell surface (5) and/or interact with the intercellular motor protein tubulin (6), chorea is induced. Involvement of different structures in the basal ganglia is supported by neuropathological (7) and MRI studies (8).

Clinical Manifestation

Classically chorea appears months after streptococcal pharyngitis (not associated with streptococcal skin infection) and often associated with hypotonia, emotional lability and regression in school performance.

The chorea typically starts with the hands but evolve to generalized involvement of face and feet; 20% of patients remain with hemichorea. Motor abnormalities distributed to the face, tongue, and eyes are well documented. Hypotonia can be severe.

Psychiatric symptoms range from crying and restlessness to increase association with obsessive-compulsive disorder (9) and attention deficit hyperactivity disorder (ADHD) (10). Chorea can be the only symptom of the rheumatic disease, but clinical carditis (28%), echocardiography carditis (63%), and arthritis (17%) are frequently present.

Diagnostic Criteria (Table 82.2)

SC is a clinical diagnosis. There are no specific blood or cerebrospinal fluid (CSF) tests for this diagnosis. Chorea is a symptom of many diseases and it is important to rule in or out other etiologies (Tables 82.1 and 82.2). Because the neurological and psychiatric manifestations are not specific, other criteria should be considered.

Evidence of Streptococcal Infection

Throat cultures are usually negative and the proof for streptococcal infection depends on the presence of specific antibodies. A rise in antistreptolysin O (ASLO) titer is seen on 80% of cases, with peak levels detected 4–5 weeks after the acute pharyngeal infection, weeks or months before the presentation of chorea. Anti-DNAse B is more sensitive marker and is elevated for a longer time; in one study (11) it was found positive in 98% of patients.

Cardiac Involvement in Sydenham's Chorea (12)

Only in 23% of patients with SC, carditis is detected clinically or by auscultation. Echocardiography helps to detect silent valvular disease in additional 40% of patients.

TABLE 82.2. Diagnostic criteria for Sydenham chorea.

1. Chorea (100%)
2. Evidence of streptococcal infection:
   –ASLO titer (76%)
   –Anti-DNAse B (98%)
3. Carditis
   –Auscultation findings (23%)
   –Echocardiographic findings (63%)
4. Exclusion of other possible etiologies (Table 82.1)
   –Serum copper
   –Ceruloplasmin
   –ANA
   –Family history (Huntington disease)

Prognosis

SC is a self-limited condition; the improvement is gradual with a mean duration of 3–6 months; sometimes it takes more than 2 years. The treatment is reserved for severe cases with a significant motor impairment.

Treatment

There are no controlled studies; however, the drug of choice is valproic acid (13). There are a number of reports on other antiepileptics and pimozide (dopamine receptor antagonist). Steroids are reserved for refractory, severe cases. There are anecdotical reports of the successful use of plasma exchange and IvIg (14). Antibiotic therapy with penicillin is recommended for at least 10 days in all cases. Antibiotic prophylaxis with penicillin should be continued until adulthood.

Chorea Gravidarum

The first description in the literature was cited in the name of Horstius in 1661; the first review was published by Wilson and Preece (15). Chorea gravidarum is a description of chorea from any cause which appears during pregnancy months. The most common causes are rheumatic fever and antiphospholipid syndrome (APS), but one should consider other causes of chorea (Table 82.1). The second trimester and the postpartum period are the most susceptible times; the treatment is directed to the underlying etiology.

Autoimmune Diseases and Chorea

Movement disorders are seen in less than 5% of patients with systemic lupus erythematosus (SLE). There is a strong association with antiphospholipid antibodies in these patients (16). Chorea is the most common movement disorder in SLE patients, treatment should be hold unless there are other indications for treatment, as chorea is a self-limited symptom.

Chorea is also seen in APS. When chorea develops during pregnancy (chorea gravidarum), after delivery or induced by oral contraceptive, one should consider the possibility of APS and look for the existence of antiphospholipid antibodies.

In 50 patients with APS (17), most (66%) presented with one episode of chorea. CT and MRI reported cerebral infarcts in 35% of patients. Patients respond to variety of medications including steroids, haloperidol, antiaggregants, anticoagulants, or combination of therapy and of course to oral contraceptive discontinuation if this was the cause.

Autoimmune chorea has also been reported in the context of paraneoplastic syndromes associated with anti-Hu and anti-CRMP5 antibodies in rare cases with small cell lung carcinoma (18, 19).

AIDS has emerged as a significant cause of chorea (1). The common causes are focal involvement of basal ganglia with toxoplasmosis, lymphoma, and progressive multifocal leukoencephalopathy (PML), but in increasing number of instances the cause remains obscure and underlying autoimmune mechanism is suggested.

References

1. Piccolo I, Sterzi R, Thiella G, et al. Sporadic choreas: Analysis of a general hospital series. *Eur Neurol* 1999; 41(No. 3): 143–149.
2. Veasy, LG, Tani, LY, Hill, HR. Persistence of rheumatic fever in intermountain area of the United States. *J Pediatr* 1994; 124: 9–16.
3. Stollerman, GH. Rheumatic fever. *Lancet* 1997; 349: 935–942.
4. Read, FE, Ciocco, A, Toussey, HB. The frequency of rheumatic manifestation among siblings, parents, uncles, aunts and grandparents of rheumatic and control patients. *Am J Hyg* 1938; 27: 719.
5. Husby, G, Van de Rijn I, Zabriskie, JB, et al. Antibodies reacting with cytoplasm of subthalamic and caudate nuclei neurons in chorea and acute rheumatic fever. *J Exp Med* 1976; 144: 1094.
6. Kirvan, CA, Cox, CJ, Swedo, Se, Cunningham, MW. Tubulin is the neuronal target of autoantibodies in Sydenham's chorea. *J Immunol* 2007; 178: 7412.
7. Lange, H, Thorner, G, Hopf, A, Schroder, KF. Morphometric studies of the neuropathological changes in choreatic diseases. *J Neurol Sci* 1976; 28: 401.
8. Giedd, JN, Rapoport, JL, Kruesi, MJ, et al. Sydnham's chorea: magnetic resonance imaging of the basal ganglia. *Neurology* 1995; 45: 2199.
9. Swedo, SE, Rapoport, JL, Cheslow, DL, et al. High prevalence of obsessive compulsive symptoms in patients with Sydenham's chorea. *Am J Psychiatry* 1989; 146: 246.
10. Maia DP, Cardoso FE, Cunningham MC, Teixeira AL. Obsessive – Compulsive behavoior and hyperactivity and attention deficit disorder in Sydenham chorea. *Neurology* 2004; 62: A203.
11. Carapetis, JR, Currie, BJ. Rheumatic chorea in northern Australia: a clinical and epidemiological study. *Arch Dis Child* 1999; 80: 353.
12. Elevli, M, Celebi, A, Tombul, T, Gokalp, AS. Cardiac involvement in Sydenham's chorea: clinical and Doppler echocardiographic findings. *Acta Paediatr* 1999; 88: 1074.
13. Dhanaraj, M, Radhakrishnan, AR, Srinivas, K, Sayeed, ZA. Sodium valporate in Sydenham's chorea. *Neurology* 1985; 35: 114.
14. Jordan LC, Singer HS. Sydenham chorea in children. *Curr Treat Options Neurol* 2003; 5: 283–390.
15. Wilson P, Preece AA. Chorea gravidarum. *Arch Intern Med* 1932; 49: 471–533.

16. Asherson, RA, Derken, RH, Harris, EN, et al. Chorea in SLE and "lupus like" disease: association with antiphospholipis antibodies. *Semin Arthritis Rheum* 1987; 16: 253.

17. Cervera, R, Asherson, RA, Font, J, et al. Chorea in the antiphospholipid syndrome. Clinical, radilogic and immunologic characteristics of 50 patients from our clinics and the recent literature. *Medicine* 1997; 76: 203–212.

18. Dorban S, Gille M, Kessler R, et al. Chorea- athetosis in the anti- Hu syndrome. *Rev Neurol (Paris)* 2004; 160: 126–129.

19. Kinirons P, Fulton A, Keoghan M, et al. Paraneoplastic limbic encephalitis (PLE) and chorea associated with CRMP- 5 neuronal antibody. *Neurology* 2003; 61: 1623–1624.

83
Autoimmune Sensorineural Hearing Loss

Aharon Kessel and Elias Toubi

Abstract   Autoimmune sensorineural hearing loss (ASNHL) is typically presented by a bilateral rapidly progressive hearing loss that may also occur suddenly. Both autoantibodies and autoreactive T cells have been implicated in the etiopathogenesis of ASNHL. However, the identity of a specific or highly relevant inner-ear self-antigen is still required. A definite diagnosis of ASNHL is usually made by excluding ototoxicity, and other factors that mimic ASNHL but most importantly by demonstrating a good therapeutic response to corticosteroid treatment.

In this chapter, we will summarize many of the current studies that have established the idea of ASNHL being autoimmune in many cases. Also, we will address the need for specific diagnostic tools to better classify/diagnose this entity. These tools may lead to the development and application of immuosuppressive therapies to prevent the deterioration of hearing loss and could possibly prevent the requirement for cochlear implantation.

Keywords   Hearing loss · autoimmunity · anti-phospholipid antibodies

Introduction

Sudden or progressive sensorineural hearing loss (SSNHL/PSNHL) is a pathology characterized by the sudden onset or progressive (over several months and some times days/weeks) of auditory impairment. It is considered idiopathic in most cases, but may have genetic or acquired factors such as viral infections, vascular diseases, ototoxic drugs and autoimmune diseases.

The possibility that part of the previously considered idiopathic SSNHL or PSNHL were autoimmune in origin was first noted by Lehnhardt in 1958. He reported a patient, in whom progressive hearing loss became bilateral when auditory deficit occurred in one ear in the past. He suggested that degeneration of inner-ear tissues in one ear led to the production of anti-cochlear antibodies that eventually damaged the second ear. This assumption challenged the theory of the inner ear being an immunologically privileged site due to a blood–labyrinthine barrier.

Further support for this assumption was derived from a seminal study by McCabe (1), in which immunosuppressive therapy with corticosteroids and cyclophosphamide improved PSNHL rapidly. He and others believed that autoimmune SNHL (ASNHL) is mediated by inner-ear specific autoreactive T cells. However, other studies provided evidences for a humoral (autoantibody)-mediated response against inner-ear antigens (2).

The recognition of autoimmunity in patients with SSNHL and PSNHL was supported by the following: (a) Sera of these patients contain reactive autoantibodies against different inner-ear proteins such as those of 28, 42 and 68 kDa (3). (b) Disease-related autoantibodies such as: anti-dsDNA, anti-thyroid (ATA), anti-cardiolipin antibodies (aCL) and rheumatoid factor (RF) were detected in sera of these patients. (c) Many trials have shown that prompt administration of corticosteroids and/or Methotrexate double the likelihood of hearing recovery. (d) Inner ear damage has been developed in animal models after immunization with heterologous cochlear antigens and immune adjuvant. (e) Inner ear pathology was documented to be part of the SLE-like phenomena, known to develop spontaneously in the MRL-lpr/lpr mice. (f) Increased infiltration of both CD4+ and CD8+ T cells were observed in patients who were highly suspected to have ASNHL.

Sudden SNHL and PSNHL were also described as a result of microthrombosis and in association with anticardiolipin antibodies, suggesting that this organ-specific defect could be a presenting symptom of a primary anti-phospholipid syndrome. In this chapter, we will

From: Y. Shoenfeld et al. (eds.): *Diagnostic Criteria in Autoimmune Diseases*, DOI: 10.1007/978-1-60327-285-8_83,
© 2008 Humana Press, Totowa, NJ

summarize the data related to the autoimmune origin of PSNHL and SSNHL, and discuss the need for a standardized evaluation of such patients, such as the creation of some diagnostic criteria that could improve the ability to decide when and how to treat these patients.

T-Cell Mediated Autoimmunity in SNHL

A role for autoreactive T cells in the pathogenesis of PSNHL was reported two decades ago by McCabe (4). He reported on leukocyte migration inhibition (LMI) in response to inner-ear membrane in activated PBMC from 54 patients in whom ASNHL was suggested. The LMI assay used to be acceptable for measuring the ability of activated antigen-specific T cells to prevent macrophage migration in vitro. This assay is not used currently, but at the time it was in use it indicated that T-cell responses to inner-ear antigens should be considered when pathogenesis of SNHL is studied.

In another previous study by Hughes et al. (5), he implicated T-cell autoreactivity in ASNHL by demonstrating that PBMCs from these patients developed proliferative responses when incubated with human inner-ear homogenate. In this study, it was shown that PBMC from 13 of 58 (22%) patients with unilateral or bilateral SNHL responded to human inner-ear antigens. In comparison, PBMC proliferation to the same antigens was demonstrated in only 1 of 15 (7%) normal control subjects. Later, the flow cytometer assay was used to analyze intracellular cytokine levels in peripheral blood from 19 patients with PSNHL and in 26 patients with Meniere's disease (MD), compared with that obtained from age and gender-matched healthy volunteers (6). The patients with PSNHL showed significantly increased levels of Th1 subsets (Interferon-gamma producing T cells) when compared with those in normal controls. The patients with MD showed significantly increased natural killer (NK) cell activity but no Th1 dominance. These results were further proofs for the role of T-cells and NK cells in the development of ASNHL.

In accordance with the above, it was shown by ELISPOT analysis that compared with normal hearing age-and sex-matched control subjects, ASNHL patients have significantly higher frequencies of circulating T cells producing either IFN-gamma ($p = 0.0001$) or IL-5 ($p = 0.03$) in response to recombinant human cochlin (7). In some patients, cochlin responsiveness involved both CD4+ and CD8+ T cells, whereas other patients showed cochlin responsiveness confined to CD8+ T cells. In this regard, the efficacy of tumor necrosis factor-alpha blockade in treating patients with ASNHL was shown by demonstrating the arrest of hearing loss, pointing to the beneficial effect of targeting cellular immunity in patients with ASNHL (8).

The inner ear-specific proteins cochlin and beta-tectorin were shown to be capable of targeting experimental autoimmune hearing loss in mice (9). Five weeks after immunization of SWXJ mice with either Coch 131–150 or beta-tectorin 71–90, auditory brainstem responses showed significant hearing loss at all frequencies tested. Flow cytometry analysis showed that each peptide selectively activated CD4+ T cells with a proinflammatory Th1-like phenotype. The adoptive transfer of peptide-activated CD4+ T cells into naïve SWXJ mice was followed by a significant hearing loss, providing a confirmation that ASNHL is a T-cell-mediated organ-specific autoimmune disorder.

The expression of Fas ligand (FasL) in some non-lymphoid tissue, as in the anterior chamber of the eye, has been hypothesized to play a role in protecting the sensitive organs from activated T-cells. Bodmer et. al. (10) showed that under resting conditions, cochlear cells express little or no Fas L. However, FasL was upregulated in adult cochlear cells after induction of a sterile labyrinthitis in vivo. The induction of FasL by inflammation may serve to limit cochlear immune responses and protect sensorineural tissue from immune and autoimmune damage. Thus defects in FasL expression could facilitate the induction of autoreactive T-cell response and the development of ASNHL.

A summary of T-cell-mediated autoimmunity is shown in Figure 83.1.

Humoral (Autoantibody) Response in SNHL

Various non-specific autoantibodies such as anti-nuclear antibodies (ANAs), anti-neutrophil cytoplasmic antibodies (ANCAs) and anti-endothelial antibodies (AEAs) were widely reported in patients with ASNHL. These antibodies were suggested to function as cross-reacting antibodies that could possibly recognize inner-ear proteins. However, looking into the autoantigens' origin in ASNHL, many specific antigens were proposed to play a role in this organ-specific autoimmune disease (Table 83.1). The inner ear (namely the endolymphatic hydrops) was already shown in earlier studies to contain several inner-ear antigens, against which specific IgG was frequently found in the sera of both SSNHL and PSNHL patients (11).

In a further attempt to identify the main target antigens for autoantibodies reactive against guinea pig inner-ear proteins, sera from 110 patients with a clinical diagnosis of either PSNHL ($n = 32$), MD ($n = 41$), SSNHL ($n = 6$) or other aetiologies of hearing loss ($n = 11$) were screened by Western blot technique (12). Forty-four percent of the patients' sera had antibodies to several inner-ear proteins, of which the 30, 42 and 68 kDa proteins were found the most reactive. These proteins were demonstrated to be the major peripheral myelin protein PO and the beta-actin protein,

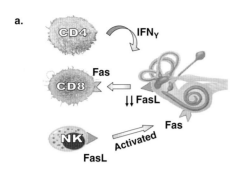

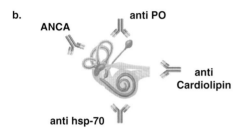

FIGURE 83.1. (a) Cochlear tissues are attacked by autoreactive T cells: Over production of IFN-gama by CD4+, cytotoxic activity of CD8+ cells due to the attenuation of Fas-L expression on cochlear membranes and the inability of eliminating T-cell invasion into inner ear tissues. NK cell activity via Fas-FasL pathway. (b) The wide range of autoreactive antibodies against inner ear antigens and also cross-reacting autoantibodies against other self-antigens.

respectively, while sequence analysis indicated that the 68-kDa protein was novel.

Furthermore, the presence of IgG antibodies against PO antigens in patients affected by sudden hearing loss and MD was evaluated in a most recent study (13). Specifically, the PO positive band was detectable in 5 of 45 patients with unilateral auditory impairment and in 5 of 5 of those with bilateral forms. Among MD patients, the PO positive band was detectable only in those with bilateral audio-vestibular impairment ($n = 10$). The positive reactions to PO in all bilateral sudden deafness patients found in this study strongly indicate that these pathologies are the result of an ongoing autoimmune process directed against specific antigens of the inner ear.

Harris and Sharp were the first to use Western blot analysis of serum from patients with bilateral PSNHL to report on the presence of non-specific autoantibody directed against a 68-kDa (heat-shock protein-70) inner-ear antigen (14). The role of these antibodies in the development of ASNHL was repeatedly shown by others. Mathews et. al. (15) presented a series of patients with clinically suspected autoimmune hearing loss in whom the presence of antibodies against bovine heat shock protein 70 (one of the many cross-reacting proteins against the inner ear in these patients) was a marker for the response to steroid treatment.

Aiming to identify whether evaluation of anti-hsp70 antibodies is an accurate diagnostic tool in patients affected by ASNHL, a most recent prospective study was designed in which all patients with a consistent suspicion of ASNHL, anti-hsp70 antibodies was determined (16). Anti-hsp70 antibodies were isolated in 52% of the study group patients, and in only 4% of the control group ($p < 0.01$). This study confirms the value of the anti-hsp70 test in the serological diagnosis of autoimmune hearing loss and suggests that this is the only available diagnostic marker that identifies an autoimmune origin of hearing loss.

SNHL and the Anti-phospholipid Syndrome (APS)

As in cutaneous and retinal manifestations of APS, it has long been suggested that a disturbed microcirculation caused by thrombosis is responsible for the development of SHNL. Measurement of the levels of anti-cardiolipin (aCL) antibody, lupus anticoagulant, and anti-β_2 GP1 are performed in order to establish the diagnosis of APS in the appropriate clinical setting.

The syndrome and its manifestations can be primary (no other autoimmune disease co-exist) or secondary (systemic lupus erythematosus being the most common associated autoimmune disease). In 1997, we reported our results on the presence of aCL in the sera of patients with SNHL (17). Low to moderate positive aCL to one or both IgG/IgM isotypes were found in 8 of 30 (27%) patients, whereas

TABLE 83.1 Summary of relevant autoantibodies in ASNHL.

Non-specific autoantibodies			
Autoantibody	Target	Association	Reference
ANA	Nucleus	Bilateral SNHL	(4, 5)
ANCA	Neutrophils	Progressive SNHL	(19)
Anti cardiolipin	Phospholipids	Sudden SNHL	(17, 18, 20)
Specific autoantibodies			
Antigens	Specificity	Association	Reference
30–42 kDa	Inner-ear proteins	Bilateral SNHL	(12)
PO antigens and beta-actine	Inner-ear proteins	Progressive SNHL	(13)
68 kDa	Heat-shock protein	Steroid-responsive SNHL	(14, 15)

none was detected in the healthy controls. In 1998, Heller et. al. (18) studied the incidence and clinical relevance of antibodies to phospholipids in patients with sudden deafness ($n = 55$) and progressive inner ear hearing loss ($n = 80$). Anti-phospholipid antibodies were demonstrated in 49% of the patients with sudden hearing loss and 50% of the patients with progressive hearing loss. Both of these studies, though they reported the association between SNHL and the existence of aCL, did not investigate their persistency over time. Whereas autoimmune aCL is of persistent character and mostly seen in conjunction with anti β_2 glycoprotein-I antibodies (anti β_2 GP1), transient aCL, in the absence of anti β_2 GP1, was reported to be the result of viral infections.

Recently, we assessed 51 patients who met the diagnostic criteria of SNHL in an extended study. We found low to moderately positive titers of aCL in 16 patients (31%) compared with 2 (6%) in the healthy controls. Six patients (12%, all aCL positive) were also positive for anti-β_2 GP1. Three months later, positive aCL persisted in 7 (14%) patients, four of whom were also positive for anti-β_2 GP1. This was consistent with the knowledge that anti-β_2 GP1 antibodies are more specifically associated with thromboembolism, thus considering some cases of SNHL to be part of primary APS (19).

In another recent study, Mouadeb et. al. investigated the possible association between anti-phospholipid antibodies and SNHL of unknown origin in a cohort of 168 patients (20). Forty-two patients (25%) had at least one elevated anti-phospholipid antibody marker. Twenty patients had two or more positive test results. Of the 42 patients, 64% ($n = 27$) met the diagnostic criteria for MD, and the remainder were diagnosed with idiopathic SNHL. Within this group of patients, 24 (57%) had unilateral hearing loss, and 18 (44%) had bilateral hearing loss. These data further support the hypothesis that anti-phospholipid antibodies are involved in the pathogenesis of some forms of inner ear dysfunction, presumably by causing microthrombosis in the labyrinthine vasculature.

Antiphospholipid antibodies may activate endothelial cells within the cochlear circulation, directly or by inducing the formation of free radicals that cause damage to the endothelium. These upregulated endothelial cells would initiate local microthrombous formation and subsequent ischemia to the inner ear. In these cases, treatment is directed toward preventing thromboembolic events. Of these medications, only warfarin has been shown to be beneficial in achieving anti-thrombotic effect. However, it is also accepted that steroid therapy, in addition to its anti-inflammatory effect, may also protect neural tissues from ischemic injury, stabilize the vascular endothelium, and restore the blood–brain barrier to normal. Although anticoagulant therapy was reported to be useful in some patients with SSNHL, it can not become a routine regimen in the absence of histological or imaging tools to demonstrate microthrombosis in the inner ear of patients with SNHL. Thus, future studies should establish clear standard approaches regarding the need to start with anti-coagulation therapy in patients who were admitted with SSNHL or PSNHL.

The wide range of autoantibodies in patients with ASNHL is summarized in Figure 83.1b

Treatment of ASNHL

Many trials have shown that prompt administration of corticosteroids can double the likelihood of recovery of hearing loss, especially when the pathology is strongly suspected to be of autoimmune origin. In this regard, Loveman et. al. (21) analyzed the disease progression and treatment outcome of ASNHL by retrospective chart review of 30 patients. All subjects were tested for anti-68 kDa antibody, and had audiometric evidence of hearing loss, and were treated with glucocorticoids. Ninety percent of subjects tested positive for anti-68 kDa antibodies. By audiometric testing, 50% of subjects were steroid-responsive; minimal improvement or no change was recorded in 12%, and worsening occurred in 39% after steroid therapy. The three anti-68 kDa antibody-negative subjects were steroid unresponsive, and one progressed to complete deafness. The authors concluded that this series of patients with ASNHL suggests a more variable and benign course with a better prognosis than that previously reported.

In accordance with the above, it was shown that the antibody to 68-kDa protein was significantly associated with hearing improvement after corticosteroid therapy (22). Patients in whom serum was positive to the presence of these antibodies were nearly three times more likely to experience improved hearing with corticosteroid treatment than those who were serum negative. Thus, antibodies to inner-ear supporting cell antigen may have value in diagnosis and treatment of patients with ASNHL.

Recent studies focused on more advanced therapeutic regimens for treating special cases of ASNHL. Therapeutic cochlear microperfusion, performed within the first 24 hours of developing severe hearing loss, immediately restored on average 24 dB ($p < 0.007$) of hearing. This suggests that cochlear microperfusion is a promising new technique for treating severe deafness caused by inflammation. The benefit may be sustained when combined with local delivery of immunosuppressive agents to the inner ear. In this regard, it was reported that local perfusion of the tumor necrosis factor-alpha blocker infliximab to the inner ear improves ASNHL. Transtympanic delivery of infliximab once weekly for 4 weeks allowed steroids to be tapered off, resulted in hearing improvement and reduced disease relapses.

Criteria for the Diagnosis of ASNHL

A definite diagnosis of ASNHL is possible when the following is available:

1. Progressive bilateral hearing loss occurs together with other symptoms of autoimmune diseases such as arthritis and skin vasculitis.
2. The presence of one or more of autoantibodies such as anti-hsp-70 antibodies, anti-nuclear, anti-neutrophil cytoplasmic antibodies, anti-endothelial cell, and anti-cardiolipin antibodies.
3. The prompt response to immunosuppressive (corticosteroids/cytotoxic) therapy.

A probable diagnosis of ASNHL could be suggested when two of the above is available.

Concluding Comments

A better understanding of the autoimmune character of SNHL, and the need for specific diagnostic assays, may lead to better application of immunosuppressive therapies for preventing the progression of hearing loss, which may be profound and require cochlear implantation. The establishment of worldwide accepted criteria for the definite diagnosis of this entity could provide us with the tools to define the prevalence of ASNHL.

References

1. McCabe BF. Autoimmune sesorineural hearing loss. Ann Otol Rhinol Laryngol 1979; 88: 585–89.
2. Solares CA, Hughes GB, Tuohy VK. Autoimmune sensorineural hearing loss: An immunologic perspective. J Neuroimmunol 2003; 138: 1–7.
3. Suzuki M, Krug MS, Cheng KC, Yazawa Y, Bernstein J, Yoo TJ. Antibodies against inner-ear proteins, in the sera of patients with inner-ear diseases. ORL J Otorhinolaryngol Relat Spec 1997; 59:10–17.
4. McCabe BF, McCormick KJ. Tests for autoimmune disease in otology. Am J Otol 1984; 5: 585–89.
5. Hughes GB, Barna BP, Kinney SE, Calabrese LH. Nalepa NL. Predictive value of laboratory tests in "autoimmune" inner ear disease: Preliminary report. Laryngoscope 1986; 96: 502–5.
6. Fuse T, Hayashi T, Oota N, et.al. Immunological responses in acute low-tone sensorineural hearing loss and Meniere's disease. Acta Otolaryngol 2003; 123: 26–31.
7. Baek MJ, Park HM, Johnson JM, Altuntas CZ, Jane-Wite D, Jaini R, Solares CA, et al. Increased frequencies of cochlin-specific T cells in patients with autoimmune sensorineural hearing loss. J Immunol 2006; 177: 4203–10.
8. Staecker H, Lefebvre PP. Autoimmune sensorineural hearing loss improved by tumor necrosis factor-alpha blockade: A case report. Acta Otolaryngol 2002; 122: 684–7.
9. Solares CA, Edling AE, Johnson JM, et.al. Murine autoimmune hearing loss mediated by CD4+ T cells specific for inner ear peptides. J Clin Invest 2004; 113: 1210–17.
10. Bodmer D, Brors D, Pak K, et.al. Inflammatory signals increase fas ligand expression by inner ear cells. J Neuroimmunol 2002; 129: 10–17.
11. Arnold W, Pfaltz CR. Critical evaluation of the immunofluorescence microscopic test for identification of serum antibodies against human inner ear tissue. Acta Otolaryngol 1987; 103: 373–78.
12. Boulassel MR, Deggouj N, Tomasi JP, Gersdorff M. Inner ear autoantibodies and their targets in patients with autoimmune inner ear diseases. Acta Otolaryngol 2001; 12: 28–34.
13. Passali D, Damiani V, Mora R, Passali FM, Passali GC, Bellussi L. P0 Antigen detection in sudden hearing loss and Meniere's disease: A new diagnostic marker? Acta Otolaryngol 2004; 124: 1145–48.
14. Haris JP, Sharp P. Inner ear autoantibodies in patients with rapidly progressive sensorineural hearing loss. Laryngoscope 1990; 97: 63–76.
15. Mathews J, Rao S, Kumar BN. Autoimmune sensorineural hearing loss: Is it still a clinical diagnosis? J Laryngol Otol 2003; 117: 212–14.
16. Bonaguri C, Orsoni JG, Zavota L, Monica C, Russo A, Pellistri I, Rubino P, et. al. Anti-68 kDa antibodies in autoimmune sensorineural hearing loss: Are these autoantibodies really a diagnostic tool? Autoimmunity 2007; 40: 73–8.
17. Toubi E, Ben-David J, Kessel A, Podoshin L, Golan TD. Autoimmune aberration in sudden sensorineural hearing loss: Association with anti-cardiolipin antibodies. Lupus 1997; 6: 540–42.
18. Heller U, Becker EW, Zenner HP, Berg PA. Incidence and clinical relevance of antibodies to phospholipids, serotonin and ganglioside in patients with sudden deafness and progressive inner ear hearing loss. HNO 1998; 46: 583–6.
19. Toubi E, Ben-David J, Kessel A, Luntz M. Immune-mediated disorders associated with idiopathic sudden sensorineural hearing loss. Ann Otol Rhinol Laryngol 2004; 113: 445–9.
20. Mouadeb, DA, Ruckenstein MJ. Antiphospolipid inner ear syndrome. Laryngoscope 2005;115: 879–83.
21. Loveman DM, de Comarmond C, Cepero R, Baldwin DM. Autoimmune sensorineural hearing loss: Clinical course and treatment outcome. Semin Arthritis Rheum 2004; 34: 538–43.
22. Zeitoun H, Beckman JG, Arts HA, Lansford CD, Lee DS, El-Kashlan HK, Telian SA, et. al. Corticosteroid response and supporting cell antibody in autoimmune hearing loss. Arch Orolaryngol Head Neck Surg 2005; 131: 665–72.

Part XI
Ocular Autoimmune Diseases

84
Autoimmune Retinopathies

Joan Giralt and Alfredo Adan

Abstract   Autoimmune retinopathies (ARs) are uncommon ophthalmic disorders in which autoantibodies directed at various retinal components damage the retina causing progressive vision loss. In most cases, an evaluation reveals an underlying malignancy, placing this condition in the category of paraneoplastic retinopathy (PR) syndromes. Specific forms of PR that have been identified include cancer-associated retinopathy (CAR) and melanoma-associated retinopathy (MAR). In rare cases, no such malignancy is found, and the patients are considered to have AR. Diffuse photoreceptor degeneration of both cones and rods are present with or without any inflammation. Symptoms usually present bilaterally, and rarely sequentially, over a period of several weeks or months before the underlying malignancy is diagnosed. The diagnosis is made on a high index of suspicion based on the clinical findings.

Keywords   Autoimmune retinopathy · cancer-associated retinopathy · melanoma associated retinopathy

Autoimmune retinopathies (ARs) are uncommon ophthalmic disorders in which autoantibodies directed at various retinal components damage the retina causing progressive vision loss. In most cases, an evaluation reveals an underlying malignancy, placing this condition in the category of paraneoplastic retinopathy (PR) syndromes. Specific forms of PR that have been identified include cancer-associated retinopathy (CAR) and melanoma-associated retinopathy (MAR). In rare cases, no such malignancy is found, and the patients are considered to have AR.

Epidemiology

In general, PR and AR are uncommon disorders; their exact prevalence is unknown. Its incidence is equal among women and men, except in MAR, where men are more commonly affected (1). It usually affects older adults. When the retinopathy is associated with cancer, the most common disorders are small-cell lung cancer, gynaecological and breast cancer, melanoma, lymphoma, pancreatic, prostate, bladder, laryngeal, or colon cancer (2, 3). CARs are the most common type of paraneoplastic syndrome seen (4).

Pathologic Features

Diffuse photoreceptor degeneration of both cones and rods are present with or without any inflammation (5). Scattered melanophages in the outer retina can also occasionally be seen. Ganglion cells in the inner retina, the optic nerve, and the geniculocalcarine pathway are all spared. Ganglion cell trans-synaptic atrophy, a marked decrease of bipolar neurons in the inner nuclear layer with normal photoreceptors cells in the outer nuclear layer, can be seen in MARs (6).

Cross-reactivity between cancerous and retinal proteins is responsible for initiating the immune-mediated cascade of events that ultimately leads to photoreceptor degeneration. The first and most commonly identified antibody in patients with CAR is directed toward recoverin, a 23-kDa retinal protein that some tumour cells also express (7). In addition to recoverin, the second most common autoimmune retinal antibody is enolasa (46-kDa), followed by a 45-kDa and a 60-kDa protein (8). Patients with MAR have immunoglobulin G (IgG) autoantibodies that react with human rod bipolar cells (9). Antibodies directed against the 35-kDa retinal Müller cell layer have been found in some patients with AR (10). The presence of anti-recovering antibody is not specific for the diagnosis of

From: Y. Shoenfeld et al. (eds.): *Diagnostic Criteria in Autoimmune Diseases*, DOI: 10.1007/978-1-60327-285-8_84,

CAR. Antibodies against recoverin and other retinal antigens of different molecular weights have been found in a wide spectrum of ARs, even in retinal degenerative diseases, such as retinitis pigmentosa (11).

Clinical Manifestation

Symptoms in both PR and AR are similar (Table 84.1). Signs and symptoms can vary depending on the retinal elements that are affected. CAR affects both rods and cones, MAR affects only rods, and AR affects Müller cells (12). Symptoms usually present bilaterally, and rarely sequentially, over a period of several weeks or months before the underlying malignancy is diagnosed (8). MAR commonly presents after the melanoma is diagnosed, often at the stage of metastases (1). Individuals with cone dysfunction have photosensitivity, prolonged glared after light exposure (hemeralopia), reduced visual acuity, and loss of colour vision. Individuals with rod dysfunction have difficulty seeing in dim illumination (nyctalopia), prolonged dark adaptation, and peripheral field loss. In either case, positive visual phenomena are often prominent, including flashing lights, flickering, smoky or swirling vision, and other entoptic symptoms. Some patients report transient dimming of vision, which may be mistaken for retinovascular disease. They may even report that their vision is better if they wear dark sunglasses (13).

Examination findings are variable. Patients with CAR usually have prominent involvement of central vision, resulting in markedly decreased visual acuity, loss of colour vision, and central scotomas. In some cases, visual field testing shows paracentral scotomas that progress to classic ring scotomas. Photostress recovery times are typically prolonged. In contrast, patients with MAR often have near-normal visual acuity, colour vision, and central visual fields, at least at presentation. Peripheral or mid-peripheral field loss can usually be demonstrated (6, 14).

Fundus findings at presentation are often normal. However, characteristic changes occur over time and include attenuation of the arterioles, with thinning and mottling of the retinal pigment epithelium (RPE) (15). In occasional cases of CAR or MAR, vitreous cells, arteriolar sheathing, and periphlebitis may be present, particularly late in the course of the disease.

Fluorescein angiography is often performed to exclude other entities as potential causes of vision loss. Findings are usually normal, but in occasional cases, fluorescein angiography may demonstrate mild peripheral vascular leakage consistent with vasculitis.

The findings from full-field (Ganzfeld) electroretinogram (ERG) are almost always abnormal; specific findings depend on the predominance of cone versus rod dysfunction. Patients with CAR usually have absent cone responses. Findings in MAR include a markedly reduced or absent dark-adapted b-wave, which indicates bipolar and Müller cell dysfunction. Multifocal ERG (MERG) may be useful in select cases in which visual field loss is localized (16). In addition, some authors have used MERG to quantify the loss of electrical activity and to correlate this finding with results of Goldmann perimetry (8).

Diagnosis

The diagnosis is made on a high index of suspicion based on the clinical findings. Early in the course of the ophthalmic diseases, findings on retinal examination may be normal, which makes diagnosis difficult. The initial workup includes a full assessment of the patient's visual function, including colour vision and visual field testing. Goldmann perimetry is preferred because it readily tests the peripheral field. Full-field ERG is crucial for localizing the disease process to the retina and for further defining the retinal layers involved (17).

A definitive diagnosis of CAR or MAR requires the demonstration of antiretinal antibodies (Table 84.2). Results of such laboratory testing are not always definitive. On occasion, individuals without clinical evidence of retinopathy have these antibodies, and, in some cases of presumed CAR, the antibodies cannot be identified with current techniques.

In any patient with suspected CAR and without a known malignancy, a chest radiograph should be obtained (Table 84.3). If the result is normal, a CT scan of the chest is appropriate. Additional imaging studies for a possible primary neoplasm include CT of the abdomen and pelvis, mammography (for women), and total body positron emission tomography (PET) (15).

Differential Diagnosis

Acute or subacute unilateral or bilateral vision loss with a normal-appearing fundus suggests the possibility of retrobulbar optic neuropathy. Specific entities include compressive orbital and intracranial lesions, demyelinating diseases, ischaemia, toxicity, and hereditary disorders. In the ideal case, the clinical findings are sufficiently distinctive to distinguish optic nerve disease from retinal disease and therefore obviate extensive neurological testing.

Hemeralopia or nyctalopia, positive visual phenomena, prolonged photostress times, and ring scotomas all suggest the possibility of retinal disease, even in the absence of funduscopic abnormalities, and prompt electrophysiological studies.

Patients with cancer-associated cone dysfunction have bilateral central vision loss with poor colour vision and central scotomas. These findings are also compatible with toxic-nutritional optic neuropathy or hereditary optic neuropathy. MERG should be effective for distinguishing optic neuropathy from maculopathy in these patients.

Metastatic disease as the cause of the vision loss should include contrast-enhanced MRI of the head and orbits and lumbar puncture for cytological examination. It may be due to infiltration of cancerous cells around the optic nerve. Some chemotherapeutic agents, such as vincristine and carmustine, can cause optic neuropathy. Patients who have received cranial radiation are also at risk of vision loss.

Bilateral diffuse uveal melanocytic proliferation is a possibility in cancers originating from the reproductive tract, retroperitoneal zone, or lungs. Patients with this proliferation develop an orange pigment deposit at the level of the RPE, shown as a diffuse pattern with round areas of hyperfluorescence on fluorescein angiography. These patients usually develop non-pigmented tumours of the iris, cataracts, and exudative retinal detachments (18).

Once it is clear that the patient's vision loss is due to photoreceptor dysfunction, the differential diagnosis is narrowed to paraneoplastic syndromes, hereditary photoreceptor degeneration (e.g., cone dystrophy, retinosis pigmentosa), and toxic retinopathy. Patients should be questioned regarding the use of potential retinal toxins, such as chloroquine or hydroxychloroquine.

Cases of acute zonal occult outer retinopathy (AZOOR) are occasionally confused with PR. The no seeing areas are sharply demarcated from the surrounding areas, the involvement is usually unilateral, and the disease has a predilection for the peripapillary area. Full-field ERG is generally normal, in distinction from PR in which ERG findings are markedly attenuated or flat early in the course of the disease. MERG demonstrates the abnormality well.

Therapy

Treatment of the underlying malignancy, steroid therapy, plasmapheresis, and administration of intravenous immunoglobulin are disappointing over all. Corticosteroids have been shown to decrease antibody titers in patients with CAR, but they do not reverse vision loss (19). These results may suggest that if the photoreceptors sustain sufficient damage, visual function is permanently altered. Current research involves methods of blocking antibody-mediated apoptosis by means of changes in intracellular calcium, and activation of recoverin-specific antitumour cytotoxic T lymphocytes. Another promising therapy involves autologous tumour cells transfected with interleukin-2 genes that are used as a vaccine to generate an immune response against the tumour cells (20).

TABLE 84.1. Symptoms and signs more commonly associated with cancer-associated retinopathies and autoimmune retinopathies.

Symptoms	Signs
Reduced vision acuity	Fundus finding normal at presentation
Loss of colour vision	Attenuation of the arterioles
Photopsias	Mottling and thinning of the RPE
Prolonged glare	Vitreous cells
Nyctalopia	Periphlebitis
Floaters	
Flickering and smoky vision	
Peripheral field loss	

RPE, retinal pigment epithelium.

TABLE 84.2. Antigen proteins in autoimmune retinopathies.

Recoverin 23 kDa (the most common in cancer-associated retinopathy)
Enolasa 46 kDa
45 kDa
60 kDa
35 kDa (in some patients with autoimmune retinopathy)
IgG (patients with melanoma-associated retinopathy)

TABLE 84.3. Frequency of malignancies associated with cancer-associated retinopathy.

Malignancy	Frequency (%)
Small-cell lung cancer	53
Non-small cell lung cancer	11
Endometrial	10
Cervical	7
Breast	6
Ovarian	5
Prostate	4
Pancreatic	4

References

1. Boeck K, Hofmann S, Klopfer M, et al. Melanoma-associated paraneoplastic retinopathy: case report and review of the literature. *Br J Dermatol* 1997; 137: 457–60.
2. Buchanan TA, Gardiner TA, Archer DB. An ultrastructural study of retinal photoreceptor degeneration associated with bronchial carcinoma. *Am J Ophthalmol* 1984; 97: 277–87.
3. Adamus G, Amundson D, MacKay C. Long-term persistence of antirecoverin antibodies in endometrial cancer-associated retinopathy. *Arch Ophthalmol* 1998; 116: 251–3.
4. Thirkill CE, Roth AM, Keltner JL. Cancer-associated retinopathy. *Arch Oftalmol* 1987; 105: 372–5.
5. Sawyer RA, Selhorst JB, Zimmerman LE. Blindness caused by photoreceptor degeneration as a remote effect of cancer. *Am J Ophthalmol* 1976; 81: 606–13.
6. Gittinger JW Jr, Smith TW. Cutaneous melanoma-associated paraneoplastic retinopathy: Histopathologic observations. *Am J Ophthalmol* 1999; 127:612–4.

7. Thirkill CE, Tait RC, Tyler NK, et al. The Cancer-associated retinopathy antigen is a recoverin-like protein. *Invest Ophthalmol Vis Sci* 1992; 33: 2768–72.

8. Keltner JL, Thirkill CE. Cancer-associated retinopathy vs. recoverin-associated retinopathy. *Am J Ophthalmol* 1998; 126: 296–302.

9. Milam AH, Saari JC, Jacobson SG, et al. Autoantibodies against retinal bipolar cells in cutaneous melanoma-associated retinopathy. *Invest Ophthalmol Vis Sci* 1993; 34: 91–100.

10. Peek R, Verbraak F, Coevoet HM, et al. Müller cell-specific autoantibodies in a patient with progressive loss of vision. *Invest Ophthalmol Vis Sci* 1998; 39: 1976–9.

11. Keltner JL, Roth AM, ChangRS. Photoreceptor degeneration. Possible autoimmune disorder. Arch Ophthalmol 1983; 101: 564–9.

12. Mizener JB, Kimura AE, Adamus G, et al. Autoimmune retinopathy in the absence of cancer. *Am J Ophthalmol* 1997; 123: 607–18.

13. Jacobson DM. Paraneoplastic diseases of neuro-ophthalmologic interest. In: Miller NR, Newman N (eds.) *Walsh and Hoyts Clinical Neuro-Ophthalmology,* 5th ed. Baltimore: Williams and Wilkins, 1998, pp. 2497–51.

14. Kiratli H, Thirkill CE, Bilgic S, et al. Paraneoplastic retinopathy associated with metastatic cutaneous melanoma of unknown primary site. *Eye* 1997; 11: 889–92.

15. Milam AH. Clinical aspects: paraneoplastic retinopathy. In: Djamgoz MBA, Archer SN, Vallerga S (eds.) *Neurobiology and Clinical Aspects of the Outer Retina.* London: Chapman and Hall, 1995, pp. 461–71.

16. Lei B, Bush RA, Milam AH, et al. Human melanoma-associated retinopathy (MAR) antibodies alter the retinal ON-response of the monkey ERG in vivo. *Invest Ophthalmol Vis Sci* 2000; 41: 262–6.

17. Matsui Y, Metha MC, Katsumi O, et al. Electrophysiological findings in paraneoplastic retinopathy. *Graefes Arch Clin Exp Ophthalmol* 1992; 230: 324–8.

18. Amin AR, Jakobiec FA, Dreyer EB, et al. Ocular syndromes associated with systemic malignancy. *Int Ophthalmol Clin* 1997; 37: 281–302.

19. Keltner JL, Thirkill CE, Tyler NK, et al. Management and monitoring of cancer-associated retinopathy. *Arch Oftalmol* 1992; 110: 48–53.

20. Palmer K, Moore J, Everard M, et al. Gene therapy with autologous, interleukin-2 secreting tumor cells in patients with malignan melanoma. *Hum Gene Ther* 1999; 10: 1261–8.

85
Autoimmune Uveitis

Francisco Assis de Andrade, Ivan Foeldvari and Roger A. Levy

Abstract Autoimmune uveitis (AU) is an important cause of blindness and should be diagnosed as early as possible and efficiently treated in order to avoid it. It can be due to an isolated type of autoimmune reaction against the uveal components, or be related to or precede a known systemic autoimmune disease. A diagnosis of a systemic autoimmune disease should be investigated and the patient's treatment should be tuned in accordance with the other organs involved. The autoimmune diseases where uveitis is most commonly seen are spondyloarthrophaties, inflammatory bowel disorders, juvenile idiopathic arthritis and Behçet's disease.

Keywords Uveitis · ocular inflammation · spondyloarthrophaties · Behçet's disease

Definition

Autoimmune uveitis (AU) is as an inflammatory process related to the presence of autoantibodies against the uvea, which constitutes the middle layer or vascular portion of the eye. The uvea encompasses the iris, the ciliary body and the choroid. During the pathogenic process of an AU, other ocular structures are also involved, such as the retina, the vitreous body and the optic nerve. This occurs due to the proximity of the ocular layers, which are in fact inseparable during the inflammatory process. Type 1 collagen α2 antigen has been identified as a target for autoimmune response in experimental AU in rodents (1). AU is an important cause of blindness all over the world. The suspicion of uveitis requires a prompt referral to an ophthalmologist, combined with an urgent diagnostic workup in order to treat and control the inflammatory process.

Clinical Picture and Classification

The clinical manifestations of the AU vary in accordance with the involved region of the eye. Therefore, the different types of AU are classified in accordance with the anatomic location of the inflammation. Anterior uveitis is by far the most common type and can be manifested as iritis, which affects only the iris and iridociclitis, which involves the ciliary body in addition to the iris. Intermediary uveitis is also know as vitritis and is characterized by the infiltration of inflammatory cells in the vitreous cavity, sometimes with the involvement of the pars plana. The posterior uveitis can be of three types: choroiditis, retinochoroiditis and chorioretinitis, also related to the involved area. Finally, there is the type called diffuse uveitis or panuveitis, which is characterized by the diffuse involvement of the whole uveal tract.

At presentation, eye redness is the major symptom, with the exemption of the juvenile idiopathic oligarticular or psoriatic arthritis, and is often accompanied by injected conjunctiva, local pain, photophobia and decreased visual acuity (blurred vision). Patients may also complain of seeing dark, floating spots along the visual field. The clinical course of the anterior uveitis can be manifested as an acute form, with sudden onset, characterized by a single episode that may last for two to three months that improves with prompt proper treatment, or may persist as a recurrent or chronic form. An AU that persists for more than three months is classified as chronic. The AU onset is usually insidious but may also have a recurrent course. The major findings are dilation of the ciliary vessels, presence of inflammatory cells in the anterior chamber and keratic precipitates (KPs) on the corneal posterior surface. These findings can be divided as granulomatous type, where the

From: Y. Shoenfeld et al. (eds.): *Diagnostic Criteria in Autoimmune Diseases*, DOI: 10.1007/978-1-60327-285-8_85,
© 2008 Humana Press, Totowa, NJ

KP is of a "mutton-fat" type or non-granulomatous, where the KPs are thinner. In accordance to the number of inflammatory cells found, the ophthalmologists refer to mild or severe forms. Complementary tests are crucial in order to differentiate the AU of those of infectious origin.

Etiology

Several conditions can be related to the development of uveitis, including systemic diseases as well as syndromes limited to the eye. In patients who present with anterior uveitis, almost one-half have a definite diagnosis confirmed, and there is a strong association with the HLA-B27 antigen presence in adults (2). The highest frequency is in children with the oligoarticular type juvenile idiopathic arthritis (JIA), where around 10–30% of patients have an anterior uveitis (3).

Seronegative Spondyloarthrophaties

Included in this group are a series of diseases that have in common the involvement of the axial skeleton with negative rheumatoid factor (RF) and no other specific serologic marker. The most prevalent disease of this group is ankylosing spondylitis (AS). Other diseases in this group are psoriatic arthritis, reactive arthritis and the arthritis related to the inflammatory bowel diseases (Crohn's disease and ulcerative colitis). There is a strong relationship with the presence of the class I antigen HLA-B27. Analyzing retrospectively a cohort of 350 patients with spondyloarthropathies in Brazil, Sampaio-Barros et al. found that 30 (14.5%) of those (207 patients) with AS presented 55 episodes of acute anterior uveitis, and there were statistically significant associations with juvenile-onset disease and Achillean and plantar enthesopathies; only one AS patient presented a single posterior uveitis episode (4).

AS affects more commonly young Caucasian males and more than 90% have the HLA-B27. In addition to low-back pain due to sacroiliitis, there is a high frequency of periarticular pain, manifested as oligoarthritis related to enthesitis. The radiographic findings of sacroiliitis may take years to appear and this may postpone the diagnosis in years. Of the extra-articular manifestations, those in the skin and the eyes are the most common ones. The most frequent ocular manifestation of AS is a non-granulomatous, unilateral anterior uveitis, characterized by acute recurrent attacks of iridociclitis and sometimes pars planitis. More rarely, there may be a chronic evolutionary course with the development of secondary glaucoma, complicated cataract and keratopathies. These complications may hamper the visual function. Uveitis may precede the diagnostic of AS in years. In reactive arthritis and psoriatic arthritis, the most common ocular

manifestation is conjunctivitis, being bilateral in the first (5). This conjunctivitis induces a scarce mucoid secretion and is usually self-limited, while in psoriatic arthritis the mucoid secretion is abundant and the course is chronic. Few cases can present iritis, iridociclitis or keratitis, which may vary from mild to severe. In children with the juvenile idiopathic psoriatic arthritis the anterior uveitis without pain and redness is a very common presentation. The laboratory tests are non-specific and related to the chronic inflammatory process. Acute-phase reactants, such as C-reactive protein, may be elevated in the plasma, as well as the level of circulating IgA. The HLA-B27 detection is not necessary for diagnosis. Local treatment for anterior uveitis in these patients is with mydriatic and corticosteroids eye drops. In refractory cases, subconjunctival or subtenonian infiltration with corticosteroids may be attempted.

Inflammatory Bowel Diseases

Ocular manifestations are found in about 2.5% of the patients with Crohn's disease and 5–12% of those with ulcerative colitis. The lesions are in general non-granulomatous, involving bilaterally the anterior uvea, and tend to be recurrent. Other ocular manifestations are conjunctivitis, peripheral corneal ulcerations, keratitis and blepharitis. Chronic posterior uveitis has also been reported in patients with inflammatory bowel diseases. The treatment of the ocular lesions in patients with inflammatory bowel diseases consists of using local or systemic corticosteroids.

Juvenile Idiopathic Arthritis

JIA is diagnosed when there is a persistent arthritis for then 6 weeks in persons less than 16 years old, once other causes of arthritis are ruled out. JIA is classified according to the type of articular involvement. The systemic type (Still's disease) is the most severe form and the less frequent, encompassing around 10% of the cases, and can be found equally in both genders; they present an intermittent fever with skin rash with symmetric arthritis and no RF. The polyarticular form accounts for 30–40% of the cases, and five or more joints are involved and most of the cases do not display RF. The RF-positive polyarticular subtype is a distinct entity and it has a similar course as rheumatoid arthritis, it presents only 5% of the JIA cases. The oligoarticular form affects 40–50% of the cases of JIA, and less then five joints are involved; around 50% of the patients are positive for antinuclear antibodies. Another subtype resembles the adult spondyloarthropathies, they are called juvenile idiopathic enthesitis-related arthritis, and the presence of sacroiliitis is not required for the diagnosis, in the pediatric cohort, enthesitis and peripheral asymmetric arthritis of the lower limb is mostly dominant (6, 7, 8).

Uveitis is rare in the systemic form and occurs around 10% in the polyarticular RF-negative form (Table 85.1). However, it is detected most frequently in the oligoarticular form (around 20% of the cases). A chronic bilateral iridociclitis due to a non-granulomatous anterior uveitis without pain and redness of the involved eye is the most typical finding. In lot of cases at the time of the diagnosis already complications like cataract or band keratopathy are present. Uveitis at time of diagnosis of JIA or before the diagnosis of JIA is bad prognostic factor (9). Uveitis in these patients is mostly painless, and that is the justification for the suggested periodic eye exam in patients with JIA according the recommendations (10). The ocular treatment includes local corticosteroids and mydriatics. For the cases of chronic iridociclitis, systemic corticosteroids as bridging agent with an immunosuppressor like methotrexate are indicated (11), and in severe cases the addition of tumor necrosis factor (TNF)-blocking agents (12) is indicated (Table 85.2).

Behçet Disease

Is a systemic vasculitic disease that involves arteries and veins of small and large calibers. It can occur in both genders usually between 20 and 40 years. There is no serologic marker of BD; however, there is as a strong association with the HLA-B51 haplotype. This genetic association is even more marked when there is ocular involvement. A pathogenic role has been imputed on Streptococcal antigens and pro-inflammatory cytokines are elevated during attacks. Several committees in different countries have proposed criteria for the diagnosis of BD. Presently, the International Study Group (ISG) criteria is the most widely used (Table 85.3) (13). The ocular involvement is present in 83–95% of the males and 67–73% of the females (14) and in general occurs 2 or 3 years after the onset of the other symptoms. The clinical manifestations of BD, including the eye involvement, can vary according to the ethnic background of the population studied. Both eyes are usually involved and non-simultaneous flares can happen. The non-granulomatous reaction can occupy all

areas of the uvea. Vasculitis of the retina is the most prominent finding. Angiofluorescein angiography is helpful for the early diagnosis of vasculitis of the retina, in spite of a normal fundoscopy.

The treatment of the uveitis seen in BD varies according to the type of finding. The treatment for iridociclitis consists of topical corticosteroids and mydriatics. Isolated posterior uveitis has been successfully treated with a combination of ciclosporin and azathioprine. Vasculitis of the retina is treated systemically with corticosteroids and immunosuppressors, usually cyclophosphamide, sometimes colchicine is also used. Infliximab has been reported to be safe for long-term use and efficacious in treating uveitis as well as retinal vasculitic in BD (15).

Kawasaki Disease

Kawasaki disease (KD) is an acute febrile disease that occurs in children under the age of 5 years. Usually there is an abrupt onset of fever followed by a bilateral subconjuctival congestion state. In the following days, dryness, fissuring and redness develop in the lips, along with painful cervical lymphadenopathy. Exanthematic lesions appear in the trunk and in palms and soles that frequently develop skin desquamation. Vasculitis of the coronary arteries is the most serious complication. Conjunctivitis is the most common ocular finding, while uveitis can happen more rarely.

Vogt–Koyanagi–Harada Syndrome

It is a multisystemic disorder that typically affects pigmented skin individuals. In the Japanese population, where the disease is more prevalent, there is a strong relationship with the presence of HLA-DR4. In addition to the eyes, typical manifestations involve the ears, the skin and the central nervous system. The characteristic presentation is a severe bilateral diffuse granulomatous uveitis with signs of meningeal irritation, bilateral neuro-sensorial dysacusia and skin alterations, such as vitiligo, alopecia and polyosis. Angiography and ultrasound exam are necessary for the

TABLE 85.1. Types of uveitis according to the anatomic area involved, manifestation and local treatment.

Type	Localization	Clinical manifestation	Treatment
1. Anterior uveitis	a – Iritis b – Iridociclitis	With or without eye redness with or without pain	Local CS and mydriatics
2. Intermediary uveitis	Vitritis, *pars planitis*	Eye redness with or without blurred vision	Systemic, peri-ocular or intra-vitreous CS/IS
3. Posterior uveitis	a – Choroiditis b – Retinochoroiditis c – Choroiretinitis	Low visual acuity	Systemic, peri-ocular or intra-vitreous CS/IS
4. Panuveitis	Diffuse uveitis	Eye redness and blurred vision	Local or intra-vitreous CS and mydriatics/IS

CS, corticosteroids; IS, immunosuppressors.

TABLE 85.2. Non-infectious systemic disorders related to uveitis.

Seronegative spondyloarthrophaties
Ankylosing spondylitis
Psoriatic arthritis
Reactive arthritis
Inflammatory bowel diseases
Juvenile idiopathic arthritis
Behçet disease
Kawasaki disease
Vogt–Koyanagi–Harada syndrome
Sarcoidosis

TABLE 85.3. International Study Group criteria for the diagnosis of Behçet disease (13).

Recurrent oral ulcerations	Minor aphthous, major aphthous or herpetiform ulceration observed by physician or patient, which recurred at least three times in 1–2 months period
Also two of the following:	
Recurrent genital ulcerations	Aphthous ulceration or scarring observed by physician and patient
Eye lesions	Anterior or posterior uveitis, or cells in vitreous on slit lamp examination or retinal vasculitis observed by an ophthalmologist
Skin lesions	Erythema nodosum observed by physician or patient, pseudofolliculitis or papulopustular lesions or acneiform nodules observed by physician in postadolescent patients not on corticosteroids
Positive pathergy sign	Read by physician at 24–48 h

ocular diagnosis. A prodromic period is followed by the uveitis phase that lasts 3–5 days or several weeks. Then a convalescence phase issues with dyspigmentation of the skin, as well as the uvea and the pigmented retinal epithelium; this phase can last for months or years. Recurrent attacks can happen during the convalescence phase. The anterior uveitis should be promptly treated with local corticosteroids and mydriatics, while the posterior form responds to periocular or intravitreous corticosteroids. As soon as the diagnosis of Vogt–Koyonagi–Harada syndrome is confirmed, systemic high-dose corticosteroids should be started along with a potent immunosuppressor agent.

Sarcoidosis

It is a multisystemic granulomatous disease characterized by deposition of $CD4^+$ cells and macrophages in the involved sites. Sarcoidosis occurs in all age groups, but is more common in persons between the ages of 20 and 50 years, with a preference for Afro descendants. Cutaneous involvement is common; in the initial phase there may be pulmonary and hepatic alterations. Of the patients with systemic disease, 27–40% present AU; isolated eye

sarcoidosis can also occur (16). In half of the cases with ocular manifestations, the presentation is an acute and self-limited granulomatous iridociclitis. The chronic presentation is mostly seen in older patients with pulmonary fibrosis and quiescent systemic disease. Alterations in the vitreous can also be seen, like posterior segment periphlebitis, retinal and choroidal granulomas and lesions of the optic nerve, in addition to lacrimary glandular and conjunctival involvement. It is important to recognize sarcoidosis as a cause of uveitis, because it imposes a systemic involvement screening as well as a proper therapeutic intervention. Chest CT scan is useful to demonstrate the hilar adenomegaly, with or without multifocal parenchymatous nodulary lesions. Gallium whole body scan is used to investigate the hypercaptation in lacrimary glands and orbital area, as well as in salivary glands and lungs; its value is enhanced when combine with the measurement of the serum angiotensin-converting enzyme level (17).

Recent Advances in the Treatment of AU

The success rate of immunosuppressors in the treatment of AU is unsatisfactory and involves serious side effects in adults. In the JIA-associated uveitis, a combination therapy of parenteral methotrexate and an anti-TNF agent seems to be promising. New modalities of local and systemic therapies that are safer and more efficient are necessary. The use of intravitreous triamcinolone has been proven to be efficacious in patients on immunosuppressants presenting side effects due to systemic corticosteroids or in those that are non-compliant. Triamcinolone injections have a short-term action and have been used in cases of BD, as well as in idiopathic vasculitis, pars planitis and panuveitis. Vitreous corticosteroids implants using a small dose of fluocinolone acetonide are indicated when an effective, safer, longer action is attained (18). A review of population-based studies of patients with AS indicates that TNF inhibitors and monoclonal antibodies (infliximab and adalimumab) prevent uveitis. On the contrary, anecdotal reports implicate etanercept as a cause of uveitis. Overall, there were more cases of uveitis associated with etanercept, than with infliximab and adalimumab (19).

References

1. Bora NS, Sohn JH, Kang SG, et al. Type I collagen is the autoantigen in experimental anterior uveitis. *J Immunol* 2004; 172: 7086–94.
2. Rivera-Cívico F, Jiménez-Alonso J, Martin-Armada M, et al. HLA-B27+ anterior uveitis with or without associated spondyloarthritis: Clinical and immunological features. *Ann Rheum Dis* 1999; 58: 721–2.

3. Grassi A, Corona F, Casellato A, Canelli V, Bardare M. Prevalence and outcome of juvenile idiopathic arthritis-associated uveitis and relation to articular disease. *J Rheumatol* 2007; 34(5): 1139–45.

4. Sampaio-Barros PD, Conde RA, Bonfiglioli R, Bértolo MB, Samara AM. Characterization and outcome of uveitis in 350 patients with spondyloarthropathies. *Rheumatol Int* 2006; 26: 1143–6.

5. Banares A, Hernández-García C, Fernández-Gutiérrez B, Jover JA. Eye involvement in the spondyloarthropathies. *Rheum Dis Clin North Am* 1998; 24: 771–84.

6. Petty RE, Southwood TR, Manners P, et al. International League of Associations for Rheumatology classification of juvenile idiopathic arthritis: Second revision, Edmonton, 2001. *J Rheumatol* 2004; 31(2): 390–2.

7. Miller M. Juvenile Rheumatoid Arthritis. eMedicine Specialties >Pediatrics >Rheumatology. 2006.

8. Ravelli A, Martini A. Juvenile idiopathic arthritis. *Lancet* 2007; 369(9563): 767–78.

9. Edelsten C, Lee V, Bentley CR, Kanski JJ, Graham EM. An evaluation of baseline risk factors predicting severity in juvenile idiopathic arthritis associated uveitis and other chronic anterior uveitis in early childhood. *Br J Ophthalmol* 2002; 86: 51–56.

10. Cassidy J, Kivlin J, Lindsley C, Nocton J. Ophthalmologic examinations in children with juvenile rheumatoid arthritis. *Pediatrics* 2006; 117(5): 1843–5.

11. Foeldvari I, Wierk A. Methotrexate is an effective treatment for chronic uveitis associated with juvenile idiopathic arthritis. *J Rheumatol* 2005; 32(2): 362–5.

12. Foeldvari I, Nielsen S, Kummerle-Deschner J, et al. Tumor necrosis factor-alpha blocker in treatment of juvenile idiopathic arthritis-associated uveitis refractory to second-line agents: Results of a multinational survey. *J Rheumatol* 2007; 34(5): 1146–50.

13. International Study Group of Behçet's Disease. Criteria for diagnosis of Behçet's disease. *Lancet* 1990; 335: 1078–80.

14. Demiroglu H, Dundar S. Effects of age, sex, and initial presentation on the clinical course of Behçet's syndrome. *South Med J* 1997; 90: 567.

15. Takamoto M, Kaburaki T, Numaga J, et al. Long-term infliximab treatment for Behçet's disease. *Jap J Ophthalmol* 2007; 51: 239–40.

16. Moller DR. Etiology of sarcoidosis. *Clin Chest Med* 1997; 18: 695–706.

17. Power WJ, Neves RA, Rodriguez A, et al. The value of combined serum angiotensin-converting enzyme and gallium scan in diagnosing ocular sarcoidosis. *Ophthalmology* 1995; 102: 2007–11.

18. Cano-Parra J, Díaz-LLopis M. New drugs in the treatment of noninfectious uveitis. *Arch Soc Esp Oftalmol* 2006; 81: 671–4.

19. Lim LL, Fraunfelder FW, Rosenbaum JR. Do tumor necrosis factor inhibitors cause uveitis? A registry-based study. *Arthritis Rheum* 2007; 56(10): 3248–52.

86
Vogt-Koyanagi-Harada Disease

Jozélio Freire de Carvalho and Joyce Hisae Yamamoto

Abstract   Vogt-Koyanagi-Harada disease (VKH) is a multisystem autoimmune disorder affecting pigmented tissues such as the eye, auditory, integumentary and central nervous systems. Patients are typically women between 20 and 50 years of age with no previous history of penetrating ocular trauma. The clinical course of VKH is divided into four phases: prodromal (mimics a viral infection), uveitic (bilateral diffuse uveitis with papillitis and exudative retinal detachment), convalescent (tissue depigmentation), and chronic recurrent (recurrent uveitis and ocular complications). Clinical, laboratorial, and experimental data corroborate to the autoimmune nature of VKH disease: a CD4+ T-cell-mediated immune response directed against self-antigens found on melanocytes in a genetically susceptible individual. HLA-DRB1*0405 is the main susceptibility allele found in patients with VKH. In accordance with the revised diagnostic criteria, the disease is classified as complete, incomplete, or probable, based on the presence of extraocular findings. The diagnosis of VKH is clinical, and differential diagnosis includes sympathetic ophthalmia, sarcoidosis, primary intraocular B-cell lymphoma, posterior scleritis, and uveal effusion syndrome. Treatment is based on initial high-dose oral corticosteroids with a low tapering during a minimum period of 6 months. Systemic immunomodulatory agents such as cyclosporine may be used in refractory or corticosteroid non-tolerant patients. Visual prognosis is usually good under a prompt diagnosis and adequate treatment.

Keywords   Uveitis · Vogt-Koyanagi-Harada · diagnostic criteria

Vogt-Koyanagi-Harada disease (VKH) is a multisystemic granulomatous autoimmune disease affecting pigmented tissues of the eye, central nervous system, internal ear, and skin. Patients with bilateral uveitis associated with poliosis, vitiligo, alopecia, and dysacusia were first described by Vogt in 1906 and then by Koyanagi in 1929 (1, 2). In 1926, Harada described a case of uveitis with exudative retinal detachment associated with pleocytosis of the cerebral spinal fluid (3).

Epidemiology

Pigmented races are more commonly affected and VKH is rare in Caucasians. Surprisingly, it is not described in sub-Saharan African descent (4). Women are affected more frequently than men and there is a clear predominance in the third to fourth decade of life, although children as young as 4-year old with VKH have been reported. VKH is more prevalent in Japan, accounting for 10.1% of all uveitis compared with 1–4% in the United States (5) and 2.5% in Brazil (6).

Pathogenesis

Although the etiology of VKH remains unknown, several evidences corroborate to the autoimmunity against melanocytes triggered by an unknown factor in a genetically susceptible individual. The prodromic manifestations point to a viral trigger such as herpes family virus (Epstein-Barr virus, cytomegalovirus). Histopathological findings as well as in vitro experiments and animal models reinforce the importance of the CD4+ T lymphocytes in the disease pathogenesis (7). Several melanocyte-derived antigens are being analyzed as the target protein of the disease mainly pointing out to tyrosinase and tyrosinase-related proteins (8). HLA-DRB1*0405 has been associated with 90% of Asian patients with VKH (9) as well as in patients from other countries (10). Autoimmunity to retinal antigens has also been found in patients with VKH.

From: Y. Shoenfeld et al. (eds.): *Diagnostic Criteria in Autoimmune Diseases*, DOI: 10.1007/978-1-60327-285-8_86,
© 2008 Humana Press, Totowa, NJ

Clinical Manifestations

VKH has four clinical phases: prodromal, uveitic, convalescent, and chronic/recurrent. Extraocular manifestations are characteristically observed in prodromal, convalescent, and chronic phases.

The prodromal phase is characterized by generalized symptoms of fever, nausea, and headache which last for 3 to 5 days. Subsequently, the uveitic phase starts, with ocular symptoms including photophobia, blurred vision, and ocular pain. On examination of the eyes a bilateral, granulomatous anterior uveitis with mutton fat keratic precipitates and iris nodules are observed. In addition, a diffuse choroiditis associated with exudative retinal detachment and optic disc hyperemia are observed. Swelling of the ciliary body may displace the lens-iris diaphragm forward with consequent shallowing of the anterior chamber, angle narrowing, and an acute increase in intraocular pressure.

In the convalescent phase, as a result of appropriate treatment, the choroiditis as well as the exudative retinal detachment gradually subsides. In this phase is observed the typical "sunset glow" fundus (orange-red fundus appearance), multiple scattered, discrete, depigmented retinal pigment epithelial lesions in the mid periphery of the fundus and retinal pigment epithelial migration, all denoting the profound melanocyte and pigmented tissue aggression. Sugiura sign is the depigmentation of limbus mainly reported by Japanese authors. In this phase, cutaneous depigmentation is observed.

Recurrence or chronicity of the uveitis may occur in 17 to 73% of patients. The recurrence is usually anterior; nevertheless signs of disease activity in the posterior pole of the eye have been recently reported, suggesting relentless melanocyte aggression (11). In the convalescent and chronic phases, ocular complications such as glaucoma, cataract, choroidal neovascular membranes, and retinal/choroidal gliosis may be observed. These long-term ocular complications may lead to final low visual acuity.

Extraocular Manifestations

Nonspecific signs such as fever and nausea can occur in the prodromal phase. The auditory system may be involved by dysacousia, tinnitus, high-frequency hearing loss, and vertigo. In the same manner, the central nervous system can be affected by headache, meningismus, and pleocytosis in the cerebral spine fluid that precede the ocular involvement by one to two weeks. Infrequently, focal neurological signs such as cranial nerve palsies and optic neuritis can develop. Diffuse manifestations such as aphasia, personality changes, loss of consciousness, and seizures characterizing encephalitis can occur. Cutaneous manifestations, commonly observed in the convalescent and chronic phases, are vitiligo of the hands, shoulders, breast, back and face, poliosis, or whitening of a patch of hair, and alopecia.

Other Conditions Observed in Patients with VKH Disease

Keratoconjunctivitis *sicca* syndrome with a few cases fulfilling diagnostic criteria for Sjögren syndrome and a frequency of 10% anti-Ro/SS-A reactivity has been described in VKH (12); Guillain-Barré Syndrome and glucose intolerance were also reported.

Pathological Features

Classical histopathological findings are a diffuse granulomatous bilateral uveitis. The choroid is remarkably thickened and infiltrated with lymphocytes, macrophages, epithelioid cells, and giant cells Another characteristic finding is the Dalen-Fuchs nodules that consisted of macrophages, epithelioid cells, lymphocytes, and altered retinal pigment epithelium cells localized between the Bruch membrane and retinal pigment epithelium. In the convalescent and chronic phases of the disease, disappearance of melanocytes of choroid is described

Laboratory Features

The diagnosis of VKH disease is basically clinical; nevertheless in atypical cases complementary examinations may be helpful. Transitory pleocytosis is observed in 72% with predominance of lymphomonocytes within the first three weeks after disease onset. UIltrasonography of the eye reveals low to medium reflective diffuse thickening of choroid with localized and extensive retinal exudative detachment, differentiating VKH from higher reflectivity of idiopathic uveal effusion and metastatic carcinoma. Fluorescein angiography in the acute phase of the disease shows typically multiple hyperfluorescent pinpoints, corresponding to choroiditis lesions, which coalesce into larger areas corresponding to the retinal exsudative detachment.

Diagnostic Criteria

In 1980, the American Uveitis Society proposed a diagnostic criteria (Table 86.1) (5) taking into consideration those previously suggested by Sugiura (Table 86.2). However, these criteria come short in making diagnosis in the acute phase as 2 of the 4 criteria occur only in the chronic phase, namely chronic bilateral iridociclytis and cutaneous signs. In an effort to unify concepts and allow the

TABLE 86.1. American Uveitis Society criteria for diagnosis of VKH.

No history of trauma or surgery and one finding from at least three of the following four groups:

1. Bilateral chronic iridocyclitis
2. Posterior uveitis: exudative retinal detachment, formed fruste of retinal detachment (disc hyperemia or edema, subretinal macular edema), and "sunset glow" fundus
3. Neurological signs: tinnitus, meningismus, cranial nerve or central nervous system problem, cerebrospinal fluid pleocytosis
4. Cutaneous signs: alopecia, poliosis, or vitiligo

TABLE 86.2. Sugiura's diagnostic criteria for VKH.

1. Acute bilateral uveitis with simultaneous involvement of both eyes. Symptoms may not be noted for 1–10 days in the second eye.
2. Circumscribed retinal edema most markedly at the posterior pole. Fluorescent angiography reveals characteristic leakage of dye through the retinal pigment epithelium into the subretinal spaces.
3. Pleocytosis of the cerebrospinal fluid is noted in the early stages of the disease. Dysacousia, vertigo, and scalp sensitivity when touching the hair are of value in early diagnosis, if present.
Floating cells in the anterior chamber, granulomatous keratic precipitates, and iris nodules are important signs that may be absent in early stages.
Hair loss and depigmentation of the eye, skin, and hair are also important signs in the convalescent stage.
Depigmentation of the corneal limbus appears earliest (Siguiura's sign), roughly 1 month after onset, and is also valuable for confirming the early diagnosis if present.

Criteria 1, 2, and 3 are major symptoms. Criteria 1 or 2, and 3 are required to diagnose VLH. Minor symptoms are noted below the major symptoms and are helpful in diagnosis, if present.

TABLE 86.3. Revised diagnostic criteria for VKH.

1. No history of penetrating ocular trauma
2. No evidence of other ocular or systemic disease
3. Bilateral ocular disease – either a or b:

a. *Early Manifestations*
   i. Diffuse choroiditis manifested as either;
      1. Focal areas of sub retinal fluid or
      2. Bullous serous retinal detachments
   ii. If equivocal fundus findings, then both of below
      1. Fluorescent angiography showing focal delayed choroidal perfusion, pinpoint leakage, pooling within sub retinal fluid, and optic nerve staining
      2. Ultrasound showing diffuse choroidal thickening without posterior scleritis

b. *Late Manifestations*
   i. History suggestive of above, and both ii and iii or multiple from iii
   ii. Ocular depigmentation
      1. Sunset glow fundus, or
      2. Sugiura sign
   iii. Other ocular signs
      1. nummular chorioretinal depigmented scars, or
      2. RPE clumping, or
      3. recurrent or chronic anterior uveitis
      4. Neurological/auditory findings
         a. Meningismus
         b. Tinnitus
         c. Cerebrospinal fluid pleocytosis
      5. Integumentary findings
         a. Alopecia
         b. Poliosis
         c. Vitiligo

Complete VKH requires 1 to 5.
Incomplete VKH requires 1 to 3 and either 4 or 5.
Probable VKH requires criteria 1 to 3 only.

comparison of results from clinical studies from different countries, the International Committee on Nomenclature proposed the Revised Diagnostic Criteria for VKH disease in 2001 (4). The Revised Diagnostic Criteria for VKH disease subdivides patients into three categories: probable, incomplete, and complete. It encompasses a broader range of patients as the ocular manifestations may be either acute or chronic to meet the criteria.

Differential Diagnosis

The principal differential diagnosis of VKH disease is sympathetic ophthalmia which prorogates the existence of previous ocular trauma or surgery. Other conditions that may mimic VKH disease are: acute posterior multi-focal placoid pigmentar epitheliopathy (APMPPE), posterior scleritis, sarocoidosis, other white-dot syndromes, other conditions related to diffuse choroiditis and intraocular primary lymphoma (Table 86.4). On the basis of this, a complete history and physical examination followed by blood tests, tuberculin test, and image should be performed in all patients.

Prognosis

Systemic steroid treatment gives to two-thirds of the patients a fair visual prognosis, retaining 20/40 or better final visual acuity. Fortunately, only the minority (11%) of these patients will have a visual acuity of 20/200 or worse.

Treatment

The standard therapy includes high dose of systemic corticosteroid besides topical medication for anterior uveitis. Prednisone should be used in a typical dosage of

TABLE 86.4. Differential diagnosis of uveitis in the set of VKH.

Sympathetic ophthalmia
Acute posterior multifocal placoid pigment epitheliopathy
Posterior scleritis
Multiple evanescent white dot syndrome
Tuberculosis
Sarcoidosis
Intraocular B-cell lymphoma
Metastatic carcinoma
Idiopathic uveal effusion syndrome

1 to 2 mg/kg/day orally. There is no evidence of superiority of intravenous to oral use of corticosteroid. Some authors recommend methylprednisolone in pulse therapy. Early steroid therapy followed by a slow taper in a period of 6 to 9 months is advised. This has shown to improve the prognosis by reducing the length of disease, the incidence of a convalescent phase, and decreasing extraocular manifestations in VKH.

In refractory cases or in those where it is necessary to withdraw the steroid administration more quickly, it is important to use systemic immunosuppressants, such as cyclosporine, which is the most commonly used. Other cytostatic agents may be used, such as cyclophosphamide, chlorambucil, azathioprine, and more recently, mycophenolate mofetil.

Choroidal neovascular membranes may be treated with traditional photocoagulation therapy or, more recently, with intraocular anti-angiogenic drug therapy. Acute angle closure glaucoma in the acute phase of the disease typically resolves after appropriate steroid treatment.

References

1. Koyanagi YD. Alopecia und poliosis bei schwerer Uveitis nicht traumatischen Ursprungs. Klin Monatsbl Augenkeikd 1929;194:194–211.
2. Vogt A. Fruhzeitiges Ergaruen der Zilien und Bemerkungen uber den sogenaten plotzlichen Eintreitt dieser Veranderung. Klin Monatsbl Augenkeikd 1906;44:228–42.
3. Harada E. Acute diffuse choroiditis. Acta Soc Ophtalmol Jpn 1926;30:356–78.
4. Read RW, Holland GN, Rao NA, et al. Revised diagnostic criteria for Vogt-Koyanagi-Harada disease: report of an international committee on nomenclature. Am J Ophtalmol 2001;131:647–52.
5. Snyder DA, Tessler HH. Vogt-Koyanagi-Harada syndrome. Am J Ophthalmol 1980;90:69–75.
6. Belfort Junior R, Nishi M, Hayashi S, et al. Vogt-Koyanagi-Harada's disease in Brazil. Jpn J Ophthalmol 1988;32:344–7.
7. Damico FM, Cunha-Neto E, Goldberg AC, et al. T-cell recognition and cytokine profile induced by melanocyte epitopes inpatients with HLA-DRB1*0405-positive and -negative Vogt-Koyanagi-Harada uveitis. Invest Ophthalmol Vis Sci. 2005;46:2465–71.
8. Yamaki K, Gocho K, Hayakawa K, et al. Tyrosinase family proteins are antigens specific to Vogt-Koyanagi-Harada disease. J Immunol 2000;165:7323–29.
9. Shindo Y, Ohno S, Yamamoto T, Nakamura S, Inoko H. Complete association of the HLA-DRB1*04 and -DQB1*04 alleles with Vogt-Koyanagi-Harada's disease. Hum Immunol 1994;39:169–76.
10. Goldberg AC, Yamamoto JH, Chiarella JM, et al. HLA-DRB1*0405 is the predominant allele in Brazilian patients with Vogt-Koyanagi-Harada disease. Hum Immunol 1998; 59:183–8.
11. Chee S-P, Chi DL, Cheng CL, et al. Visual function in Vogt-Konayagi-Harada patients. Graefe's Arch Clin Exp Ophthalmol 2005;243; 785–790
12. M Shinzato, JH Yamamoto, CE Hirata, et al, Anti-SS-A/Ro reactivity in patients with Vogt-Koyanagi-Harada syndrome-Lupus 2004;13, 279–80.

87
Orbital Myositis

Sergio Prieto and Josep M. Grau

Abstract Idiopathic orbital myositis (IOM) represents a subtype of nonspecific inflammation related to the clinical entity known as inflammatory pseudotumour, which affects one or more of the external extrinsic ocular muscles. Although its aetiology is unknown, an immunological process is suspected because of the association of the syndrome wirh other autoimmune diseases. Young women are predominantly affected, with unilateral orbital pain which worsens with ocular movements being the main complaint. Imaging by ultrasonography, CT-scan or magnetic resonance are useful for the diagnosis. In all of them, an usually single muscular enlargement can be demonstrated. Systemic corticosteroids represent the treatment of choice with quick and effective clinical response in most patients.

Keywords Orbital · myositis · inflammatory pseudotumour

Idiopathic orbital myositis is an autoimmune process characterized by unilateral orbital pain due to isolated inflammation of the extrinsic ocular musculature. Its natural course can evolve to a definitive ophthalmoplegia, particularly in the cases with a significant delay in the initiation of therapy with steroids.

Epidemiology

The main demographic group affected are middle-aged women with a ratio of 2:1 with respect to men and an average age of 35 years (range 3–80 years) (1). There are no data on the incidence, prevalence or geographical distribution. Influenza-like syndrome and streptococcal pharyngitis have been proposed as possible triggers of the disease (2,3).

History

In 1954, Tolosa (4) reported a case of a man with unilateral retrorbital pain, III, IV and VI cranial nerve palsies and diminution of corneal reflex, which resolved in three years. Necropsy disclosed a granulomatous lesion in the cavernous sinus affecting the cranial nerves. Seven years later, Hunt (5) reported six similar cases without pathological studies. The eponym Tolosa-Hunt syndrome was therefore used for cases with coexistant ocular pain and paralysis. Only in the past decade and with the use of CT-scan or magnetic resonance imaging could the different orbitary structures be defined, thereby allowing the clear differentiation between orbital myositis and the remaining inflammatory conditions affecting orbital tissues.

Clinical Manifestations

The most important signs and symptoms of the disease are reflected in Table 87.1, categorized as localized (orbital) and systemic (6–9). Unilateral orbital pain that worsens with ocular movements is the cardinal symptom. Ophthalmoparesis does occur but later in the clinical evolution. The disease onset is usually acute, but it may be subacute or even chronic. In more than two-third of the cases, only one muscle is involved, with the rectus external or internal being the most frequently affected. Participation of the obliquous muscle or bilaterality is considered as exceptional (10).

As in other autoimmune diseases, orbital myositis may be associated with other immunological processes shown in Table 87.2 (11).

From: Y. Shoenfeld et al. (eds.): *Diagnostic Criteria in Autoimmune Diseases*, DOI: 10.1007/978-1-60327-285-8_87,

TABLE 87.1. Clinical presentation of idiopathic orbital myositis.

Localized	Systemic
Periorbital pain	Headache
Diplopia	Fever
Palpebral edema	Vomiting
Exophthalmos	Anorexia
Conjunctival chemosis	Lethargy
Palpebral ptosis	Abdominal pain
Palpable orbitary mass	Odinophagia

TABLE 87.2. Autoimmune diseases associated with orbital myositis.

Crohn's disease
Sytemic lupus erythematosus
Rheumatoid arthritis
Type I diabetes
Polyarteritis nodosa
Dermatomyositis
Ankylosing spondylitis
Giant cell myocarditis

TABLE 87.3. Diagnostic criteria[a] for orbital myositis.

1. Unilateral orbital pain (+/– ophthalmoparesia).
2. Positive image test of muscle involvement (+/– tendinous) without bone compromise.
3. Satisfactory response to corticosteroid therapy.
4. Compatible pathological examination .

[a] Fullfiling the first three criteria a probable case is admitted, and with the fourth item a definite form.

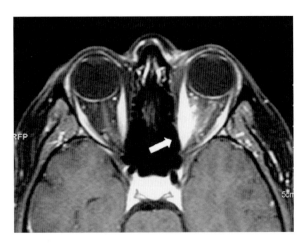

FIGURE 87.1. Orbital CT-scan showing the thickening of an isolated ocular muscle. Orbital myositis.

Biochemical Features

All the standard biochemical parameters are within normal values except for a raised ESR and mild eosinophilia in some cases. Antinuclear autoantibodies can be detected in a percentage of patients with an unspecific pattern and in low titers. There are no abnormalities in thyroid function tests and it is useful in the differential diagnosis.

Pathological Features

Nonspecific inflammatory infiltrate mainly composed of mononuclear cells, plasma cells, polynuclear cells and some eosinophils is the rule in the affected muscles.

Diagnosis

There are no definitive criteria for the diagnosis of orbital myositis. This diagnosis may be admitted when at least three of the four proposed criteria are present (Table 87.3). They consist in suggestive clinical findings, an imaging test demonstrating muscle involvement and satisfactory response to steroid treatment. The histological approach is reserved for selected cases. Ultrasonography, magnetic resonance and CT-scan are all valid techniques, but CT-scan is preferred because of its better sensitivity, specificity and lower cost. The characteristic finding is an isolated thickened extraocular muscle, with or without tendinous involvement (this is a typical but not a constant finding), but without bone

participation (Figure 87.1). Muscle biopsy is performed only in selected cases when the diagnosis is confusing or when the case is refractory to therapy, because the procedure may aggravate the inflammatory phenomenon (10).

Because there are no established criteria for the diagnosis of this disease, we suggest four different items (Table 87.3). With three of these criteria, a probable form could be considered while a definite case would require all four criteria.

Differential Diagnosis

Table 87.4 describes the pathological conditions that can mimic an orbital myositis (3,12). Among them, Grave's disease is the most important to be ruled out becuase it is the first cause of thickened extraocular muscle involvement (13).

Therapy

Systemic corticosteroids are the treatment of choice with a positive response rate over 70%, complete clinical response over 30% and recurrences in about 40% of the cases. (14). The recommended dose is 1–2 mg/kg body weight for the first two weeks with a decreasing doses for the following two months. To optimize the results, treatment should be started within the first 2 weeks of clinical

TABLE 87.4. Orbital myositis. Differential diagnosis.

1. Systemic inflammatory conditions:
   Autoimmune thyroid disease
   Sarcoidosis
   Wegener's Granulomatosis
   Churg-Strauss syndrome
   X Histiocytosis
   Giant cell arteritis
   Polyarteritis nodosa
   Systemic sclerosis
   Sclerosing cholangitis
2. Neoplastic diseases
   Lymphoproliferative disorders
   Rhabdomiosarcoma
   Choroidal malignant melanoma
   Metastasis
3. Congenital malformations
4. Infectious diseases
5. Trauma

TABLE 87.5. Recurrence related factors in orbital myositis.

Male gender.
Several muscles involved.
Bilateral involvement.
Lack of exophthalmos.
Poor initial response to treatment.
Lack of tendinous involvement.

presentation (6,15,16). Factors related to a high proportion of recurrences have been identified and are shown in Table 87.5 (14,17).

Intravenous immunoglobulins (18), radiotherapy (13) and other immunosuppressive agents have been used, albeit in anecdotal reports.

References

1. Scott IU, Siatkowski RM. (1997) Idiopathic orbital myositis. *Curr Opin Rheumatol* **9**, 504–12.
2. Furcell JJ Jr, Taulbee WA. (1981) Orbital myositis after upper respiratory tract infection. *Arch Ophthalmol* **99**, 434.
3. Lutt JR, Lim LL, Phal PM, Rosebaum JT. Orbital Inflammatory Disease. (2008) *Semin Arthritis Rheum* **37**, 207–22.
4. Tolosa E. (1954) Periarteritic lesions of carotid siphon with clinical features of carotid infraclinoidal aneurysm. *J Neurol Neurosurg Psychiatry* **17**, 300.
5. Hunt WE, Meagher JN, LeFever HE, Zeman W. (1961) Painful ophthalmoplegia: Its relation to indolent inflammation of the cavernous sinus. *Neurology* **11**, 56.
6. Slavin ML, Glaser JS. Idiopathic orbital myositis: Report of six cases. (1982) *Arch Ophthalmol* **100**, 1261.
7. Trokel SL, Hilal SK. (1979) Recognition and differential diagnosis of enlarged extraocular muscles in computed tomography. *Am J Ophthalmol* **87**, 503.
8. Mottow-Lippa L, Jakobiec FA. Idiopathic inflammatory orbital pseudotumor in childhood: I. Clinical characteristics (1978). *Arch Ophthalmol* **96**, 1410.
9. Mottow-Lippa L, Jakobiec FA, Smith M. Idiopathic inflammatory orbital pseudotumor in childhood: II. Results of diagnostic tests and biopsies. (1981) *Ophthalmology* **88**, 565.
10. Siatkowski RM, Capo H, Byrne SF, Gendron EK, Flynn JT, Munoz M et al. (1994) Clinical and echographic fingdings in idiopathic orbital myositis. *Am J Ophthalmol* **118**, 343–50.
11. Le Gal G, Ansart S, Boumediène A, Tonnelier JM, Tilly-Gentric A, Pennec YL (2001). Idiopathic orbital myositis. *Rev Med Interne* **22(2)**, 189–93.
12. Gordon LK. Orbital inflammatory disease: a diagnostic and therapeutic challenge (2006) *Eye* **20(10)**, 1196–206.
13. Mombaerts I, Koornneef L. (1997) Current status in the treatment of orbital myositis. *Ophthalmology* **104**, 402–8.
14. Mombaerts I, Koornneef L. (1997) Current status in the treatment of orbital myositis. *Ophthalmology* **104**, 402.
15. Bullen CL, Younge BR.(1982) Chronic orbital myositis. *Arch Ophthalmol* **100**, 1749.
16. Weinstein GS, Dresner SC, Slamovitis TL, Kennerdell JS. (1983) Acute and subacute orbital myositis. *Am J Ophthalmol* **96**, 209.
17. Bullen CL, Younge BR. (1982) Chronic orbital myositis. *Arch Ophthalmol* **100**, 1749–51.
18. Shambal S, Lindner A, Zierz S. (1998) Succesful treatment of orbital myositis with intravenous inmunoglobulins. *Muscle Nerve* **21**, 1359.

Part XII
Renal Autoimmune Diseases

88

IgA Nephropathy

Jordi Ara i del Rey

Abstract   Primary IgA nephropathy (IgAN) is a mesangial proliferative glomerulonephritis characterized by diffuse mesangial deposition of IgA and is always diagnosed by performing a renal biopsy. This entity is now recognized as one of the commonest forms of glomerulonephritis worldwide and normally affects young adults with a male predominance. The clinical presentation of primary IgAN ranges from asymptomatic forms with microhematuria without proteinuria, microhematuria with different grades of proteinuria, chronic renal failure (CRF) or forms that present with acute renal failure, nephritic syndrome or malignant hypertension. Its evolution is very variable but is generally considered as a disease that progresses slowly to renal failure with about of 15% of patients progressing to CRF in 10 years and 30% in 20 years of follow-up. The most important clinical risk factors of progression are age, proteinuria, renal function at diagnosis, hypertension and significant glomerulosclerosis or chronic tubulointerstitial lesions in renal biopsy. At present, the treatment of IgAN is still not clearly defined. Concerning the pharmacological treatment, all proteinuric patients must receive ACEI or ARA II with the intention to keep blood pressure below 125/75 mmHg, as well as statins in case of dyslipaemia. If proteinuria persists above 1 g/day with normal or scarcely altered renal function, treatment with prednisone may be administered for 6 months. In case of rapidly progressive renal failure, the addition of cyclophosphamide–prednisone shall be taken into consideration. Fish oil treatment may be useful in some patients. In cases of severe CRF with creatinine >2.5 mg/dl, only conservative treatment and dialysis or subsequent kidney transplant will be indicated.

Keywords   IgA nephropathy · clinical features · diagnosis · treatment

Introduction

IgA nephropathy (IgAN) was first described in 1968 by Berger and Hinglais and is now recognized as one of the commonest forms of glomerulonephritis worldwide. This nephropathy may present in different ways and its evolution is also very variable, with about 15% of patients progressing to chronic renal failure (CRF) in 10 years and 30% in 20 years of follow-up. The clinical manifestation of this condition is very variable and ranges from asymptomatic forms that present with microhaematuria without proteinuria, microhaematuria with different grades of proteinuria with or without hypertension and renal failure, or forms that present with acute renal failure, rapidly progressive glomerulonephritis or nephrotic syndrome.

Primary IgAN is a mesangial proliferative glomerulonephritis characterized by diffuse mesangial deposition of IgA and is unique among glomerular disease in being defined by the presence of immune reactant rather than by any other morphologic feature found on renal biopsy.

Many other diseases are also associated with glomerular IgA deposits (secondary IgAN) and the most common of these is Schönlein–Henoch purpura. The histologic features of Schönlein–Henoch purpura nephritis are indistinguishable from those of primary IgAN and may represent a systemic form of the disease process (see Table 88.1).

Epidemiology

IgAN may affect persons of all ages but it normally affects young adults (second to third decade of life) with a male predominance of 2–3:1. This entity occurs with greatest frequency in Asians and Caucasians and is relatively rare in blacks. The frequency of the disease varies substantially

From: Y. Shoenfeld et al. (eds.): *Diagnostic Criteria in Autoimmune Diseases*, DOI: 10.1007/978-1-60327-285-8_88,

TABLE 88.1. Disease reported in association with IgA nephropathy.

Schönlein–Henoch purpura
Hepatic disease (nonalcoholic cirrhosis, alcoholic liver disease)
Intestinal diseases (Crohn's disease ulcerative colitis, celiac disease)
HIV infection
Glomerulonephritis (lupus nephropathy, minimal change disease, membranous nephropathy)
Skin diseases (psoriasis, dermatitis herpetiformis)
Systemic/immunological disorders (systemic lupus erythematosus, rheumatoid arthritis, ankylosing spondylitis, Reiter's syndrome, uveitis, Bechet's syndrome, Takayasu's syndrome, myasthenia gravis, sicca syndrome)
Malignancy (small cell carcinoma, lymphoma, Hodgkin's disease, T-cell lymphomas including mycosis fungoides, IgA monoclonal gammopathy)
Respiratory disease (tuberculosis, bronchiolitis obliterans, sarcoidosis)
Infections (B hepatitis, brucellosis, leprosy)

between countries. In the USA, the incidence ranges from 5 (1979) to 12 (1990) new cases per million inhabitants per year, whereas in France, Germany and Italy the rate is two- or three-fold higher. Japan has the highest frequency, with approximately 140 new cases per million inhabitants per year, probably due to widespread screening of school-aged children for urinary abnormalities.

In most studies, the prevalence of this entity is expressed as the percentage of all the biopsies conducted. The greatest prevalence is found in Asia (40–50% of all biopsies examined), followed by Europe (20–25%), North America (12%), Central and South America (6%) and South Africa (1%) (2). According to the data from the Spanish Glomerulonephritis Register, actually the percentage of IgAN in respect of the total number of biopsies was about 17%. There are also specific geographical areas with very high (Native Americans of New Mexico) or low prevalence (Polynesian of New Zealand).

The differences in the incidence and prevalence observed between the different territories may of course be explained by genetic differences between different populations but also by the different criteria used for the conducting of kidney biopsies. The incidence is higher in areas where there are screening programmes for urinary abnormalities and subsequent biopsies are conducted than in populations who are not systematically screened or in areas where renal biopsies are not recommended for mild microhaematuria and proteinuria and only conducted in patients with major proteinuria or deterioration of renal function.

Clinical Features

The clinical presentation of primary IgAN varies greatly and depends on the population studied. Table 88.2 shows the clinical–analytical data at the time of diagnosis as shown in the different series published in the literature.

For practical purposes, the different clinical presentations of this entity may be divided in the following manner:

Macroscopic Haematuria

Approximately 40–50% of patients present with one or recurrent episodes of gross haematuria, usually following an upper respiratory infection. In contrast to a 10- to 14-day delay in onset in patients with post-streptococcal glomerulonephritis, the urine becomes red 1–2 days after the first infectious symptoms. Some patients also describe loin pain, which usually reflects stretching of renal capsules, low-grade fever, malaise or myalgia. Hypertension and peripheral oedema are rare. The macroscopic haematuria resolves spontaneously over the course of a few days and episodes can recur months or years later with febrile illness or extreme exercise. This presentation typically occurs in patients under 40 years of age.

Asymptomatic Haematuria and Proteinuria

Asymptomatic urine testing identifies 30–40% of patients with IgAN. Such patients are often adults and they rarely experience macroscopic haematuria. Proteinuria is usually under 2 g day and the percentage of patients with arterial hypertension (AHT) is variable. The percentage of patients diagnosed with this presentation depends very much on the biopsy criteria used in the region.

Nephrotic Syndrome

Nephrotic syndrome is uncommon and represents only 5% of all patients with IgAN. This presentation may be due to two different situations: (a) nephrotic syndrome with normal urinary sediment and normal renal function, and (b) high proteinuria selectivity and histologic features similar to minimal change disease but with diffuse mesangial staining for IgA or patients with advanced renal disease clinically presenting with CRF, nephrotic proteinuria and hypertension. In this case, chronic tubulointerstitial and glomerular lesions predominate histologically and the evolution is not favourable.

Acute Renal Failure

Rarely, patients develop acute renal failure. This may be due to:

a) heavy glomerular haematuria leading to tubular occlusion and damage by red cells. The latter is usually reversible.
b) crescentic IgAN

Malignant HTA

Rarely, IgAN may present with malignant hypertension.

Table 88.2. Clinical features at presentation and 10 years actuarial survival [modified from ref (5)].

Author	Number of patients	Mean age (years)	High creatinine (%)	HTA	Proteinuria >3 g/24 h (%)	Macroscopic haematuria (%)	Follow-up (months)	10 years renal survival
D'amico (1986) Europe (e)	365	29	24	36	7	55	79	85
Droz (1987) (e)	280	–	–	6	10	37	60	85
Velo (1987) (e)	153	22	–	–	1	78	60	81
Bogenschutz (1990) (e)	239	–	34	19	–	26	59	81
Rekola (e) (1990)	209	25	16	11	1	64	76	83
Alamartine (e) (1991)	282	28	2	9	3	27	96	94
Johnston (e) (1992)	220	30	28	26	32	–	65	83
Gaddes (e. glasgow) 2003	112	37	46 (creatinine clearance <75 ml/min)	Mean arterial blood pressure 105	–	–	86	64
Gaddes (e. Helsinky) 2003	123	35	17 (creatinine clearance <75 ml/min)	Mean arterial blood pressure 102	–	–	123	96
Nichols 1984 Australia (a)	244	32	36	43	6	39	60	87
Ibels 1994 (a)	121	39	36	31	16	40	107	93
Gaddes 2003 (a)	73	33	% creatinine clearance <75 ml/min 42%	Mean arterial blood pressure 103	–	–	73	61%
Katafuchi Asia (as) 1994	225	32	36	22	16	20	48	74
Yoo (as) 1986	151	27	6	33	4	24	65	82
Koyama (as) 1997	448	–	19	29	3	24	142	85
Wyatt 1984 America (am)	58	27	–	–	–	–	60	78
Radford 1997 (am)	148	39	59	47	30	–	45	67
Hass 1997 (am)	109	40	Mean creatinine 2.2 mg/dl	49	33	35	>18	57
Gaddes 2003 Canada	274	37	% creatinine clearance <75 ml/min 48%	Mean arterial blood pressure 105	–	–	53	62

Chronic Renal Failure

Some patients have renal impairment, proteinuria and hypertension when first diagnosed. The smaller size of the kidneys renders kidney biopsy more difficult. These patients tend to be older and it is probable that they have a longstanding disease which was not detected earlier because the patient did not have haematuria or undergo routine analysis.

Other Diseases with IgA Deposition

Schönlein–Henoch Purpura

Schönlein–Henoch purpura is an IgA-mediated small-vessel vasculitis affecting the skin, joints, gut and kidney in which the glomerular disease may be indistinguishable from IgAN. Furthermore, Schönlein–Henoch purpura

and IgAN are currently considered to be a related disease because both can be encountered consecutively in the same patient; they have been described in identical twins and present identical pathological and biological abnormalities. IgAN seems to be a kidney-restricted form of Schönlein–Henoch purpura. Apart from the typical systemic signs of vasculitis (skin, joints, gut), the clinical differences between the two entities are:

a) peak age lower in Schönlein–Henoch purpura (<15 years old) than in IgAN (>15 years old)
b) acute haematuria and/or massive proteinuria is much more common in Schönlein–Henoch purpura than in IgAN
c) Schönlein–Henoch purpura is more often described in association with drug hypersensitivity
d) Schönlein–Henoch purpura is much less frequently associated with other diseases than IgAN

Secondary Forms of IgA Nephropathy

In the vast majority of cases, IgAN is an isolated disease (primary IgAN) but it may be associated with various clinical disorders. Cirrhosis, celiac disease and HIV infection are all associated with a high frequency of glomerular IgA deposition. IgAN has been infrequently associated with a variety of other diseases, including glomerulonephritis (minimal change disease, membranous nephropathy), intestinal diseases (Crohn's disease, ulcerative colitis), skin diseases (psoriasis, dermatitis herpetiformis), systemic/immunological disorders (systemic lupus erythematosus, rheumatoid arthritis, ankylosing spondylitis), small cell carcinoma, lymphoma (Hodgkin's disease, T-cell lymphomas including mycosis fungoides), tuberculosis and bronchiolitis obliterans. For more information, see Table 88.1

Pregnancy and IgAN

The effects of pregnancy on the course of IgAN are not well established, nor are the maternal–foetal risks of the pregnancy in women with this disease. From the point of view of perinatal mortality, this appears to be increased in pregnant women with IgAN and renal failure compared with a healthy population or compared with patients with IgAN but with no renal failure (14% vs 3%). Higher perinatal mortality was also observed in women with IgAN plus hypertension compared with normotensive patients. In a study with a 5-year follow-up, no adverse influence of gestation on the natural course of IgAN was detected.

Histology

Immunofluorescence Findings

Histologically, IgAN (as its name suggests) is characterized by the presence of diffuse mesangial IgA deposits that are visible by immunofluorescence techniques. At the same time, c3 (90% of cases), IgG (40% of cases) and IgM (40% of cases) deposits may also be observed, but c1q deposits are not found. On some occasions, IgA deposits may also be observed in the capillary wall, though this is much more typical in Schönlein–Henoch purpura nephropathy than in primary IgAN. When it does appear in cases of IgAN, it is associated with a poorer prognosis. The disappearance of the IgA deposits after a long remission period has been described in a paediatric series. This fact has not been confirmed in an adult population.

Light Microscopy

There is great variation in the histological lesions that may be observed under light microscope in IgAN. These findings may span from practically normal glomeruli, to the most common form characterized by various levels of focal or diffuse mesangial hypercellularity, to forms similar to focal and segmental glomerulosclerosis. The latter form often appears in cases of patients who have suffered the disease for many years, where the biopsy is usually taken when there is already CRF with major proteinuria, and the above glomerular lesions are often accompanied by chronic tubulointerstitial lesions (interstitial infiltrate, interstitial fibrosis, tubular atrophy). It has been observed that the lesions detected by light microscopy in this disease are not well correlated topographically with the IgA deposits localized by immunofluorescence.

With light microscopy, there are also other types of histological presentations which correspond to special clinical presentations. These are:

a) necrotizing glomerulonephritis with crescent formation (acute renal failure);
b) tubular occlusion by red cells without glomerular injury (acute renal failure);
c) malignant hypertension;
d) optically normal glomeruli with fusion of the pedicles of the podocytes under electronic microscopy and mesangial IgA deposits (minimal change disease like) (nephrotic syndrome).

A number of classifications of IgAN based on light microscopic findings have been proposed (Haas, Lee), but their ability to predict prognosis and guide therapeutic decision making is uncertain. An international consensus of the pathologic classification of IgAN is being developed by the international IgAN network with the Renal Pathology Society under the auspices of the International Society of Nephrology. It is expected that the consensus statement will be issued in 2008.

Electronic Microscopy

The most frequent observation is electron-dense deposits that are localized in the areas of mesangial deposits of IgA. In the ultrastructural description of the capillary wall, focal thinning of the glomerular basement membrane (GBM) is appreciated increasingly. Consistent and widespread GBM thinning indistinguishable from that described in thin membrane nephropathy has also been described in IgAN. The significance of this association has not yet been clarified.

Other Entities with Mesangial Deposits of IgA

There are entities other than IgAN that may present with mesangial deposits of this immunoglobulin. IgA deposits may be observed in cases of lupus nephritis, but IgG deposits are more prominent. Moreover, whereas in IgAN the complement is activated by the "alternative pathway," in the case of lupus, it is the classic pathway (c1q). Renal mesangial deposits of IgA may also be seen in patients with chronic alcohol-induced liver disease, IgA monoclonal gammopathy and schistosomial nephropathy.

Histological Differences Between IgAN and Schönlein–Henoch Purpura Nephropathy

Histologically, Schönlein–Henoch purpura nephropathy is differentiated from primary IgAN in that the former usually presents necrotizing glomerular lesions and usually has a higher percentage of crescents and more diffuse endocapillary proliferation and fibrosi.

Clinical Evolution and Progression Factors

The evolution of IgAN is very variable and spans from very benign forms to forms that present rapidly progressive renal impairment. This entity is generally considered as a disease that progresses slowly to renal failure as demonstrated by the fact that approximately 15% of patients diagnosed will enter haemodialysis programmes after 10 years and after 20 years of follow-up; 40% of patients will have CRF (50% in haemodialysis). As it is most frequently diagnosed in the second or third decade of life, this fact has greater importance.

There is a series of factors that affect the natural evolution of IgAN which include geographical location, age and the clinical presentation of the disease. There are significant differences between the renal survival percentages observed according to the geographical location.

Ten-year renal survival rates in European and Asian series is around 80–90%, whereas in American series this is lower (60–70%). Apart from possible genetic factors, this fact is also due to different biopsy policies in different regions. Patients undergoing biopsies in the USA had a higher proportion of proteinuria >3 g, hypertension and CRF at diagnosis.

The clinical course also varies depending on the age of the patient when the disease presents, with lower renal survival in adults than in children over the same follow-up period. In the paediatric population (<15 years), the percentage of complete remission according to some series is high and only 4% developed CRF (7-year follow-up).

The type of clinical presentation has also been seen to be important in the evolution of the disease. Patients with IgAN with only microhaematuria or microhaematuria with minimal proteinuria have a very good long-term prognosis, while those with major proteinuria, hypertension or renal failure at diagnosis have the worst prognosis. Despite this, a recent study demonstrated that a subgroup of patients with an "apparent" good prognosis (microhaematuria with minimal proteinuria) may also have an unfavourable outcome. In this study, 33% of these patients developed proteinuria of >1 g after 7 years, 26% AHT and 7% CRF (Cr >1.4 mg/dl).

Five-year studies were conducted with repeated biopsies in patients with IgAN who had microhaematuria and variable levels of proteinuria at the time of diagnosis. These indicated that a histological deterioration was observed in up to 55% of patients and a reduction in glomerular filtration in 33% of patients (much more marked in patients with higher proteinuria) with this type of clinical presentation.

There are data that suggest that the risk of progression to CRF is proportional to the proteinuria at 1 year of follow-up: patients with proteinuria <0.5 g daily have a 0% risk of progression to CRF at 5 years of follow-up, patients with proteinuria between 0.5 and 1.5 g/day have a 13% risk, those with proteinuria between 1.5 and 3 g/day have a 25% risk and, finally, patients with proteinuria of >3 g have a 60% risk of progression to CRF.

A retrospective study of a large series of patients with this disease enabled us to establish the factors that are considered key to the progression of the disease. The factors that are unquestionably linked to a poor prognosis from a clinical point of view are: (a) elevated creatinine at diagnosis, (b) hypertension (c) and proteinuria >500 mgs/1 daily. Histologically, the following are considered as poor prognostic factors: (a) a significant percentage of glomerulosclerosis, (b) chronic tubulointerstitial lesions, (c) Haas or Lee class IV–V and (d) the presence of significant extracapillary proliferation. Other classic factors that were for many years considered as associated with poor prognosis are now thought to carry less prognostic weight (older age at diagnosis, male sex, no history of macrohaematuria, mesangial hypercellularity and expansion, marked arteriolar hyalinosis and IgA deposits in capillaries).

Based on the poor clinical prognostic factors, some attempts have been made to stratify patients into risk groups for the evolution of CRF. The scores used to calculate if a patient belongs to the high-risk group as proposed by Magistroni are the following: 2 points for creatinine >1.4 mg/dl, 1 point for proteinuria >1 g daily and 1 point for age >30 years. Patients with scores between 0–2 would be included in the low-risk group (91% renal survival after 10 years) and those with scores of 3–5 would be included in the high-risk group (35% renal survival after 10 years).

IgAN Evolution Following a Kidney Transplant

There are few studies on the progression of IgAN following a kidney transplant. Disease recurrence is relatively common despite the immunodepressant medication that transplant patients receive. Neither classic immunosuppressors nor the new immunosuppressors appear to be capable of preventing the recurrence of the disease. Various series have demonstrated a very variable percentage recurrence ranging between 13 and 60%. In series where biopsies are only performed in cases of suspected clinical relapse (no protocol biopsies), the percentage of relapse is about 20%. The course of recurrent IgAN in transplant patients is relatively benign with percentages of graft dysfunction and graft failure of 11–23%/2–16% in function of the different series. Analysis of actuarial renal survival of transplant patients due to IgAN demonstrates that the percentage survival is very similar to that of patients receiving a transplant for any other cause.

Although some studies question it due to the high relapse rates, more recent data indicate that transplants from live donors is not contraindicated in this situation.

Diagnosis

IgAN is always diagnosed by performing a renal biopsy. Although a compatible clinical picture would be highly suggestive, it is insufficient for a diagnosis. Same is the case for high serum IgA levels, a finding that is observed in about 30% of patients. No analytical or immunologic data have demonstrated high diagnostic sensitivity or specificity. Once the renal biopsy is performed, the patient must be classified as having primary or secondary disease (see Table 88.1).

The main problem is to decide the most appropriate time to conduct the biopsy. An aggressive approach with the biopsy criteria (microhaematuria alone or microhaematuria with minimal proteinuria) would increase the cases diagnosed but would have little relevance on changes in therapeutic attitudes, and would also increase the number of patients undergoing kidney biopsies and the inherent risks.

Although there is no global agreement on the indication, it would appear reasonable to consider a kidney biopsy in patients with clinical suggestive signs and:

a) microhaematuria with proteinuria >1 g daily;
b) microhaematuria with proteinuria and renal failure.

Given that the forms of the disease with good prognostic criteria (isolated haematuria or haematuria with minimal proteinuria) do have some risk of progression, clinical control of these unbiopsied patients is recommended as well as a change of attitude if the above criteria are met.

The aim with this policy is to adjust and limit the number of biopsies to those cases where the patient would benefit from immunosuppressive treatment.

Treatment

Although this is a prevalent glomerular disease, at present the treatment of IgAN is still not clearly defined and there is no unanimous consensus on how to treat it. There are few well-designed studies on this subject and those that do exist generally contain small sample sizes. In addition, as the onset of the nephropathy is very slow, it may take years to reach the end-points being studied (CRF/duplication of creatinine). This has greatly limited the quantity and quality of the existing studies and has hindered the reaching of definitive conclusions on the usefulness of the different treatment modalities. Some of the existing trials, generally with short follow-ups, use proteinuria as the end-point assuming that the risk of CRF is proportional to the intensity of the proteinuria.

The treatment of this entity may be divided into two sections: conservative non-immunosuppressive treatment and immunosuppressive treatment.

Non-immunosuppressive Treatment

Non-immunosuppressive treatment of chronic proteinuric nephropathies includes antihypertensive and antiproteinuric treatments as well as the control of cholesterol fractions with statins. These treatments are beneficial due to the effects on reducing cardiovascular risk, which is very high in the population with CRF. The antihypertensive treatment is based mainly on the use of ACEI/ARA II alone or in combination with reducing blood pressure to at least 125/75 mmHg and reducing proteinuria as far as possible. The use of an ACE inhibitor (enalapril) or ARA II (valsartan) to treat this entity has been shown to slow down progression of CRF. The addition of ACEI + ARA II may contribute even further to the stabilization or reduction of the loss of renal function in this entity. The Cooperate study demonstrated that the pharmacological combination of ACEI plus ARA II reduces the advance of chronic renal impairment in a group of patients with chronic proteinuric nephropathies of non-diabetic origin and has a greater antiproteinuric effect than the administration of these two drugs separately. Of the 263 patients recruited for this study, all Japanese, 50% had IgAN.

Lipid abnormalities are very common in proteinuric patients. Statins have been shown to have a beneficial effect based on the reduction of the cardiovascular risk, and they may also have a beneficial effect on the progression of CRF.

There is some controversy on the efficacy of the administration of fish oils to reduce the advance of CRF in

IgAN. A meta-analysis encompassing five controlled trials (two with positive results and three with negative results) was incapable of providing statistical evidence of the beneficial effects of this therapeutic approach and recommended further studies. A substudy of this meta-analysis suggests that fish oils may be useful in patients with proteinuria >3 g daily.

Immunosuppressive Treatment

Prednisone

A recent meta-analysis has been conducted on the risks and benefits of immunosuppressive treatment in IgAN. This study included 13 clinically controlled randomized trials including 623 patients. The conclusions of this study (that focused solely on immunosuppressive treatment ignoring traditional treatment) were that the optimal treatment has yet to be defined. The studies that exist are small with less than optimal methodological quality and tend to highlight favourable results lacking detailed information of the harmful effects of the treatments. Despite all these drawbacks, the meta-analysis indicated that prednisone is useful in the treatment of this disease.

Considering the six studies that included prednisone versus placebo and which included 341 subjects, the meta-analysis suggests that treatment with prednisone reduces proteinuria, stabilizes renal function and reduces the risk of going on dialysis compared with the placebo.

Specifically analysing the studies, we may conclude that steroids alone may have a beneficial effect in case of IgAN in two situations:

a) Young patients with an abrupt onset of nephrotic syndrome without hypertension or renal function disturbances and with a histology compatible with minimal change disease with IgA deposits. In these cases, the doses of prednisone that should be used are the same as those used in nephrotic syndrome with minimal lesions and the treatment response, as in this entity, is good.
b) Patients with IgAN with Cr <1.5 mg/dl and proteinuria between 1 and 3 g. Prednisone, at variable doses depending on the study, may reduce proteinuria and prevent deterioration of renal function. There is greater debate on the use of steroids in this patient group as some studies overlook the effects of ACE inhibitors, as some do not comply with current recommendations on strict blood pressure control and because not all studies obtained results as positive as those of Pozzi et al. In this study, the patient group treated with prednisone obtained a 10-year renal survival of 97% compared with 53% in the placebo group.

In terms of the secondary effects observed with these regimens, the available information is scarce. In the studies in which the secondary effects were specified, the percentage oscillated between 0 and 40%.

Prednisone/Cyclophosphamide or Azathioprine

With the meta-analysis, it was not possible to clearly demonstrate the usefulness of this drug combination in the treatment of IgAN. It is therefore clear that this combination is not useful when applied in a general manner in patients with low risk, but it appears that it may be very useful in a subgroup of patients:

a) creatinine >1.5 and <2.5 mg/dl;
b) patients where inverse creatinine would suggest that that they will require haemodialysis in less than 5 years;
c) a 15% increase of creatinine in the past year;
d) >10% epithelial crescents in the renal biopsy.

Clinically, these patients often present nephrotic proteinuria. Although experience is lacking, there are various papers that support the use of regimens with sequential cyclophosphamide–azathioprine + steroids, cyclophosphamide bolus + steroids or azathioprine + steroids in this disease as a clearly better renal survival was attained. Survival of the treated group and the control group in two of the most relevant studies were 72% versus 6% (sequential CF-AZA + prednisone vs conservative treatment. 5 years of follow up) and 90% vs 55% [CF-Pd vs conservative treatment (retrospective group) 3 years of follow-up]. As is to be expected, these treatment regimens are accompanied with an appreciable percentage of adverse effects.

Mycophenolate

This is the latest drug to be used to treat this entity. Experience is still scarce, it does not appear in the meta-analyses and there are few data available to ascertain its real usefulness. From the few studies available, it would appear that this immunosuppressive agent is not useful in IgAN with major renal function impairment and histologic chronicity data. In contrast, there are promising results in reducing proteinuria in one study where it was used as a rescue therapy in patients with IgAN with sustained proteinuria (>1 g) despite optimal blood pressure control with ACE inhibitors. There are insufficient data on long-term follow-up regarding renal function to reach definitive conclusions.

Intravenous Immunoglobulin

High-dose intravenous immunoglobulin has been tried in severe IgAN, characterized by heavy proteinuria and a relatively rapid decline in glomerular filtration rate

TABLE 88.3. Treatment recommendations for IgA nephropathy.

Recurrent macroscopic haematuria with low or without proteinuria and normal renal function
No specific treatment
Microhaematuria + proteinuria <1 g
No specific treatment. Consider ACEI/ARA II
If HTA ACEI/ARA II (target 125/75)
Microhaematuria + proteinuria 1–3 g/24 h
ACEI/ARA II (target 125/75)
If proteinuria >1 g 24 h and creatinine <1.5 mg/dl after 6 months, consider prednisone (6 months)
If proteinuria >1 g 24 h and creatinine <1.5 mg/dl after treatment with prednisone, consider to add azathioprine
If proteinuria > 3 g and serum creatinine >1.5 mg/dl, consider fish oil 12 g daily for 6 months
Very high risk patients
Proteinuria > 3 g day and creatinine >1.5 and <2.5 mg/dl
or
patients where inverse creatinine would suggest that that they will require haemodialysis in less than 5 years
or
a 15% increase of creatinine in the past year
or
10% epithelial crescents in the renal biopsy/crescentic IgA glomerulonephritis
Consider to treat with sequential cyclophosphamide–azathioprine + steroids, cyclophosphamide bolus + steroids or azathioprine + steroids (similar to small vessel vasculitis)
Nephrotic syndrome with normal renal function and minimal change disease with mesangial IgA deposits in renal biopsy
Prednisone 1 mg/kg 4 weeks, ½ mg/kg 4 week and slow dose decrease (the same treatment of menial change disease without IgA deposits)
Acute tubulary necrosis
Supportive measures only
Chronic renal failure creatinine >2.5 mg/dl
Consider treatment of chronic renal failure, ACEI and fish oil

(GFR). In a single study, it was shown to reduce proteinuria, stabilize renal function and improve the inflammatory condition and the IgA deposit in a control biopsy. The benefit of intravenous immunoglobulin needs to be confirmed prospectively in a large number of patients.

Although the optimal treatment is yet to be defined, with all the available data one possible treatment algorithm could be that outlined in Table 88.3.

References

1. Berger J, Hinglais N. Les depots intercapillaires dIgA-IgG. *J Urol Nephrol* 74: 694–5, 1968.
2. Donadio JV, Grande JP. IgA nephropathy. *N Engl J Med* 347: 738–48, 2002.
3. Rai A, Nast C, Adler S. Schönlein-Henoch purpura nephritis. *J Am Soc Nephrol* 10: 2637–44, 1999.
4. Davin JC, Ten Berge IJ, Weening JJ. What is the difference between IgA nephropathy and Henoch-Schönlein purpura nephritis? *Kidney Int* 59: 823–34, 2001.
5. D'Amico G. Natural history of idiophatic IgA nephropathy; role of clinical and histological prognostic factors. *Am J Kidney Dis* 36: 227–37, 2000.
6. Donadio JV, Grande JP. IgA nephropathy. *N Engl J Med* 347: 738–48, 2002.
7. Floege J, Feehally J. IgA nephropathy: Recent developments. *J Am Soc Nephrol* 11: 2395–403, 2000.
8. Geddes C, Rauta V, Gronhagen-Riska C, Bartosik L, Jardine A, Ibels LL, Pei Y, Cattran D. A tricontinental view of IgA nephropathy. *Nephrol Dial Transplant* 18: 1541–48, 2003.
9. Ying B, Mao Chan T, Lai Lo S, Kei Lo S, Neng K. Renal transplantation in patients with primary IgA nephropathy. *Nephrol Dial Transplant* 18: 2399–404, 2003.
10. Barrat J, Feehally J. Treatment of IgA nephropathy. *Kidney Int* 69: 1934–44, 2006.
11. Russo D, Minutolo R, Pisani A. Esposito R, Signoriello G, Andreucci M, Balletta MM. Coadministration of losartan and enalapril exerts additive antiproteinuric effect in IgA nephropathy. *Am J Kidney Dis* 38: 18–25, 2001.
12. Nakao N, Yoshimura A, Morita H, Takada M, Koyano T, Ideura T. Combination treatment of ARA II and ACEI in non-diabetic renal disease (COOPERATE): A randomized controlled trial. *Lancet* 361: 117–24, 2003.
13. Dillon JJ. Fish oil therapy for IgA nephropathy: Efficacy and inter-study variability. *J Am Soc Nephrol* 8: 1739–44, 1997.
14. Ballardie FW, Roberts ASN. Controlled prospective trial of prednisolone and cytotoxics in progressive IgA nephropathy. *J Am Soc Nephrol* 13: 142–8, 2002.
15. Tumlin JA, Lohavichan V, Hennigar R. Crescentic, proliferative IgA nephropathy: Clinical and histological response to methylprednisolone and intravenous cyclolphosphamide. *Nephrol Dial Transplant* 18: 1321–9, 2003.
16. Goumenos DS, Davlouros P, El vahas Am, Ahuja M, Shortland JR, Vlachorjannis JG, Brown CD. Prednisolone and azathioprine in IgA nephropathy-a ten year follow up study. *Nephron Clin Prac* 93: c58–68, 2003.

17. Samuels JA, Strippoli GF, Craig JC, Schenna FP, Molony DA. Immunosuppressive treatments for IgA nephropathy: A meta-analysis of randomized controlled trials. *Nephrology (Carlton)* 9: 177–85, 2004.

18. Apple GB, Walkman M. The IgA nephropathy treatment dilemma. *Kidney Int* 69: 1939–44, 2006-11-05.

19. Ballardie FW. IgA nephropathy treatment 25 years on: Can we halt progression? The evidence base. *Neprhol Dial Tranplant* 19: 1041–6, 2004.

20. Laville M, Alamartine E. Treatment options for IgA nephropathy in adults: A proposal for evidence-based strategy. *Nephrol Dial Transplant* 19: 1947–51, 2004.

89
Membranous Nephropathy

Ziv Paz and Yehuda Shoenfeld

Abstract   Membranous nephropathy (MN) is a glomerular disease characterized by nephrotic syndrome and typical changes on renal biopsy. MN could be idiopathic or secondary to other conditions. Both idiopathic form and secondary forms are mediated by autoantibodies supporting the autoimmunity base of this disease. The underlying pathogenesis of the idiopathic form is still obscure, but diagnostic criteria based on clinical presentation and renal biopsy are suggested in this chapter, provide us diagnostic and therapeutic tool and help us to assess one prognosis.

Keywords   Membranous nephropathy · nephrotic syndrome · renal biopsy · subepithelial deposits · in situ autoantibodies

Membranous nephropathy (MN) is one of the glomerular diseases; as in other glomerular diseases, the name arises from the histopathological appearance in biopsy.

MN is accounting for one-third of biopsy results taken from adult patients present with nephrotic syndrome (1).

On light microscopy, one can see a glomerular basement membrane thickening with no proliferation or infiltration (2).

MN is mediated by different autoantibodies and immune complexes deposition with subsequent complement system activation.

MN could be secondary to different conditions (Table 89.1), but it is most often idiopathic; the scope of this chapter is to define diagnostic criteria for idiopathic MN.

Epidemiology

In the past, the majority of adult patients with nephrotic syndrome had the biopsy diagnosis of MN. Presently only one-third of patients with nephrotic syndrome are diagnosed with MN with increase diagnosis of focal segmental glomerulosclerosis especially in the black population (1).

MN distributes evenly in all races and in both sexes; the idiopathic type is more common in white male over the age of 40 years. When a young woman is diagnosed with MN, we have to suspect lupus as the underlying cause.

When the disease is diagnosed in children (represent less then 5% of nephrotic syndrome in this population), one

TABLE 89.1. Major secondary causes of membranous nephropathy (MN).

SLE (WHO class V)
Hepatitis B virus
Hepatitis C virus
Malignancy (commonly solid tumors: lung and GI)
Renal transplantation
Bone marrow transplantation
Sarcoidosis
Sjögren's syndrome
Tertiary syphilis
Malaria
Schistosomiasis
In association of other glomerular diseases
Drugs
Gold salts
Penicillamine
NSAIDS (diclofenac is most commonly associated)
Anti-TNF therapy (infliximab, etanercept, adalimumab)
Bucillamine
Tiopronin
Captopril

should look for hepatitis B infection (3). Still the majority of MN cases are idiopathic (75%).

Pathology

The classical appearance on light microscopy is diffusely distributed glomerular basement membrane thickening without significant cellularity (2). In early stage, the

From: Y. Shoenfeld et al. (eds.): *Diagnostic Criteria in Autoimmune Diseases*, DOI: 10.1007/978-1-60327-285-8_89,

glomeruli may appear normal, but in late stages, one will see diffuse sclerosis associated with tubulointerstitial changes. There are different classifications and staging systems of MN biopsy results, which have no effect on patient management and prognosis.

Diffuse granular pattern of IgG and C3 along the glomerular basement membrane (GBM) is seen in immunofluorescence microscopy. In electron microscopy, characteristic findings are subepithelial dense deposits located on the outer aspect of the GBM, effacement of podocytes foot processes and deposition of extracellular matrix between deposits (spikes).

The pathological findings described above are common both to idiopathic and secondary MN, but there are subtle differences that help to differentiate between idiopathic and secondary forms of GN.

In idiopathic MN, the deposits seen in EM are located subepithelial compared with secondary forms, where the deposits could be seen also in the mesangium and subendothelium.

In the idiopathic form there are no tubuloreticular structures inside the glomerular endothelium, characteristic findings of lupus MN.

Pathogenesis

In the past, MN was thought to be a presentation of chronic serum sickness. With research evolvement, MN like other glomerular diseases is now thought to be an autoimmune disease (4).

Heymann and colleague (5) described the first model of MN in rats called Heymann nephritis; this model is the base of our understanding of MN pathogenesis.

In immune complex-mediated process, one expect to see deposits in the mesangium or subendothelium (like in lupus MN), but in the idiopathic form of MN, there are isolated deposits in the subepithelial area.

Couser et al. (6) showed that subepithelial deposits result from direct in situ binding of IgG antibodies against self-antigens presented on podocytes foot processes.

The IgG deposits are IgG4 in the idiopathic form compared with other immunoglobulins and different complement deposits seen in the secondary forms; IgG4 is produced in type 2 immune response of Th2 lymphocytes (7). The antigen that involved in the idiopathic form of MN needs to be found. But there is a single report (8) on antibodies developed against podocyte neutral endopeptidase that lead to MN. In the secondary forms of MN, there are several known antigens described by Ronco et al. (9).

The glomerular injury is mediated by complement activation (10). C5b-9 stimulates podocytes to produce catalytic enzymes and to secrete different cytokines leading to podocytes dysfunction and barrier insufficiency with subsequent massive proteinuria.

Clinical Manifestations

Most patients present with a nephrotic syndrome (80%). In 70% of patients, the blood pressure is normal and there are no signs of renal failure unless there is an associated glomerular disease or one of the secondary causes of MN that can lead to a renal failure in different mechanism, keeping in mind that nephrotic syndrome by itself is a hypercoagulable state that can lead to a renal vein thrombosis with a further insult to renal function.

Urinary Findings (Table 89.2)

Proteinuria can range from a non-nephrotic range (<3 g/ 24 h urine collection) to a dozen of grams per day. The proteinuria is non-selective. In urine microscopy one can see fatty casts, oval fat bodies and lipid droplets. RBC casts are rare, but microscopic hematuria is seen in 50% of cases. Sometimes glycosuria is seen in normoglycemic patients.

Biochemical Findings (Table 89.2)

Hypoalbuminemia and severe hyperlipidemia are seen in most cases.

Diagnostic Criteria (Table 89.3)

The diagnosis of idiopathic form of MN is based on three criteria: renal biopsy (Table 89.4), appropriate clinical presentation (Table 89.2) and excluding an alternative diagnosis. In every patient with MN or nephrotic range

TABLE 89.2. Urinalysis and blood biochemistry in idiopathic membranous nephropathy (MN).

Non-selective proteinuria	100%
Nephrotic range proteinuria	80%
Microscopic hematuria	50%
Glycosuria	>50%
Urine microscopy	
Fatty casts	up to 90%
RBC casts	rare (consider other diagnosis)
Blood biochemistry	
Hypoalbuminemia	>90%
Hyperlipidemia	>90%
Azotemia	rarely

TABLE 89.3. Diagnostic criteria for idiopathic MN.

1. A nephrotic syndrome
2. The classic pathological picture in renal biopsy (Table 89.4)
3. Exclusion of other possible etiologies (Tables 89.1 and 89.5)

All criteria must be met.

TABLE 89.4. Renal biopsy findings in idiopathic membranous nephropathy (MN).

Light microscopy: Basement membrane thickening without a significant cellularity.
Immunofluorescence: Diffuse granular pattern of IgG 4 and C3 along the GBM.
Electron microscopy: Isolated subepithelial deposits.

No tubuloreticular structures inside the glomerular endothelium.
No subendothelial or mesangial deposits.

TABLE 89.5. Laboratory tests ordered in membranous nephropathy (MN).

ANA
Complement levels
Hepatitis B serology
Hepatitis C serology
Routine screening for malignancy (e.g., colonoscopy in patients over the age of 50 years) unless there are directing signs and symptoms.

proteinuria, different laboratory tests are ordered (Table 89.5) to rule in or out other diagnosis. Even though the autoimmunity nature of MN is well established by biopsy findings, immunohistochemistry studies and significant response to an immunosuppressive therapy, the underlying mediating antibodies need to be found and specific autoantibodies are not considered part of MN diagnosis.

Prognosis

MN has a benign course; spontaneous remission occurs in 30% of patients. It happens mostly in the first 2 years but can occur at any time along the course of the disease. Schieppati et al. (11) studied the natural history of the idiopathic form of MN. In this study, 37 patients with MN were followed for 5 years and 65% had a complete or partial remission without the use of steroids or other immunosuppressive drugs. The prognosis in this study was related to the level of proteinuria, with a worse prognosis in cases present with massive proteinuria.

Louis et al. (12) reviewed the literature, listing the prognostic factors that can help to identify the patients at risk of an end-stage kidney disease, who can benefit from an early immunosuppressive intervention. Their review concluded that age, glomerular stage on biopsy and hypertension are not useful as predictors. In contrast, young females with normal plasma creatinine, without tubulointerstitial changes or sclerosis, and without nephrotic syndrome or massive proteinuria (the most important prognostic factor) have very good prognosis. Cumulative prognostic factors that are sensitive and specific enough and help to direct the treatment and to assess disease activity are urinary levels of C3dg, C5b-9, IgG and B2

microglobulin. These tests are not available in most clinical laboratories.

Treatment

To treat or not to treat is a significant question asked in every patient with idiopathic MN, especially when considering the possibility of spontaneous remission in 30% of patients and the significant adverse effects of the immunosuppressive therapy (13).

The questions need to be asked are: When to treat? and with what to treat? Obviously patient with several risk factors for an end stage kidney disease will benefit from the therapy but for most patients the decision is complicated and depends mostly on the knowledge and experience of the treating physician.

In the secondary forms of MN, the therapy is directed to the underlying cause.

In any patient with a nephrotic syndrome including those with MN, our goals are to treat the edema, control blood pressure, to lower blood cholesterol and to employ angiotensin-converting enzyme inhibitors to reduce proteinuria.

The risk for progression to an end-stage kidney disease is assessed and patients are assigned to different risk groups. The low-risk group (normal plasma creatinine, proteinuria <4 g) is treated conservatively.

Two therapeutic approaches are considered beneficial in the medium risk group (normal plasma creatinine, proteinuria between 4 and 8 g on a maximal conservative treatment). Monthly cycling of corticosteroids and cyclophosphamide on alternate months over 6 months period is one accepted approach (14); the other alternative is using cyclosporine as a single drug for 6 months period (15). The high-risk group (deteriorating renal function and or proteinuria more then 8 g) will benefit from a combined therapy with steroids and cytotoxic drugs. Few cytotoxic drugs are suggested in this indication, including chlorambucil, cyclosporine and cyclophosphamide.

New therapies have been used with a great success in resistant cases, including mycophenolate mofetil (16) and rituximab (17).

The conditions of 30% of the patients deteriorate on therapy and few of them depend on dialysis or undergo kidney transplantation. The advances in understanding of autoimmunity will provide us better understanding of this disease and help us to help these patients.

References

1. Braden, GL, Mulhern, JG, O'Shea, MH, et al. Changing incidence of glomerular diseases in adults. *Am J Kidney Dis* 2000; 35: 878–884.

2. Austin, HA 3d, Antonovych, TT, Mackay, K, et al. NIH Conference. Membranous nephropathy. *Ann Intern Med* 1992; 116: 672–680.

3. Johnson, RJ, Couser, WG. Hepatitis B infection and renal disease: Clinical, immunopathogenetic and therapeutic considerations. *Kidney Int* 1990; 37: 663–670.

4. Couser, WG. Membranous nephropathy: A long road but well traveled. *J Am Soc Nephrol* 2005; 16: 1184–1187.

5. Heymann, W, Hackel, DB, Harwood, S, Wilson, SG, Hunter, JL. Production of nephrotic syndrome in rats by Freund's adjuvants and rat kidney suspensions. *Proc Soc Exp Biol Med* 1959; 100: 660–664.

6. Couser, WG, Salant, DJ. In situ immune complex formation and glomerular injury. *Kidney Int* 1980; 17: 1–13.

7. Hirayama, K, Ebihara, I, Yamamoto, S, Kai, H, Muro, K, Yamagata, K, Kobayashi, M, Kyoma, A. Predominance of type-2 immune response in idiopathic membranous nephropathy. Nephron 2002; 91: 255–261.

8. Debiec, H, Guigonis, V, Mougenot, B, Decobert, F, Haymann, JP, Bensman, A, Deschenes, G, Ronco, PM. Antenatal membranous glomerulonephritis due to anti-neutral endopeptidase antibodies. *N Engl J Med* 2002; 346: 2053–2060.

9. Ronco, P, Debiec, H. Molecular pathomechanism of membranous nephropathy: from Heymann nephritis to alloimmunization. *J Am Soc Nephrol* 2005; 16: 1205–1213.

10. Nangaku, M, Shankland, SJ, Couser,WG. Cellular Response to injury in Membranous Nephropathy. *J Am Soc Nephrol* 2005; 16: 1195–1204.

11. Schieppati, A, Mosconi, L, Perna, A, et al. Prognosis of untreated patients with idiopathic membranous nephropathy. *N Engl J Med* 1993; 329: 85.

12. Reichert, LJM, Koene, RAP, Wetzels, JFM. Prognostic factors in idiopathic membranous nephropathy. *Am J Kidney Dis* 1998; 31: 1–11.

13. Cattran, D. Management of membranous nephropathy: When and what for treatment. *J Am Soc Nephrol* 2005; 16: 1188–1194.

14. Ponticelli, C, Piccoli, G, Lupo, A, Segagni, S, Antonucci, F, Dugo M, Minari M, Scalia A, Pedrini L, Pisano G, Grassi C, Farina M, Bellazzi R. A randomized study comparing methylprednisolone plus chlorambucil versus methylprednisolone plus cyclophosphamide in idiopathic nephropathy. *J Am Soc Nephrol* 1998; 9: 444–450.

15. Cattran, DC, Appel, GB, Hebert, LA, Hunsicker, LG, Pohl, MA, Hoy, WE, Maxwell, DR, Kunis, CL; North American Nephrotic Syndrome Study Group. Cyclosporine in patients with steroid resistant membranous nephropathy: A randomized trial. *Kidney Int* 2001; 59: 1484–1490.

16. Miller, G, Zimmerman, R, Radhakrishnan, J, Appel, G. Use of mycophenolate Mofetil in resistant membranous nephropathy. *Am J Kidney Dis* 2000; 36: 250–256.

17. Ruggenenti, P, Chiurchiu, C, Brusgen, V, Abate M, Perna A, Remuzzi G: Rituximab in idiopathic membranous nephropathy: A one year prospective study. *J Am Soc Nephrol* 2003; 14: 1851–1857.

90
Minimal Change Nephropathy

Pilar Arrizabalaga Clemente

Abstract   Minimal Change Nephropathy (MCN) is the basic primary glomerulonephritis subsisting under the Idiopathic Nephrotic Syndrome (INS), which is characterized by massive selective proteinuria, hypercholesterolemia and generalized edema. MCN is present in more than 80% of children with INS and in less than 10% of adult patients with INS. Familial forms of NS are caused by genetic defects. Clinical and experimental data including production of several cytokines from circulating T cells and disturbances of the podocyte antigens support autoimmune pathogenesis in non-familial forms of MCN. The natural history of the disease may vary widely, but proteinuria is the cardinal prognosis factor in renal outcome.

Keywords   Primary glomerulonephritis · idiopathic nephrotic syndrome · podocyte

Minimal Change Nephropathy (MCN) is the basic primary glomerulonephritis subsisting under the Idiopathic Nephrotic Syndrome (INS), which is defined by urinary protein level exceeding 3.5 g/day in adults or 40 mg/h/m^2 in children and hypoalbuminemia (<3 g/dl). Hypovolemia due to reduced plasma oncotic pressure stimulates the renin–angiotensin–aldosterone. Salt and water retention leading to generalized edema and primary dysfunction in sodium tubule reabsorption contribute to its persistence. The NS is accompanied by hypercholesterolemia and a wide range of comorbidities: thromboembolic tendency, protein malnutrition, disorders of vitamin D and hypocalcemia, and susceptibility to infection, especially pneumococcal in children and the elderly.

Epidemiology

MCN is the most common histological picture in children with INS, accounting for more than 80% in children younger than 10 years of age and 50% in older children. MCN affects less than 10% of adults with INS (1) and can also affect elderly patients in whom there is a higher tendency for microhematuria, hypertension and acute renal failure.

History

In 1913, Munk (2) described massive proteinuria under the histological picture called "lipoid nephrosis" because of the fat bodies in the urine and fatty changes in the tubules seen at autopsy. Since the 1960s, the application of percutaneous renal biopsy introduced MCN as descriptive term under NS responding to steroid therapy (3). Abnormalities in both humoral and cell-mediated immunity from clinical and experimental data support autoimmune pathogenesis over the visceral epithelial cells or podocyte (4) in MCN.

Pathology

MCN shows no changes under light microscopy and no immunodeposition under fluorescence microscopy. The histological finding, as detected by electron microscopy, consists of loss or effacement of the foot processes as a result of condensation of the actin microfilaments constituting the podocyte cytoskeleton. This change leads to a leak in the glomerular barrier to proteins and highly selective proteinuria, mainly albumina.

From: Y. Shoenfeld et al. (eds.): *Diagnostic Criteria in Autoimmune Diseases*, DOI: 10.1007/978-1-60327-285-8_90,
© 2008 Humana Pressm, Totowa, NJ

Pathogenesis

MCN has been associated with disturbances in the immune system.

History of hypersensitivity such as atopy and allergy, favorable response of NS to steroids and immunosuppressive drugs, increased serum levels of IgE, and expanded CD8-positive T-cells during relapse suggest activation of both B and T cells in MCN.

In vitro studies of mitogen-stimulated production of cytokines by peripheral blood monocyte cells and T-cells from MCN under NS have shown an increase of cytokines such as interleukin (IL)-1, IL-2 and tumor necrosis factor (TNF)-α (5). Moreover, increased IL-12 and IL-13 point to activation of T-helper with Th2-mediated immunity.

Advances in molecular biology have recently recognized that nephrin, a major functional molecule in the slit diaphragm, is reduced in the glomeruli of MCN, but its significance is uncertain. MCN is the consequence of podocyte injury that may result from damage of immune origin because of: (a) a circulating lymphocyte-derived permeability factor, (b) intra or extracellular stimulus directed to α3β1 integrin and integrin-linked kinase that are linked to the actin (6).

Clinical Manifestations

The primordial clinical manifestation looking for medical attention is the edema as consequence of the relatively abrupt onset of massive proteinuria and hypoalbuminemia. In some patients, the edema is only of minimal discomfort but in most patients the generalized edema causes substantial morbidity. The nephrotic proteinuria, the hypoalbuminemia, and the comorbidities are responsible for signs and symptoms listed in Table 90.1.

There are some differences in clinical features between children and adults with MCN. Non-familial MCN is usually primary or idiopathic in children, but in some children there is a history of respiratory infection, allergy, or vaccines.

In adults, MCN is usually associated with other conditions, including both viral and parasitic infections,

TABLE 90.1. Symptoms and signs of MCN at presentation.

	Prevalence	
	Children (%)	Adults (%)
Fatigue	>70	>70
Edema	100	100
Anasarca	>80	<60
High blood pressure	No	30
Arterial thrombosis	1	3
Vein thrombosis	1	>30
Infections	>30	<15

medications (no steroidal anti-inflammatory drugs, lithium, gold, interferon alpha, ampicillin, rifampicin, captopril, etc.), leukemia and lymphoma (Hodgkin disease), solid tumors (carcinoma and sarcoma) and allergy (food, bee stings, and pollen). Hypertension, sometimes severe, as well as renal insufficiency is more common in adults (7). In fact, failure renal has been reported in up to 20% of elderly patients. Acute renal failure can be reversible when involving both hypovolemia and interstitial nephritis due to diuretic treatment. But evidence of atherosclerosis and tubular epithelial features compatible with ischemic failure may be present in patients older than 60 years (8).

Thromboembolic episodes occur in 20 to 44% (9) of the adult patients with NS, in particular, those with deep venous thrombosis and renal vein thrombosis. Factors such as flank pain, hematuria, and renal failure are useful in predicting the presence of renal vein assessed as increased kidney size by imaging diagnostic techniques. Pulmonary embolism has been reported as 20%, but 15% of adult patients with NS and no symptoms of pulmonary thrombosis show positive results on ventilation/perfusion scans, so that may be even higher.

It has been reported that the patients with NS are at a substantially increased relative risk of 5.5 compared with the general population for coronary artery disease (10). However, hyperlipemia and hypercoagulability as well as others factors of cardiovascular risk, e.g. smoking, hypertension, or hereditary factors, contribute to making the association between NS and atherosclerosis uncertain.

The prevalence of bacterial infections ranges from 10 to 40% in children, principally peritonitis as the result of Streptococcus pneumoniae. Other complications are sepsis, cellulites, urinary tract infection, and osteomyelitis. The infections are notable during episodes of relapse (11) and are associated to IgG levels profoundly decreased.

In non-responder children, MCN progress to advanced stages, complications can result of long-lasting minerals and vitamins leading to both malnutrition and reduction in bone density with features of osteopenia and osteoporosis. These last can account through long steroids treatment.

Biochemical Features

MCN is characterized by nephrotic proteinuria (>3.5 g/day in adults or 40 mg/h/m² in children), hypoalbuminemia (<3 g/dl), and hypercholesterolemia. Other laboratory abnormalities observed in MCN are listed in Table 90.2.

The primary defect is loss of selective protein in the urine. The liver reacts to the fall in serum albumen levels by increasing albumen synthesis, but the response in NS is inadequate. The alteration in serum globulins and lipoproteins in MCN is the consequence of the hypoalbuminemia that would increase the synthesis of cholesterol and

TABLE 90.2. Laboratory findings in MCN. The semiquantitative (↑↑) system indicates the extent of the observed abnormalities in plasma and serum.

Biochemical feature	Changes
Lipid abnormalities	
Cholesterol	↑↑↑↑
LDL/VLDL	↑↑
Apolipoproteins apo B, C-II, E	↑↑
Triglyceride	↑↑
Coagulation abnormalities	
Antithrombin III	↓↓↓
Factors IX, XI, XII	↓↓
Plasma plasminogen	↓↓
Factors II, V, VII, VIII, X, XIII	↑↑
Plasma fibrinogen	↑↑
Binding proteins	
Metal: iron, copper, zinc	↓↓
Vitamin D: 25 (OH), 1–25 (OH)$_2$	↓↓
Transferrin	↓↓
Serological feature	
α2-globulin/β-globulin	↑↑
γ-globulin	IgG ↓↓↓ / IgA /IgM/IgE ↑ or =
Factor B /C$_3$	↓↓

TABLE 90.3. Patterns of response of MCN to corticosteroid treatment. The percentage values are given in brackets.

Initial response	Outcome
Complete remission	*Permanent remission*
Children (90%)	Children (20%)
Adults (75%)	Adults (65%)
Partial remission	*Infrequent relapses*
Proteinuria > 0.3 g/day in adults or > 4 mg/h/m^2 in children	One relapse in the first 6 months after initial response
Steroid-induced remission	*Frequent relapses*
No response to relapse	More than one relapses a year
Steroid resistance	*Steroid dependency*
Children (< 10%)	Children (50%)
Adults (25%)	Adults (20%)

lipoproteins in liver. Hyperlipidemia is also due to diminished catabolism.

The hypercoagulability leading to thrombosis in NS is multifaceted (12). Causes such as platelet hyperaggregability, urinary loss of small clotting factors, increased hepatic synthesis of clotting factors, decreased fibrinolysis, and especially decreased levels of antithrombin III are being implicated.

Diagnostic Criteria

MCN prevalence is cardinal in young children. The most children with MCN are steroid responsive. Therefore, the current practice is to perform renal biopsies those who are steroid unresponsive within 4- to 6-week course of prednisone or develop clinical features suggesting other diagnosis than MCN.

In adults, the prevalence of MCN compared with other causes of NS (1) is tenuous. Thus, the renal biopsy is always required in adults and in elderly patients.

Prognosis

Ninety percent children and 70% adults with MCN are corticosensitive at the presentation and respond with disappearance of proteinuria (<0.3 g/day in adults or <4 mg/h/m^2 in children). Adults with MCN are more steroid resistant than the children. On the contrary, children have more frequent relapsing NS than adults (Table 90.3). Finally, a half of children, who present relapses during

tapering of steroids or within 2 weeks after withdrawal, becomes steroid dependent and requires additional therapy aimed at minimizing the complications of corticosteroid treatment.

Prediction

Genetic defects that affect the function and the composition of the glomerular capillary wall, in particular of the visceral epithelial cells called podocytes, have been recognized as the cause of familial forms of NS, which can be predicted (13).

The insight in the non-familial forms of NS such as MCN is limited. The renal function is conserved at the presentation of the disease. The proteinuria is the principal prognosis factor in MCN. A large body of evidence indicates that patients with MCN and persistent nephrotic proteinuria have a poor prognosis and that its reduction by treatment is the best indicator of long term outcome (7, 14, 15). In fact, the prognosis of the MCN is good, in particular in the corticosensitive patients.

Therapy

The treatment of MCN is directed to three standard goals:

- To lower proteinuria and thereby slow rate of deterioration in renal function
- To decrease the number of relapses of NS
- To renoprotection and whole protection by active treatment of all comorbid conditions.

Prednisone at a dose of 60 mg/m^2/day in children and 1 mg/kg body weight (not exceeding 80 mg/day) in adults is the initial cardinal treatment. This therapy results in a complete disappearance of proteinuria within 4 to 6 weeks, and must be continued to alternate-day prednisone during at least other 4 weeks. If the dose is changed to alternate-day when remission has occurred, the tapering regimen of

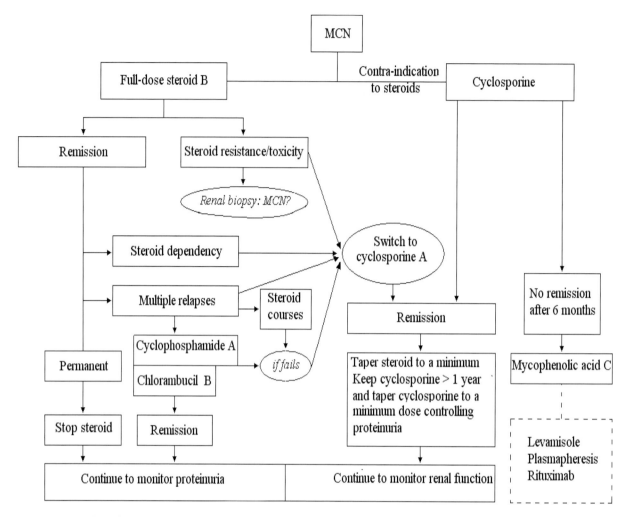

FIGURE 90.1. Algorithm of treatment pathway in MCN. The therapeutic recommendation rank based on evidence is expressed as A, B, and C.

prednisone must be slow because sudden withdrawal may prompt a release. The corticosteroid treatment and immunosuppressor agents can be considered in both relapsing and steroid-dependent MCNs. This last steroid-sparing treatment is important, in particular, in children and young patients. Generally, cyclophosphamide at a dose of 2 mg/kg for 8 to 12 weeks leaves patients free of proteinuria for 2 years in up to 75% of patients. The use of chlorambucil in doses of 0.1 to 0.2 mg/kg/day in an 8-week course can also produce stable remission (16). Both cyclophosphamide and chlorambucil have profound side-effects such as bone marrow suppression, life-threatening infection, gonadal dysfunction, hemorrhagic cystitis, and risk of leukemia.

Cyclosporine at a dose of 100–150 mg/m^2/day in children and 4–5 mg/kg body weight in adults induces remission of proteinuria in 80% of corticosensitive patients with MCN (17). Cyclosporine has been found effective in MCN corticoresistant patients, in those for whom corticosteroid treatment is overly toxic, and those patients who are resistant to alkylating agents (18). Mycophenolic acid-derived agents are an encouraging alternative approach to the treatment in MCN (19). Finally, other agents including levamisole, plasmapheresis, and rituximab (20) have been used in patients resistant to treatment with corticosteroids, alkylating agents, and calcineurin inhibitors, but evidence is still limited. Figure 90.1 is an algorithm of the specific management of MCN notifying the therapeutic recommendation rank based on evidence. Edema is currently treated with thiazide diuretics and furosemide for moderate to severe NS. At present, hepatic hydroxy-methylglutariyl-coenzyme A (HMG-CoA) reductase inhibitors appear to be the treatment of choice in hyperlipidemia.

References

1. Rivera F, López-Gómez JM, Pérez-García R. Spanish Registry of Glomerulonephritis. Clinicopathologic correlations of renal pathology in Spain. Kidney Int 2004; 66: 898–904.

2. Munk F. Die Nephrosen. Med Klin 1946; 12: 1019.

3. Blainey JD, Brewer DB, Hardwicke J, Soothill JF. The nephrotic syndrome. Diagnosis by renal biopsy and biochemical and immunological analyses related to the response to steroid therapy. Q J Med 1960; 29: 235–56.

4. Wiggins RC. The spectrum of podocytopathies. A unifying view of glomerular diseases. Kidney Int 2007; 71: 1207–14.

5. Van Den Berg JG, Weening JJ. Role of the immune system in the pathogenesis of idiopathic nephrotic syndrome. Clin Sci 2004; 107: 125–36.

6. Arrizabalaga P, Mampaso F. Integrins and Glomerulonephritis. In Inflammation and Chronic Disease. Esbrit P and Alvarez-Arroyo MV (eds). Transworld Research Network 2006, 67–87.

7. Tse KC, Lam MF, Yip PS et al. Idiopathic minimal change nephrotic syndrome in older adults: steroid responsiveness and pattern of relapses. Nephrol Dial Transplant 2003; 18: 1316–20.

8. Smith JD, Hayslett JP. Reversible renal failure in the nephrotic syndrome. Am J Kidney Dis 1992; 19: 201–13.

9. Cameron JS. Nephrotic syndrome in the elderly. Semin Nephrol 1996; 16: 319–29.

10. Ordonez JD, Hiatt RA, Killebrew EJ, Fireman BH. The increased risk of coronary heart disease associated with nephrotic syndrome. Kidney Int 1993; 44: 638–42.

11. Cavagnaro F, Lagomarsino E. Peritonitis as a risk factor of acute renal failure in nephrotic children. Pediatr Nephrol 2000; 15: 248–51.

12. Rabelink TJ, Zwaginga JJ, Koomans HA, Sixma JJ. Thrombosis and hemostasis in renal disease. Kidney Int 1994; 46: 287–96.

13. Arrizabalaga P. Slit diaphragm of glomerular filtration: diagnostic and therapeutic approach in nephrotic syndrome. Nephrología 2005; 4: 17–23.

14. Hodson EM, Knight JF, Willis NS, Craig JC. Corticosteroid therapy for nephrotic syndrome in children. Cochrane Database of Systematic Reviews 2005, Issue 1. Art. No.: CD001533. DOI: 10.1002/14651858.CD001533.pub3.

15. Hodson EM, Habashy D, Craig JC. Interventions for idiopathic steroid-resistant nephrotic syndrome in children. Cochrane Database of Systematic Reviews 2006, Issue 2. Art. No.: CD003594. DOI: 10.1002/14651858.CD003594.pub3.

16. Arrizabalaga P. Consideraciones patogenéticas en el tratamiento del síndrome nefrótico por lesiones mínimas. Clínica Nefrológica y Trasplante Renal 2006; 1: 3–7.

17. Meyrier A, Condamin AC, Broneer D. Treatment of adult idiopathic nephrotic syndrome with cyclosporin A: minimal-change disease and focal-segmental glomerulosclerosis. Collaborative Group of the French Society of Nephrology. Clin Nephrol 1991; 35 Suppl. 1: S37–42.

18. Ponticelli C, Edefonti A, Ghio L et al. Cyclosporin versus cyclophosphamide for patients with steroid-dependent and frequently relapsing idiopathic nephrotic syndrome: A multicentre randomized controlled trial. Nephrol Dial Transplant 1993; 8: 1326–32.

19. Mendizabal S, Berbel O, Sanahuja MJ, Fuentes J, Simon J. Mycophenolate mofetil in steroid/cyclosporine-dependent/resistant nephrotic syndrome. Pediatr Nephrol 2005; 20: 914–19.

20. Bagga A, Sinha A, Moudgil A. Rituximab in Patients with the Steroid-Resistant Nephrotic Syndrome. N Engl J Med 2007; 356: 2751–2.

91
Focal and Segmental Glomerulosclerosis

José A. Ballarín, Cristina Cabrera, Carlos Quereda and Montserrat Díaz

Abstract Focal and segmental glomerulosclerosis (FSGS) is a common cause of Nephrotic Syndrome in adults. Its most typical course runs from NS to progressive loss of renal function and may recur in the graft after renal transplantation. Current evidence favors prolonged corticosteroid therapy (6 months or longer) to induce remission of proteinuria. Steroid-dependent and steroid-resistant patients may benefit from treatment with cyclosporine or cyclophosphamide. Angiotensin-converting enzyme inhibitors (ACEIs) and angiotensin receptor blockers (ARBs) are effective in reducing proteinuria and are recommended in all patients with FSGS, particularly those with nonnephrotic proteinuria. FSGS can be idiopathic or secondary to glomerular hyperfiltration and high intraglomerular capillary pressure or to viral or toxin-mediated damage. The characteristic lesion is a segmental solidification of the glomerular tuft.

Keywords Focal and segmental glomerulosclerosis · classification · treatment

Introduction

Focal and segmental glomerulosclerosis (FSGS) is a nonspecific pattern of glomerular injury, defined by a segmental solidification of the glomerular tuft owing to collapse of the capillary wall, affecting some glomeruli only. It is one of the main causes of nephrotic syndrome in adults and is characterized by a high incidence of progression to end-stage renal disease. The best predictor of outcome is remission of proteinuria, and because adult nephrotic patients may respond to an aggressive course of corticosteroids, a trial of therapy is recommended. Steroid-dependent and steroid-resistant patients may benefit from treatment with cyclosporine or cyclophosphamide.

FSGS can be idiopathic or secondary to glomerular hyperfiltration (including disorders with a reduced renal mass), viral infections or drug toxicity. Secondary forms usually present with nonnephrotic proteinuria, and primary forms with nephrotic syndrome. Several genetic abnormalities involving proteins of the glomerular epithelial cell cytoskeleton and cell junction proteins have been described in patients with familial NS; in some others, a factor increasing glomerular permeability has been identified (1, 2).

There has been a long debate as to whether Minimal Change Disease and FSGS are part of the same disease spectrum. Some patients with biopsy-proven minimal change disease later progress to FGS: in both, the response to corticosteroids is the major prognostic factor for progression to renal insufficiency and the same genetic defects have been described in both entities (3).

Epidemiology

In the past 20 years, the incidence of FSGS has increased considerably. It is the most common cause of NS, accounting for 35% of cases (33% for membranous nephropathy) in the general population, for more than 50% of cases in black adults and for 67% of such cases in black adults younger than 45 years of age. There has been an eleven-fold increase (United States Renal Data) of it as a cause of ESRD during a 20-year period (1980–2000) and it is now the most common cause of ESRD owing to primary glomerular disease in both black and white populations. In contrast, in other countries, the incidence of FSGS has not varied in the past years as shown by data from Europe.

The peak decade of life for ESRD incidence is 40 to 49 years in black subjects and 70–79 years in white individuals. Men have 1.5- to 2-fold greater risk than women (4, 5, 6).

From: Y. Shoenfeld et al. (eds.): *Diagnostic Criteria in Autoimmune Diseases*, DOI: 10.1007/978-1-60327-285-8_91,
© 2008 Humana Press, Totowa, NJ

Pathogenesis

The podocyte constitutes a major portion of the glomerular filtration barrier that separates blood from the urinary space and has a pivotal role not only in genetic but also in many acquired forms of FSGS. The podocyte dysfunction may be caused by a primary T-cell disorder leading to the presence of circulating toxin (perhaps cytokines) or a genetic disease with mutations in genes that encode proteins which are localized to the slit diaphragms or which interact with the actin cytoskeleton. These proteins are vital for an intact glomerular barrier.

One gene located on chromosome 19q13 has been linked with familial autosomal dominant FSGS. It codes for nephrin, a major component of the slit diaphragm of the podocytes. NPHS2, a gene that codes for the protein podocin localized to the slit-diaphragm, is responsible of some recessive and sporadic forms (20–30% of steroid-resistant forms). It has been mapped to chromosome 1q25–31. The patients are heterozygotes for mutations in NPHS2 and compound heterozygotes for a nonconservative R229Q amino acid substitution in the same gene. Mutations that codes for other proteins, such as α-actin-4, CD2AP, and TRPC6 have also been identified in some cases of autosomal dominant forms of the disease. These forms present later and progress more slowly than recessive forms (7, 8) Table 91.1.

In others cases, a "circulating factor" of T-cell origin that is able to alter glomerular permeability has been hypothesized. This idea derives from the following observations: the frequent and immediate recurrence of proteinuria after renal transplantation in 30–40% of the corticosteroid-resistant cases, the beneficial effect of plasmapheresis or protein A immunoabsorption in these cases, and the transmission from mother with FSGS to fetus of the increase of the glomerular permeability. However, the identity of that plasma factor has not yet been discovered (9).

When a circulating factor is present, steroids and/or immunosuppressive agents may have a beneficial effect and recurrence after renal transplantation is frequent. The inherited forms do not respond convincingly to cyclophosphamide or cyclosporin A (CsA) and the disease does not recur after transplantation.

However, the difference between the genetic forms and those due to a circulating factor is not so clear and it has been hypothesized that idiopathic NS may be a multifactorial disease, including both pathogenic mechanisms, because in some patients with NPHS2, immunosuppressive drugs have a beneficial effect and in some others FSGS recurs after renal transplantation (10).

In addition to idiopathic forms, FSGS can be observed in a variety of secondary settings. In these cases, the histological injury results from an adaptive response to glomerular hypertrophy or hyperfiltration or from scarring of previous injury. This adaptative response occurs in diseases with nephron loss or renal vasodilatation (1).

Clinical Presentation

Most patients (60–75%) present with acute onset of the nephrotic syndrome. In addition, hypertension (45–65%) and microscopic hematuria (30–50%) are also commonly seen. The level of kidney function may vary (renal insufficiency in 25–50% of the cases). Slowly increasing, often nonnephrotic proteinuria and renal insufficiency over time are characteristic of the secondary disorders (1, 2) Table 91.2.

Histological Variants

The typical lesion of FSGS is a segmental solidification of the glomerular tuft owing to obliteration of the glomerular capillary lumen by a relative acellular matrix material on light microscopy and a diffuse epithelial foot process fusion on electron microscopy. The glomeruli not involved in the sclerotic lesion and the remaining part of the tuft of the glomeruli involved in the segmental lesion appear normal. Immunofluorescence microscopy only reveals nonspecific binding of IgM and complement (C3 and variably C1) in sclerotic lesions and very weak mesangial deposition of IgM.

Recently, five histopathological variants have been included in the diagnosis of primary FSGS (11) Figure 91.1:

1. classic FSGS or "NOS" (not otherwise specified) with the above-described typical histological lesion,
2. perihilar variant: Sclerosis and hyalinosis are perihilar. This variant is frequently observed in the secondary forms.
3. cellular variant: characterized by segmental hypercellularity in some glomeruli and "classic" lesions in others.
4. tip variant: the lesion occurs at the "tip" of the glomerulus near the beginning of the proximal tubule. This variant presents with a high incidence of NS and absence of chronic tubulointerstitial injury. It could include two conditions, one an early form of classic FSGS, and the other closely related to MCN.
5. collapsing variant: the entire glomerular tuft is collapsed and sclerosed. This variant may be primary or due to HIV infection, presents with NS, is often resistant to therapy and has the worst outcome of all the histological variants.

However, there is no significant difference in the response to steroid treatment among the patients with these different histopathological subsets (12), and it does not seem that this new classification will help in selecting treatment protocols.

Natural History

Rates of remission of proteinuria and progression to ESRD were reported in a recent systematic review where data from 380 adult patients with FSGS and NS were analyzed (13). Two hundred and four (54%) patients were treated with steroids and different immunosuppressive drugs, and 138 (46%) were untreated. Fifty-five percent of treated patients ($n = 113$) achieved partial (22%) or complete remission (33%), only 20% ($n = 28$) achieved partial (17%) or complete remission (3%) ($p < 0.001$). The overall renal survival varies from 58 to 85.2% at 5 years and from 25 to 58% at 10 years. In patients without NS, the 10-year renal survival varies from 83 to 92% (14, 15).

Patients with FSGS are initially treated with corticosteroids and, irrespective of histological variant, steroid responsiveness is the best predictor of outcome in nephrotic patients. Failure to obtain remission is associated with a 50–60% likelihood of ESRD and complete remission is associated with no risk (12).

More recently, it has been demonstrated that even partial remission improves long-term renal survival (16).

Others predictors of outcome are nephrotic-range proteinuria and presence of interstitial fibrosis on biopsy. FSGS is more frequent and more severe in black and Hispanic men, both in adults and in children (12).

Relapse on Transplanted Kidney

Primary FSGS may recur in the renal allograft with a rate that varies from 30 to 56%. Recurrence is of rapid onset (during the first month in 66% of the cases) and results in a high rate of graft loss (13).

There is no difference in the frequency of recurrence between living, related or cadaveric transplants.

The inherited forms have very low recurrence rates (10% in the case with podocin mutations).

Reported risk factors for recurrence include age at onset of proteinuria (less than 20 years), recurrence in a prior allograft (the rate of recurrence is 80%), rapid deterioration from initial diagnosis to end-stage renal disease and mesangial hypercellularity in the native kidney (17).

Because of the risk of graft loss in recurrent disease, aggressive therapy including plasmapheresis or immunoadsorption is recommended. This approach improves graft survival (13).

Treatment

Clinically, it is important to distinguish secondary from primary FGS, because the treatment is different.

There have been no randomized clinical trials of steroid therapy in primary FSGS. In two systematic reviews, it was concluded that treatment with prednisone should be considered for patients with FSGS and NS (13, 18). Full dose (1 mg/kg/day with a maximum dose 50 to 80 mg/day) is

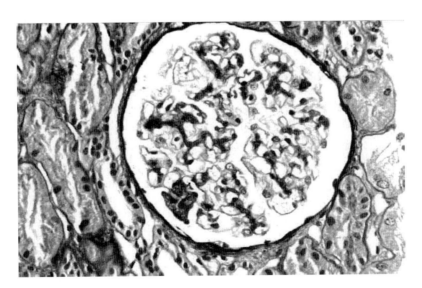

FIGURE 91.1. Focal and segmental Glomerulosclerosis (FSGS): Glomerular segmental sclerosis and collapsed with presence of hyaline. Silver Staining.

TABLE 91.1. Hereditary forms of FSGS.

Primary
Secondary
  Hyperfiltration/reduced nephron mass
    Reflux interstitial nephropathy
    Morbid obesity
    Solitary kidney
    Glomerulopathies
  Toxic agents
    Heroin
    Pamidronate
  Viral infections
    HIV-associated nephropathy
    ParvovirusB19
    Cytomegalovirus
  Hereditary forms

given for 12–16 weeks followed, in case of even partial remission, by a slow tapering schedule over months (6–8 months) to avoid a rebound effect. The treatment must be sufficiently long (4 months at 1 mg/kg/day) before declaring the patient steroid resistant (1). The efficacy of steroids in patients with decreased kidney function is unclear and they are not indicated in case of nonnephrotic proteinuria. Only 50% of the patients achieve a complete remission of the proteinuria with such a protocol, 25% a partial remission, and 25% do not respond.

Cyclophosphamide and chlorambucil have been used since the 1950s and the best results are obtained in the cases with steroid dependency. Steroid resistance is highly predictive of resistance to alkylating agents (13).

Randomized controlled trials and uncontrolled studies have demonstrated the effectiveness of cyclosporine in reducing proteinuria in steroid-dependent and steroid-resistant FGS. The initial dose is approximately 5 mg/kg/day adjusted to 12-h levels of 100–150 ng/mL. CsA is discontinued at 3 months if there is no response. CsA dependency is observed but the likelihood of relapse appears to be lower if the cyclosporine treatment is prolonged up to one year or longer after remission is induced, and then gradually tapered and discontinued (13, 18).

Angiotensin-converting enzyme inhibitors (ACEIs) and angiotensin receptor blockers (ARBs) reduce proteinuria but remission is rarely attained. In addition, it is well

TABLE 91.2. Classification of FSGS.

Gene	Protein	Disease	Inheritance
NPHS1	Nephrin	Congenital NS Finish type	Autosomal recessive
NPHS2	Podocin	Steroid resistant NS	Autosomal recessive
CD2AP	CD2AP	Proteinuria in adolescence and early adulthood, chronic renal failure	Autosomal dominant
ACTN4	alpha-actin 4	Proteinuria in adolescence and early adulthood, chronic renal failure	Autosomal dominant

known that they slow the rate of progression to ESRF. They are recommended in all patients with FSGS (19, 20).

References

1. Meyrier, A. (2004) Nephrotic focal segmental glomerulosclerosis in 2004: An update. *Nephrol Dial Transplant* **19**, 2437–2444.
2. D'Agati, V. (1994) The many masks of focal segmental glomerulosclerosis. *Kidney Int* **46**, 1223–1241.
3. Ahmad, H., Tejani, A. (2000) Predictive value of repeat renal biopsies in children with nephrotic syndrome *Nephron* **84**, 342–346.
4. Haas, M., Meehan, SM., Karrison, TG., Spargo, BH. (1997) Changing etiologies of unexplained adult nephrotic syndromes: a comparison of renal biopsy findings from 1976–1979 and 1995–1997 *Am J Kidney Dis* **30**, 621–631.
5. Kitiyakara, C., Eggers, P., Kopp, JB. (2004) Twenty-one-year trend in ESRD due to focal segmental glomerulosclerosis in the United States *Am J Kidney disease* **44**, 815–825.
6. Rivera, F., Lopez-Gomez, JM., Perez-Garcia, R. (2004) Spanish Registry of Glomerulonephritis. Clinicopathologic correlations of renal pathology in Spain. *Kidney Int* **66**, 898–904.
7. Weber, S., Gribouval, O., Esquivel, EL., Morinière, V., Tête, MJ., Legendre, C., Niaudet, P., Antignac, C. (2004) NPHS2 mutation analysis shows genetic heterogeneity of steroid-resistant nephrotic syndrome and low post-transplant recurrence *Kidney Int* **66**, 571–579.
8. Winn M. (2003) Approach to the evaluation of heritable renal disease and update on familial focal segmental glomerulosclerosis *Nephrol Dial Transplant* **18**, 4–20.
9. Dantal J., Bigot, E., Bogers, W. et al. (1994) Effect of plasma protein adsorption on protein excretion in kidney-transplant recipients with recurrent nephrotic syndrome. *N Engl J Med* **330**, 7–14.
10. Ruf, R., Lichtenberg, A., Karl, SM. (2004) Patients with mutations of podocin don't respond to standard steroid treatment of nephrotic syndrome *J Am Soc Nephrol* **15**, 722–732.
11. D'Agati, VD. (2004) Pathological classification of focal segmental glomerulosclerosis: A working proposal *Am J Kidney Disease* **43**, 368–382.
12. Chun, MG., Korbet, SM., Schwartz, MM., Lewis, EJ. (2004) Focal segmental glomerulosclerosis in nephrotic adults: presentation, prognosis and response to therapy of histologic variants *J Am Soc Nephrol* **15**, 2169–2177.
13. Quereda, C., Ballarin, J., Galeano, C., García Lopez, F., Praga, M. (2007) Immunosupresive therapy of primary focal sclerosing glomerulonephritis in the adult a systematic review *Nefrologia* **27**, 249–260.
14. Velosa, JA., Holley, KE., Torres, VE., Offord, KP. (1983 Sep) Significance of proteinuria on the outcome of renal function in patients with focal segmental glomerulosclerosis *Mayo Clin Proc* **58 (9)**, 568–77.
15. Stirling, CM., Mathieson, P., Boulton-Jones, JM., Feehally, J., Jayne, D., Murray, HM., Adu, D. (2005) Treatment and outcome of adult patients with primary focal segmental glomerulosclerosis in five UK renal units *QJM* **98(6)**, 443–9.

16. Troyanov, S., Wall, CA., Miller, JA., Scholey, JW., Cattran, DC. Toronto Glomerulonephritis Registry Group (2005) Focal and segmental glomerulosclerosis: definition and relevance of a partial remission *J Am soc nephrol* **16**, 1061–1068.

17. Pardon, A., Audard, V., Caillard, S., Molin B., Desvaux, D., Bentaarit, B., Remy, P., Sahali, D., Roudot-Thoraval, F., Lang, P., Grimbert, P. (2006) Risk factors and outcome of focal and segmental glomerulosclerosis recurrence in adult renal transplant recipients *Nephol Dial Transplant* **21**, 1053–1059.

18. Burgess, E. (1999) Management of focal and segmental glomerulosclerosis: evidence based recommendations *Kidney Int* **55 (S70)**, S26–S32.

19. Praga, M., Hernandez, E., Montoyo, C., Andres, A., Ruilope, LM., Rodicio, JL. (1992) Long-term beneficial effects of angiotensin-converting enzyme inhibition in patients with nephrotic proteinuria *Am J Kidney Dis.* **20**, 240–248.

20. Delucchi, A., Cano, F., Rodriguez, E., Wolf, E., Gonzalez, X., Cumsille, MA. (2000) Enalapril and prednisone in children with nephrotic-range proteinuria *Pediatr Nephrol* **14**, 1088–1091.

92
Membranoproliferative or Mesangiocapillary Glomulonephritis

Montserrat M. Díaz, Laia Sans, Yolanda Arce and José Ballarin

Abstract   Membranoproliferative glomerulonephritis (MPGN), also called mesangiocapillary glomerulonephritis, is a complex and uncommon cause of glomerular disease. Its name describes the most relevant histological characteristics of this entity: thickening of glomerular basement membrane due to immune complexes deposition and cell proliferation caused by mesangial cell and influx of inflammatory cells, mainly monocytes. Identification of circulating antibodies against some complement substrates supports the autoimmune pathogenesis of this disease.

MPGN accounts for 4–5% of all glomerular diseases. The outcome is usually poor; the estimated renal survival ranges from 60 to 65% after 10–15 years from the initial renal biopsy, regardless of treatment. Signs of prognostic value are: nephrotic syndrome, renal impairment, high blood pressure, crescents and tubulointerstitial involvement in biopsy. Corticosteroids are the only treatment that has shown prognostic improvement of this disease in children, not in adults.

Keywords   Mesangial proliferation · immune deposits · complement antibody · nephritic factor

Membranoproliferative or mesangiocapillary glomerulonephritis (MPGN) is caused by an abnormal, immune response with deposits of antibodies in the kidneys resulting in chronic inflammation and finally ESRD. MPGN is a pathological definition of a very complex entity. Its main characteristic features are: (a) immune deposits in different structures of glomerular basement membrane, (b) intense glomerular hypercellularity due to mesangial proliferation involving cells and matrix with interposition of mesangial cells into the capillary wall. (c) Influx of inflammatory cells, mainly monocytes (1).

Classification

MPGN can be primary (or idiopathic) and secondary. The primary form, less common in industrialized countries, is divided into three subcategories: types I, II and III. These entities can be differentiated by the location of the immune deposits: subendothelial (Type I), intramembranous dense deposits (type II) and subendothelial and subepithelial deposits, both at the same time (type III) as well as by the pathogenesis: activation of the classical complement-mediated pathway by immune complex (Type I), alternative pathway mediated by an antibody (the Nephritic Factor) (Types II and III) (1, 2, 3).

Epidemiology

MPGN is a chronic nephritis that occurs most commonly in children and young adults and is more frequent between the ages of 5 and 15 years, but it can be diagnosed at any age. Some studies suggest a slight increase of frequency in men, but in most of them the gender ratio is close to one. Its overall incidence is progressively decreasing in developed countries, accounting for around 7–12% of glomerular disease diagnosed by kidney biopsy. In underdeveloped areas or developing countries, it still represents a high proportion of glomerulopathies. The real incidence is difficult to ascertain, because a kidney biopsy is required for diagnosis and this procedure is not available routinely in most of the underdeveloped areas (4, 5, 6).

Pathogenesis

Immune complex formation that activates the classical complement pathway may be the mechanism involved in most cases of MPGN type I, but the antigen or antigens that trigger this immune response remain unknown. A cause-effect relationship is difficult to invoke because neither the complement level nor the presence of the C3

From: Y. Shoenfeld et al. (eds.): *Diagnostic Criteria in Autoimmune Diseases*, DOI: 10.1007/978-1-60327-285-8_92,

nephritic factor antibody (C3NeF) is related with the disease severity or outcome. In the case of MPGN type II and III, the alternative pathway is impaired, because an autoantibody against the C3 convertase has been identified that stabilizes the enzyme to become resistant to H factor inactivation; in addition, the stability of the convertase is greater than the one produced by binding to properdin, and is properdin independent. Another mechanism is the genetic absence or dysfunction of H factor. Some cases of MPGN type III have been related to a circulating nephritic factor, which is properdin dependent, and which affects the terminal loop of the alternative pathway (2, 7, 8, 9).

Clinical Manifestations

The clinical features of this disease are variable. It can have an asymptomatic course, with persistent hematuria and/or proteinuria detected in a screening programme of Japanese schoolchildren. Nephrotic syndrome is present in roughly 50% of cases, ranging from 24 to 69%, hypertension in about 40% and renal impairment at time of presentation is highly variable, between 15 and 44% (6, 7). This is summarized in Table 92.2.

Pathology

The classification of MPGN in three histological types, based on serological and histological differences, is currently accepted.

TABLE 92.1. Classification of MPGN.

Idiopathic form (Immune complex or antibody-mediated without identifiable cause)
    MPGN type I
    MPGN type II or dense deposits disease
    MPGN type III
Secondary MPGN or with identifiable association
  Chronic infection:
    Viral: (hepatitis B, hepatitis C)
    Bacterial: Endocarditis, Infected ventriculoatrial shunt, leprosy
    Protozoal: Malaria, schistosomiasis
    Others: Mycoplasma
Autoimmune diseases: Systemic SLE, Sjögren's syndrome, Inherited complement deficiencies, cryoglobulinemia, also described in Rheumatoid Arthritis,
Thrombotic Microangiopathies: Antiphospholipids Syndrome, Sickle cell anemia, polycythemia,
Malignant neoplasm: Lynphoma, Leukemia, Carcinoma, also described in hydatidiform mole.
Paraprotein deposition disease: Waldeström's macroglobulinemia, immunotactoid glomerulopathy, fibrilary glomerulopathy
Miscellaneous: chronic liver disease, a1-antitrypsin deficiency, transplant glomerulopathy, radiation nephritis, familial partial lipodystrophy (Type II)

TABLE 92.2. Symptoms and Signs of MPGN at presentation.

Symptoms or Signs	%
Minimal urinary abnormality (hematuria and/or non nephrotic proteinuria)	20–30
Nephrotic Syndrome	50 (24–69)
Acute Nephritic syndrome	16–30
Renal impairment	15–40
Hypertension	40
Recurrent episodes of gross hematuria	10–20

The percentage presented in the table come from data published (6, 7) by six different authors and 342 patients.

TABLE 92.3. Serological features by type of MPGN.

MPGN Complement:	C3	C4	C5	C6-C9	P	NF
Type pattern						
Type I (A, B, C)	↓/N	↓↓	↓/N	↓/N	↓/N	50% (NF$_a$/NF$_t$)
Type II (B)	↓↓↓	↓/N	N	N	N	80% (NF$_a$)
Type III (C)	↓/↓↓↓	N	↓	↓↓↓	↓↓	* (NF$_t$)

(A) classical pathway, (B) Alternative pathway (C3 activation), (C) Alternative pathway (terminal pathway activation). Nephritic Factor (NF), Properdin (P).
*There are not enough data to estimate the frequency of NF$_t$ in MPGN type III.

Type I: predominant presence of subendothelial deposits; in 15–20% of cases subepithelial "hump-like" deposits. Mesangial cells and matrix proliferation and in some cases, exudative leukocytes, cause interposition along the membrane; this gives the morphological appearance of "double contour." Matrix and cell proliferation can be prominent, producing a lobular aspect (Figure 92.1). The composition and distribution of the deposits are variable: C3 is almost always present, C4 and C1q in 50% of cases, IgG and IgM in one-third of the cases. The deposits have a granular appearance (1).

Type II, also called dense deposits disease (DDD), is characterized by homogeneus dense deposits along the basement membrane and in the mesangium. They can also involve Bowman's capsule and tubular basement membrane. The C3 immune deposits are described as ribbon-like, linear or sublinear, granular or nodular (8).

Type III can be differentiated from type I only by the subepithelial deposits always present in type III and by the complement pattern. The characteristic lesion of MPGN type III consists of interruptions of lamina densa, associated with subendothelial and subepithelial deposits, sometimes confluent, and combined with multiple layers of new basement membrane (3).

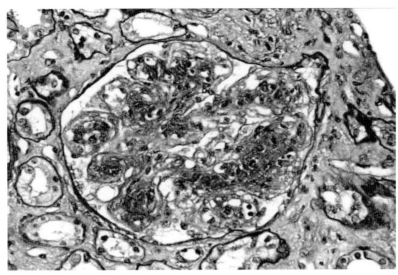

• Membranoproliferative glomerulonephritis with glomerular hypercellular lobular appearance, endocapillary and mesangial proliferation, presence of double contours. PAS.staining

FIGURE 92.1. 40 X.

Serological Features

Hypocomplementemia and presence of nephritic factor are the most relevant serological features of this disease. In MPGN type I, three different patterns of complement activation may be present (a) nephritic factor of amplification loop (NFa); in this case, C3 is very low and the earlier components of the complement cascade are normal, (b) nephritic factor of the terminal pathway (NF_t), characterized by a decrease in the last complement component (C6–C9); C3 is low in variable degree and properdin is also decreased. (c) The last and more common pattern is immune complex-mediated classical pathway activation with decrease of C1q, C2 in variable extent. The MPGN type III complement pattern is similar to that of the terminal pathway described earlier. MPGN type II is characterized by C3 depression and the presence of C3 nephritic factor in 80% of cases (3, 9). ANAS, Rheumatoid Factor, and viral serology for HBV and HCV should be investigated, but they are negative in primary forms of this disease.

Diagnostic Criteria

There are no clinical criteria for diagnosis and the clinical presentation is diverse. To reach a diagnosis, some histological criteria need to be fulfilled, namely, the presence of: (a) Diffuse or segmental thickening of glomerular membrane and (b) hypercellularity, mainly due to mesangial proliferation.

Prognosis

Long term prognosis of this disease is poor, and this has been confirmed in most studies carried out to analyze its outcome. Renal survival is variable but large series estimate a mean of 60–65% survival at 10 years, with or without treatment, the worst prognostic features being nephrotic syndrome, renal impairment at time of presentation and interstitial fibrosis. Patients with normal interstitial space remain with normal ir slightly altered renal function in 63% of cases; this proportion decreases to 13–25% when interstitial fibrosis or renal impairment is present. The degree of glomerular involvement does not worsen the prognosis, but as in most renal diseases the presence of crescents in the biopsy decreases the probability of maintaining renal function. Eighty-seven percent of these patients die; they are in need of dialysis or renal transplantation (5, 7). Relapse after transplantation is around 30% in MPGN type I, but is highly variable by series, ranking between 9%, as reported by Cameron and 53% in O'Meara's series (10). The recurrence of MPGN type II is hard to estimate, fluctuating from 18 to 100% by series; a recent report estimates recurrence in 40% of patients, but is a cause of graft loss in less than 10% (11).

Treatment

The low incidence of this disease makes it very difficult to design clinical trials with new immunosuppressant drugs. All randomized studies were carried out during the 1980s.

In children with impaired renal function, with or without nephrotic proteinuria, treatment with high doses of prednisone (40 mg/m² in every other day during 6–12 months) has been advocated (12, 16). Immunosuppressive drugs (cylophosphamide and chlorambucil) are not effective in changing the disease's natural history. In adults, treatment with aspirin plus Dypiridamol in patients with renal function impairment and/or nephrotic proteinuria is widely accepted. Corticosteroids and immunosuppressant drugs are not effective (13, 14, 15, 16).

References

1. D'Amico G. and Ferrario F. (1992) Mesangiocapillary Glomerulonephritis. *J. Am. Soc. Nephrol.* **2**, S159–S166.
2. Varade W.S., Foristal J., West.C. (1990) Patterns of Complement Activation in Idiopathic Membranoproliferative Glomerulonephritis, Type I, II, III. *Am. J. Kidney Dis.* **XVI(3)**, 196–206.
3. Braun MC, West CD, Strife CF. (1999) Differences between Membranoproliferative Type I and III in Long-Term Response to an Alternate-Day Prednisone Regimen. *Am. J. Kidney Dis.* **34(6)**, 1022–1032.
4. Spanish Society of Nephrology (1989). Progressively decreasing incidence of membranoproliferative glomerulonephritis in Spanish adult population: A multicentre study of 8545 cases of primary glomerulonephritis. *Nephron* **52**, 370–371.
5. Schmitt Hans, Bohle Adalbert, Reineke Torsten, Mayer-Eichberger Dieter, Vogl Wolfgang.(1990). Long Term of Membranoproliferative Glomerulonephritis Type I. Significance of Clinical and Morphological Parameters: An Investigation of 220 Cases. *Nephron* **55**, 242–250.
6. West Clark D. (1986) Childhood membranoproliferative glomerulonephitis: An Approach to management. *Kidney Int.* **29**, 1077–1093.
7. Cansick Janette C, Lennon Rachel, Cummins Carole L, Howie Alexander J, McGraw Mary E, Saleem Moin A, Tizard E. Jane, Hulton Sally-Anne, Milford David V, Taylor C. Mark (2004) Prognosis, treatment and outcome of childhood mesangiocapillary (membranoproliferative) glomerulonephritis. *Nephrol Dial Transplant* **19**, 2769–2777.
8. Gerald B. Appel, H. Terence Cook, Gregory Hageman, J. CharlesJennette, Michael Kashgarian, Michael Kirschfink, John D. Lambris, Lynne Lanning Hans U. Lutz, Seppo Meri, Noel R. Rose, Dvid J. Salant, Sanjeev Sethi, Richard J.H. Smith, William Smoyer, Hope F. Tully, San P. Tully, Patrick Walker, Michael Welsh, Reinhard Würzner and Peter F. Zipfel. (2005) Membranoproliferative Glomerulonephritis Type II (Dense Deposit Disease). *An Update. J. Am. Soc. Nephrol.* **16**, 1392–1403.
9. West Clark D and McAdamas J. (1999) Glomerular Paramesangial Deposits: Association with Hypocomplementemia in Membranoproliferative glomerulonephritis Type I and III. *Am. J. Kidney Dis.* **32(1)**, 56–63.
10. Andresdottir MB, Assmann K, Hoitsma AJ, Koene R, Wetzels J. (1997) Recurrence of type I membranoproliferative glomerulonephritis after renal transplantation. Analysis of the incidence, risk factors and impact on graft survival. *Transplantation* **63(11)**, 1628–1633.
11. Braun MC, Stablein DM, Hamiwka LA, Bell L, Bartosh SM, Strife CF(2005). Recurrence of Membranoproliferative Glomerulonephritis Type II in Renal Allograft: The North American Pediatrics Renal Transplant Cooperative Study Experience. J. Am. Soc. Nephrol. **16**, 2225–2233.
12. Tarshish P., Bernstein J., Tobin JN., Edelmann CM Jr. (1992) Treatment of mesangiocapillary glomerulonephritis with alternative day prednisone: A report of the international study of kidney disease in children. *Pediatr. Nephrol.* **6**, 123–130.
13. Donadio JV. Jr, Anderson CF., Mitchell JC. III, Holley KE, Ilstrup DM, Valentin Fuster MS, Chesebro JH. (1984) Membranoproliferative Glomerulonephritis. A Prospective clinical trial of platelet inhibitors therapy. *N. Engl. J. Med.* **310**, 1421–1426.
14. Zauner I., Bohler J., Grupp C., Heering P., Schollmeyer P. (for the collaborative Glomerulonephritis therapy study group(CGTS)). (1994) Effect of Aspirin and Dipiridamol on proteinuria in idiopathic Membranoproliferative Glomerulonephritis: a multicenter prospective clinical trial. *Nephrol Dial. Transplant.* **9**, 619–622.
15. Cattran DC., Cardella CJ., Roscoe JM., Charron RC., Rance PC., Ritchie SM., Corey PN. (1985) Result of a controlled drug trial in membranoproliferative glomerulonephritis. *Kidney Int.* **27**, 436–441.
16. Levin A. (1999) Management of Membranoproliferative Glomerulonephritis: Evidence-based recommendations. *Kidney Int.* **55**, Suppl. 70 S41–S46.

Part XIII
Hematologic Autoimmune Diseases

93
Autoimmune Hemolytic Anemia

Urs E. Nydegger

Abstract   Autoaggressive targeting of red blood cells (RBCs) including complement (C) activation hits an erythron, the total cell surface of which in an adult adds up to one of the largest destinations for any autoimmune process. New developments in diagnostic precision, such as Coombs tests completed by cytofluorometry and specific diagnostic monoclonal antibodies (mAbs), bring us closer to understanding autoimmune hemolytic anemia (AIHA) triggers. The rituximab (mAb anti-CD20) landslide has also reached AIHA treatment; improved treatment of underlying diseases in secondary AIHA guides ways to curative AIHA treatment. The acute phase of AIHA, often lethal in former times, if readily diagnosed, can now be stopped using plasma exchange, extracorporeal immunoadsorption and/or RBC transfusion with donor RBCs devoid of the autoantibody target antigen. Genotyping blood groups (http://www.bloodgen.com) and narrowing down the blood-type subspecificities with diagnostic mAbs help to define the triggering autoantigen and to select well compatible donor RBC concentrates which thus escape recognition by the autoantibodies.

Keywords   Autoimmune hemolytic anemia · Coombs test · antiglobulin test · immunoglobulin · complement

Anemia occurs by reduced red blood cell (RBC) production or increased destruction, the latter being the case in autoimmune hemolytic anemia (AIHA). Hemolysis involves a shortening of the half-life time of RBC, from normally ~100 days down to a few days in overt cases. With other autoimmune diseases, AIHA shares the offence of the hosts' immune system against his/her own tissue, in this case the erythron (1). The antibody and complement (C)-offended RBC either lyses or becomes phagocytosed by Fc- and C-receptor bearing cells. Some authors compare AIHA with aplastic anemia, caused by autoreactive T lymphocytes, which suppress or destroy hematopoietic cells – an aggression against the erythron at an early stage of maturation brought about by early stages of (auto-) immune responses indeed.

There is no preselection of demographic groups or life age for AIHA although children with primary immunodeficiency disease (PID) are commonly affected; because PID is rare, this association does not tip the balance to pediatrics. Different forms of AIHA can be distinguished based on serologic characteristics of involved autoimmune process with autoantibodies maximally active at body temperatures or at cooler ranges referred to as warm-type AIHA or cold agglutinin disease. An alternate classification of AIHA is based on the presence/absence of underlying disease; in the latter case the condition is termed primary or idiopathic AIHA. Secondary AIHAs may be associated with lymphoproliferative disorders (e.g., Hodgkins disease, lymphoma), rheumatic disorders, primarily SLE, certain infections (2), nonlymphoid neoplasma (e.g., ovarian tumors), certain chronic inflammatory diseases (e.g., ulcerative colitis) or certain drugs (e.g., α-methyldopamin, alemtuzumab, mycophenolate).

The Diagnosis of AIHA

The diagnosis of AIHA must go beyond the clinical triad of anemia, splenomegalia and jaundice, the latter two with signs of inconsistent presence (Table 93.1). It is the Coombs test, often referred to as direct antiglobulin test, which ends up to be the most powerful diagnostic tool after a long train of deductions for AIHA. If AIHA still remains idiopathic in many patients, currently many forms come to light as secondary form for different reasons related to modern diagnostic criteria.

AIHA has been noted with increased incidence in patients receiving uridine nucleoside analogues for hematologic malignancies. Upon hematopoietic stem cell transplantation, recipients of ABO-mismatched products can

From: Y. Shoenfeld et al. (eds.): *Diagnostic Criteria in Autoimmune Diseases*, DOI: 10.1007/978-1-60327-285-8_93,
© 2008 Humana Press, Totowa, NJ

TABLE 93.1. Signs and symptoms of autoimmune hemolytic anemia in percentage.

	Percent cases with this sign	Circumstance	Reference number
Breath shortage	60–70	Relates to acute cases	
Pallor	100	Hb <80 g/l	
Splenomegaly	20	Ultrasound diagnosis required	
Jaundice	60		(3)
Rapid heart rate	50	Upon physical effort	

receive, becoming self in the posttransplant life, non-self-anti-RBC antibodies, transferred by passenger lymphocytes from the donor; fortunately, AIHA in these cases is generally transient, even upon severe hemolysis (4). Venous thromboembolism is a little-recognized, though likely common, complication of AIHA and in some instances may be related to coexistent antiphospholipid antibodies (5).

Monoclonal antibody (mAb) therapy of an ever-increasing number of labeled indications can induce, in rare instances, AIHA (6) because of formation of soluble immune complexes involving mAb. With the Coombs test, antibody avidity, or strength of bonding, and distribution and concentration of accessible antigens on the RBC surface differentiate the agglutination responses. Thermodynamics is the first factor: complexes of Coombs antibodies and their antigen on or adsorbed in the form of previously soluble immune complexes (7) to RBCs are unable to form strong bridges, requiring the intervention of rabbit anti-human antibodies to link and agglutinate the RBCs. While most cold antibodies are IgM class, Donath-Landsteiner antibodies are IgG: they bring C to the surface at warm temperatures and leave the RBC <25°C with C left back on the cell surface. To the immunohematologist, "cold" is <30°C already and for patients suffering from this type of AIHA, exposure to cold air or food can suffice to trigger a AIHA crisis. The diagnosis of mixed-type AIHA is based on demonstrating the presence of "warm" IgG autoantibody and "low titer" (<64 at 4°C), "high thermal amplitude" (reacting at/or >30°C) and "cold" IgM autoantibody. While mixed-type AIHA on the same patient is uncommon, large groups of AIHA patients classify to different temperature spectra of anti-RBC antibody reactivity. RBC agglutination on the peripheral blood film is a common finding in mixed-type AIHA and can lead, initially, to a misdiagnosis of cold agglutinin disease.

A reactive Coombs test should be sought by all means and, if reactive, rarely proves to be capable of bearing another interpretation than AIHA. The distinction between primary and secondary AIHA is more of a scholarly problem because the former is an exclusion diagnosis and must remain one during the follow-up care of the patient. Presence of anti-RBC autoantibodies with a reactive Coombs test are the mainstays of AIHA. Using

agglutination tests and/or flow cytometry, IgG, proteolytic fragment of C (mainly C3 and C4) or both are found on the thus damaged RBCs. The blood film exhibits polychromasia and spherocytosis, the latter a blood film hallmark of the disease visible not only at microscopic inspection but detectable also by the CellAVision® device (8). Indirect hyperbilirubinemia, increased urinary urobilinogen and serum lactate dehydrogenase and increased serum haptoglobin are variably present but not necessary for the diagnosis.

Laboratory Tests

Laboratory tests, if fully detached from clinical pictures, must be reviewed critically (Table 93.2): the importance of the Coombs test, while rock-solid, should not be overestimated because Coombs-test-negative AIHA exists (10). To stretch diagnostic inference too far with Coombs tests may mislead physician and patient. Thus the antiglobulin serum used to detect RBC-bound IgG may fail because it might not be reactive with IgA anti-RBC. Coombs test results may become reactive only when C protein fragments cover the RBC surface brought about by C-activating antibodies, albeit non-C-activating antibodies are inducing AIHA with identical fierceness, as recently confirmed with a well-established mouse model (11) in which erythrophagocytosis by Kupffer cells was also evaluated. Accordingly, the quality/composition of RBC-reactive immune complexes has been shown as of relevance in human medicine (12) IgG2 containing IgM–IgG immune complex being innocuous to RBCs. Evidence is accruing that the Coombs test will more frequently become completed by, instead of reading agglutination patterns, performing flow cytometry (FC). In 33 Chinese patients with AIHA who were found to have RBC-bound IgG, both the mean fluorescence intensity (MFI) and percentage of fluorescence-activated RBCs were remarkably increased and results

TABLE 93.2. Laboratory findings bearing strong evidence for autoimmune hemolytic anemia.

	Percent cases with this finding (approx)	Circumstance
Hyperbilirubinemia	80	Indirect, prehepatic bilirubin increased (3)
Increased serum lactate dehydrogenase	100	Iso-form 5
Reticulocytosis	100	
Mean reticulocyte hemoglobin content	reduced	
Coombs test	90% (revealed by agglutination)	95% revealed by FC[a] (9)

[a] Flow cytometry.

TABLE 93.3. Serological markers of autoimmune hemolytic anemia.

Antibody property	Particularity	Reference number
Anti-RBC autoantibodies	Often with Rhesus D specificity	(17)
Association auto- with alloantibodies	15–47% of cases	[Meta-analysis, (18)]
Circulating immune complexes	Defective composition	Other than IgG2 subclass in mixed IgM–IgG complexes
		(12)
Anti-phospholipid antibodies	Part of antiphospholipid syndrome part of disease cluster	(5)
Cold agglutinins	20% of cases	
Donath-Landsteiner	5% of cases	
Erythrophagocytosis	In the presence/absence of opsonizing antibodies	

of both were considered positive (13). In anemic patients with negative Coombs test, the results of FC were always negative. FC performed in suspected AIHA cases can be reactive whilst conventional, agglutination-based Coombs test remained negative (14). In this study, there was poor correlation between strength of Coombs test and MFI by FC. Preliminary evidence suggests that FC-based Coombs test is more sensitive test than the hemagglutination-based and helps in the serological diagnosis of hemagglutination-based Coombs negative AIHA. In resource poor settings, the hemagglutination-based Coombs test remains state of the art.

The quantity of IgG subclass bound to the surface of RBCs can be estimated (15). A mean number of 80,000–120,000 molecules of IgG1/RBC were detected. The mean concentration of IgG2a autoantibodies was lower ~40,000 molecules/RBC. In humans, the healthy RBC normally carries several thousands of IgG molecules because in the normal state, RBCs transport physiological immune complexes (7), but cut-offs of both Coombs tests and CF need to be set such that these normal amounts do not show up as pathological. This might not be the end of increasing the sensitivity of the Coombs principle. Single-cell analysis that avoids loss of information associated with ensemble averaging of large cell numbers is now possible: a micro-fluidic device lets one manipulate, lyse, label, separate and quantify protein contents of single cells using molecule fluorescence counting – if such technology will perhaps not help to improve patient care, at least it could help us to better understand development of AIHA at the molecular level (16). Other researchers use the activity of phagocytes to ingest damaged RBCs with the erythro-phagocytosis assay that has the advantage of revealing function (Table 93.3). Such system may help identification of AIHA patients with negative Coombs test as well (19).

Predictive Values

Predictive values for AIHA do exist but because this disease may or may not express itself in a number of underlying immunopathological disorders, their exchange for corroboration of diagnosis is relatively weak – too many

criteria must act in concert to boost positive prediction of laboratory criteria.

There exists a susceptibility of AIHA in case of underlying diseases. Thus, in contrast to the NZLB/W mouse, whose SLE is preceded by AIHA, in humans, AIHA is a well known but not obligatory complication of overt SLE. However, AIHA remains a rare complication of any of the cited underlying diseases such that a Positive Predictive Value is way from reaching significance. A reactive Coombs test in individuals without clinical overt AIHA cannot be used to predict development of AIHA. The frequency of healthy blood donors with a positive direct Coombs test was approximately 1 in 3000 in a recent study (9). None of the donors had hemolysis. Hence, Coombs test reactive donors can be a reason for incompatibility results upon RBC donor/recipient compatibility testing.

If there is one disease that cannot be predicted, it is AIHA. There is no familial hereditary component, there is no age preselection, nor have we identified genetic background making an individual susceptible to develop AIHA.

Therapy

Therapy of diseases that sometimes resolve spontaneously, such as AIHA, is often deferred to stages at which measures become urgent. This is certainly so, when RBC transfusions become necessary, often on Friday or Saturday nights. Many years ago, Mueller-Eckhardt and his disciples have taught us that RBC concentrate transfusions should not be withheld to severely anemic AIHA patients with reactive Coombs tests. Compatibility testing is the standard protocol that identifies suitable blood for patients requiring transfusion. Where autoantibodies or non-clinically significant alloantibodies compromise the indirect Coombs test, the supply of RBC transfusions will delay the supply of blood to the patient. No adverse reactions were reported in a recent study where "suitable" blood was provided after a serologically mismatched Coombs testing.

Glucocorticoids are effective in slowing the rate of hemolysis. Because speculation exists that the spleen is the principal producer of anti-RBC autoantibodies, splenectomy may become indicated for patients who require an unacceptable high maintenance of prolonged administration of steroids, but these cases should first go through other options than surgeon's knife. Intravenous immunoglobulins (IVIgs) and rituximab may provide short-term control of hemolysis, especially in children, and immunosuppressive drugs and danazol have been used with success in refractory adults. With anti-RBC antibodies of known specificity, novel approaches in therapy might prove useful for some patients. Thus, anti-A/B antibodies are increasingly depleted using absorber technology (http://www.absorber.se). Prior to removing such antibodies by plasma exchange or absorption, a careful diagnosis now involves such techniques as Luminex or XM-ONE™ of AbSorber, whose commercially available product is based on beads (magnetic nanoparticles) carrying synthetic blood group A and B antigens. By adding patient sera to the beads, the presence of blood group antibodies can be measured by flow cytometry. The most common measurement methods today are hemagglutination or ABO-ELISA. Measurement results are unreliable in that they vary from time to time and from clinic to clinic.

For paroxystic nocturnal hemolysis, the mAb eculizumab (Alexion Pharmaceutcal's Soliris®) may be efficient and colleagues have begun to look at the efficacy of rituximab (anti-CD20) in treating selected cases of AIHA in adults as well (20).

References

1. Petz LD, Garratty G. *Immune Hemolytic Anemias*. New York, Churchill Livingstone, 2004.
2. Agrawal N, Naithani R, Mahapatra M. Rubella infection with autoimmune hemolytic anemia. *Indian J Pediatr* 2007; 74(5): 495–496.
3. Naithani R, Agrawal N, Mahaptra M, Kumar R, Pati HP, et al. Autoimmune hemolytic anemia in children. *Pediatr Hematol Oncol* 2007; 24(4): 309–315.
4. Stussi G, Mueller RJ, Passweg J, Schanz U, Rieben R, Seebach JD. ABO blood group incompatible haematopoietic stem cell transplantation and xenograft rejection. *Swiss Med Wkly* 2007; 137(1–2): 13–20.
5. Krause I, Leibovici L, Blank M, Shoenfeld Y. Clusters of disease manifestations in patients with antiphospholipid syndrome demonstrated by factor analysis. *Lupus* 2007; 16(3): 176–180.
6. Elimelakh M, Dayton V, Park KS, Gruessner AC, et al. Red cell aplasia and autoimmune hemolytic anemia following immunsuppression with alemtuzumab, mycophenolate, and declizumab in pancreas transplant recipients. *Haematologica* 2007; 92(8): 1029–1036.
7. Nydegger UE. Immune complex pathophysiology. *Ann N Y Acad Sci* 2007; 1109: 66–83
8. Ceelie H, Dinkelaar RB, van Gelder W. Examination of peripheral blood films using automated microscopy: Evaluationof Diffmaster Octavia and Cellavision DM96. *J Clin Pathol* 2007; 60(1): 72–79.
9. Bellia M, Georgopoulos J, Tsevrenis V, Nomikou E, Vgonza N, et al. The investigation of the significance of a positive direct antiglobulin test in blood donors. *Immunohematol* 2002; 18(3): 78–81.
10. Sachs UJ, Roder L, Santoso S, Bein G. Does a negative direct antiglobulin test exclude warm autoimmune haemolytic anaemia? A prospective study in 504 cases. *Br J Haematol* 2006; 132(5): 655–656.
11. Baudino L, Fossati-Jimack L, Chevalley C, Martinez-Soria E, Shulman MJ, Izui S. IgM and IgA anti-erythrocyte autoantibodies induce anemia in a mouse model through multivalency-dependent hemagglutination but not through complement activation. *Blood* 2007; 109(12): 5355–5562.
12. Stahl D, Sibrowski W. IgG2 containing IgM-IgG immune complexes predominate in normal human plasma, but not in plasma of patients with warm autoimmune hemolytic anemia. *Eur J Haematol* 2006; 77(3): 191–202.
13. Wang Z, Shi J, Zhou Y, Ruan C. Detection of red blood cell-bound immunoglobulin G by flow cytometry and its application in the diagnosis of autoimmune hemolytic anemia. *Int J Hematol* 2001; 73(2): 188–193.
14. Chaudhary R, Das SS, Gupta R, Khetan D. Application of flow cytometry in detection of red-cell-bound IgG in Coombs-negative AIHA. *Hematology* 2006; 11(4): 295–300.
15. Mazza G, Day MJ, Barker RN, Corato A, Elson CJ. Quantitation of erythrocyte-bound IgG subclass autoantibodies in murine autoimmune haemolytic anaemia. *Autoimmunity* 1996; 23(4): 245–255.
16. Huang B, Wu H, et al. Counting low-copy number proteins in a single cell. *Science* 2007; 315: 81–84.
17. Iwamoto S, Kamesaki T, Oyamada T, et al. Reactivity of autoantibodies of autoimmune hemolytic anemia with recombinant rhesus blood group antigens or anion transporter band3. *Am J Hematol* 2001; 68(2): 106–114.
18. Ahrens N, Pruss A, Kahne A, Kiesewetter H, Salama A. Coexistence of autoantibodies and alloantibodies to red blood cells due to blood transfusion. *Transfusion* 2007; 47(5): 813–816.
19. Biondi CS, Cotorruelo CM, Ensinck A, Racca AL, Racca LL. Use of erythrophagocytosis assay for predicting the clinical consequences of immune blood cell destruction. *Clin Lab* 2004; 50(5–6): 265–270.
20. D'Arena G, Califano C, et al. Rituximab for warm-type idiopathic autoimmune hemolytic anemia: a retrospective study of 11 adult patients. *Eur J Haematol* 2007; 79(1): 53–58.

94
Pernicious Anemia

Mario García-Carrasco, Mario Jiménez-Hernández, Claudia Mendoza-Pinto,
Alejandro Ruiz-Argüelles and Salvador Fuentes-Alexandro

Abstract   Pernicious anemia (PA) is the most common manifestation of vitamin B_{12} deficiency, in which an autoimmune pathogenesis is supported by (a) the presence of mononuclear-cell infiltration into gastric mucosa with loss of parietal cells, (b) autoantibodies to parietal cells and intrinsic factor, (c) autoreactive T cells, (d) regeneration of parietal cells after therapy with corticosteroids or immunosuppressive drugs, (e) familial predisposition and (f) association with other autoimmune diseases. The progression of the chronic atrophic gastritis to gastric atrophy and clinical anemia is likely to span 20 to 30 years. The presence of serum antibodies to gastric parietal-cells predicts autoimmune gastritis. Immune suppression with corticosteroids or azathioprine appears to be the best treatment in early stages of the disease.

Keywords   Pernicious anemia · vitamin B_{12} deficiency · type A gastritis

Pernicious anemia (PA) also known as *Biermer's anaemia, Addison's anaemia* or *Addison-Biermer anaemia*, is a form of megaloblastic anemia due to vitamin B_{12} (Cbl) deficiency; it is an autoimmune disease resulting from antibodies against intrinsic factor (IF) and gastric parietal cells (1); gastric atrophy probably resulting from immune destruction of the acid and pepsin-secreting portion of the gastric mucosa.; PA is considered as a chronic illness in which there is impaired absorption of vitamin B_{12} in the terminal ileum because of a lack of IF (secreted by the parietal cells of the gastric mucosa) (2); its usual course is slowly progressive and is the most common cause of vitamin B_{12} deficiency and, at the end stage, of the type A atrophic gastritis influencing the fundus and body of the stomach (3).

than was previously recognized. Accordingly, reports of small case series of Chinese PA patients have emerged: Wun Chan et al. (5) recently found that 224 of 296 (76%) Chinese with megaloblastic anemia had PA. In fact the incidence is increasing in women and older adults because the diagnosis is unusual before 35 years of age, although typical pernicious anemia can be seen in children under 10 years of age (juvenile pernicious anemia) (3) and the overall prevalence of undiagnosed PA over age 60 years of age is 1.9% (4). In general, the prevalence is 80 cases per 100,000 individuals and the prevalence is highest in women (2.7%), particularly in black women (4.3%) and is less common in southern Europeans and Asians (6).

Epidemiology

Traditionally, pernicious anemia was believed to occur predominantly in people of northern European descent as well as in older populations because multiple epidemiological studies have shown that the average age of onset of pernicious anemia is greater than 60 years, with an increasing frequency with advancing age. Moreover, Carmel et al. (4) in a population survey found that 1.9% of persons more than 60 years of age have undiagnosed pernicious anemia. Nowadays, it has become apparent that the occurrence of PA in all racial and ethnic groups is more common

History

Pernicious anemia was first described in 1849 by the English physician Thomas Addison; later on, Austin Flint in 1869 linked the anemia with alterations of the stomach. (7) The name "pernicious anemia" was coined in 1872 by the German physician Anton Biermer. The studies of George H. Whipple on the effects of feeding liver in anemia followed by those of George R. Minot and William P. Murphy on the effects of feeding liver specifically in pernicious anemia led to the cure of pernicious anemia and to their receiving the Nobel Prize in 1934. As a result, it was suggested that the anemia was caused by lack of an

From: Y. Shoenfeld et al. (eds.): *Diagnostic Criteria in Autoimmune Diseases*, DOI: 10.1007/978-1-60327-285-8_94,

extrinsic factor found in liver that was vitamin B-12 and an intrinsic factor in gastric secretion. Afterward, a serum inhibitor factor of intrinsic factor and autoantibodies to parietal cells were discovered (8) giving an immunological explanation of the underlying gastritis that caused pernicious anemia. Also in the 1950s and 1960s, the Schilling test became established.

Pathogenesis

A genetic predisposition to PA is suggested by clustering of the disease and of gastric autoantibodies in families, and by the association of the disease and gastric autoantibodies with the autoimmune endocrinopathies. About 20% of the relatives of patients with PA have PA. These relatives, especially first-degree female relatives, also have a higher frequency of gastric autoantibodies than normal. Recently, Junca et al. (8) detected early abnormalities in gastric function in first-degree relatives of patients with PA. About 23% of these relatives had parietal-cell antibodies. The disease is associated with HLA types A2, A3, A7, and B12 and with blood group A (9). The pathological process associated with type A gastritis appears to be directed toward the gastric parietal cells, shown by pathologic lesions restricted to parietal cells and the presence of autoantibodies to parietal cells and to their secretory product, intrinsic factor, in the serum and gastric juice. Evidence has shown that H^+/K^+-ATPase is the antigen recognized by parietal-cell autoantibodies (10). This enzyme has a highly conserved catalytic (α) subunit that is phosphorylated during reaction cycles. Gastric H^+/K^+-ATPase is responsible for secretion of hydrogen ions by parietal cells in exchange for potassium ions. Autoantibodies to parietal cells bind to both the 100-kd catalytic (α) subunit and the 60-to-90-kd glycoprotein (β) subunit of gastric H^+/K^+-ATPase. Although parietal-cell autoantibodies can fix complement and lyse parietal cells in vitro, it is unlikely that these autoantibodies are pathogenic in vivo, because gastric H^+/K^+-ATPase is not accessible to circulating antibodies. The importance, if any, of an early observation that passive transfer of parietal cell autoantibodies to rats resulted in reduction in parietal-cell mass without an inflammatory response is therefore uncertain. This particular finding could reflect that cell loss is due to antibody-triggered apoptosis, as has been forwarded for other pathophysiological conditions (11). A report describing autoantibodies that bind to the gastrin receptor was not confirmed. The results of studies showing reactivity of parietal-cell autoantibodies with the surface membranes of parietal cell in vitro may be explained by the loss of cell polarity after cellular dissociation (12). Pathogenic CD4+ T cells are reactive to the parietal cell autoantigen, H^+/K^+ ATPase, and are controlled by CD4+CD25+ T cells in an immunosuppressive cytokine-independent manner. Comparison of CD4+CD25+ T cell-mediated suppression in other autoimmune models shows inconsistencies with respect to requirements of cytokines for immunosupression. More recent data, however, indicate that the evidence for requirement of IL-10 and TGF-β could be due to the complex nature of the T cells causing the disease, as well as the role of induced regulatory T-cell populations. Evidence from this model indicates that immune responses must be initiated and then CD4+CD25+ T cells are recruited to control the quality of the immune response (10, 12). Finally, anemia, the principal feature of PA is caused by malabsorption of vitamin B_{12} in the terminal ileum due to intrinsic-factor deficiency.

Clinical Manifestations

The classic triad of weakness, sore tongue, and paresthesias may be elicited but usually is not the chief symptom complex, because the onset of PA is insidious and unclear and progresses slowly. Generally, the anemia is often well tolerated in this disease and many patients are ambulatory. The median age at diagnosis is 60 years; however, childhood PA has been reported associated with genetic failure to secret intrinsic factor or the secretion of a defective intrinsic factor (13). Symptoms of anemia are the usual presentation, but asymptomatic patients can be identified by routine hematologic investigation. Generally, the presentation of pernicious anemia resembles that of any other form of anemia. Mainly, neurological complications secondary vitamin B_{12} deficiency are developed which may cause peripheral neuropathy (paresthesias and numbness) and lesions in the posterior (loss of vibration and position sense, sensory ataxia) and lateral columns (limbs weakness, spasticity, and extensor plantar response) of the spinal cord and in the cerebrum. These lesions progress from desmyelination to axonal degeneration and eventual neuronal death (14). Megaloblastic madness is less common and can be manifested by delusions, hallucinations, outbursts, and paranoid schizophrenic ideation. Identifying the cause is important because significant reversal of these symptoms and findings can occur with vitamin B-12 administration. Also, patients with PA may develop several abnormalities of the digestive tract such as atrophic glossitis characterized by smooth and beefy, tongue megaloblastosis of the epithelial cells of the small intestine that results in diarrhea and malabsorption. Instestinal metaplasia is a risk factor for adenocarcinoma (15). Achlorhydria and bacterial overgrowth may also lead to the formation of carcinogenic nitrosoamines. The cardiovascular system is also affected; cardiac output is usually increased with hematocrit less than 20%, and the heart rate accelerates; therefore, in patients with preexisting heart disease, coronary insufficiency and congestive heart failure can occur. On the contrary, PA has been associated with common

TABLE 94.1. Clinical manifestation of PA.

Clinical Manifestation	Prevalence %
Anemia	30–60
Neurological complications	10–28
Peripheral neuropathy	0.6
Degeneration of cord	2.8
Dementia	5
Gastrointestinal complication	15
Glositis	1–3
Gastric carcinoma	

variable immunodeficiency and low serum immunoglobulin concentrations. Prevalence of clinical manifestations is shown in Table 94.1. PA may be associated with other autoimmune diseases such as autoimmune thyroiditis, insulin-dependent diabetes mellitus, Addison's disease, primary ovarian failure, primary hypoparathyroidism, Grave's disease, vitiligo, myasthenia gravis, and the Lambert-Eaton syndrome.

Pathological Features

Chronic atrophic gastritis is recognized macroscopically by loss of gastric mucosal folds and thinning of the gastric mucosa. It can be classified into two types according to whether the lesion affects the gastric antrum. Type A (autoimmune) gastritis involves the fundus and the body of the stomach and spares the antrum. It is associated with PA, autoantibodies to gastric parietal cells and to intrinsic factor, achlorhydria, initial low serum gastrin concentrations, that later result in hyperplasia of gastrin-producing cells. Type B gastritis is usually associated with *Helicobacter pylori* infection (10). The most common lesion in gastric-biopsy specimens from PA patients are mononuclear cellular infiltrates in the submucosa extending into the lamina propria between the gastric glands; extension of the cellular infiltrate into the mucosa is accompanied by degenerative changes in parietal cells and zymogenic cells. The cellular infiltrate includes plasma cells and T cells (16). Thereafter, the mucosa becomes atrophic, containing few pepsin-secreting and parietal cells, and then intestinal metaplasia is established. The chronic atrophic gastritis in PA is also associated with an increased risk of intestinal-type gastric cancer and gastric carcinoid tumors. The latter are presumably due to prolonged achlorhydria resulting from parietal-cell loss, compensatory hypergastrinemia, and argyrophilic cell hyperplasia. The bone marrow biopsy and aspirate usually shows that erythroid precursors are large and often oval. The nucleus is large and contains course motley chromatin clumps, having a checkerboard appearance. Nucleoli are visible in the more immature erythroid precursors. Giant metamyelocytes and bands are present, and the mature neutrophils and eosinophils are hypersegmented. The bone marrow histology is similar

in both folic acid and Cbl deficiency. The megaloblastic changes due to Cbl deficiency can be reversed by pharmacological doses of folic acid but not otherwise. (17).

Hematologic Features

Laboratory abnormalities found in PA with established megaloblastic anemia are summarized in Table 94.2. The most important laboratory finding observed in PA is erythrocytic macrocytosis which is obvious when the mean cell volume (MCV) is greater than 100 fL (1, 17). The MCV and mean corpuscular hemoglobin (MCH) are increased, with a mean corpuscular hemoglobin concentration (MCHC) within the reference range. In addition, the peripheral blood usually shows a mild leukopenia and thrombocytopenia or pancytopenia, which parallel the severity of the anemia because vitamin B12 deficiency affects all hematopoietic cell lineages (10). Examination of the marrow is not indicated if the diagnosis is unequivocal; the earliest sign of megaloblastosis reflected in the peripheral blood smear is hypersegmentation of the polymorphonuclear leukocytes followed by the appearance of oval macrocytes, and anisopoikilocytosis (17).

Serological and Biochemical Features

Diagnosis of PA is supported by measuring blood levels of Cobalamin (Cbl) and folate; Cbl is low in most but not all patients with cobalamin deficiency. Patients with vitamin B12 deficiency will have serum levels $<170\,pg/mL$, with symptomatic patients usually having levels $<100\,pg/mL$. The diagnosis is best confirmed by finding an elevated level of serum methylmalonic acid ($>1000\,nmol/L$); in fact, two metabolic markers, plasma methylmalonic acid (MMA) and plasma total homocysteine (tHC), are generally considered as more sensitive indicators of vitamin B12 status than plasma cobalamin levels. MMA and tHC are elevated in vitamin B12 deficiency (17). Normal MMA and

TABLE 94.2. Hematological findings in PA patients.

Peripheral blood
Macrocytosis with hypersegmented polymorphonuclear leucocytes.
Anemia
Leukopenia
Thrombocytopenia or
Pancytopenia
Bone marrow
Megaloblasts
Large myeloid precursors ("gyant metamyelocytes")
Low serum vitamin B_{12} concentrations
Normal serum folate concentrations
Positive Schilling test
Low serum holotranscobalamin concentrations

TABLE 94.3. Prevalence of autoantibodies to gastric parietal cells in several situations.

Patients with pernicious anemia	90%
Patients with simple atrophic gastritis	60%
Nonanemic first-degree relatives of patients with PA	30%
Normal subjects in the third decade	2.5%
Normal subjects in the eight decade	9.6%

homocysteine levels rule out cobalamin deficiency with 100% confidence, and normal homocysteine levels suggest that megaloblastic anemia is not caused by folate deficiency, since only tHC is elevated in folic acid deficiency (18). However an increased concentration of plasma methylmalonic acid (P-MMA) does not predict clinical manifestations of vitamin B_{12} deficiency and should not be used as the only marker for diagnosis of B_{12} deficiency. A Schilling test will confirm that vitamin B_{12} deficiency is the results of intestinal malabsorption due to intrinsic-factor deficiency. The Shilling test assay for cobalamin absorption consists of measuring urinary radioactivity after an oral dose of radioactive cobalamin is given: Absorption is low in PA, and it increases if radioactive vitamin B_{12} is administered along with intrinsic factor (17). In patients with PA, serum antibodies that recognize the H^+/K^+-ATPase occur. Table 94.3 shows the prevalence of autoantibodies in PA. Antiparietal cell antibodies also occur in a significant percentage of patients with thyroid disease (1), and conversely, patients with PA have a higher than expected prevalence of antibodies against thyroid epithelium, lymphocytes, and renal collecting duct cells. Serum antibodies to gastric parietal cells can be detected by indirect immunofluorescence with unfixed, air-dried, frozen sections of mouse stomach in which the antibodies stain parietal cells. Antibodies to intrinsic factor ("type I" or "blocking," antibodies) or the intrinsic factor–cobalamin complex ("type II" or "binding," antibodies) are highly specific to PA patients. Type I autoantibodies are demonstrable in the serum of about 70% of patients with PA. Type II autoantibodies are found in the serum of about 35–40% of patients, and rarely occur in the absence of type I antibodies. Both types of autoantibodies can be detected more frequently in gastric juice than in serum (16).

Diagnostic Criteria

There are no diagnostic criteria for PA; however the presence of hematologic disorders, such as megaloblastic anemia, with positive Schilling test and type A chronic atrophic gastritis with loss of gastric parietal cells can support the diagnosis.

Prognosis

PA is a silent disease until its advanced or end stage. The prognosis depends of the stage of the disease when the diagnosis is made. Neurological complications may not be reversed even when the treatment is begun. On the contrary, if gastric cancer or gastric carcinoid tumors are developed, the prognosis will also depend on the early diagnosis and treatment. Because PA is associated with achlorhydria there is a 3-fold likelihood of developing gastric carcinoma; therefore periodic endoscopy is recommended approximately every 5 years, even in asymptomatic cases, to rule out gastric polyps or gastric carcinoma.

Predicting Role of Autoantibodies

The presence of serum gastric parietal cells predicts autoimmune gastritis. Anti parietal cells and anti-intrinsic factor antibodies are rarely measured in individuals with megaloblastic anemia, even though the anti-intrinsic factor antibodies in particular could be of considerable diagnostic value. Anti-intrinsic factor antibody is highly specific for PA (although its sensitivity is only modest), and its presence in megaloblastic anemia makes the diagnosis of PA almost certain.

Therapeutic Management

The first standard treatment widely used was a regular monthly intramuscular injection of at least 1 mg of vitamin B12 to correct the vitamin deficiency (4). Therapeutic management is summarized in Table 94.4. However, nowadays there are different proposed schedules:

(a) Therapy consisting of five to six intramuscular injections of hydroxocobalamin (1 mg each) over a 3-week period. Patients are then given 1 mg intramuscularly every 3 months for life (19). This regimen corrects the hematological abnormalities and replaces B12 stores.
(b) Therapy consisting of intramuscular injection of hydroxocobalamin 1 mg three times a week for two weeks and then once every 3 months for life. Daily dosing is given initially if there is neurological involvement (20).

These two treatments correct the anemia and may correct the neurological complications if given soon after their onset.

There is little evidence of a satisfactory hematological, biochemical, and clinical short-term response for oral B12 replacement in some randomized controlled trials. The evidence derived from limited studies suggests that high oral doses of B12 (1000 and 2000 mg daily) could be as effective as intramuscular administration in achieving hematological and neurological responses (21). Accordingly, high doses of oral vitamin B12 (1000 mg) initially

TABLE 94.4. Pharmacological treatment of pernicious anemia.

	Acute treatment	Dose	Duration	Maintenance	Dose	Duration
A	Hydroxocobalamin	100 mcg IV every other day	3 weeks	Hydroxocobalamin	100 mcg IV	Every 3 months for life
B	Hydroxocobalamin	100 mcg IV 3 times a week	2 weeks	Hydroxocobalamin	100 mcg IV	once every 3 months for life
C	Hydroxocobalamin	1000–2000 mg VO daily	120 days	Not available data		
D	Hydroxocobalamin	1000 mg VO		Not available data		

daily, thereafter weekly, and then monthly, are as effective as intramuscular vitamin B12 (22).

In the meantime, for newly diagnosed patients with vitamin B12 deficiency secondary to pernicious anaemia, who have an intact terminal ileum, an initial intramuscular dose of vitamin B12 followed by a trial of oral replacement may be considered (21). This recommendation is based on the observation that about 1% of vitamin B12 is absorbed by mass action in the absence of intrinsic factor.

A further large, pragmatic trial in primary care is needed to determine whether oral vitamin B12 is effective in patients with pernicious anaemia in primary care settings, but this therapy should not be used in hospitalized/critical patients.

Precautions in the therapy replacement of B12 deficiency should be considered:

– Administration of folic acid in a patient with vitamin B12 deficiency may induce a hematological response but will worsen any neurological symptoms, and can actually precipitate subacute combined degeneration of the cord (19).
– Patients with pernicious anaemia should also be given oral iron, because most will soon exhaust their iron stores (20).

References

1. Kumar V. Pernicious anemia. MLO Med Lab Obs 2007 Feb;39(2):28, 30–1.
2. Andres E, Federici L, Affenberger S, Vidal-Alaball J, Loukili NH, Zimmer J, Kaltenbach G. B12 deficiency: A look beyond pernicious anemia. J Fam Pract 2007 Jul; 56(7): 537–42.
3. Toh BH, Van Dreil IR, Gleeson PA. Pernicious anemia. N Engl J Med 1997;337:1441–48.
4. Carmel, R. Prevalence of undiagnosed pernicious anemia in the elderly. Arch Intern Med 1996;156:1097.
5. Wun Chan JC, Yu liu HS, Sang Kho BC, Yin Sim JP, Hang Lau TK, Luk YW, Chu RW, Fung Cheung FM, Tat Choi FP, Kwan Ma ES. Pernicious anemia in Chinese. Medicine 2006; 85:129–38.
6. Castle WB. Development of knowledge concerning the gastritis intrinsic factor and its relation to pernicious anemia. N Eng J Med 1953;249:603–14.
7. Taylor KB. Inhibition of intrinsic factor by pernicious anemia sera. Lancet 1959;2:1347–52.
8. Junca J, de Soria PL, Granada ML, Flores A, Márquez E. Detection of early abnormalities in gastric function in first-degree relatives of patients with pernicious anemia. Eur J Haematol 2006;77:518–22.
9. Ungar B, Matthews JD, Tait BD, Cowling DC: HLA-DR patterns in pernicious anaemia. Br Med J 1981;282:768.
10. Ban-Hock, van Driel, Ian R, Gleeson, Paul A. Mechanisms of Disease: Pernicious Anemia. N Engl J Med 1997 Nov 13; 337(20):1441–8.
11. Ruiz-Argüelles A, Jímenez-Brito G, Reyes-Izquierdo P, Pérez-Romano B, Sánchez-Sosa S. Apoptosis of melanocytes in vitiligo results from antibody penetration. J Autoimmun; 2007;29:281–6.
12. McHuhgs RS. Autoimmune gastritis is a well-defined auto-immune disease model for the study of the CD4+ CD25+ T cell-mediated suppression. Curr Top Microbiol Immunol 2005;293:153–77.
13. McIntyre OR, Sullivan LW, Jeffries GH, Silver RH. Pernicious anemia in childhood. N Eng J Med 1965;272:981–86.
14. Stabler SP, Allen RH, Savage DG, Lindenbaum J. Clinical spectrum and diagnosis of cobalamin deficiency. Blood 1990;76:871–81.
15. Hsing AW, Hansson L-E, McLaughllin JK, et al. Pernicious anemia and subsequent cancer: A population-based cohort study. Cancer 1993;71:745–50.
16. Kaye MD, Whorweel PJ, Wright R. Gastric mucosal lymphocyte subpopulations in pernicious anemia and in normal stomach. Clin Immunol Immunopathol 1983; 28: 431–40.
17. Anne-Mette Hvas et al. Diagnosis and treatment of vitamin B$_{12}$ deficiency: An update. Haematologica 2006;91:1506–12.
18. Goringe A, Ellis R, McDowell I, Vidal-Alaball J, Jenkins C, Butler C, et al. The limited value of methylmalonic acid, homocysteine and holotranscobalamin in the diagnosis of early B12 deficiency. Haematologica 2006;91:231–4.
19. Provan D, Weatherall D. Red cells II: Acquired anaemias and polycythaemia. Lancet 2000;355:1260–8.
20. Ballinger A. Gastroenterology and Anaemia. Medicine 2007;35(3):142–6.
21. Butler CC, Vidal-Alaball J, Cannings-John R, McCaddon A, Hood K, Papaioannou A, Mcdowell I, Goringe A. Oral vitamin B12 versus intramuscular vitamin B12 for vitamin B12 deficiency: A systematic review of randomized controlled trials. Fam Pract 2006;23(3):279–85.
22. Bolaman Z, Kadikoylu G, Yukselen V, Yavasoglu I, Barutca S, Senturk T. Oral versus intramuscular cobalamin treatment in megaloblastic anemia: A single-center, prospective, randomized, open-label study. Clin Ther 2003;25:3124–34.

95
Idiopathic Aplastic Anemia

Baraf Lior and Levy Yair

Abstract Aplastic anemia, an uncommon hematological disease, is the paradigm of the human bone marrow failure syndromes. The pathophysiology is immune mediated in most cases, with activated type 1 cytotoxic T cells implicated. The molecular basis of the aberrant immune response and deficiencies in hematopoietic cells is now being defined genetically; examples are telomere repair gene mutations in the target cells and dysregulated T-cell activation pathways. Almost universally fatal just a few decades ago, aplastic anemia can now be cured or ameliorated by stem-cell transplantation or immunosuppressive drug therapy. Immunosuppression with antithymocyte globulins (ATGs) and cyclosporine is effective at restoring blood-cell production in the majority of patients, but relapse and especially evolution of clonal hematologic diseases remain problematic. Allogeneic stem-cell transplant from histocompatible sibling donors is curative in the great majority of young patients with severe aplastic anemia; the major challenges are extending the benefits of transplantation to patients who are older or who lack family donors.

Keywords Aplastic anemia · pancytopenia · CD34$^+$

Definition

The term "aplastic anemia" was introduced by Vaquez and Aubertin in the year 1904. The word "aplastic" is derived from the Greek "a" and "plasso" meaning "without form." "Anemia" is a potentially misleading term, as patients with aplastic anemia fail to form blood cells from all three lineages. The combination of peripheral cytopenias with a decreased or absent bone marrow precursor cells characterizes aplastic anemia. Although there are many known etiologies (Table 95.1), the cause of aplastic anemia is generally difficult to determine in an individual patient, and in the vast majority of cases, no causal etiology can not be found. At times, multiple risk factors can be uncovered in a given patient (Table 95.1).

Epidemiology

A large, prospective study conducted in Europe and Israel between 1980 and 1984 that required stringent case definition and pathologic confirmation reported an annual incidence of aplastic anemia of 2 new cases per 1 million population per year (1). Aplastic anemia occurs two- to three-fold higher in the Far East than in the West. This geographic variation likely stems from environmental rather than genetic risk factors, because the Japanese population in Hawaii manifests similar rates of aplastic anemia as other Americans (2). Studies have not been able to attribute the increased risk of aplastic anemia in the Far East to specific agents, such as chloramphenicol, widely used in Asia (3).

The incidence of acquired aplastic anemia varies bimodally with age, with one peak between ages 15 and 25 years and another peak at older than 60 years of age (4). Aplastic anemia occurs with equal frequency in both genders (1, 2).

Pathophysiology

An immune mechanism was implied decades ago from the recovery of hematopoiesis in patients who failed to engraft after stem-cell transplantation, when renewal of autologous blood-cell production was credited to the conditioning regimen. Also suggestive was that the majority of syngeneic transplantations in which bone marrow was

From: Y. Shoenfeld et al. (eds.): *Diagnostic Criteria in Autoimmune Diseases*, DOI: 10.1007/978-1-60327-285-8_95,
© 2008 Humana Press, Totowa, NJ

TABLE 95.1. A classification of aplastic anemia.

Acquired aplastic anemia
Secondary aplastic anemia
  Irradiation
  Drugs and chemicals
    Regular effects
      Cytotoxic agents
      Benzene
    Idiosyncratic reactions
      Chloramphenicol
      Nonsteroidal anti-inflammatory drugs
      Antiepileptics
      Gold
      Other drugs and chemicals
  Viruses
    Epstein–Barr virus (infectious mononucleosis)
    Hepatitis virus (non-A, non-B, non-C, non-G hepatitis)
    Parvovirus (transient aplastic crisis, some pure red cell aplasia)
    Human immunodeficiency virus (acquired immunodeficiency
      syndrome)
  Immune diseases
    Eosinophilic fasciitis
    Hypoimmunoglobulinemia
    Thymoma and thymic carcinoma
    Graft-versus-host disease in immunodeficiency
  Paroxysmal nocturnal hemoglobinuria
  Pregnancy
Idiopathic aplastic anemia
Inherited aplastic anemia
Fanconi's anemia
Dyskeratosis congenita
Shwachman–Diamond syndrome
Reticular dysgenesis
Amegakaryocytic thrombocytopenia
Familial aplastic anemias
Preleukemia (e.g., monosomy 7)
Nonhematologic syndromes (e.g., Down, Dubowitz, Seckel)

infused without conditioning failed (5). The responsiveness of aplastic anemia to immunosuppressive therapies remains the best evidence of an underlying immune pathophysiology: the majority of patients show hematologic improvement after only transient T-cell depletion by antithymocyte globulins (ATGs).

In early laboratory experiments, removal of lymphocytes from aplastic bone marrows improved colony numbers in tissue culture and their addition to normal marrow inhibited hematopoiesis in vitro (6). The effector cells were identified by immunophenotyping as activated cytotoxic T cells expressing Th1 cytokines, especially interferon-γ. In general, patients at presentation demonstrate oligoclonal expansions of a few subfamilies of those T cells, which diminish or disappear with successful therapy. Original clones re-emerge with relapse, sometimes accompanied by new clones, consistent with spreading of the immune response. Occasionally, a large clone persists in remission, perhaps evidence of T-cell tolerance (7). The impact of T-cell attack on marrow can be modeled in vitro. It has been shown that interferon-γ in increasing doses reduces

numbers of human hematopoietic progenitors assayed by inducing apoptosis in CD34 target cells (8).

A number of hypothesis have been made for the unclear activation of T cells in aplastic anemia patients, most of whom are associated with alterations in nucleotide sequence (e.g., polymorphisms in cytokine genes like interferon-γ) or in gene regulation: SAP gene encodes a small modulator protein that inhibits interferon-γ production whose levels are markedly diminished in a majority of acquired aplastic anemia cases (9). Perforin gene which is an important cytolytic, T cell mediated, APCs is diminished and assumptually responsible in the uncontrolled expansion of cytotoxic T cells and CD34 destruction in few idiopathic aplastic patients.

The aforementioned process in which hematopoietic cells are immunely T-cell mediated and destroyed leads to marrow failure. The pallor of the marrow biopsy core or empty spicules of an aspirate, few or no CD34 cells on flow cytometry, and minimal numbers of colonies derived from committed progenitors in semisolid media all reflect the severe reduction in hematopoietic cells that defines the disease. The few hematopoietic cells that are seen in the marrow of aplastic patients experience cell destruction through apoptotic mechanisms. The same process was reproduced in normal CD34 cells exposed to interferon-γ (10).

One peculiar feature of white blood cells in aplastic anemia is telomeres length. Telomeres are short in one-third to one-half of patients (11). The first hypothesis that blamed telomere shortening on stem-cell exhaustion was dismissed by the discovery of mutations in genes that repair and protect telomeres. The working premise in these days is that those mutations are genetic risk factors in acquired aplastic anemia, probably because they confer a quantitatively reduced hematopoietic stem-cell compartment that may also be qualitatively inadequate to sustain immune-mediated damage.

Finally, to date, there is no satisfying mechanism to explain clonal escape evolving to other hematologic diseases that are characterized by proliferation of distinctive cell clones, as in paroxysmal nocturnal hemoglobinuria (PNH) or myelodysplasia (MDS).

Clinical Manifestations

The patient with aplastic anemia occasionally comes to medical attention because of the fatigue and even cardiopulmonary compromise associated with progressive anemia. However, more common presentations are recurrent infections due to profound neutropenia or mucosal hemorrhage due to thrombocytopenia. Increased menstrual flow is a common complaint in premenopausal women. Major hemorrhage from any organ can occur in aplastic anemia but is usually not seen until late in the course of the disease and is generally associated with infections, or traumatic therapeutic procedures (e.g., intravenous line placements).

The infections in aplastic anemia patients are typically bacterial, including sepsis, pneumonia, and urinary tract infection. However, invasive fungal infection is a common cause of death, especially in subjects with prolonged and severe neutropenia.

The physical examination is generally unremarkable except for bruising and petechiae, as noted above. Hepatosplenomegaly and lymphadenopathy are usually absent.

Diagnosis

Signs and symptoms at presentation are illustrated in Table 95.2.

The possible presence of aplastic anemia is suggested by the complete blood count, which reveals pancytopenia along with absolute reticulocytopenia, suggestive of bone marrow failure. The red blood cells are usually normocytic but occasionally may be macrocytic. Examination of the peripheral blood smear shows that the remaining elements, while reduced, are morphologically normal.

Aspiration and biopsy of the bone marrow, along with cytogenetic analysis, are pathognomonic and usually provide sufficient information to establish the diagnosis: in most cases the marrow shows hypocellularity with a decrease in all elements, although significant residual cellularity is present in some patients because of lymphocytes.

In those few patients in whom there is a discordant relationship between cellularity and peripheral blood findings, cellularity often diminishes rapidly and a second evaluation will reveal the classic marrow picture. The marrow space is composed mostly of fat cells and marrow stroma. The residual hematopoietic cells are morphologically normal and there is no malignant infiltrates or fibrosis. Bone marrow cytogenetics is typically normal for patients initially presenting with aplastic anemia. In contrast, cytogenetic abnormalities are frequently found in myelodysplastic bone marrows and may be helpful in distinguishing aplastic anemia from hypoplastic MDS.

TABLE 95.2. Presenting symptoms of aplastic anemia.

Symptoms	Number of patients
Bleeding	41
Anemia	27
Bleeding and anemia	14
Bleeding and infection	6
Infection	5
Routine examination	8
Total	101

Adapted from Williams DM, Lynch RE, Cartwright GE. Drug induced aplastic anemia. *Semin Hematol* 1973; 10: 195.

The severity of aplastic anemia was classified (12) in an effort to make possible the comparison of diverse groups of patients and different therapeutic approaches. Diagnosis of severe aplastic anemia requires that the patient have a marrow biopsy showing <25% of normal cellularity or marrow showing <50% normal cellularity, in which fewer than 30% of the cells are hematopoietic and at least two of the following are satisfied: a granulocyte count <500/μl, a platelet count <20,000/μl, and an absolute reticulocyte count <40,000/μl. Very severe aplastic anemia is further defined by a granulocyte count <200/μl.

Treatment: Curative Treatment

Immunosuppression

For aplastic anemia that is severe, as defined above, definitive therapies are immunosuppression or stem-cell transplantation.

Immunosuppressive therapies are most widely used because of lack of histocompatible sibling donors, patient age, and the immediate cost of transplantation. The most acceptable immunosuppression regimen today is an ATG used in combination with cyclosporine (13). ATGs, which are produced by immunizing animals against human thymocytes, probably are immunomodulatory as well as lymphocytotoxic, perhaps by producing a state of tolerance by preferential depletion of activated T cells. Cyclosporine's selective effect on T-cell function is due to direct inhibition on the expression of nuclear regulatory proteins, resulting in reduced T-cell proliferation and activation. Although severe aplastic anemia can respond to cyclosporine alone, it is less effective than ATG alone or ATG plus cyclosporine.

Reported hematologic response rates vary, at least in part due to lack of consensus on parameters (transfusion independence, absolute or relative improvement in blood counts) and defined landmarks. Improvement in blood counts, so that the criteria for severity are no longer met, highly correlates with termination of transfusions, freedom from neutropenic infection, and better survival (14). By this standard, about 60% of patients are responders at 3 or 6 months after initiation of ATG treatment (15). Responders have much better survival prospects than do non-responders and the outcomes are related to patient age: 5-year survival of >90% of children has been reported in recent trials, compared with about 50% survival for adults older than 60 years in the collective European experience (16).

Relapse, defined as a requirement for additional immunosuppression, is not uncommon, occurring in 30–40% of responding patients. Reinstitution of cyclosporine usually reverses declining blood counts, and when required, a second round of ATG is usually effective. As much as it known today, relapse does not confer a poor prognosis.

Molecular analysis of T cell suggests that the major reason for relapse is incomplete eradication of pathogenic clones by ATG.

The addition of other immunosuppressive agents (mycophenolate mofetil, sirulimus) to the ATG–cyclosporine regimen has not shown any superiority in hematologic response, relapse, or evolution rates.

Hematopoietic Stem Cell Transplantation

Allogeneic transplant from a matched sibling donor cures the great majority of patients with high 5-year survival rates (17). Despite this, graft-versus-host disease (GVHD) remains a serious problem for older patients (40–45% > 20 years of age), even with routine cyclosporine prophylaxis. Chronic GVHD rises the risk of death and often requiring years of immunosuppressive therapy (18). Even with resolution, chronic GVHD remains a risk factor for late complications such as growth and endocrine system effects, pulmonary disease, cataracts, neurological dysfunction, and secondary malignancy. Addition of ATG and more recently its substitution by alemtuzumab (monoclonal antibody against CD52, which is found on mature lymphocyts) (18) may reduce the frequency and severity of acute GVHD, a predictor of chronic GVHD.

As the outcome in aplastic patients who have failed a single round of ATG has been poor and the matched sibling donor available is only 20–30% of cases, alternative sources of hematopoietic stem cells have been sought. The outcomes of 318 alternative donor transplants performed from 1988 to 1998 recently have been summarized for the European registry (19): the rejection rate was 15%, the GVHD 2–4 grades, 48%, and 5-year survival was estimated at 39%. The mortality rate is about twice that observed in matched sibling transplants. On the contrary, retrospective analysis from the Japan Marrow Donor Program suggested that patients with the most favorable characteristics and conditioned with a minimal dose of radiation might anticipate survival comparable with matched sibling transplants (20). In current practice, unrelated transplant is offered for children who have failed a single course of immunosuppression and to adults who are refractory to multiple courses of ATG and alternative therapies such as androgens. Studies with longer follow-up of larger numbers of patients are crucial to establish the optimal conditioning regimen and to define which patients will benefit and especially how early unrelated transplantation should be performed.

Very few clinical trials have specifically addressed moderate disease in which the course and treatment are less clear. As for the course, some patients progress to severe disease, whereas others remain stable and may not require intervention. The two most acceptable modes of treatment options are immunosuppressive and androgen therapies.

Supportive Care

The initial management in the majority of aplastic anemia patients consists of blood transfusions, platelet concentrates, and treatment and prevention of infection. All blood products should be filtrated to reduce the risk of alloimunization and irradiated to prevent grafting of live donor lymphocyte.

Although it is generally accepted that prophylactic platelet transfusions can reduce the risk of hemorrhage, the guidelines for such treatments remain an area of controversy. Multicenter, randomized trials in newly diagnosed acute myelocytic leukemia (AML) patients found no significant difference in risk of major bleeding between patients randomized to receive prophylactic platelet transfusions at threshold platelet counts of $20,000/\mu l$ versus $10,000/\mu l$. Use of the lower platelet threshold significantly reduced platelet use. Platelet transfusions at platelet counts below $5000–10,000/\mu l$ in stable outpatients with chronic severe aplastic anemia were feasible and safe in recent studies (21). In practice, the decision for platelet transfusion must be individualized and take into account the number of platelets, the personal tendency of the patient to bleed, and whether is the patient at increased risk of bleeding (e.g., fever, infection). Whereas severe granulocytopenia may last for years, the cellular immune functions of aplastic anemia patients remain intact. Neutropenia (and perhaps monocytopenia) increases the risk of bacterial infection in aplastic anemia. Because neutropenia precludes the development of an inflammatory response, signs and symptoms of infection can be deceptively minimal. Despite all of that, the use of prophylactic antibiotics has no demonstrated role in the otherwise well patient with aplastic anemia. In the context of fever and neutropenia, complete evaluation and cultures of all possible sites should generally be followed by the administration of broad-spectrum parenteral antibiotics until the fever abates and all cultures are negative. Deficiency of hemopoietic growth factors (such aserythropoietin) is not the cause of the bone-marrow failure in aplastic anaemia; concentrations of hemopoietic growth factors are very high in patients with the disorder, in a compensatory attempt to increase blood production. Hence, these factors should not be used routinely.

References

1. Kaufman D, Kelly J, et al. The drug etiology of agranulocytosis and aplastic anemia. New York: Oxford University Press, 1991: 259.
2. Aoki K, Fujiki N, Shimizu H, Ohno Y. Geographic and ethnic differences of aplastic anemia in humans. In: Najean Y (ed.), *Medullary Aplasia*, Vol 79. New York: Masson, 1980.

3. Issaragrisil S, Kaufman DW, Anderson T, et al. Low drug attributability of aplastic anemia in Thailand. The Aplastic Anemia Study Group. *Blood* 1997; 89: 4034–9.

4. Young N. Acquired aplastic anemia. In: NS Y (ed.), *Bone Marrow Failure Syndromes*. Philadelphia: WB Saunders, 2000: 1–46.

5. Hinterberger W, Rowlings PA, Hinterberger-Fischer M, et al. Results of transplanting bone marrow from genetically identical twins into patients with aplastic anemia. *Ann Intern Med.* 1997; 126: 116–22.

6. Young NS. Hematopoietic cell destruction by immune mechanisms in aquired aplastic anemia. *Semin Hematol.* 2000; 37: 3–14.

7. Young NS, et al. Current concepts in the pathophysiology and treatment of aplasticanemia. *Blood* 2006 October 15; 108(8): 2509–19. Epub 2006 June 15. Review.

8. Maciejewski JP, Selleri C, Anderson S, Young NS. Fas antigen expression on CD34_ human marrow cells is induced by interferon-gamma and tumor necrosis factor-alpha and potentiates cytokine – mediated hematopoietic suppression in vitro. *Blood.* 1995; 85: 3183–90.

9. Zeng W, Chen G, Kajigaya S, et al. Gene expression profiling in CD34 cells to identify differences between aplastic anemia patients and healthy volunteers. *Blood* 2004; 103: 325–32.

10. Zeng W, Miyazato A, Chen G, Kajigaya S, Young NS. Interferon-_-induced gene expression in CD34 cells: identification of pathologic cytokinespecific signature profiles. *Blood* 2006; 107: 167–75.

11. Brummendorf TH, Maciejewski JP, Young NS, Lansdorp PL. Telomere length in leukocyte subpopulations of patients with aplastic anemia. *Blood* 2001; 97: 895–900.

12. Rozman C, Marin P, Nomdedu E, Montserrat E. Criteria for severe aplastic anemia. *Lancet* 1987; 2: 955.

13. Marsh J, Schrezenmeier H, Marin P, et al. Prospective randomized multicenter study comparing cyclosporin alone versus the combination of antithymocyte globulin and cyclosporin for treatment of patients with nonsevere aplastic anemia: a report from the European Blood and Marrow Transplant (EBMT) Severe Aplastic Anemia Working Party. *Blood* 1999; 93: 2191–5.

14. Young NS, Calado RT, Scheinberg P. Current concepts in the pathophysiology and treatment of aplastic anemia. *Blood* 2006; 108: 2509–19.

15. Rosenfeld S, Follman D, Nunez O, Young NS. Antithymocyte globulin and cyclosporine for severe aplastic anemia: Association between hematologic response and long-term outcome. *JAMA* 2003; 289: 1130–5.

16. Tichelli A, Socié G, Henry-Amar M, et al. Effectiveness of immunosuppressive therapy in older patients with aplastic anemia: The European Group for Blood and Marrow Transplantation Several Aplastic Anaemia Working Party. *Ann Intern Med* 1999; 130: 193–201.

17. Horowitz MM. Current status of allogeneic bone marrow transplantation in acquired aplastic anemia. *Semin Hematol* 2000; 37: 30–42.

18. Gupta V, Ball SE, Sage D, et al. Marrow transplants from matched unrelated donors for aplastic anaemia using alemtuzumab, fludarabine and cyclophosphamide based conditioning. *Bone Marrow Transplant* 2005; 35: 467–71.

19. Passweg JR, Perez WS, Eapen M, et al. Bone marrow transplants from mismatched related and unrelated donors for severe aplastic anemia. *Bone Marrow Transplant* 2006; 37: 641–9.

20. Kojima S, Matsuyama T, Kato S, et al. Outcome of 154 patients with severe aplastic anemia who received transplants from unrelated donors: The Japan Marrow Donor Program. *Blood* 2002; 100: 799–805.

21. Sagmeister M, Oec L, Gmur J. A restrictive platelet transfusion policy allowing long-term support of outpatients with severe aplastic anemia. *Blood* 1999; 93: 3124–6.

22. Frickhofen N, Rosenfeld SJ. Immunosuppressive treatment of aplastic anemia with antithymocyte globuilin and cyclosporine. *Semin Hematol.* 2000; 37: 56–68.

23. Deeg HJ, Leisenring W, Storb R, et al. Long-term outcome after marrow transplantation for severe aplastic anemia. *Blood* 1998; 91: 3637–45.

96
Acquired Adult Pure Red Cell Aplasia

Hedi Orbach, Gisele Zandman Goddard, Asher Winder and Yehuda Shoenfeld

Abstract   Pure red cell aplasia (PRCA) is a selective non-regenerative erythroid cell line disease characterized by anemia with the arrest of erythropoiesis, severe reticulocytopenia and absence of bone marrow erythroblasts. Primary adult PRCA is an isolated disease. The etiology of secondary disease includes exogenic triggers as drugs mainly recombinant erythropoietin (EPO), infections (parvovirus B19) incompatible ABO bone marrow transplantation, autoimmune diseases, malignancies (mainly hematological and thymoma), and pregnancy. In most of the cases, the red cell aplasia is immunologically mediated. The diagnosis is made in severe symptomatic normochromic normocytic anemia. In our opinion, anemia with almost complete absence of erythroblasts in the bone marrow with normal development of the myeloid and megakaryocytic lines is diagnostic. The treatment includes blood transfusions and therapy of the primary disease, and if the anemia persists despite multiple blood transfusions, immunomodulation by corticosteroids is warranted. In resistant cases, other options are used: cyclophosphamide, azathioprine, cyclosporine, anti-thymocytic globulin and high-dose intravenous immunoglobulin (IVIg). Plasmapheresis, EPO, interferon and monoclonal antibodies against CD20 and CD52, splenectomy and allogeneic stem cell transplantation after cyclophosphamide conditioning are anecdotal therapies.

Keywords   Pure red cell aplasia · anemia · reticulocytopenia · erythroblasts · diagnostic criteria · large granular lymphocytes · erythropoietin · parvovirus

Pure red cell aplasia (PRCA) is characterized by anemia with severe reticulocytopenia caused by selective failure of erythropoiesis (1). This disease was first described by Kaznelson in 1922 (2).

Epidemiology

PRCA is a rare disorder. The incidence rate is not known. It affects all age groups in all parts of the world without known ethnic or racial predisposition (3).

Classification of PRCA (Table 96.1)

The congenital form of PRCA known as Diamond-Blackfan anemia is a genetic disease with chromosomal and physical abnormalities (4). Transient erythroblastopenia of childhood is a heterogeneous disease with unclear etiology (5).

The causes of acquired PRCA of the adult (Table 94.1) include a primary disorder (isolated PRCA) or secondary PRCA. The most common etiologies of acquired PRCA are manifold: exogenic triggers include drugs, infections and ABO-incompatible bone marrow transplantation (6). Drugs induce disease [recently the main drug is human serum albumin-free recombinant erythropoietin (EPO) (7) administered subcutaneously to dialysis treated patients]. Infections induce PRCA mainly parvovirus B19. PRCA is a rare manifestation of autoimmune diseases as systemic lupus erythematosus (8) and rheumatoid arthritis (9). Malignancies include hematological malignancies as chronic lymphocytic leukemia [B-cell, T-cell or large granular lymphocyte (LGL) leukemia], lymphomas and solid tumors mainly thymoma (10) (and rarely other solid tumor malignancies) and pregnancy rarely induce PRCA. There is not enough information in the literature on the percentage of the different primary causes of PRCA.

From: Y. Shoenfeld et al. (eds.): *Diagnostic Criteria in Autoimmune Diseases*, DOI: 10.1007/978-1-60327-285-8_96,
© 2008 Humana Press, Totowa, NJ

TABLE 96.1. Classification of acquired adult PRCA by associated disease.

A.	Primary pure red cell aplasia
B.	Secondary red cell aplasia
1.	Exogenic triggers
	I. Drugs: Recombinant human erythropoietin, phenytoin, trimethoprim–sulfamethoxazole, zidovudine, chlorpropamide, mycophenolate mofetil
	II. Infections: B19 parvovirus, human immunodeficiency virus, viral hepatitis, Epstein–Barr virus
	III. ABO-incompatible bone marrow transplantation
2.	Autoimmune diseases: Systemic lupus erythematosus, rheumatoid arthritis, mixed connective tissue disease, Sjögren's syndrome, autoimmune hemolytic anemia
3.	Malignancies
	I. Hematological malignancies: Chronic lymphocytic leukemia (B-cell, T-cell, large granular lymphocyte type), lymphoma, myeloma, chronic myeloid leukemia, agnogenic myeloid metaplasia with myelofibrosis, prodrome of myelodysplastic syndrome
	II. Solid tumors: Thymoma, adenocarcinoma of breast, squamous cell carcinoma of lung
4	Pregnancy

Pathophysiology of PRCA

The mechanism of B19 parvovirus-induced PRCA is by direct damage. The virus destroys proerythroblasts by attacking the blood group P antigen receptor. Severe anemia occurs usually in patients with hemolytic anemia or immune compromised patients (11). Most of the other cases are immunologically mediated red cell aplasia.

In vitro studies show that PRCA bone marrow responds to EPO or normal plasma, but incubation with the patient's plasma causes often inhibition in heme synthesis. The inhibitor disappears in PRCA remission (12).

Antibody-Mediated PRCA

IgG antibodies are complement binding or directly cytotoxic to erythroblasts (13). The antibodies inhibit burst-forming unit erythroid (BFU-E) and colony-forming unit erythroid (CFU-E) colony formation. In rare cases, EPO-specific antibodies were identified, mainly in epoietin α (Eprex)-induced PRCA (7). Other possible targets are the EPO receptor or other red cell signaling pathway factors (1).

In EPO-induced PRCA, the underlying cause may be connected to the stabilizer polysorbate 80 in rubber-coated pre-filled syringes and poor handling of the syringes, producing organic compounds that act as an adjuvant resulting in anti-EPO antibodies. More than 200 dialysis patients treated with EPO α subcutaneously developed PRCA, mainly between the years 2001 and 2003. Afterwards the rate declined because of new instructions in order to prevent this complication (7).

T-cell-Mediated PRCA

Lymphocytes from patients with PRCA secondary to chronic lymphocytic leukemia (CLL), lymphomas, thymoma, and infection with EBV and HTLV1 suppress erythropoiesis in colony assays (14). Expansion of LGLs and LGL leukemia are most commonly associated with PRCA (1).

Clinical Manifestations

Because the course of disease is slow, symptoms of anemia appear only in advanced stage. Physical examination reveals pallor and signs of anemia. After long-term red cell transfusion and glucocorticoid therapy, physical findings compatible with hemosiderosis and iatrogenic cushingoid state appear. In secondary PRCA the findings are usually consistent with the primary disease.

Laboratory Findings (Table 96.2)

A significant normocytic normochromic anemia, usually requiring recurrent blood transfusions, is found in PRCA patients. The blood smear reveals severe reticulocytopenia. Bone marrow analysis depicts normal myelopoiesis, lymphopoiesis and megakaryopoiesis, but only few, if any, erythroid precursors. The levels of vitamin B_{12}, folic acid, serum iron, transferrin and ferritin are normal.

Differential Diagnosis (Table 96.2)

The differentiation of PRCA from other diseases associated with red cell aplasia is usually not difficult and is based mainly on bone marrow findings. In myelodysplastic syndrome (MDS) patients, the bone marrow usually reveals dysplastic features in two or more blood linages. Moreover, the marrow is hypercellular. Cytogenetic abnormalities are frequent in MDS. In aplastic anemia, pancytopenia with hypoplasia or aplasia of all three lines is the hallmark in bone marrow.

In order to exclude the diagnosis of lymphoid malignancies (B, T, or LGL CLL), immunophenotyping of the lymphocytes by flow cytometry or T-cell receptor gene rearrangement are performed (3).

In parvovirus B19 infection-related PRCA, usually giant proerythroblasts with vacuolated cytoplasm and pseudopodia exist in bone marrow. Elevated liters of IgM antibodies confirm the diagnosis, but in chronic infection, in an immune compromised host, further diagnosis is needed with demonstration of the presence of viral DNA in the serum (1).

Chest CT scan is mandatory to exclude thymoma.

Diagnostic Criteria (Table 96.3)

The diagnosis of PRCA is established in severe normochromic normocytic anemia, with reticulocytopenia and almost complete absence of erythroblasts in the bone marrow with normal development of myeloid and megakaryocytic lines.

There are no formal validated diagnostic criteria based on studies reporting sensitivity and specificity, because PRCA is a rare disease with heterogeneous etiologies.

According to Casadevall et al., the current standard diagnostic criteria for PRCA are listed in Table 96.3 (15). The limit of erythroblast percentage is 0.5% (3) or <5% erythroblasts (15); all the other features are consistent in the literature. In our opinion for the diagnosis, anemia with the findings in bone marrow of less than 1% erythroblasts with normal myeloid cells and megakaryocytes are sufficient. It is required to exclude secondary PRCA according to the classification.

Therapy

According to clinical criteria, blood transfusions should be given for symptomatic anemia, and supplement with Vit B_{12} or folic acid in case of deficiency. Once the etiology is known, specific therapy should be given. Medications that might cause PRCA should be discontinued. Thymectomy is recommended in patients with thymoma.

In cases of primary PRCA or secondary PRCA that is not responding to the therapy of the primary disorder, the recommended treatment is based on case series.

Corticosteroids, usually prednisone 1 mg/kg, are prescribed until remission, which occurs in 40% of patients usually after 4 weeks. It is not recommended to continue more than 12 weeks in non-responders. In responders, after reaching hematocrit of 35%, the dose is tapered gradually and prednisone is discontinued after 3–4 months.

Patients who do not respond to prednisone after 2–3 months are candidates for immunosuppressive therapy including cyclophosphamide, azathioprine, cyclosporine, anti-thymocytic globulin and a course of high-dose intravenous immunoglobulin (IVIg) (16) in the dosage recommended for other autoimmune diseases.

The choice of therapy is based on the primary disease, age, kidney function and fertility status.

Other successful therapies reported in refractory cases include plasmapheresis (17), EPO (8), interferon and reports of successful therapy in resistant PRCA with rituximab and alemtuzumab (18), splenectomy and allogeneic stem cell transplantation after cyclophosphamide conditioning (19).

In the immune compromised host, particularly in AIDS patients with chronic or severe cases of PRCA due to parvovirus infection, IVIg therapy is recommended with good results and few side effects (16).

TABLE 96.2. Diagnostic procedures in acquired PRCA.

	PRCA	Other diseases
Blood smear	Normocytic normochromic anemia, normal white cells and platelets	MDS: macrocytic anemia, dysplastic features of white cells, sometimes monocytosis or Pelger–Huët anomaly Aplastic anemia: pancytopenia CLL: lymphocytosis
Bone marrow biopsy	<0.5–5% erythroblasts with normal myeloid and megakaryocytic lines	MDS: hypercellular with dysplastic myelopoiesis, shift to the left and ↑blasts and mononuclear megakaryocytes. Erythroblasts >5% with megaloblastoid features Aplastic anemia: hypoplasia or aplasia of all 3 lines Parvovirus B19: giant proerythroblasts with vacuolated cytoplasm and pseudopodia
Reticulocyte count	<1%	Usually >1% except of aplastic anemia
Vitamin B_{12}, folic acid	Usually normal	
Erythropoietin serum level	↑Except of in presence of anti erythropoietin antibodies (↓)	
Cytogenetic tests	Normal	MDS: frequent abnormalities
Immune phenotyping of lymphocytes	Normal	CLL: monoclonal proliferation
Parvovirus B19, IgM, PCR or viral DNA	Negative IgM	Parvovirus: IgM↑, in immune compromised patients: PCR or viral DNA detected.
Chest CT scan	Normal	Thymoma: mediastinal mass
Erythroid colony assay	CFU-E and BFU-E usually present. ↓Between CFU-E and proerythroblast. In 60%, IgG in serum inhibits growth of erythroid progenitors	

BFU-E, burst-forming unit erythroid; CFU-E, colony-forming unit erythroid; CLL, chronic lymphocytic leukemia; MDS, myelodysplastic syndrome; PRCA, pure red cell aplasia.

TABLE 96.3. Diagnostic criteria for PRCA (15).

1.	Fall in red cell count of about 1%/day
2.	Reticulocyte count below 1%
3.	No major changes in white cell count, platelet count, or differential leukocyte count
4.	Normal cellularity of bone marrow, less than 1% erythroblasts (occasionally up to 5% proerythroblasts or basophilic erythroblasts)
5.	Normal myeloid cells and megakaryocytes in bone marrow

In order to diagnose PRCA, anemia with the 4th and 5th criteria is suffice.

Prognosis

Five to ten percent of patients remit spontaneously. The majority of patients (68%) enter remission with the common immunosuppressive therapy, but up to 80% are at risk to relapse in 2 years, part of them will need low-dose maintenance immune suppressive treatment for 1–2 years. The estimated median survival of primary PRCA patients is 14 years (20).

Refractory cases diagnosed as primary PRCA may develop leukemia usually the LGL type. The prognosis of secondary PRCA is dependent on the prognosis of primary disease (3).

References

1. Fisch, P., Handgretinger, R., and Schefer, H. E. (2000) Review, pure red cell aplasia *Br J Haematol* 111, 1010–22.
2. Kaznelson, P. (1922) Zur Entstehung der blut Plättchen *Verh Dtsch Ges Inn Med* 34, 557–8.
3. Dessypris, E. N. (2005) Pure red cell aplasia. In: Hoffman R (ed.), *Hematology: Basic Principles and Practice*, 4th edn. New York: Churchill Livingstone, 27, 429–36.
4. Ball, S. E., McGuckin C. P., Jenkins G., and Gordon-Smith, E. C. (1996) Diamond-Blackfan anaemia in the U.K.: Analysis of 80 cases from a 20-year birth cohort. *Br J Haematol* 94, 645–53.
5. Skeppner, G., Kreuger, A., and Elinder, G. (2002) Transient erythroblastopenia of childhood: Prospective study of 10 patients with special reference to viral infections. *J Pediatr Hematol Oncol* 24, 294–8.
6. Gmur, J. P., Burger, J., Schaffner, A., et al. (1990) Pure red cell aplasia of long duration complicating major ABO-incompatible bone marrow transplantation. *Blood* 75, 290–5.
7. Bennett, C. L., Luminari, S., Nissenson, A. R. et al. (2004) Pure red-cell aplasia and epoetin therapy. *N Engl J Med* 351, 1403–8.
8. Orbach, H., Ben-Yehuda, A., Ben-Yehuda, D., Manor, D., Rubinow, A., and Naparstek, Y. (1995) Successful treatment of pure red cell aplasia in systemic lupus erythematosus with erythropoietin. *J Rheumatol* 22, 2166–9.
9. Dessypris, E. N., Baer, M. R., Sergent, J. S., and Krantz, S. B. (1984) Rheumatoid arthritis and pure red cell aplasia. *Ann Intern Med* 100, 202–6.
10. Thompson, C. A. (2007) Pure red cell aplasia and thymoma. *J Thorac Oncol* 2, 263–4.
11. Brown, K. E. and Young, N. S. (1995) Parvovirus B19 infection and hematopoiesis. *Blood Rev* 9, 176–82.
12. Djaldetti, M., Blay, A., Bergman, M., Salman, H., and Bessler, H. (2003) Pure red cell aplasia – A rare disease with multiple causes. *Biomed Pharmacother* 57, 326–32.
13. Krantz, S. B. and Kao, V. (1969) Studies on red cell aplasia. II. Report of a second patient with an antibody to erythroblast nuclei and a remission after immunosuppressive therapy. *Blood* 34, 1–13.
14. Young, N. S. (2006) Pure red cell aplasia. In: Lichtman, M. A., Beutler, E., Kipps, T. J., et al. (eds.), *William's Hematology*, 7th edn, New York: McGraw-Hill, 437–47.
15. Casadevall, N., Cournoyer, D., Marsh, J., et al. (2004) Recommendations on haematological criteria for the diagnosis of epoetin-induced pure red cell aplasia. *Eur J Haematol* 73, 389–96.
16. Mouthon, L., Guillevin, L., and Tellier, Z. (2005) Intravenous immunoglobulins in autoimmune- or parvovirus B19-mediated pure red-cell aplasia. *Autoimmun Rev* 4, 264–9.
17. Choi, B. G. and Yoo, W. H. (2002) Successful treatment of pure red cell aplasia with plasmapheresis in a patient with systemic lupus erythematosus. *Yonsei Med J* 43, 274–8.
18. Robak, T. (2004) Monoclonal antibodies in the treatment of autoimmune cytopenias. *Eur J Haematol* 72, 79–88.
19. Muller, B. U., Tichelli, A., Passweg, J. R., Nissen, C., and Wodnar-Filipowicz, A. (1999) Successful treatment of refractory acquired pure red cell aplasia (PRCA) by allogeneic bone marrow transplantation. *Bone Marrow Transplant* 23, 1205–7.
20. Clark, D. A., Dessypris, E. N., and Kranz S. B. (1984) Studies on pure red cell aplasia. XI. Results of immunosuppressive treatment of 37 patients. *Blood* 63, 227–86.

97
Myelodysplastic Syndromes

Laura F. Newell and Joseph M. Tuscano

Abstract   The myelodysplastic syndromes comprise a heterogeneous cluster of hematological stem cell disorders. Patients typically present with cytopenias that often manifest with a variety of symptoms, ranging from asymptomatic to the sequel of anemia, infections, bruising, or bleeding. Classification is based on the FAB and WHO criteria. Abnormalities in cytogenetics, apoptosis, and in the hematopoietic microenvironment are involved in the development of the MDS phenotype. The role of autoimmune pathogenesis is suggested by clonal expansion of cytotoxic T cells, as well as the response in many patients to immunosuppressive therapy. Treatment options are supportive care, growth factors, DNA modifiers, immunomodulatory drugs, and hematopoietic stem cell transplantation.

Keywords   Myelodysplastic syndromes · hematopoiesis · dysplasia

The myelodysplastic syndromes (MDSs) are a heterogeneous group of conditions with widely different biological features and clinical manifestations. MDS defines a spectrum of clonal myeloid disorders marked by ineffective hematopoiesis, cytopenias, qualitative disorders of blood cells and their precursors, clonal chromosomal abnormalities, and a variable predilection to evolve into acute myelogenous leukemia (AML) (1). There are a number of overlapping diseases that include myeloproliferative disease, AML, and those with autoimmune elements including aplastic anemia (AA), paroxysmal nocturnal hemoglobinuria (PNH), pure red cell aplasia, and large granular lymphocytosis (Figure 97.1) (2).

History

MDS was first described as a "pseudo-aplastic anemia" by Luzzatto in 1907, and in 1949 Hamilton-Paterson used the term "preleukemic anemia" to describe patients with refractory anemia antecedent to AML development. It was not until 1975 at a conference in Paris that it was classified as a separate disease (3).

Epidemiology

There are an estimated 10,000–15,000 new cases every year and the incidence is increasing. This may be due to the aging population (median age at diagnosis is 65–70), improved recognition and diagnostic capabilities, and secondary MDS due to prior treatment with chemotherapy (3).

Pathogenesis

MDS affects the development of immature blood cells (blasts), resulting in a disproportionate number of blasts remaining in the bone marrow. A hypercellular bone marrow is present in 90% of cases; in the blood, circulating mature blood cells are fewer in number and may not function properly because of dysplasia. A hypocellular marrow is present in approximately 10% of cases and must be distinguished from AA (1). Ineffective hematopoiesis results from a complex interaction between hematopoietic progenitors and their maturing progeny. Several biological features drive the MDS phenotype. These include chromosomal and epigenetic DNA abnormalities, accelerated apoptosis, impaired responses to cytokines, and defects in the bone marrow microenvironment such as stromal dysregulation and medullary angiogenesis (4, 5, 6). Accelerated apoptosis of hematopoietic progenitors and abnormal regulation of apoptosis in their progeny represent important mechanisms underlying the development of MDS. Studies indicate that large numbers of hematopoietic cells are rapidly proliferating in the bone marrow but are also undergoing apoptosis, a process mediated by cytokines such as TNF-α, IL-1β, IL-6, and others.

From: Y. Shoenfeld et al. (eds.): *Diagnostic Criteria in Autoimmune Diseases*, DOI: 10.1007/978-1-60327-285-8_97,
© 2008 Humana Press, Totowa, NJ

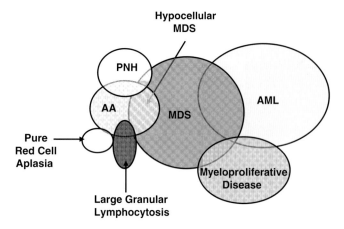

FIGURE 97.1. A number of diseases share biological features and clinical manifestations; however, treatment and prognosis can be very different. Paroxysmal nocturnal hemoblobinuria (PNH) aplastic anemia (AA), pure red cell aplasia, and hypoplastic MDS all may respond to immunosupressive therapy. However, AML, most MDS, and myeloproliferative diseases may also present with cyopenia but in frequently will respond to immunosupressive therapy.

Excessive apoptosis is a plausible hypothesis that can explain how a clonal expansion of marrow progenitor cells could result in ineffective hematopoiesis and peripheral cytopenias (5). In addition, the presence of stromal cell apoptosis and the altered distribution of cell types in the marrow suggest an underlying abnormality in the stroma. Aberrant cytokine production and altered interactions of hematopoietic cells within the extracellular matrix have both been demonstrated in MDS (5).

The Role of Autoimmunity in the Pathogenesis of MDS

Immune-mediator cells, particularly T cells, are part of the hematopoietic microenvironment regulating both hematopoietic proliferation and differentiation. The response of some cytopenic MDS patients to immunosuppressive treatment led to the hypothesis that MDS may be in part, autoimmune mediated. MDS patients exhibit high percentages of CD8+, CD28−, and CD57+ T cells, a phenotype consistent with mature cytotoxic T cells. In many autoimmune disorders such T cells have been found to differentiate either from antigen-specific naïve or memory T cells. These T cells have limited T-cell receptor (TCR) repertoire representation, suggesting expansion of dominant T-cell clones. Clonal expansions are not always necessarily a manifestation of a malignant process; they may also represent clonal or oligoclonal expansion of autoreactive T cells. The increase in CD57 expression by CD8+ cells and the demonstration of expanded TCR variable beta

chain families expressing CD57 are characteristic features of diseases attributable to an activated immune environment such as acute graft-versus-host disease, multiple sclerosis, and rheumatoid arthritis (7). Recent findings in patients with MDS have led to the hypothesis that MDS may be the result of an autoimmune reaction directed against marrow stem cells. However, we still lack proof of an antigen-driven T-cell process, not to mention identification of the causal antigen. A high percentage of researchers subscribe to the popular concept of immune system involvement in the pathogenesis of MDS; evidence supporting this theory was found in a prospective study identifying an autoimmune inflammatory manifestation (AIM) in 22% of MDS patients (8). While the observed associations are extremely variable and not specific, taken together with the clonal expansion of cytotoxic T cells and the response in many patients to immunosuppressive therapy, these associations give support to the autoimmune hypothesis.

Clinical Manifestations

Approximately half of the individuals are asymptomatic at the time of initial diagnosis and are usually diagnosed after a routine blood count. Progressive hematopoietic failure leading to anemia, thrombocytopenia, and leukopenia, either alone or in any combination, is the dominant finding in MDS. Anemia is an almost universal characteristic at the time of initial diagnosis; more than 80% of patients present with a hemoglobin concentration below 10 g/dl. Fatigue and/or exertional dyspnea as a clinical manifestation of anemia may develop insidiously, often exceeding 6–12 months. The reticulocyte count is usually reduced. Peripheral blood leukocyte count is low in ~25–30% of individuals with MDS. Granulocytes may exhibit reduced segmentation and either diminished or absent granulation. Approximately one-third of individuals have recurrent infections. These occur not only because of quantitative neutropenia, but also as a result of qualitative defects in neutrophil function including impaired chemotaxis and reduced phagocytic activity. Signs of bleeding, such as petechiae, gingival bleeding, or hematoma following trivial injuries, are surprisingly uncommon, given the frequency of thrombocytopenia. Fewer than 10% of patients will initially present with serious bleeding (9).

Classification

In 1982, the French–American–British (FAB) Cooperative Group classified five subentities of MDS: refractory anemia (RA), refractory anemia with excess of blasts (RAEB),

TABLE 97.1. The FAB and WHO classification of the myelodyplastic syndromes.

FAB				WHO			
Category	Description	BM Blasts (%)	Median Survival (mo)	Category	Description	BM blasts (%)	Median survival (mo)
RA	Refractory anemia	<5	37	RA	Unilineage erythroid dysplasia	<5	69
RARS	RA + >15% ringed sideroblasts	<5	49	RARS	RA + > 15% ringed sideroblasts	<5	69
RAEB	RA with excess blasts	5–20	9	RCMD	RARS+ multilineage dysplasia	<5	33
RAEB-t	RAEB in transformation	21–29	6	RCMD-RS	RCMD + > 15% ringed sideroblasts	<5	32
CMML	Chronic Myelo-monocytic leukemia	5–20	22	REAB-1	RA with excess blasts	5–9	18
				RAEB-2	RA with excess blasts	10–20	10
				MDS 5q-	MDS + isolated 5q-	<5	116
				MDS-U	MDS unclassifiable	<5	–

refractory anemia with excess of blasts in transformation (RAEB-T), refractory anemia with ringed sideroblasts (RARS), and chronic myelomonocytic leukemia (CMML) (10). This classification based on morphological criteria was recently revised, resulting in the World Health Organization (WHO) classification (Table 97.1). While the FAB grouping provides prognostic information, the WHO classification incorporates cytogenetics, subcategories for subentities (i.e. better prognosis of patients with an isolated cytogenetic aberration at 5q), and changes in AML diagnostic criteria (11). Secondary MDS is a term that is used to differentiate the subtype of MDS resulting from exposure to a mutagen, occurring either as a consequence of therapy for another disease (treatment-related MDS), or as an exposure to a toxic material such as benzene.

Karyotypic and Molecular Abnormalities

The cytogenetic changes found in MDS are not unique to the disease. Both structural and numerical cytogenetic changes may occur. The most frequent chromosomal abnormalities in MDS involve deletions of chromosomes 5, 7, 11, 12, and 20 and/or trisomy 8 (Table 97.2) (9). The incidence of chromosomal abnormalities is about 30–50% in primary MDS and 80% in mutagen-related MDS. The latter often features complex changes that involve deletions of chromosomes 5 and/or 7. Translocations are rare in MDS. MDS-related chromosomal deletions imply alterations in tumor suppressor genes or DNA repair genes. Usually such changes require two hits: mutation of the target gene and loss of the second allele through deletion, duplication, or recombination.

TABLE 97.2. Most frequent karyotypic abnormalities.[a]

Numerical	Translocations	Deletions
+8 (19%)	inv 3 (7%)	del 5q (27%)
−7 (15%)	T(1;7)(2%)	del 11q (7%)
+21 (7%)	t(1;3) (1%)	del 12q (5%)
−5 (7%)	t(3;3) (1%)	del 20q (5%)
	t(6;9) (<1%)	del 7q (4%)
	t(5;12) (<1%)	del 13q (2%)

[a] Symbols, loss of chromosome.
+, additional chromosome.
inv, inversion.
t, translocation.
del, chromosomal deletion.

Prognosis

Based on the substantial clinical heterogeneity of MDS, there have been many attempts to identify prognostic factors that allow for an accurate prediction of clinical outcome and response to therapy. The most widely adopted is the International Prognostic Scoring System (IPSS). This system generates a score that is based on the number of cytopenias, karyotype, and percentage of blasts in the bone marrow (Table 97.3). The total score predicts median survival and the risk of transformation to AML. Scores ranging from 0 to ≥2.5 predict a median survival from 5.7 to 0.4 years, respectively. Using IPSS to stratify patients in clinical trials has allowed for better prediction of therapeutic efficacy (12). The presence of a PNH phenotype, i.e. CD55 and CD59 negative granulocytes and erythrocytes, is of pathogenetic and prognostic importance. A significant increase in PNH-type cells has been detected in 18% of patients with RA. These patients may exhibit distinct clinical features, such as "less-pronounced" red cell dysplasia, more severe thrombocytopenia, a lower incidence of clonal cytogenetic

TABLE 97.3. International prognostic scoring system.

Prognostic variable	Score value				
	0	0.5	1.0	1.5	2.0
Bone marrow blast (%)	<5	5–10	–	11–20	21–30
Karyotype[a]	Good	Intermediate	Poor	–	–
# of cytopenias[b]	0/1	2/3	–	–	–
Total score	0	0.5–1.0	1.5–2.0	>2.5	–
Median survival (yr)	5.7	3.5	1.2	0.4	–
Median time to AML[c](yr)	9.4	3.3	1.1	0.2	–

[a] Good = normal, -Y, del(20), del(5q).
[b] Hgb,10 g/dl, ANC < 1800/μl, plt < 100 K.
[c] when 25% of patients with this score will develop AML.
Intermediate = other karyotypic abnormalities.
Poor = complex (≥ 3 abnormalities) or chromosome seven abnormalities.

abnormalities (4.8% vs 32.8%) and a lower incidence of progression to AML (0% vs 6.2%). They also demonstrate a higher probability of responding to immunosuppressive therapy.

Treatment

Until recently, the treatment of MDS has been primarily supportive. However, within the past several years a number of agents have been approved by the FDA and several other promising investigational agents are in different stages of development. New and emerging therapies have mediated a change in the treatment goals from supportive care to active therapy, and may change the natural history of this disease. Active therapeutic options for patients include epigenetic DNA modifiers, immunosuppressive therapy, immune modulators/anti-angiogenics, bone marrow/stem cell transplantation, and numerous investigational agents.

Supportive Care

Supportive care remains an essential component of MDS patient management, even in those that are receiving active and/or intensive therapy. The primary goal of supportive therapy is to reduce morbidity and mortality from cytopenia(s) while providing an acceptable quality of life (QoL). Anemia, the most common clinical manifestation, is supported with packed red cell transfusions and erythropoietic stimulating agents (ESAs). Transfusions can provide reliable and immediate relief, but may be associated with a number of complicating issues including iron and fluid overload, alloimmunization, and transfusion reactions. ESAs have reduced the need for red cell transfusion, but only a minority of patients has significant hematological benefit. On average, only 16% of patients have a significant response to ESA; however, rates

can vary widely from 7 to 74% depending on serum erythropoietin levels (above or below 100–500 U) and prior transfusion requirements (above or below 2 units/month). The addition of low dose myeloid growth factors (G/GM-CSF) can enhance the erythropoietic response to ESA (13).

Epigenetic DNA Modifiers

Based on the propensity for cytogenetic deletions, it has been hypothesized that tumor suppressor genes play a dominant role in the pathogenesis of MDS. Hypermethylation is common in MDS and methyltransferase inhibitors (MTIs) promote hypomethylation of DNA, allowing expression of previously silenced genes. Two MTIs have recently been approved by the FDA for the treatment of MDS: 5-azacitabine (Vidaza^{TM}) and decitabine (Dacogen^{TM}). 5-Azacitabine was the first to be approved by the FDA; in a pivotal randomized trial comparing this agent to best supportive care (BSC), 5-azacitabine generated an overall response rate of 60% compared with 5% in the BSC arm, with 7% being complete remissions (CRs) and 45% becoming transfusion independent. Decitabine has produced similar overall response rates (38–70%); however, CRs were 21–48%. Similar to 5-azacitabine, the median survival of patients treated with decitabine was 22 months (14, 15).

Immunosuppressive Therapy

Evidence of immune dysfunction includes abnormal CD4:CD8 ratios and increased activated cytotoxic and oligoclonal T cells in MDS patients compared with controls. Immunotherapeutic agents that inhibit these immune mechanisms play an important role in the management of some patients with MDS. Antithymocyte globulin (ATG) has been demonstrated to produce clinically meaningful responses in patients with MDS. Approximately 34–44% of unselected patients with RA or RAEB can be expected to become transfusion independent within 8 months of a single 4-day course of ATG. HLA-DR2 and HLA-DR15 frequencies have been shown to be higher in patients with RA and aplastic anemia; in some studies, both appear to be associated with clinically significant positive responses to ATG or cyclosporine (2, 7, 9, 15).

Immune Modulators/Anti-angiogenics

Immunomodulatory drugs (IMiDs) have an effect on extrinsic factors in the bone marrow microenvironment that are hypothesized to drive the MDS phenotype. These agents modulate ligand-induced responses to inflammatory cytokines, immune responses, and medullary angiogenesis to both improve erythropoiesis and suppress IMiD-sensitive MDS clones. Thalidomide (Thalomid™), which displays both anti-angiogenic and TNFα inhibitory properties, represents the first agent investigated in this class of therapeutics. In a Phase II trial of thalidomide, 15 of 83 (18%) patients experienced either red blood cell transfusion independence (TI) or a >50% decrease in transfusion burden, whereas improvement in non-erythroid lineages was uncommon. Lenalidomide (Revlamid™), a much more potent analog, produced dramatic responses in patients with the del(5q) cytogenetic abnormality. Eighty-three percent of patients with a deletion of 5q31.1 had an erythroid response, compared with 57% of patients with normal karyotypes, and 12% of patients with other cytogenetic abnormalities; nearly 50% of patients with del(5q) became TI. What was most striking was that cytogenetic responses occurred in 55% of patients with a clonal cytogenetic abnormality; of note, 83% of patients who had del(5)(q31.1) achieved cytogenetic response, with 75% achieving complete cytogenetic remission. A subsequent study confirmed the striking activity in patients with del(5q) with 67% achieving TI and 77% having a cytogenetic response, 45% being complete. A larger study assessed the response to lenalidomide in patients without del(5q), in whom 43% achieved a erythroid response or become TI (25%). Cytogenic responses were considerably lower (20% with 9% being complete), although considering the difficulty of treating this disease, the data in the non-del(5q) patients is quite remarkable (14, 15).

Hematopoietic Stem Cell Transplantation

Autologous and allogeneic hematopoietic stem cell transplantation (HSCT) has been extensively investigated in MDS. Autologous HSCT in MDS is theoretically feasible in only a small proportion of patients who achieve a complete remission after induction chemotherapy and in whom a suitable autologous harvest can be collected. A successful autograft is restricted by a limited potential for peripheral blood stem cell (PBSC) collection, graft contamination, delayed engraftment, and a high relapse risk of up to 72%, with a 2-year disease-free survival of only 25% for patients 40 to 63 years of age. On the basis of this, enthusiasm for this approach is limited. Although conventional myeloablative allogeneic HSCT has a significantly lower relapse rate than autografts at 28–48%, the transplant-related mortality (TRM) can be substantial (39% to 54%). Transplant-related complications include graft-versus-host disease (GVHD), which increases in frequency and severity with advancing age. Allogeneic HSCT is the

only therapeutic modality at present that may be delivered with curative intent in MDS: recipient dysplastic hematopoiesis is replaced with healthy donor hematopoiesis and an immune system with an attendant graft-versus-leukemia (GVL) effect. Its applicability, however, is limited by the availability of a suitable HLA-matched donor and by the toxicity of the conditioning regimens, which is directly proportional to the age of the recipient. Most patients with MDS are of advanced age, with only about 25% of patients younger than 60 years. Often with concurrent medical conditions that effectively preclude standard conditioning for allogeneic HSCT, various strategies have been adopted in order to attempt to reduce the toxicities associated with the transplant procedure. At present, there is considerable interest in reduced-intensity or "non-myeloablative" conditioning, which can result in stable donor hematopoietic engraftment, without the toxicity associated with conventional HSCT (14, 15).

Promising Investigational Approaches

A clearer understanding of the biology of MDS has provided important new therapeutic strategies for active treatment of these diseases. New treatment approaches currently under investigation are reversal of epigenetic gene silencing, apoptosis inhibition, suppression of the malignant MDS clone, immune modulation, histone deacetylase inhibition, farnesyl transferase inhibition, and more specific and potent angiogenesis inhibition (9, 14, 15).

References

1. Hofmann WK, Lubbert M, Hoelzer D, Koeffler PH. Myelodysplastic syndromes. *Hemtol J* 2004;5(1):1–8.
2. Young NS. Acquired aplastic anemia. *Ann Intern Med* 2002;136(7):534–46.
3. List AF in Wintrobe's Clinical Hematology Copyright © 2003 Lee RG (eds) Williams & Williams.
4. List AF. New Approaches to the treatment of myelodysplasia. *Oncologist* 2002;7,Suppl. 1:39–49.
5. Parker JE and Mufti GJ. The myelodysplastic syndromes: a matter of life and death. *Acta Haematol* 2004;111(1–2):78–99.
6. Cilloni D, Messa E, Messa F, Carturan S, Defilippi I, Arruga F, Rosso V, Catalano R, Bracco E, Nicoli P, Saglio G. Genetic abnormalities as targets for molecular therapies in myelodysplastic syndromes. *Ann NY Acad Sci.* 2006;1098: 411–23.
7. Martin Stern, Andreas S. Buser, Andreas Lohri, André Tichelli, Catherine Nissen-Druey. Autoimmunity and malignancy in hematology—More than an association. *Crit Rev in Onc/Hematol.* 2007;63:100–110.
8. S. Giannouli, M. Voulgarelis, E. Zintzaras1, A. G. Tzioufas and H. M. Moutsopoulos. Autoimmune phenomena in

myelodysplastic syndromes: a 4-yr prospective study. 2004; *Rheumatology*;43:626–32.

9. Hofmann K-K and Koeffer PH. Myelodysplastic syndromes. *Annu Rev Med*. 2005;56:1–16.

10. Bennett JM, Catovsky D, Daniel MT, Flandrin G, Galton DA, Gralnick HR, Sultan C. Proposals for the classification of the myelodysplastic syndromes. *Br J Haematol* 1982;51(2): 189–99.

11. James W. Vardiman, Nancy Lee Harris, and Richard D. Brunning. The World Health Organization (WHO) classification of the myeloid neoplasms. *Blood* 2002;100(7): 2292–302.

12. Greenberg P, Cox C, LeBeau MM, Fenaux P, Morel P, Sanz G, Sanz M, Vallespi T, Hamblin T, Oscier D, Ohyashiki K, Toyama K, Aul C. Ghulam Mufti, and John Bennett. International scoring system for evaluating prognosis in myelodysplastic syndromes. *Blood* 1997;89(7) 2079–88.

13. Bowden D. Culligan D, Jowitt S, Kelsey S, Mufiti G, Oscier D, Parker J. Guidelines for the diagnosis and therapy of adult myelodysplastic syndromes. *Br J Haematol* 2003;120(2):187–200.

14. Schiffer C. Myelodysplasis: The good, the fair, and the ugly. *Best Prac & Reserch Clin Haematol* 2007;20(1): 49–55.

15. Mufti G, List AF, Gore SD, and Ho AYL. Myelodysplastic syndrome. *Hematology Am Soc Hematol Educ Program*. Copyright 2002 Hematology online by The American Society of Hematology. Print Issue:1520–4391.

98
Autoimmune Lymphopenia

Amani Mankaï, Sophie Hillion, Valérie Devauchelle-Pensec, Alain Saraux, M. Eric Gershwin and Pierre Youinou

Abstract   Lymphocyte cytotoxic antibodies (Abs) are encountered in a number of pathological conditions, particularly nonorgan-specific autoimmune diseases, and most particularly systemic lupus erythematosus (SLE). The basic test systems to detect these autoAbs are the microlymphocytotoxic test and Western blotting. As a target, CD45 is of special interest, given the role of this phosphatase in the signal transduction of lymphocytes. Lymphopenia may be associated with opportunistic infections, renal failure, and central nervous system complications in SLE. Their relevance to the disease remains nonetheless elusive.

Keywords   Lymphocyte · autoantibody · lymphocytotoxin

Lymphocyte cytotoxic antibodies (LCAs) were first identified in sera from women immunized by pregnancy and recipients of repeated transfusions (1). They were subsequently acknowledged as autoantibodies (Abs) during the course of systemic lupus erythematosus (SLE). Among them, cold lymphocytotoxins (CLTs) resulting from nonallogenic stimuli have been described in patients with infectious disease, and characterized in that they have a temperature optimum of 15°C and present as inherently IgM. In contrast, autologous cytotoxicity reacts at 37°C, and, for most part, is due to IgG. Interestingly, these autoAbs bind to T cells rather than to B cells, recognize activated T lymphocytes, and target different isoforms of CD45 (2). Not only have reduced lymphocyte counts been selected as a diagnostic criterion in SLE (3), but this abnormality also exists in rheumatoid arthritis (RA) and primary Sjögren's syndrome (SS). Lymphopenia is indeed a poorly studied but recognized feature or RA (4), while Ab to CD4 is a frequent finding in patients with primary SS (5). Idiopathic CD4 lymphocytopenia (ICL) refers to a decrease of CD4 T lymphocytes below 300 cells/μL on two separate points, 6 weeks apart, with no evidence of human immunodeficiency virus (HIV) infection. Both groups of lymphopenia may be relevant to basic mechanisms underlying immunological dysfunction in autoimmune diseases.

Pathogenesis

Owing to its unusually high expression on hematopoietic cells, the leukocyte common antigen CD45 is of special interest in this process. All blood cells except erythrocytes harbor one or several CD45 isoforms generated by alternative splicing of 5 variable exons encoding sequences at the NH$_2$ terminal domain of the molecule. They vary both in size with a molecular weight ranging from 180 to 240 kiloDaltons (kDa) from CD45RA through CD45RO, and in glycosylation with N- and/or O-linked polysaccharides. Their function has been defined best in T lymphocytes, and these tyrosine phosphatases shown to be critical regulators of signaling thresholds in immune cells. However, questions concerning the physiological significance of the findings obtained still remain.

Lymphopenia may be induced by LCAs, and, in return, the system is open to a breach of tolerance to the self. The phenotype of the latter sequence involves a marked decline of CD4 cells, and a less pronounced decrease of CD8 cells. Little research has, however, tried to dissect such a heterogeneous syndrome. That is, all we know is that disturbed differentiation of stem cells contributes to some cases, and that progressive loss of CD4 cells may rather be due to specific autoAbs (6). A group of CD45 autoAbs have even the capacity to neutralize activated T lymphocytes through anergy and apoptosis (7). There is also evidence to suggest

From: Y. Shoenfeld et al. (eds.): *Diagnostic Criteria in Autoimmune Diseases*, DOI: 10.1007/978-1-60327-285-8_98,

that some antinuclear Abs might have LCA effect, as supported by the close association of anti-Ro/sicca syndrome (SS) A and anti-La/SSB Abs with lymphopenia in SLE (8) and primary SS (9). In yet another group of SLE patients, IgG anti-ribosomal P protein Abs bind to a lymphocyte membrane-associated 38-kDa molecule apparently identical to the ribosomal protein (10). Anti-P Abs might also penetrate cells by an unknown mechanism.

Irrespective of the mechanism, lymphopenia accounts for homeostatic expansion of naïve T cells, and thereby for the generation of autoimmunity (11). This complication is normally prevented by CD4+CD25+ regulatory T cells (Treg). The seminal transfer experiments implicating critical roles for Treg in the control of homeostatic T-lymphocyte expansion have established that naïve T cells induce autoimmune colitis, whereas memory T cells do not (12).

Consanguineous relatives to SLE and RA patients may possess LCAs, suggesting that their production is genetically controlled. Eroglu and Köhler (13) have reported a microlymphocytotoxic (MCL) assay positive for 83% of the SLE patient group, 50% in the consanguineous relative group, 11% in the nonconsanguineous relative group, and 5% in the healthy control group.

Clinical Presentation

A number of pathological settings are associated with LCAs (Table 98.1). These include nonorgan-specific and organ-specific autoimmune conditions, infectious diseases, malignancies, drug side-effects and all sorts of immune-mediated disturbances.

Bacteria, such as *Mycobacterium tuberculosis* or typical mycobacteria, and viruses, such as HIV, or cytomegalovirus, may depress CD4 cell counts. Reciprocally, lymphocytopenia typically becomes apparent through the manifestation of opportunistic infections (Table 98.2), ranging from asymptomatic to severe complications. These include *Pneumocystis carinii* pneumonia, *histoplasma*-induced brain abscess, and cryptococcal meningitis (14).

Bermas et al. have reported association of lymphopenia with increased activity of SLE (15). Furthermore, LCAs accompany active lupus nephritis concomitant with a reduction in the circulating CD45RA population, a diminished plasma complement level, and a high titer of circulating anti-double-stranded (ds) DNA Ab. Diverging titers of anti-dsDNA from LCAs suggest different mechanisms for their production. The association of cold-reactive IgM LCAs with lymphopenia and disease flares in SLE (16) and increased acute phage response in RA (17) suggests that these autoAbs may play a role in T-cell depletion.

Several studies also present relationships between the presence of LCAs and the development of nervous complications in patients with SLE. LCAs have finally been

TABLE 98.1. Pathological settings of lymphocytotoxic antibodies.

- Nonorgan-specific autoimmune conditions
  - Systemic lupus erythematosus
  - Rheumatoid arthritis
- Organ-specific autoimmune conditions
  - Autoimmune thyroiditis
  - Multiple sclerosis
  - Primary biliary cirrhosis
  - Myasthenia gravis
  - Autoimmune haemolytic anemia
- Infectious diseases
  - Infectious mononucleosis
  - Rubeola
  - Acquired immunodeficiency syndrome
- Immune-mediated disturbances
  - Graft-versus-host reactions
  - Organ transplantation
- Malignancies
  - Non-Hodgkin lymphoma
  - Mycosis fungoide
  - Aplastic anemia
  - Myelodysplastic syndrome
- Drugs side-effects
  - Corticosteroids
  - Immunosuppressants
  - Cephalosporins

TABLE 98.2. Clinical features of autoimmune lymphopenia.

- Opportunistic infection
- Glomerulonephritis
- Neurological complications
- Spontaneous pregnancy loss

suspected to be involved in reproductive failure in these patients.

The Serological Concerns

Special care has to be taken to minimize the ambiguity inherent in such experiments, by ruling out interactions of Fc-gamma in the serum sample with Fc-gamma receptors on the lymphocyte membrane.

In the MLC assay, the presence of LCA-mediated complement cytolysis is tested using peripheral blood lymphocytes from healthy donors. Several parameters need attention. First, the reaction has to be conducted at 15°C to ensure the binding of all Ab classes. Second, the source of complement is critical. In this way, rabbit sera which contain heterologous LCAs should be avoided as source of complement. If human sera are used, autologous LCAs have to be dismissed first. Third, fresh cells, instead of frozen ones, are preferred to avoid cell susceptibility to lysis and false-positive results. The usual cutoff to define a positive test is set at 10% but may vary according to the laboratory.

The MLC test presents several disadvantages. Viable cells are required. Activation of complement is necessary, leading to the inability to detect noncomplement fixing Abs. All determinants may not be present on lymphocyte-like antigens (Ags) that are temporarily expressed, induced by activation. Differentiation between IgA and IgG is possible with the standard MLC assay. Then, several techniques were introduced as an alternative to the MLC test to overcome MLC's pitfalls. These are based on immunofluorescence, enzyme-linked immunosorbent assay (ELISA) and flow cytometry (FACS), and immunoblotting.

The ELISA test permits the presenting of purified Ags, instead of living lymphocytes, as target for the binding of Abs. This method permits furthermore to differentiate IgG versus IgM Abs. The FACS Ab screen detects Ab binding independently from the complement activation and also detects small amount of Abs and thus is more sensitive. Discrimination between IgM and IgG may be also done. Use of Ag-coated microparticles as targets may be used for the Ab specificity determination. By immunoblotting, crude lymphocyte preparations can confirm the presence of Abs to Ags of defined size.

Anti-dsDNA Abs may be identified bound to T-cell surface membrane (18). Their specificity is not restricted to T cells, because they bind different cell lines. Other anti-lymphocyte Abs are specific for B cell (17) (Table 98.3). Perplexingly, those RA patients with the shared epitope have lower numbers of circulating CD19+ B cells than those without it. Lupus autoAbs can also recognize CD45 on B cells, in particular Abs encoded by VH4.34, which are greatly expanded in SLE, and appear to have special tropism for B cells (19).

Thus, patients with various conditions develop LCAs. Part of them are specific for T lymphocytes, or even CD4+ T lymphocytes, while others are specific for B cells. It is interesting that natural Abs (20) include LCAs, notably those reacting with thymocytes. The rationale for such a process is unknown. Additional studies are currently under way to dissect the mechanisms and actual consequences of these autoAbs.

TABLE 98.3. Anti-lymphocyte antibodies specificities.

Target	Isotype	Cells	Effect	Disease
CD45 (desialyl O-link)	IgM, G	T-cells	ADCC	SLE
B2 microglobulin, HLA class I/II	IgM, IgG	B-cells	Unknown	Alloimmunization
CD45 (N-acetyl galactosamin)	IgM, G (V$_H$4034)	naïve B cells	Apoptosis	SLE
TCR/CD3	IgG	T cells	Repress IL-2 synthesis	SLE

ADCC: Antibody-dependent cell cytotoxicity; SLE: Systemic lupus erythematosus; TCR: T-cell receptor; IL: interleukin.

Acknowledgments. Simone Forest is gratefully acknowledged.

References

1. Mittal KK, Rossen RD, Sharp JT, Lidsky MD, Butler WT. Lymphocyte cytotoxic antibodies in SLE. Nature 1970; 225: 1255–6

2. Mimura T, Fernsten P, Jarjour W, Winfield JB. Autoantibodies specific for different isoforms of CD45 in SLE. J Exp Med 1990; 172: 653–6

3. Tan EM, Cohen AS, Fries JF, et al. The 1982 revised criteria for the classification of systemic lupus erythematosus. Arthritis Rheum 1982; 25: 1271–7

4. Symmons DP, Farr M, Salmon M, Bacon PA. Lymphopenia in rheumatoid arthritis. J R Soc Med 1989; 82: 462–3

5. Mandl T, Bredberg A, Jacobsson LT, Manthorpe R, Henriksson G. CD4+ T-lymphocytopenia, a frequent finding in anti-SSA antibody seropositive patients with primary Sjögren's syndrome. J Rheumatol 2004; 31: 726–8

6. Mamoune A, Saraux A, Delaunay JL, Le Goff P, Youinou P, Le Corre R. Autoantibodies to CD45 in systemic lupus erythematosus. J Autoimmun 1998; 11: 485–8

7. Mamoune A, Kerdreux S, Durand V, et al. CD45 autoantibodies mediate neutralization of activated T cells from lupus patients through anergy or apoptosis. Lupus 2000; 9: 622–31

8. Wenzel J, Gerdsen R, Uerlich M, Bauer R, Tueting T, Bieber T. Lymphocytopenia in lupus erythematosus: close in vivo association to autoantibodies targeting nuclear antigens. Br J Dermatol 2004; 150: 994–8

9. Henriksson G, Manthorpe R, Bredberg A. Antibodies to CD4 in primary Sjogren's syndrome. Rheumatology (Oxford) 2000; 39: 142–7

10. Stafford HA, Chen AE, Anderson CJ, et al. Anti-ribosomal and 'P-peptide-specific autoantibodies bind to T lymphocytes. Clin Exp Immunol 1997; 109: 12–19

11. King C, Ilic A, Koelsch K, Sarvetnick N. Homeostatic expansion of T cells during immune insufficiency generates autoimmunity. Cell 2004; 117: 265–77

12. Powrie F, Leach MW, Mauze S, Caddle LB, Coffman RL. Phenotypically distinct subsets of CD4+ T cells induce or protect from chronic intestinal inflammation in C. B-17 scid mice. Int Immunol 1993; 5: 1461–71

13. Eroglu GE, Kohler PF. Familial SLE: the role of genetic and environmental factors. Ann Rheum Dis 2002; 61: 29–31

14. Schattner A, Friedman J, Bentwich Z. Opportunistic infection due to unexplained CD4+ lymphocytopenia and associated Sjogren's syndrome. Rheumatology (Oxford) 2004; 43: 111–2

15. Bermas BL, Petri M, Goldman D, et al. T helper cell dysfunction in systemic lupus erythematosus : relation to disease activity. J Clin Immunol 1994; 14: 169–77

16. Winfield JB, Mimura T, Fernsten PD. Autoantibodies to CD45 in systemic lupus erythematosus. Int J Clin Lab Res 1992; 21: 292–5

17. Wagner U, Kaltenhauser S, Pierer M, Wilke B, Arnold S, Hantzschel H. B lymphocytopenia in rheumatoid arthritis is associated with the DRB1 shared epitope and increased acute phase response. Arthritis Res 2002; 4: R1

18. Shoenfeld Y, Zamir R, Joshua H, Lavie G, Pinkhas J. Human monoclonal anti-DNA antibodies react as LCA. Eur J Immunol 1985; 15: 1024–8

19. Cappione AJ, Pugh-Bernard AE, Anolik JH, Sanz I. Lupus IgG VH4.34 antibodies bind to a 220-kDa glycoform of CD45/B220 on the surface of human B lymphocytes. J Immunol 2004; 172: 4298–307

20. Hardy RR, Hayakawa K. Development of B cells producing natural autoantibodies to thymocytes and senescent erythrocytes. Springer Semin Immunopathol 2005; 26: 363–75

99
Autoimmune Neutropenia

Pierre Youinou, Amani Mankaï, Sophie Hillion, Yehuda Shoenfeld Christian Berthou
and Ibtissem Ghedira

Abstract   Neutropenia is defined by a reduction in the number of circulating polymorphonuclear neutrophils (PMNs) below 1.5×10^9/L. This may occur as a primary condition, or as a complication of systemic autoimmune diseases or hematological neoplasms. The autoantibodies are particularly difficult to identify. Granulocyte colony-stimulating factor is the first-line therapy, but should be restricted to patients with total absence of PMNs and/or severe infections.

Keywords   Polymorphonuclear neutrophil · autoantibody

Neutropenia denotes blood polymorphonuclear neutrophil (PMN) count below 1.5×10^9/L for at least 6 months. By definition, this disorder is autoimmune when the excessive destruction of PMNs proceeds from the harnessing of their plasma membrane with antibodies (Abs). Given the controversy over the role of immune complexes (ICs), such autoAbs have, however, proved extremely difficult to charge with the pathophysiology of the disease (1). Primary autoimmune neutropenia (AINs) occur as isolated clinical entities, especially in infancy, where the frequency is 1 in 100,000 newborn babies. Secondary AINs are more common and set against a background of connective tissue disease, e.g., primary Sjögren's syndrome (SS), systemic lupus erythematosus (SLE), and rheumatoid arthritis (RA), or a background of hematological neoplasms, e.g., large granular lymphocyte (LGL) leukemia, autoimmune lymphoproliferative syndrome (ALPS), and even Hodgkin's disease. Insights have recently been gained into the pathogenesis of these confusing settings.

number of apoptotic PMNs in the circulation of patients with SLE (4), this source might be the release of antigens (Ags) by injured cells. There is no definite evidence of the exact mechanism and location of cell destruction. Unlike autoimmune hemolytic anemia and idiopathic thrombopenic purpura where complement-mediated or Ab-dependent cell cytotoxicity operate, these anti-PMN Abs generate opsonic activity favoring the phagocytosis of sensitized cells by the reticulohistiocytic system. However, although the patients show features of a survival defect, the degree of neutropenia does not square with the level of autoAb. Not only is the clearance of PMNs offset by a commensurate raise in the production of PMNs, but such response can also be inverted. That is, a subset of anti-PMN Abs have the capacity to rescue senescent cells from spontaneous apoptosis, through the synthesis of granulocyte colony-stimulating factor (G-CSF) and granulocyte-macrophage colony-stimulating factor and the resulting downregulated expression of *Bax* in PMNs (5).

Pathogenesis

Approximately one-third of adult patients (2) and almost 80% of newborn babies with AIN (3) present with anti-PMN Abs in their serum. These autoAbs have to be set apart from Fc-gamma receptor (FcγR)II and FcγRIIIb-bound ICs in the former population, and from neonatal alloimmune Abs in the latter. The source of immunization is currently unknown. Consistent with the heightened

Clinical Presentation

The clinical course of primary AIN is relatively benign. AINs occur much more frequently than originally stated, because of two biases. On one side, asymptomatic individuals do not give rise to investigation. On the other side, PMN counts vary considerably from day to day, so that cases described as cyclic neutropenia are possibly AINs (6). Conversely, a normal PMN count can be

From: Y. Shoenfeld et al. (eds.): *Diagnostic Criteria in Autoimmune Diseases*, DOI: 10.1007/978-1-60327-285-8_99,

TABLE 99.1. Infections present at the time of diagnosis.

Infection	Frequency (%)
Upper respiratory infections	20
Otitis media	17
Pyoderma	12
Fever of unknown origin	12
Abscess	10
Gastroenteritis	10
Pneumonia	8

Based on References (2) and (8).

maintained, despite the presence of anti-PMN autoAb, through accelerated turn-over of the cells. AutoAbs may, however, lead to qualitative defects by impairing the function of the cells (7).

It has been recognized that the degree and length of neutropenia augment the risk of infection. The most frequent complications are listed in Table 99.1: various Gram-positive and Gram-negative bacterial infections and fungal infections with *Candida* and *Aspergillus* have been reported in infants (8), as well as in adults (2). In secondary AINs, infections have been noticed to be worse during relapse of the underlying pathology. With respect to autoimmune settings, the messages are that neutropenia is rarely seen in patients with primary SS (9), detected in up to half of those with SLE (10), and associated with RA and variable splenomegaly (11) in the Felty's syndrome (FS). AIN can also coexist with hematological diseases, and one-fourth of the LGL leukemia patients who experience RA resemble those with FS (12). There is an obvious need for clarification of the relationship between these two diseases, because they are just distinguished by T-cell clonality which exists in LGL leukemia, but not in FS. The clinical features in common are presented in Table 99.2. Of note, rheumatologic manifestations are more severe in FS compared with RA. Another condition associated with PMN and platelet autoAbs is ALPS (13). In this intriguing disease, it is uncertain as to why blood cells seem to be such a common target for anti-self responses, and not the various organ systems, as seen in RA or SLE, for example.

TABLE 99.2. Clinical features associated with large granular lymphocyte leukemia.

Clinical feature	Frequency (%)
Age > 50 years	70
Male : female	1
Recurrent infection	20–40
Splenomegaly	20–50
Fever, night sweats, and weight loss	20–30
Bone marrow involvement	25–80
Hepatomegaly	<20
Lymphadenopathy	<5

Based on Reference (12).

Hematological Findings

Laboratory findings are summarized in Table 99.3. Around 60% of the patients have isolated neutropenia, while the remaining 40% combine their neutropenia with anemia and/or thrombocytemia (2, 8). Most of them show normal or increased cellularity in the bone marrow (BM), with a normal or low number of mature PMNs. Phagocytosis of PMNs by BM macrophages is occasionally observed.

Serological Tests

Given that no single method can pick up all possible anti-PMN autoAbs, a number of assays have been devised. The screening procedure should include a minimum of two of them (15): viz the granulocyte agglutination test (GAT) and the granulocyte immunofluorescence test (GIFT), both based on the use of PMNs from blood donors as the substrate. Formal quality assurance schemes have recently confirmed that, although the GAT has low sensitivity compared with the GIFT, it is the only reliable method for detecting particular PMN-specific autoAbs (16). Most of them act against human neutrophil Ags (HNA) HNA-1a, HNA-1b, and HNA-1c on FcγRIIIb referred to as CD16, FcγRII referred to as CD32, complement receptor 1 referred to as CD35, and HNA-4a and HNA-4b on CD11b and CD11a, respectively (8, 14). Recourse to the monoclonal Ab immobilization of granulocyte Ag assay is indicated in cases in which there are complex mixtures of Abs, or in which confirmatory tests are required (16).

PMN Abs have also been detected using an indirect immunofluorescence flow (IIF) cytometric test, coupled with an enzyme-linked immunosorbent assay (ELISA) with recombinant FcγRIIIb as a capture agent; such autoAbs have been detected in half of the patients with primary SS, and the sera categorized on the basis of positivity for the two methods as IIF+ELISA+, IIF+ELISA- and IIF-ELISA+ (17). Their presence does not necessarily imply that the patients are neutropenic. More recently, autoAbs to myeloid precursors have been recognized in pure white-cell aplasia (18), and autoAbs against G-CSF

TABLE 99.3. Hematological features in primary autoimmune neutropenia.

Finding	Frequency (%)
Isolated neutropenia	60
Neutropenia + anemia and/or thrombocytopenia	40
Normal bone marrow	30
Reduced no. of mature neutrophils	15
Hypercellular with reduced no. of mature neutrophils	20

Based on References (2), (8) and (14).

TABLE 99.4. Polymorphonuclear neutrophil-specific antibodies in primary autoimmune neutropenia.

Autoantibody specificity	Glycoprotein	Frequency (%)
CD16	FcγRIIIb	30
CD11b		25
CD35	CR1	15
CD32	FcγRII	5

Based on References (2) and (8).

identified in neutropenic patients with SLE or FS (19). In some other patients, there is evidence for anti-Ro/Sicca syndrome A cross-reacting with PMN membrane Ags in patients with SLE or primary SS (20).

Therapy

Steroids exert little effect. To date, G-CSF is the sole therapy allowing recovery of the circulating PMN count and better control of infection in primary AIN and FS. This treatment should be all the more restricted to cases with severe infections, that RA and SLE patients can flare on G-CSF. Remission was also obtained using the humanized monoclonal anti-CD52 Ab Campath-1 H. Parenthetically, although it can induce neutropenia, intravenous immunoglobulin has met transient remission. It stands to reason that control of the underlying disease in secondary AINs is of utmost importance in secondary AINs.

In conclusion, there is a need for standardization of the tests for anti-PMN autoAbs. These may accompany numerous pathological settings, such as BM or organ transplantation, treatment with Rituximab or fludarabine, and infection with parvovirus B19 or human immunodeficiency virus. Still, several issues remain areas of intense investigation.

Acknowledgments. Thanks are due to Cindy Séné and Simone Forest for excellent secretarial assistance.

References

1. Boxer LA, Greenberg MS, Boxer GJ, Stossel TP. Autoimmune neutropenia. N Engl J Med 1975; 293:748–53
2. Logue GL, Shastri KA, Laughlin M, *et al.* Idiopathic neutropenia: antineutrophil antibodies and clinical correlations. Am J Med 1991; 90:211–16
3. Lalezari P, Khorshidi M, Petrosova M. Autoimmune neutropenia of infancy. J Pediatr 1986; 109:764–9
4. Courtney PA, Crockard AD, Williamson K, Irvine AE, Kennedy RJ, Bell AL. Increased apoptotic peripheral blood neutrophils in systemic lupus erythematosus: relations with disease activity, antibodies to double stranded DNA, and neutropenia. Ann Rheum Dis 1999; 58:309–14
5. Durand V, Renaudineau Y, Pers JO, Youinou P, Jamin C. Cross-linking of human FcgammaRIIIb induces the production of granulocyte colony-stimulating factor and granulocyte-macrophage colony-stimulating factor by polymorphonuclear neutrophils. J Immunol 2001; 167:3996–4007
6. Dale DC, Hammond WP 4th. Suppression of in vitro granulocytopoiesis by captopril and penicillamine. Exp Hematol 1988; 16:674–80.
7. Durand V, Pers JO, Renaudineau Y, Saraux A, Youinou P, Jamin C. Differential effects of anti-Fc gamma RIIIb autoantibodies on polymorphonuclear neutrophil apoptosis and function. J Leukoc Biol 2001; 69:233–40
8. Bux J, Behrens G, Jaeger G, Welte K. Diagnosisand clinical course of autoimmune neutropenia in infancy: analysis of 240 cases. Blood 1998; 91:181–6
9. Friedman J, Klepfish A, Miller EB, Ognenovski V, Ike RW, Schattner A. Agranulocytosis in Sjögren's syndrome: two case reports and analysis of 11 additional reported cases. Semin Arthritis Rheum 2002; 31:338–45
10. Nossent JC, Swaak AJ. Prevalence of haematological abnormalities in patients with lupus. Q J Med 1991; 80:605–12
11. Spivak JL. Felty's syndrome: an analytical review. Johns Hopkins Med J 1977; 141:156–62
12. Burks EJ, Loughran TP Jr. Pathogenesis of neutropenia in large granular lymphocyte leukemia and Felty syndrome. Blood Rev 2006; 20:245–66
13. Kwon SW, Procter J, Dale JK, Straus SE, Stroncek DF. Neutrophil and platelet antibodies in autoimmune lymphoproliferative syndrome. Vox Sang 2003; 85:307–12
14. Capsoni F, Sarzi-Puttini P, Zanella A. Primary and secondary autoimmune neutropenia. Arthritis Res Ther 2005; 7:208–14
15. Bux J, Chapman J. Report on the second international granulocyte serology workshop. Transfusion 1997; 37:977–83
16. Lucas G, Rogers S, de Haas M, Porcelijn L, Bux J. Report on the Fourth International Granulocyte Immunology Workshop: progress toward quality assessment. Transfusion 2002; 42:462–8
17. Lamour A, Le Corre R, Pennec YL, Cartron J, Youinou P. Heterogeneity of neutrophil antibodies in patients with primary Sjogren's syndrome. Blood 1995; 86:3553–9
18. Levitt LJ, Ries CA, Greenberg PL. Purewhite-cell aplasia. Antibody-mediated autoimmune inhibition of granulopoiesis. N Engl J Med 1983; 308:1141–6
19. Hellmich B, Csernok E, Schatz H, Gross WL, Schnabel A. Autoantibodies against G-CSF in Felty's syndrome and neutropenic systemic lupus erythematosus. Arthritis Rheum 2002; 46:2384–91
20. Kurien BT, Newland J, Paczkowski C, Moore KL, Scofield RH. Association of neutropenia in systemic lupus erythematosus (SLE) with anti-Ro and binding of an immunologically cross-reactive neutrophil membrane antigen. Clin Exp Immunol 2000; 120:209–17

100
Autoimmune Thrombocytopenic Purpura

Nurit Rosenberg, Yulia Einav and Boris Shenkman

Abstract   Immune thrombocytopenic purpura (ITP) is a common acquired autoimmune disorder characterized by a low platelet count caused by antibodies against platelet surface antigens, mostly glycoproteins IIb/IIIa and Ib/IX. ITP can be present as acute (mainly in children 1–7 years old) and chronic (mainly more than 10 years old). Platelet destruction is triggered by antibodies, but complement-mediated lysis and T-cell cytotoxicity could be involved. Disturbance in megakaryocytes maturation and platelet production, as well as apoptosis were also described. ITP is a diagnosis of exclusion. The diagnostic approach is based primarily on clinical history and physical examination. The first indication of ITP is reduction of platelet count without a change in other cell types. Detection of antiplatelet antibody supports an immune nature of the disease rather than contributing to ITP diagnosis. Treatment of ITP includes steroids, IV immunoglobulin, Rho(D)Ig, anti-CD20 antibody, splenectomy, immunosuppressive drugs, and thrombopoietin.

Keywords   ITP · bleeding disorder · platelet antibodies

Definition

Immune (idiopathic) thrombocytopenic purpura (ITP) is a common acquired autoimmune disorder characterized by a low platelet count caused by antibodies against platelet surface antigens. The antiplatelet antibodies are mainly IgG, but IgA and IgM were also found. The epitopes against the antibodies are lying mostly in GPIIb/IIIa and GPIb/IX complexes, but antibodies against GPIa/IIa or GPIV were also described, and antibodies that react with multiple platelet antigens are common. The specific platelet antibodies considered causing accelerated platelet destruction. ITP can be classified based on the absence or presence of other diseases (primary or secondary), patient age (adults or children), and duration (acute or chronic). Considerable heterogeneity in ITP definition exists in the literature: platelet count thresholds ranged from 100 to 150×10^9/l; duration of thrombocytopenia (TP) before chronic disease is developed ranged from 6 weeks to 3–6 months. The presence of antiplatelet antibody in the plasma is not required for ITP definition. The consensus in definition of ITP is low platelet count, normal hemoglobin level and white blood cell count, no changes in blood smear (except TP), and the absence of other causes of TP.

Epidemiology

ITP is relatively common in children with estimated prevalence of 5:100,000 and somewhat lower in adults; an equal incidence in both males and females in the 1- to 7-year-old age patients with acute ITP is documented (Table 100.1). This is different from the adults who are more likely to have chronic ITP (1) with a female preponderance (1.7:1) (2). Women of age 20–40 years are afflicted most often and outnumber men by a ratio of 3:1 (3).

The trigger for ITP in children is assumed to be a viral infection (Epstein–Bar virus, cytomegalovirus, varicella, rubella, mumps, and parvovirus); most of the children recover within few weeks to 1 year, but about 15% of them remain chronically thrombocytopenic (4). Predisposing conditions in adults are infections such as human immunodeficiency virus, hepatitis C, and *Helicobacter*

From: Y. Shoenfeld et al. (eds.): *Diagnostic Criteria in Autoimmune Diseases*, DOI: 10.1007/978-1-60327-285-8_100,
© 2008 Humana Press, Totowa, NJ

TABLE 100.1. Acute and chronic immune thrombocytopenic purpura (ITP).

	Acute	Chronic
Age (mostly)	1–7 years	>10 years
Lasting period	<3–6 months	>3–6 months
Sex	F:M = 1:1	F:M = 1.7:1
Incidence	After viral infection, vaccination, allergy	Primary or secondary
Association between platelet count and bleeding	Mild	Strong
Presence of IgM antiplatelet antibodies	Frequent	Rare
Need of therapy with platelet count	$<10 \times 10^8/l$	$<30 \times 10^8/l$
Preferential therapy	Anti-D, IVIg	Steroids, IVIg, splenectomy
Recovering	2 months	Years

pylori or presence of other diseases such as systemic lupus erythematosus (SLE) or cancer.

History

ITP was first described in the mid 16th century by Amatus Lusitanus as an exanthema in a disease called "flea-like without fever." Lazarus Riverius (1658) observed bleedings, which come out at the nose. A hundred years later, in 1735, Paul Gottlieb Werlhof reported a disease called "morbus maculosus hemorrhagicus." In 1808, Robert Willan described various types of purpura. Joseph Denys found in 1887 that purpura was associated with low platelet count. Name Kaznelson (1916) hypothesized that spleen was the site of platelet destruction and performed the first splenectomy in a TP patient. William Harrington (1951), who transfused plasma from ITP patients into normal volunteers, which was followed by a rapid fall in platelet counts, presented first evidence for humoral factors causing TP. The immune nature of the disease was suspected when Shulman in 1965 showed that the factor absorbed by platelets was present in the IgG-rich plasma fraction. Since the 1970s, the identification of platelet antigens led to definition of specific platelet autoantibodies causing TP.

Pathogenesis

The pathogenesis of ITP is accelerated platelet destruction as a result of antiplatelet antibodies. Interaction of autoantibodies with platelet surface antigens leads to platelets clearance by the reticuloendothelial system, mostly by the spleen, via Fcγ receptors, or to platelet destruction by complement-mediated lysis. The T-cell cytotoxicity is not excluded. Disturbance in megakaryocytes maturation and

platelet production was also described (5). Electron microscopic studies showed that 50–75% megakaryocytes in ITP had extensive damage, with abnormalities of the membrane system. Other studies showed extensive apoptosis and an increased proportion of megakaryocytes with activated caspase-3 (6). In some cases, thrombopoietin level was found to be inappropriately low in patients with ITP, and plasma of patients with ITP suppressed in vitro production or maturation of megakaryocytes and platelet production. Although antibodies appear to mediate these effects, other mechanisms as altering the cytokine milieu of the bone marrow may alternatively be the cause. Transforming growth factor (TGF)-β1 secreted by T cells is a potent inhibitor of megakaryocyte maturation and its level inversely correlates with disease activity. Recently, a role of platelet apoptosis in the pathogenesis of ITP was suggested; accelerated platelet apoptosis in response to anti-GPIIb antibody was demonstrated in a murine model of ITP (7).

The trigger for the autoantibody production is not clear. In acute childhood ITP, molecular mimicry has been proposed as the pathogenetic mechanism, although only few reports showed cross-reactivity between viral antibodies and platelets (e.g., varicella zoster). In chronic adults' ITP, molecular mimicry was suggested for *H. pylori* and GPIIIa, but in most cases the antibodies are directed against "cryptic" epitopes or neoantigens that become visible to the immune system. Recent studies show that apoptotic cells cause exposure of hidden antigens to the immune system by redistribution of intracellular autoantigens into cell surface blebs or by generating neoantigens. Existence of "cryptic" antigen could be explained also by increased expression of HLA-DR and CD40-ligand by platelets of ITP patients. In summary, the pathogenesis of ITP is associated with different immune defects triggered by external events cooperating with genetic factors and environment.

Clinical Manifestations

ITP in adults usually has an insidious onset and is presented as a chronic disorder. In contrast, ITP in children at an age 1–7 years follows viral or another illness and typically is presented as an acute disorder. Children older than 10 years may be more likely to have a chronic course. Symptoms of ITP are variable and range from mild bruising and mucosal bleeding to massive hemorrhage. Local abnormalities in different systems may increase the risk of bleeding. Generally, bleedings are associated with reduction of platelet count below $30 \times 10^9/l$. Children with severe TP (below $10 \times 10^9/l$) suffer from mild hemorrhage, and only few of them have serious symptoms including intracranial hemorrhage. During normal pregnancy, within the third trimester, platelet count tends to fall, usually with no bleeding risk to mother or infant. However, ITP in pregnant women is dangerous to infants due to transmission of antibodies across the placenta causing fetal or neonatal TP and hemorrhage. This type of neonatal TP must be distinguished from alloimmune TP, in which mothers become sensitive to platelet membrane antigens present on fetal platelets.

Diagnostic criteria

ITP presents as primary (idiopathic) or secondary disorder. The latter is associated with lymphoma, leukemia, HIV infection, hepatitis C, myelodysplastic syndrome, and other disorders. In children, a preceding illness, mostly viral infection or other immunogenic factors, such as allergic reaction, insect bite, or vaccination, may be a trigger for development of ITP. The diagnostic approach for ITP is based primarily on clinical history and physical examination (8, 9). ITP is a diagnosis of exclusion. First of all, the physician should distinguish the type of bleeding due to primary (platelet-type) or secondary (coagulation-type) hemostasis disorder. Pseudo-TP and other pathologies, such as microangiopathic drug-induced TP, and those associated with bone marrow failure should be ruled out. In young children (within a few weeks of birth), a possibility of congenital disorders, such as Wiskott Aldrich syndrome and Bernard–Soulier syndrome, should be considered. In older children, aplastic anaemia and acute leukaemia must not be missed.

The first indication of ITP is reduction of platelet count without a change in other cell types, found on a routine blood count. The blood film serves also to exclude other abnormalities. If atypical findings are present, additional investigations are desired to perform.

Despite many studies have been undertaken regarding definitive search for platelet autoantibodies, this issue still remains a diagnostic challenge. Measurement of platelet-associated IgG by fluorescence flow cytometry is sensitive but lacks specificity. Assay of serum-containing antibodies, especially when a pool of normal platelets is used for antibodies binding, has a higher specificity but lacks sufficient sensitivity. Measuring autoantibodies against specific platelet targets, including glycoproteins (GP) IIb/IIIa, Ib/IX, IV, and Ia/IIa, is promising but still possess low sensitivity. Among them, the anti-GP IIb/IIIa antibodies are the most common. Currently, monoclonal antibody immobilization of platelet antigen (MAIPA) and radioactive immunobead assays are used. But such assays are available in a limited number of platelet laboratories. Even when the specific antibodies are assayed, they can be demonstrated in only 60–65% of ITP patients. The causes of "absent" specific antiplatelet antibody may be the presence of antibody against other platelet surface proteins, presence of anti-idiotype antibodies, T-cell-mediated platelet destruction, immunosuppressive therapy, or methodological detection problems. Hence, to date, detection of antiplatelet antibody supports an immune nature of the disease rather than contributing to ITP diagnosis. However, in the case that the third-line treatment is considered, the determination of anti-platelet antibodies may be of use.

Bone marrow examination for the diagnosis of ITP is not recommended providing that thorough clinical history and physical examination are undertaken and that the blood count and smear show no abnormalities apart from TP. Bone marrow analysis is recommended to perform in patients who are older than 60 years, or have atypical findings, or poor response to first line treatment, or in whom splenectomy is being considered. In children, bone marrow examination should be reserved for those having atypical clinical and laboratory features (10). It is performed usually before steroid therapy is given.

Special assays such as thrombopoietin level and the presence of reticulated (young) platelets may be informative, but they are restricted to limited number of laboratories. Based on the role of *H. pylori* in initiating ITP, it is worthwhile to detect the microorganism, at least in patients who are refractory to the common therapy.

Prediction

In patients with TP whose peripheral blood film revealed only low platelet count, several laboratory findings allow prediction of ITP and discrimination from other disorders: increased platelet-associated and serum anti-platelet antibodies, finding of platelet antibody-producing B cells, elevated percentage of reticulated platelets, and normal or slightly increased plasma thrombopoietin level. Three or more of these signs were found at presentation in 96% patients later diagnosed as ITP (11).

Therapy

Treatment of ITP should be considered on the basis of platelet count, bleeding severity, and general clinical status (12). The requirement for treatment is tailored to the individual patient. In adults, therapy is not indicated in those patients having platelet count greater than $30 \times 10^9/l$ or without signs of bleeding. If there is a need for maintenance therapy, platelet count of more than $30 \times 10^9/l$ must be achieved.

Children with acute ITP and mild clinical disease may be managed with supportive advice, but platelet count should be monitored until resolution of clinical symptoms. The asymptomatic pregnant women with ITP and platelet count higher than $20 \times 10^9/l$ do not require treatment until delivery is imminent. Platelet count of $50 \times 10^9/l$ is regarded safety for both vaginal delivery and Caesarian section (8).

The treatment of ITP aimed to interfere with antibody-mediated platelet destruction, to inhibit the function of macrophage Fcλ receptors and antibody production by B cells. The first-line therapy includes corticosteroids and intravenous immunoglobulin (IVIg). About two-thirds of patients respond well to corticosteroids, but the drug should be stopped in non-responding patients after 4 weeks of therapy. In about 75% patients, IVIg therapy is followed by rapid elevation of platelet count that lasts about 3–4 weeks. The mechanism of action of IVIg involves blockade of Fc receptors on macrophages, immune suppression, and possibly the presence of anti-idiotype antibodies in the pooled human Ig. It is the decision of the physician not to treat ITP, treat with one of these two drugs or with the combination of drugs, and to define the duration of the treatment.

Splenectomy belongs to the second-line therapy, and in two-thirds of patients significant increase of platelet count occurs, which is often sustained without additional therapy. Patients failing to respond to the first- and second-line therapies can be treated with interferon-α, anti-CD20 antibody (rituximab), Rho(D) immunoglobulin (for Rhesus-positive patients), or cytotoxic drugs modulating or inhibiting B-cell antibody production and T-cell cytotoxicity. Repeated protein A immunoadsorption alone or in combination with corticosteroids is effective in patients with refractory ITP. Thrombopoietin or nonimmunogenic thrombopoietic peptides represent a new strategy for treatment of ITP patients who are refractory to second- and third-line therapies.

References

1. Nugent, D. J. (2006) Immune thrombocytopenic purpura of childhood, *Am Soc Hematol Educ Program* **1**, 97–103.

2. Zhou, B., Zhao, H., Yang, R. C., and Han, Z. C. (2005) Multi-dysfunctional pathophysiology in ITP. *Crit Rev Oncol/Hematol* **54**, 107–16.

3. Kravitz, M. S. and Shoenfeld, Y. (2005) Thrombocytopenic conditions-autoimmunity and hypercoagulability: Commonalities and differences in ITP, TTP, HIT, and APS. *Am J Hematol* **80**, 232–42.

4. Imbach, P., Kühne, T., Müller, D., et al. (2006) 12 months follow-up data from the prospective registry I of the Intercontinental Childhood ITP Study Group (ICIS). *Pediatr Blood Cancer* **46**, 351–6.

5. McMillan, R. and Nugent, D. (2005) The effect of antiplatelet autoantibodies on megakaryocytopoiesis. *Int J Hematol* **81**, 94–9.

6. Catani, L., Fagioli, M. E., Tazzari, P. L., et al. (2006) Dendritic cells of immune thrombocytopenic purpura (ITP) show increased capacity to present apoptotic platelets to T lymphocytes. *Exp Hematol* **34**, 879–87.

7. Leytin, V., Mykhaylov, S., Starkey, A. F., et al. (2006) Intravenous immunoglobulin inhibits anti-glycoprotein IIb-induced platelet apoptosis in a murine model of immune thrombocytopenia. *Br J Haematol* **133**, 78–82.

8. British committee for standards in Haematology (2003) Guidelines for the investigation and management of idiopathic thrombocytopenic purpura in adults, children and in pregnancy. *Br J Haematol* **124**, 574–96.

9. Bussel, J. B. (2007) Immune thrombocytopenia purpura. Chapter 46 in Platelets (edt) Elsevier Science (USA).

10. Ahmad, Z., Durrani, N. U., and Hazir, T. (2007) Bone marrow examination in ITP in children: Is it mandatory? *J Coll Physicians Surg Pak* **17**, 347–9.

11. Kuwana, M., Okazaki, Y., Satoh, T., et al. (2005) Initial laboratory findings useful for predicting the diagnosis of idiopathic thrombocytopenic purpura. *Am J Med* **118**, 1026–33.

12. Bromberg, M. E. (2006) Immune thrombocytopenic purpura – The changing therapeutic landscape. *N Engl J Med* **355**, 1643–5.

101
Thrombotic Thrombocytopenic Purpura and Other Thrombotic Microangiopathic Hemolytic Anemias

Boris Shenkman, Yulia Einav and Ophira Salomon

Abstract Thrombotic microangiopathies (TMAs) include several diseases, most prominently thrombotic thrombocytopenic purpura (TTP) and hemolytic uremic syndrome (HUS) characterized by profound thrombocytopenia and microangiopathic hemolytic anemia. Usually congenital TTP is due to mutations in the gene ADAMTS13 or idiopathic when autoantibodies against ADAMTS13 are defined. The differential diagnosis of TTP from other TMAs can be sometimes challenging even with the discovery of ADAMTS13 for more than a decade. The presence of ADAMTS13 activity does not rule out TTP and ultra-large von Willebrand factor (ULVWF) multimers not always present in plasma of patients with TTP. Pathogenesis of TTP is related to massive intravascular aggregation of platelets as a result of lack of degradation of ULVWF multimers because of a lack of ADAMTS13 or secretion of excessive ultra-large multimers by endothelial cells. Diagnostic criteria of TTP are based on clinical features of neurological and renal disfunction along with hemolytic anemia, severe thrombocytopenia, low ADAMTS13 activity, and mutation in ADAMTS13 gene when congenital TTP is suspected. The standard treatment of TTP includes plasma exchange or plasma infusion. Splenectomy, protein A immunoadsorbtion, immunosuppressive drugs, and CD20 antibodies against B cells like rituximab are also used. Recombinant ADAMTS13 in congenital TTP is still to be used only in clinical trials. In HUS plasmapheresis is not efficient. Treatment of other TMA diseases is based on their underlying conditions.

Keywords Thrombotic thrombocytopenic purpura · hemolytic uremic syndrome · thrombotic microangiopathies · ADAMTS13 · von Willebrand factor

Definition

Thrombotic microangiopathy (TMA) is the term for diseases in which disseminated microthrombi composed of agglutinated platelets occluding arterioles and capillaries. Thrombotic thrombocytopenic purpura (TTP) and hemolytic uremic syndrome (HUS) are the two main diseases associated with TMA and characterized by severe thrombocytopenia, erythrocyte fragmentation, and organ failure. TMA is the result of immune-mediated phenomenon as in idiopathic TTP or direct endothelial activation or toxicity following chemotherapy and/or radiotherapy (Table 101.1). TTP can be congenital or idiopathic depending on whether it is the result of mutation in ADAMTS13 or acquired by development of autoantibodies directed against ADAMTS13. Other TMA types include TTP-like syndromes that occur after bone marrow transplantation, occur in disseminated malignancy, catastrophic antiphospholipid syndrome, or sepsis, or are drug induced.

Epidemiology

The incidence of TTP in the USA is estimated at 4 to 11 cases per million people. The incidence is lower in congenital TTP. Females before the age of 50 are at greater risk than male with a ratio of about 2:1 but become equal after the age of 60 (1). Congenital TTP often present between neonatal period and 5 years in contrast to idiopathic TTP with peak incidence between 30 and 50 years. *Escherichia coli* is the most common cause of HUS, which is slightly less common than TTP and is distributed throughout childhood.

History

TTP was first described in 1924 by Eli Moschovitz as "an acute febrile pleomorphic anemia with hyaline thrombi in arterioles and capillaries" (2). Clinical link of TTP to von Willebrand factor (VWF) was made in 1982 by Moake,

From: Y. Shoenfeld et al. (eds.): *Diagnostic Criteria in Autoimmune Diseases*, DOI: 10.1007/978-1-60327-285-8_101,
© 2008 Humana Press, Totowa, NJ

TABLE 101.1. Etiology, epidemiology, and pathogenesis of thrombotic microangiopathy (TMA).

	Congenital TTP	Acquired TTP	HUS
Etiology	ADAMTS13 mutation	Antibody to ADAMTS13, endothelial cell activation	*Escherichia coli* or other microorganisms
Epidemiology	≤1 case per year per million	5–10 cases per year per million	1–5 cases per year per million, mainly in children
Pathogenesis	Defective cleavage of VWF multimers, massive secretion of ULVWF multimers, increased platelet deposition under shear condition, occlusion of blood vessels in microcirculation		Intoxication with Shiga-like toxin, damage of endothelial cells, enterohemorrhagic colitis, renal disorder

HUS, hemolytic uremic syndrome; TTP, thrombotic thrombocytopenic purpura; ULVWF, ultra-high VWF; VWF, von Willebrand factor.

who found that plasma of patients with chronic relapsing TTP contained ultra-large VWF (ULVWF) multimers (3). He postulated that deficiency of depolymerase is responsible for the ULVWF multimers. But only in 1996, the two groups had isolated from normal plasma a metal-dependent protease that cleaves VWF multimers in the A2 domain at the peptide bond between tyrosine at position 1605 and the methionine at position 1606 (4, 5). In 1998, patients with idiopathic TTP were reported to develop autoantibodies against VWF-cleaving protease, but in children with congenital TTP, the activity of this metalloprotease was absent (6). In 2001, Zheng et al. identified the protease as a new member (the thirteenth) of "a disintegrin and metalloprotease with thrombospondin type 1 repeats" (ADAMTS13), which was involved in TTP (7). At the same time Levy et al. identified the ADAMTS13 locus by linkage analysis in families suffering from congenital TTP, and mutations in the ADAMTS13 were defined (8). In subsequent clinical trials, the association between congenital and idiopathic TTP and severe deficiency of ADAMTS13 activity was established.

Pathogenesis

Factors that trigger TTP are poorly understood, but there is an accumulation of ULVWF multimers due to the absence or substantial reduce of ADAMTS13 activity. As a result, intravascular aggregation of platelets occurs occluding arterioles and capillaries. The microcirculation of each organ can be affected with microthrombi leading to ischemia and even to infarction with organ dysfunction. In TTP the involvement of the brain is almost usual. Despite similar clinical picture of different TMA types, etiology and pathogenesis is not unique. Only "classical" TTP is associated with profound deficiency of ADAMTS13 activity and accumulation of ULVWF multimers in blood circulation. However, recent studies suggest that ADAMTS13 deficiency is not sufficient for development of the disease. Regarding acquired TTP, it is not known what factors trigger the formation of antibodies against ADAMTS13 or insult the endothelial cells to secrete large

quantities of ULVWF multimers. HIV infection, pregnancy, antiplatelets, antibodies and immunosuppressive drugs were found to be the candidates.

The etiology of HUS is usually associated with ingestion of *E. coli*, which produces Shiga-like toxin (verotoxin) (9). This type of TMA does not have a severe reduction in plasma ADAMTS13 activity.

Clinical Manifestations

Typical TTP is distinguished from other TMA types by a pentad: severe thrombocytopenia (≤10,000/μl), hemolytic anemia with schistocytosis (≥3%), fever, and neurological and renal abnormalities. However, neurological abnormalities occur in only 50–75% of the patients, and renal disfunction is not severe as in HUS. Children with congenital TTP usually present with thrombocytopenia, hemolytic anemia, and unconjugated hyperbilirubinemia. In contrast to idiopathic TTP, they tend to have chronic relapses. HUS is characterized by the prodromic diarrhoea and severe renal dysfunction.

Diagnostic Criteria

The diagnosis of TTP may be difficult because the symptoms are not specific. The values of the measuring of ADAMTS13 antigen and ADAMTS13 activity and inhibitor remain uncertain. Although undetectable levels of ADAMTS13 can direct the diagnosis, not all cases of TTP present with low titers of ADAMTS13 activity. The presence of ADAMTS13 mutation identified those with congenital TTP. The diagnosis is still depended on laboratory evidence of anemia and thrombocytopenia in the absence of leukopenia. The anemia is "Coombs" negative hemolytic anemia manifested by fragmented red cells (schistocytes) and polychromatophilic red cells (reticulocytes) in peripheral smear, increased serum levels of indirect bilirubin, reduced or absent haptoglobin, and elevated serum levels of lactate dehydrogenase. In TTP there is no evidence of disseminated intravascular coagulation. The clinical symptoms of TTP usually are manifested as fluctuating

TABLE 101.2. ADAMTS13-related parameters in thrombotic microangiopathy (TMA).

	Congenital TTP	Acquired TTP	Other TMA
Antigen	Very low or absent	Low or variable	Normal or moderately decreased
Activity	≤5%	≤5% or variable	30–100%
Inhibitor	No	Mostly yes	No

neurological dysfunction at presentation or during follow-up and renal dysfunction with increased serum creatinin and microhematuria with proteinuria. Other symptoms reflected the organ in which microvascular thrombosis is involved. Although neurological disorder at presentation is substantially more common in TTP and renal failure in HUS, these differences are not sufficient to distinguish between them. In typical HUS, the prodromic manifestation is diarrhea followed by severe renal failure. In this circumstance, a search for infection producing Shiga toxin or other infection is mandatory. The diagnosis of secondary TMA is based on the existence of underlying condition such as lupus anticoagulant in catastrophic antiphospholipid syndrome.

The role of ADAMTS13 in the pathogenesis of TTP triggered development of different assays for determination of ADAMTS13 level and activity and the presence of the ADAMTS13 inhibitor (Table 101.2). Based on the observations that shear stress accelerates and enhances proteolysis of ULVWF multimers by ADAMTS13, Dong et al. proposed a physiological method for measuring ADAMTS13 activity under shear condition (10). In this method, the ability of plasma to detach platelets to ULVWF strings on endothelial cell cultures is assayed using a plate perfusion system. However, this assay is very complex and therefore could not be used as a routine test. A simple and specific screening test for acute TTP was proposed by Shenkman et al. based on the ability of TTP plasma to increase normal whole blood platelet deposition under shear stress (11). Furthermore, addition to this mixture of BaCl$_2$ initiating ADAMTS13 activity in citrated blood allowed discrimination of TTP with the presence or absence of ADAMTS13 inhibitor in the patient plasma (12). This method uses the Impact-R device [Cone and plate(let) analyzer] intended to assess platelet function in different diseases under shear condition and to monitor anti-platelet therapy (13).

Prognosis

Acute TTP was mostly fatal until introduction of plasma therapy in the 1970s. Recent studies have shown that TTP with severe ADAMTS13 deficiency (<5%) has a good response to plasma exchange with relatively low mortality rate (8–19%). TMA patients with mild ADAMTS13 deficiency have a higher mortality rate (18–56%) due to other underlying conditions (14).

Therapy

The standard therapy of idiopathic TTP is based on removing autoantibodies against ADAMTS13 by plasma exchange. Daily plasma exchange with replacement of 1 to 1.5 times the predicted plasma volume should be continued according to the British guidelines for a minimum of 2 days after platelet count reaches 150,000 and above. Cryo-supernatant lacking the larger VWF multimers has been used as replacement fluid instead of plasma. However, cryo-supernatant has not been shown to be mandatory in subsequent randomized studies. Plasma infusion is suitable in patients with congenital TTP. Other modalities of treatment are based on depleting B lymphocytes producing the autoantibodies against ADAMTS13, like rituximab that has been used in treatment of lymphoma. Splenectomy is performed in patients who are refractory to conventional treatment or having multiple relapses.

Following cloning of ADAMTS13, recombinant active form of the protease was produced. The recombinant protease has been found to correct the defective degradation of VWF multimers in vitro, but more studies are required in order to analyze its efficacy in patients with TTP especially in those with hereditary TTP.

Protein A immunoabsorption can remove IgG against ADAMTS13.

Aspirin and other antiaggregants are not useful because platelet aggregation induced by ULVWF is not inhibited by them. Moreover, there is concern about the risk of increasing bleeding because of severe thrombocytopenia and tendency to bleed in TTP patients.

Plasma therapy is not helpful in E. coli-associated HUS. Supportive therapy including renal dialysis is required. For patients with drug-induced TTP, removal of the offending drug is the first step to apply. In patients who develop TMA following transplant, the decision as to stop or decrease the dose of immunosuppressive drug like cyclosporine can be difficult. Ticlopidine or clopidogrel is different from other offending drugs because in the serum of those patients, no activity of ADAMTS13 was detected and inhibitors were present. Plasmapheresis is not helpful in TTP developed after bone marrow transplantation or in cancer patients because ADAMTS13 activity is normal or moderately decreased.

References

1. Sadler, J. E., Moake, J. L., Mijata, T., and George J. N. (2004) Recent advances in thrombotic thrombocytopenic purpura Hematology (Am Soc Hematol Educ Program) 1, 407–23.

2 Moschovitz, E. (1925) An acute febrile pleiochromic anemia with hyaline thrombosis of the terminal arterioles and capillaries. *Arch Intern Med* **36**, 89–93.

3. Moake, J. L., Rudy, C. K., Troll, J. H., and Weinstein, M. J. (1982) Unusually large plasma factor VIII: von Willebrand factor multimers in chronic relapsing thrombotic thrombocytopenic purpura. *N Engl J Med* **307**, 1432–5.

4. Furlan, M., Robles, R., and Lammle, B. (1996) Partial purification and characterization of a protease form human plasma cleaving von Willebrand factor to fragments produced by in vivo proteolysis. *Blood* **87**, 4223–34.

5. Tsai, H. M. (1996) Physiologic cleavage of von Willebrand factor by a plasma protease is dependent on its conformation and requires calcium ion. *Blood* **7**, 4235–44.

6. Tsai, H. M. and Lian, E. C. (1998) Antibodies to von Willebrand factor-cleaving protease in acute thrombotic thrombocytopenic purpura. *N Engl J Med* **339**, 1585–94.

7. Zheng, X., Chung, C., Takayama, T. K. et al. (2001) Structure of von Willebrand factor cleaving protease (ADAMTS 13), a metalloprotease involved in thrombotic thrombocytopenic purpura. *J Biol Chem* **276**, 41059–63.

8. Levy, G. A., Nichols, W. C., Lian, E. C. et al. (2001) Mutations in a member of the ADAMTS gene family cause thrombotic thrombocytopenic purpura. *Nature* **413**, 488–94.

9. Moake, J. L. (2002) Thrombotic thrombocytopenic purpura and the hemolytic uremic syndrome. *Arch Pathol Lab Med* **126**, 1430–3.

10. Dong, J. F., Moake, J. L., Nolasco, L., et al. (2002) ADAMTS-13 rapidly cleaves newly secreted ultralarge von Willebrand factor multimers on the endothelial surface under flowing condition. *Blood* **100**, 4033–9.

11. Shenkman, B., Inbal, A., Tamarin, I., et al. (2003) Diagnosis of thrombotic thrombocytopenic purpura based on modulation by patient plasma of normal platelet adhesion under flow condition. *Brit J Haematol* **120**. 597–604.

12. Shenkman, B., Budde, U., Angerhaus, D., et al. (2006) ADAMTS-13 regulates platelet adhesion under flow. A new method for differentiation between inherited and acquired thrombotic thrombocytopenic purpura. *Thromb Haemost* **6**, 160–6.

13. Savion, N. and Varon, D. (2006) Impact – the cone and plate (let) analyzer: Testing platelet function and anti-platelet drug response. Pathophysiology of Haemostasis and Thrombosis, 19-th international congress on thrombosis, Tel-Aviv, 83–8.

14. Zheng, X. L., Kaufman, R. M., Goodnough, L. T., and Sadler, J. E. (2004) Effect of plasma exchange on ADAMTS13 metalloprotease activity, inhibitor level, and clinical outcome in patients with idiopathic and nonidiopathic thrombotic thrombocytopenic purpura. *Blood* **103**, 4043–9.

102
Heparin-Induced Thrombocytopenia

Gowthami M. Arepally and Douglas B. Cines

Abstract   Heparin-induced thrombocytopenia (HIT) is an acquired hypercoagulable disorder caused by drug-dependent antibodies that recognize complexes of platelet factor 4 (PF4) and heparin. The clinical syndrome manifests as thrombocytopenia and/or thrombosis in temporal association with heparin therapy. Owing to the frequent occurrence of asymptomatic PF4/heparin antibodies in patients receiving heparin, current approaches to the diagnosis of HIT rely on clinical criteria with additional support provided by laboratory testing for heparin-dependent antibodies. This chapter will address the clinical and laboratory diagnostic features of HIT.

Keywords   Heparin · platelet factor 4 (pf4) · heparin-induced thrombocytopenia · hit · thrombocytopenia · thrombosis

Introduction

Heparin-Induced Thrombocytopenia (HIT) is a prothrombotic autoimmune disorder typically triggered by exposure to unfractionated heparin (UFH) or low-molecular weight heparin (LMWH). HIT develops in defined temporal association with heparin therapy and manifests either as an unexplained thrombocytopenia (isolated HIT) or thrombocytopenia complicated by thrombosis (HITT). In a small subset of patients, the clinical syndrome develops days to weeks after drug exposure has ceased, which is referred to as "delayed HIT". The propensity for recurrent thrombosis distinguishes HIT from other common drug-induced thrombocytopenias.

The autoantibodies in HIT recognize a complex composed of two normal constituents, Platelet Factor 4 (PF4), a cationic platelet protein released from platelet alpha-granules upon activation, and negatively charged glycosaminoglycans (GAGs, such as heparin and heparin-like molecules), that line the vascular endothelium and hematopoietic cells. The inciting events leading to PF4/heparin autoantibody formation are not well understood. However, it is well established that in approximately 1–3% of patients exposed to drug, pathogenic autoantibodies develop and elicit disease by activating platelets and monocytes through their Fcγ receptors and possibly by inducing endothelial cell injury. Cellular activation culminates in a profound hypercoagulable state associated with platelet activation/consumption leading to thrombocytopenia, accompanied by intense thrombin generation promoting thrombosis. Unless specified, the term heparin will be used in this chapter to encompass UFH, LMWH, and other heparin-like anticoagulants, because PF4/heparin autoantibodies triggered by all agents appear clinically and biologically indistinguishable.

This chapter will focus on the challenges related to the clinical recognition and laboratory diagnosis of HIT. For a comprehensive discussion of the pathogenesis and/or management of HIT, the reader is referred to recent reviews (1).

Incidence of HIT

HIT occurs in 0.8–3% of all patients exposed to UFH and 0.2–1% of patients exposed to LMWH (2) for a minimum of 5 days. Certain patient populations, such as general medical and surgical patients, appear to be more susceptible to developing clinical complications than others, such as obstetric, pediatric, and chronic hemodialysis patients (1). The reasons for the variable risk of disease are not understood.

The incidence of asymptomatic seroconversion is high in patients exposed to heparin, which frequently confounds the laboratory diagnosis of HIT (see below). Anti-PF4/heparin antibodies can be detected in ~8–17% of general medical

From: Y. Shoenfeld et al. (eds.): *Diagnostic Criteria in Autoimmune Diseases*, DOI: 10.1007/978-1-60327-285-8_102,
© 2008 Humana Press, Totowa, NJ

and surgical patients treated with UFH, 2–8% of those treated with LMWH, and in 1–2% of patients treated with fondaparinux (1). Heparin sensitization occurs in ~50% of patients undergoing cardiac surgery. The determinants that convert antibody-positive asymptomatic individuals into patients with thrombosis are unknown but in part may be related to development of high titers of IgG antibodies in the context of underlying cardiovascular disease marked by endothelial dysfunction and platelet activation.

Clinical Features of HIT

The two cardinal clinical manifestations of HIT are a substantial fall in the platelet count and/or thrombosis occurring in the setting of recent heparin therapy. An unexplained fall in the platelet count (>40%) or thrombocytopenia is evident at presentation in approximately two-thirds of patients and becomes evident in >95% of patients with serologically confirmed disease (3). Thrombocytopenia is defined in most studies as either an absolute (<150,000/μL) or relative decrease (by 30–50%) in platelets (3). The fall in platelet count may precede, occur coincidentally, or less commonly follow the thrombotic event. Platelet counts infrequently fall below 10,000/μL in the absence of extensive ischemic tissue damage or comorbidities, and hemorrhagic complications are rare.

Thrombocytopenia serves as a surrogate marker for increased thrombotic risk. Recent prospective and retrospective series suggest that ~25% of patients with isolated HIT are at risk of developing thrombotic complications within four weeks of diagnosis (4, 5). Several studies have shown a correlation between IgG antibody titer, severity of thrombocytopenia, and risk of thrombosis (3).

Approximately 60% of patients with HIT present with thrombosis (3), which affects any vascular bed including both large vessels and the microvasculature. Venous thromboses are more common (2:1) in most clinical populations, with the exception of patients undergoing cardiovascular surgery, who appear to be at higher risk for peripheral arterial occlusion (3). Sites of vascular injury caused by cannulation are especially vulnerable to thrombosis. Thrombosis in the absence of thrombocytopenia is more characteristic of atypical presentations, e.g. heparin-induced skin necrosis, venous limb gangrene, or anaphylactic-type reactions (6). Thrombotic complications are associated with significant morbidity and considerable mortality (~8–20%), notwithstanding the recent introduction of alternative forms of anticoagulation with direct thrombin inhibitors (see below) (5).

Diagnostic Criteria: Clinical

Clinical evaluation of HIT is difficult. Many hospitalized patients, especially in the intensive care setting, are routinely exposed to heparin, and often develop thrombocytopenia

from other causes such as infection, medications (e.g. GPIIb/IIIa inhibitors, antibiotics), mechanical devices (balloon pumps), and/or end-stage multiorgan failure. The laboratory diagnosis of HIT is also problematic, as there is no readily available test that can be relied upon to affirm or exclude HIT in the absence of clinical information. Therefore, current approaches to diagnosis rely on establishing probability of disease integrating clinical criteria with laboratory analysis of heparin-dependent antibodies for confirmation.

The clinical diagnosis of HIT is established by documenting the development of thrombocytopenia and/or thrombosis in temporal association with heparin therapy, excluding other causes of thrombocytopenia and affirming the diagnosis by demonstrating a recovery in platelet counts after heparin has been discontinued (see Table 102.1). The most reliable and available among these criteria is the temporal relationship between thrombocytopenia and/or thrombosis and heparin exposure. In heparin-naive individuals or in patients with remote exposure (>120 days (7)), disease manifestations typically develop 5–10 days after exposure to heparin. Thrombocytopenia and/or thrombosis can occur more abruptly (<24 hrs) in patients with recent drug exposure (<120 days) because of the presence of circulating PF4/heparin antibodies (7). Rarely, patients develop delayed HIT, with the onset of thrombocytopenia and/or thrombosis 1–2 weeks after cessation of heparin.

Diagnosing HIT in patients with cardiac bypass surgery is especially challenging, as the prevalence of heparin-dependent antibodies is high (~30–>50% (8, 9)), post-surgical thrombocytopenia is common, fever and hypotension are frequent, indwelling intravascular devices are used commonly and patients are often exposed to other medications that can be implicated. Most patients who develop HIT after cardiac bypass surgery show a triphasic

TABLE 102.1. Patients presenting with thrombocytopenia in association with heparin therapy should be carefully assessed for the above clinical criteria (19).

Clinical Criteria for HIT
1. Temporal association of thrombocytopenia +/– thrombosis with recent heparin therapy
a. Classic presentation: 5–10 days in heparin naive individuals or with remote history of heparin use (>120 days)
b. Acute/rapid onset: <24 hours in patients with recent heparin exposure (<120 days)
c. Delayed HIT: >10 days after heparin exposure
2. Exclusion of other causes of thrombocytopenia
a. Drugs (glycoprotein IIb/IIIa inhibitors, vancomycin, quinine, bactrim, prostacyclin agents)
b. Infection (bacterial/viral/fungal)
c. Mechanical devices (intra-aortic balloon pump, ventricular assist devices)
d. Organ dysfunction (liver failure, hepato- or splenomegaly, marrow disease)
e. Other immune thrombocytopenias (thrombotic thrombocytopenic purpura, immune thrombocytopenia, systemic lupus erythematosus)
3. Recovery in platelet counts

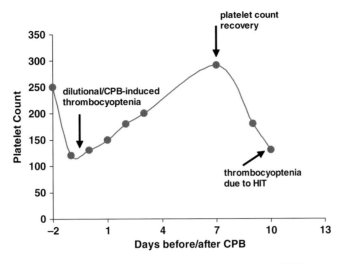

FIGURE 102.1. Biphasic pattern of platelet count recovery in patients with post-bypass HIT.

pattern of platelet counts after surgery. Platelet counts initially decline for 2–4 days after surgery, rebound into the normal range or beyond, and then fall once again ((8, 9), Figure 102.1). In others, a failure of the platelet count to recover by 3–5 days of surgery prompts the diagnosis to be considered. In one study, short cardiac bypass and an interval of 5 days or longer between surgery and the re-development of thrombocytopenia were useful predictors of HIT (8).

Several algorithms have been developed to stratify patients for risk based on clinical criteria. The most widely studied has been Dr. Warkentin's "4T's" algorithm, which assigns pre-test probability scores (0–2) to various criteria, including: (a) severity of thrombocytopenia, (b) timing of fall in platelet count, (c) presence of thrombosis, and (d) exclusion of other causes. The clinical probability based on cumulative scores is defined as high (6–8 points), intermediate (4–5 points), or low (≤3 points). In a recent prospective study of 336 patients enrolled in two major medical centers, the clinical utility of the 4T's algorithm was compared with results of laboratory testing as the gold standard in patients suspected of HIT (10). An excellent correlation was observed between low pretest probability and negative serology, suggesting that low clinical scores have a high negative predictive value (NPV). However, the clinical algorithm was less useful in predicting the presence of disease, demonstrating significant clinician-dependent differences in assessment based on experience (10). Clinical algorithms have also proved less useful in the post-cardiac bypass setting where diverse addition causes of thrombocytopenia and thrombosis are common.

Diagnostic Criteria: Laboratory

Although PF4/heparin antibodies are detected in almost all patients with a clinical diagnosis of HIT, not all PF4/heparin antibodies trigger clinically overt disease (11).

Thus, the challenge of laboratory testing lies in distinguishing patients with seemingly pathogenic PF4/heparin antibodies from those found in patients who are and are likely to remain asymptomatic. Recent studies indicate that affected patients are more likely to have high titers of IgG antibodies that possess platelet-activating potential (4, 11, 12). However, developing narrowly defined criteria that can be applied prospectively to an individual patient has not been possible, given the clinical and serological overlap among symptomatic and asymptomatic presentations and lack of a "gold standard" laboratory assay for diagnosis.

Heparin-dependent antibodies can be detected using immunological assays that measure antibody binding to PF4/"heparin" or functional assays that detect heparin-dependent platelet activation (See Table 102.2). Commercial immunological assays, such as the PF4/heparin ELISA or gel-particle immunoassays currently in use measure IgG, IgA, and IgM antibodies concurrently; assays specific for IgG-specific antibodies have recently been developed but there is less published experience with reliance on outcome. Antigen-based assays are technically easy to perform and are more widely available than functional assays (see below). Immunoassays offer excellent sensitivity (>98%), and therefore, carry an excellent negative predictive value for excluding the diagnosis of HIT (11). However, the specificity of immunoassays (50–74%) is compromised by the frequent detection of PF4/heparin antibodies in asymptomatic individuals and those in whom other causes of thrombocytopenia are more likely (11, 13). The frequency of PF4/heparin antibodies, particularly among cardiac surgery patients, considerably diminishes the positive predictive value of immunoassays as stand-alone tests (39–50%) in this setting where the diagnosis of HIT is often considered (11, 14). Although the specificity of immunoassays may be slightly improved (by >15%) by

TABLE 102.2. Sensitivity and Specificity of Laboratory Tests in HIT[a].

Test	Sensitivity	Specificity	PPV	NPV	References
A. Immunological assays:					
Heparin/PF4 ELISA	>95%	50–74%	39%	100%	(11, 13, 14)
Gel-particle immunoassay	95%	92%	57%	99%	(14).
B. Functional assays:					
[14]C Serotonin Release Assay (SRA)	88–100%	95–100%	100%	81%	(14, 18).
Platelet Aggregation Test (PAT) or Heparin-Induced Platelet Aggregation (HIPA)	37–91%	77–100%	89%	81%	(18, 19)
Functional flow cytometric assay (microparticles or platelet activation marker)	83–95%	92–100%	ND	ND	(20)

[a]Assays included only if validated by multiple laboratories/multiple investigators; tests reported only by individual laboratories, such as lumi-aggregometry, gel-particle assay, HPLC (high-pressure liquid chromatography) not included; ND = not determined.

measuring IgG antibodies alone (11, 13), this is still often insufficient to be relied upon clinically.

Functional assays detect heparin-dependent IgG antibodies capable of activating platelets through FcγRII receptors, though complement-fixing lytic antibodies are found in some occasions. The most frequently used functional assays include the platelet aggregation test (PAT), heparin-induced platelet activation assay (HIPA), flow cytometric detection of platelet activation (P-selectin and/or annexin V), and the ^{14}C-serotonin release assay (SRA). Owing to platelet donor variability and/or possibly the influence of antibody titers (12), the sensitivity of functional assays is generally lower (35–90%) than their specificity (95–100% (15)). In some reports, the sensitivities of the functional assays have been improved to >95% through technical refinements, including use of radioactivity, responsive donor platelets, and optimization of buffer conditions (11, 13). PPVs of functional assays are higher than immunoassays (89–100% (1)), but the technical expertise required limits their availability in real-time.

Because immunoassays are more widely available than functional assays, various approaches have been described to improve their diagnostic utility. These approaches include integrating the results of immunological assays with functional assays and/or clinical algorithms (14, 16). A recent prospective study examined the utility of "4T's" clinical algorithm in conjunction with the SRA and gel-particle immunoassays. As expected, for patients assigned to a low-risk or high-risk clinical category, functional and immunoassays were concordant, yielding high NPVs and PPVs, respectively. For patients assigned to an intermediate risk category, a negative immunoassay lowered the pre-test probability score from 11% to <0.4%, whereas a positive immunoassay in this clinical category increased the pre-test probability from 11% to only 45% on post-test analysis (14).

On the basis of these observations, the following diagnostic approach has been proposed by some for patients suspected of HIT in settings where functional assays are not routinely available. For patients with a low clinical probability of HIT, testing is not advised, as this group of patients has an extremely low likelihood of disease (10, 14) and a positive ELISA is not diagnostic in this setting. Serological testing for PF4/heparin antibodies is recommended where the clinical suspicion of HIT is intermediate or high. For patients with a high pre-test probability of HIT and who have a strongly positive ELISA, no further diagnostic evaluation is required, as the PPV of the immunoassay in this setting is high. Patients with negative serologies who are at high or intermediate clinical probability for disease should be evaluated for an alternative diagnosis, as negative immunoassays are associated with a very low likelihood of disease (14). For patients who are in an intermediate risk category and whose ELISA is positive, functional testing is recommended because of its high PPV in this setting (11, 14).

Therapy of HIT

If the diagnosis of HIT is suspected based on clinical criteria, it is imperative to discontinue all exposure to heparin and initiate alternative anticoagulant therapy while awaiting the results of laboratory testing. In addition to discontinuing therapeutic or prophylactic administration of heparin, patients must be evaluated for occult exposures in the form of heparin-locks, heparin-bonded catheters, including dialysis lines and arterial lines, as well as cell-saver devices, and heparin-containing infusion solutions, among others. The use of LMW heparin is ill advised because of antibody cross-reactivity and warfarin is contraindicated in active disease, as it can exacerbate the hypercoagulable state by lowering protein C. Screening for occult thrombosis, e.g. Doppler studies of the legs, is advisable in some settings.

Only two classes of anticoagulants have been shown to be effective in the clinical management of HIT. The heparinoids, a family of heparin-like molecules with anti-factor Xa activity, are available in Canada, Europe, and Australia, but not in the United States (1). Heparinoids are administered subcutaneously, have long half-lives, and are monitored based on anti-factor Xa activity (1). The direct thrombin inhibitors ('DTIs') inactivate thrombin without need for anti-thrombin. In general, DTIs have short half-lives (<1 h), are not recognized by HIT antibodies, and therapy is monitored with the aPTT (17). Three DTIs (lepirudin, argatroban and bivalirudin) are available in the United States and have been approved by the Food and Drug Administration for various indications in HIT. The DTIs differ with respect to their half-lives, mechanisms of clearance (renal vs. hepatic), and effect on the prothrombin time.

The risk of thrombosis remains high for 2–4 weeks in patients with isolated HIT (5, 7). Therefore, anticoagulation with warfarin is recommended for 4 weeks even in the absence of overt thrombosis. The transition to oral anticoagulants should be undertaken only after control of the disease, i.e. resolution of thrombosis and platelet counts that some recommend reach a stable plateau of >100 K, while others recommend waiting until the platelet count has normalized. Treatment of HIT-induced thrombosis requires more extended therapy.

References

1. Arepally, G. M., Ortel, T. L. (2006) Heparin-Induced Thrombocytopenia N Engl J Med 355, 809–17.
2. Martel, N., Lee, J., Wells, P. S. (2005) Risk for heparin-induced thrombocytopenia with unfractionated and low-molecular-weight heparin thromboprophylaxis: A meta-analysis Blood 106, 2710–15.
3. Greinacher, A., Farner, B., Kroll, H., Kohlmann, T., Warkentin, T. E., Eichler, P. (2005) Clinical features of heparin-induced thrombocytopenia including risk factors for thrombosis. A retrospective analysis of 408 patients Thromb Haemost 94, 132–5.
4. Zwicker, J. I., Uhl, L., Huang, W.-Y., Shaz, B. H., Bauer, K. A. (2004) Thrombosis and ELISA optical density values in hospitalized patients with heparin-induced thrombocytopenia J Thromb Haemost 2, 2133–7.
5. Hirsh, J., Heddle, N., Kelton, J. G. (2004) Treatment of heparin-induced thrombocytopenia: A critical review Arch Intern Med 164, 361–9.
6. Warkentin, T. E., Roberts, R. S., Hirsh, J., Kelton, J. G. (2005) Heparin-induced skin lesions and other unusual sequelae of the heparin-induced thrombocytopenia syndrome: A nested cohort study Chest 127, 1857–61.
7. Warkentin, T. E., Kelton, J. G. (2001) Temporal aspects of heparin-induced thrombocytopenia N Engl J Med 344, 1286–92.
8. Lillo-Le Louet, A., Boutouyrie, P., Alhenc-Gelas, M., Le Beller, C., Gautier, I., Aiach, M., Lasne, D. (2004) Diagnostic score for heparin-induced thrombocytopenia after cardiopulmonary bypass J Thromb Haemost 2, 1882–8.
9. Pouplard, C., May, M. A., Regina, S., Marchand, M., Fusciardi, J., Gruel, Y. (2005) Changes in platelet count after cardiac surgery can effectively predict the development of pathogenic heparin-dependent antibodies Br J Haematol 128, 837–41.
10. Lo, G. K., Juhl, D., Warkentin, T. E., Sigouin, C. S., Eichler, P., Greinacher, A. (2006) Evaluation of pretest clinical score (4 T's) for the diagnosis of heparin-induced thrombocytopenia in two clinical settings J Thromb Haemost 4, 759–65.
11. Greinacher, A., Juhl, D., Strobel, U., Wessel, A., Lubenow, N., Selleng, K., Eichler, P., Warkentin, T. E. (2007) Heparin-induced thrombocytopenia: a prospective study on the incidence, platelet-activating capacity and clinical significance of antiplatelet factor 4/heparin antibodies of the IgG, IgM, and IgA classes J Thromb Haemost 5, 1666–73.
12. Alberio, L., Kimmerle, S., Baumann, A., Taleghani, B. M., Biasiutti, F. D., Lammle, B. (2003) Rapid determination of anti-heparin/platelet factor 4 antibody titers in the diagnosis of heparin-induced thrombocytopenia. Am J Med 114, 528–36.
13. Warkentin, T. E., Sheppard, J.-A. I., Moore, J. C., Moore, K. M., Sigouin, C. S., Kelton, J. G. (2005) Laboratory testing for the antibodies that cause heparin-induced thrombocytopenia: How much class do we need? J Lab Clin Med 146, 341–6.
14. Pouplard, C., Gueret, P., Fouassier, M., Ternisien, C., Trossaert, M., Regina, S., Gruel, Y. (2007) Prospective evaluation of the "4T's" score and particle gel immuno-assay specific to heparin/PF4 for the diagnosis of heparin-induced thrombocytopenia J Thromb Haemost 5, 1373–9.
15. Greinacher, A., Amiral, J., Dummel, V., Vissac, A., Kiefel, V., Mueller-Eckhardt, C. (1994) Laboratory diagnosis of heparin-associated thrombocytopenia and comparison of platelet aggregation test, heparin-induced platelet activation test, and platelet factor 4/heparin enzyme-linked immunosorbent assay Transfusion 34, 381–5.
16. Pouplard, C., Amiral, J., Borg, J. Y., Vissac, A. M., Delahousse, B., Gruel, Y. (1997) Differences in specificity of heparin-dependent antibodies developed in heparin-induced thrombocytopenia and consequences on cross-reactivity with danaparoid sodium Br J Haematol 99, 273–80.
17. Warkentin, T. E., Greinacher, A. (2003) Heparin-induced thrombocytopenia and cardiac surgery. Ann Thorac Surg 76, 2121–31.
18. Pouplard, C., Amiral, J., Borg, J. Y., Laporte-Simitsidis, S., Delahousse, B., Gruel, Y. (1999) Decision analysis for use of platelet aggregation test, carbon 14-serotonin release assay, and heparin-platelet factor 4 enzyme-linked immunosorbent assay for diagnosis of heparin-induced thrombocytopenia Am J Clin Pathol 111, 700–6.
19. Chong, B. H., Burgess, J., Ismail, F. (1993) The clinical usefulness of the platelet aggregation test for the diagnosis of heparin-induced thrombocytopenia Thromb Haemost 69, 344–50.
20. Tomer, A. (1997) A sensitive and specific functional flow cytometric assay for the diagnosis of heparin-induced thrombocytopenia Br J Haematol 98, 648–56.

103
Autoimmune Coagulopathies

Fabio Tucci and Rolando Cimaz

Abstract   Acquired inhibitors to Factor VIII (not related to treatment for hemophilia) are autoantibodies that, although rare, may cause significant and often life-threatening hemorrhage. They occur, predominantly in older individuals, in association with autoimmune disorders, lymphoproliferative disorders, solid tumors, medications, and during post-partum. However, in almost half of the cases they develop spontaneously without an underlying medical condition. Laboratory diagnosis is made by performing the aPTT clotting time in conjunction with a mixing study, and subsequently with specific clotting assays. Treatment varies depending upon the underlying medical condition, the titer of the inhibitor, and the clinical presentation. Acutely bleeding patients with high titers of autoantibodies may respond well to infusions of Factor VIII concentrate. Extracorporeal plasmapheresis with exchange will also rapidly reduce circulating antibodies and can be used in conjunction with Factor infusions and/or intravenous immunoglobulins (IVIg). Long-term treatment for reduction of autoantibodies will include immunosuppressants.

Acquired inhibitors to other coagulation factors, e.g. Factor IX, XI, XIII, vWF protein, and the vitamin K-dependent proteins, can arise but are extremely rare. The principles of their therapy mirror those applied to the management of Factor VIII autoantibodies.

Keywords   Coagulopathies · autoimmune · Factor VIII · inhibitors

Coagulopathies and bleeding disorders can be secondary to autoimmune processes; some of those (i.e. anti-phospholipid-related and autoimmune thrombocytopenic purpura) are dealt with elsewhere in this book, and are therefore not discussed in this chapter. It is just worth noting that anti-phospholipid antibodies are usually related to thrombosis, but hemorrhagic episodes and significant coagulopathy can occur in the so-called lupus anticoagulant-hypoprothrombinemia syndrome, with positive lupus anticoagulant and decreased Factor II (prothrombin) activity. This phenomenon is linked to the presence of non-neutralizing antibodies directed against Factor II. This is a rare clinical entity, which can occur in association with SLE, transient viral infections, drug reactions, or even in healthy individuals.

We will briefly review the current knowledge of acquired inhibitors of the clotting cascade.

Acquired Factor VIII Inhibitors

Hemophilia A is classically caused by a congenital deficiency of Factor VIII, but an acquired form due to inhibitors typically presents later in life. Patients who develop such inhibitors may have catastrophic bleeding episodes despite no prior history of a bleeding disorder.

In congenital hemophilia, patients treated with Factor VIII will develop alloantibodies in 20–40% of cases. In contrast, acquired inhibitors/autoantibodies against Factor VIII in non-hemophiliacs occur in only about one case per million/year (1). In acquired hemophilia, autoantibodies are non-complement fixing, non-precipitating immunoglobulins from the IgG family that binds FVIII in a time- and temperature-dependent manner (2). The responsible antibody has been identified as belonging to the IgG4 subclass, and the epitope that binds to Factor VIII has also been identified.

Acquired hemophilia differs from congenital hemophilia as it occurs both in men and women, and as it is more frequent in adulthood, even if pediatric cases have been described. The median age at presentation is during the seventh decade of life, but a wide age range has been reported, with a small pediatric series of six children (3, 4) and a patient as young as 2 years of life (5).

The onset is often acute and severe: in a series of 215 patients, 87% of cases needed red blood cell transfusion

From: Y. Shoenfeld et al. (eds.): *Diagnostic Criteria in Autoimmune Diseases*, DOI: 10.1007/978-1-60327-285-8_103,

for post-hemorrhagic anemia (6). Mortality rates have been described ranging from 8 to 22% of cases.

Hemarthroses are the hallmark of congenital hemophilia, while they are rare in the acquired form, which typically presents with purpura or soft tissue bleeding. Moreover, severe muscle bleeding, hematuria, epistaxis, gastrointestinal bleeding, and even intracerebral bleeds are seen more frequently than are hemarthroses.

An association with autoimmune diseases has been found in almost 20% of cases, mainly in systemic lupus erythematosus, rheumatoid arthritis, diabetes, and Sjogren's syndrome. Cutaneous disorders such as pemphigus, epidermolysis bullosa, and pustular psoriasis have also been reported with acquired hemophilia. The interesting association of Factor VIII inhibitors with autoimmune lymphoproliferative syndrome (ALPS) has also been reported (7). In a study, the frequency and specificity of acquired coagulation inhibitors in 511 patients with inflammatory and malignant gastrointestinal diseases were reported (8). An increased incidence of coagulation factor inhibitors was found in patients with gastrointestinal inflammatory and malignant diseases compared with the healthy population. In particular, 15 patients acquired inhibitors to the following coagulation factors: factor IX (four patients), factor X (three patients), factor XII (three patients), factor VIII (two patients), factor XI (two patients), and factor V (one patient). Only one patient, with factor VIII inhibitor, presented with severe bleeding and was treated with recombinant human activated factor VII, while the others had no complications.

Among physiological conditions that have been associated with acquired hemophilia, a transient postpartum form has been described, with a favorable outcome in the vast majority of cases. Of note, when the inhibitor develops during pregnancy there is a risk of transplacental passage of the antibody and of neonatal hemorrhage (9).

The diagnosis is based on the following points:

- Isolated prolongation of aPTT, with normal PT and normal platelet count;
- Absence of aspecific inhibitors (Lupus anticoagulant, heparin);
- Lack of correction of the prolonged aPTT by the addition of normal plasma (indicating the presence of an inhibitor);
- When suspecting a Factor VIII inhibitor, the mixing has to be incubated at 37°C for 1 or 2 hours;
- The antibody has to be measured in Bethesda Units (BU). However, results from a Bethesda assay often require several days because samples are referred to specialty laboratories, and ELISA systems have been designed, with good results as a screening system (10).

Treatment

In order to increase Factor VIII levels (milder cases), DDAVP (vasopressin) as in von Willebrand disease can be administered, as well as Factor VIII concentrate. To bypass Factor VIII, in the presence of high levels of inhibitor (>5BU), activated prothrombin complex concentrates and recombinant Factor VII can be administered. If the inhibitor removal is desired, this can be accomplished with plasmapheresis or immunoadsorption (Staphylococcal A protein). Pharmacological treatment relies on immunosuppression with corticosteroids (prednisone 1 mg/Kg/day), which results in improvement in 30% of cases, with or without the addition of cytotoxics such as cyclophosphamide (the combined treatment leads to higher rates of improvement).

However, the inhibitor often poses a serious problem because any infused factor will be rapidly neutralized and will not be available to induce hemostasis. For the eradication of the inhibitor, rituximab (anti-CD20) has also been suggested (3, 11, 12, 13, 14). If no benefit is obtained, other immunosuppressants can be considered, including mycophenolate mophetil, cyclosporine A; azathioprine, and vincristine. 2-Chlorodeoxyadenosine, an immunosuppressant that is thought to act through the Fas-Fas ligand pathway with subsequent activation of cellular apoptosis, has also been tried with satisfactory results (15).

Intravenous immunoglobulin (IVIg) therapy for acquired coagulation inhibitors, including factor VIII inhibitor, and for acquired von Willebrand syndrome has been considered in 44 published reports (16). Among 35 patients with factor VIII inhibitor, the efficacy of IVIg therapy alone was about 30%, whereas the response to combination therapy with IVIg plus immunosuppressive agents (e.g. corticosteroids, cyclophosphamide) seemed to be better (approximately 70%) than with IVIg alone. The response to IVIg therapy appears to occur rapidly, and coagulation inhibitors seem to be neutralized immediately.

Acquired Von Willebrand Syndrome

In this disorder, laboratory findings are similar to those present in congenital von Willebrand disease. However, no personal or family history of bleeding is present (17). It has been described in association with autoimmune hemolytic anemia, lymphoproliferative, myeloproliferative, and cardiovascular disorders.

Other Inhibitors

Factor V is an essential component of the prothrombinase complex, which activates prothrombin to thrombin. Antibodies against Factor V have been reported to appear after the administration of bovine thrombin in a surgical setting. In fact, acquired inhibitors of coagulation factors, particularly to Factor V and thrombin, have been described after topical bovine thrombin exposure during or after surgery, and may result in clinically important coagulopathies (18). Bovine thrombin can be antigenic by itself, but it is also thought that impurities during its preparation may be responsible for the adverse reactions (19). Usually, these antibodies are IgG that bind to the C2 domain of the Factor V light chain; however, an IgA antibody has also been described. Hemorrhagic symptoms linked to the presence of these inhibitors are variable: the most frequent symptoms are represented by hematuria and bleeding during surgical procedures (20), but in some cases no clinical symptoms appear. In this condition laboratory findings show abnormalities both in the PT (prothrombin time) and in the aPTT.

This inhibitor has been described after administration of bovine thrombin during surgical procedures, or after human thrombin administration after endoscopy for gastric ulcer (21). These inhibitors have also been found in association with autoimmune diseases, such as in one case of Hashimoto's thyroiditis, primary biliary cirrhosis, and membranous nephropathy (22).

References

1. Hay CR. Acquired haemophilia. Bailleres Clin Haematol 1998; 11: 287–303.
2. Cohen AJ, Kessler CM. Acquired inhibitors. Bailleres Clin Haematol 1996; 9: 331–54.
3. Ma AD, Carrizosa D. Acquired Factor VIII Inhibitors: Pathophysiology and treatment. Hematology Am Soc Hematol Educ Program 2006; 432–7;
4. Moraca RJ, Ragni MV. Acquired anti-FVIII inhibitors in children. Haemophilia 2002; 8: 28–32.
5. Mazzucconi MG, Peraino M, Bizzoni L, Bernasconi S, Luciani M, Rossi GD. Acquired inhibitor against factor IX in a child: Successful treatment with high-dose immunoglobulin and dexamethasone. Haemophilia 1999; 5: 132–4.
6. Green D, Lechner K. A survey of 215 non-hemophilic patients with inhibitors to Factor VIII. Thromb Haemost 1981; 45:200–3.
7. Fang BS, Snellen MC, Straus SE, Frenkel L, Dale JK, Rick ME. Report of a factor VIII inhibitor in a patient with autoimmune lymphoproliferative syndrome. Am J Hematol 2000: 64: 214–17.
8. Kyriakou DS, Alexandrakis MG, Passam FH, Foundouli K, Matalliotakis E, Koutroubatis IE, et al. Acquired inhibitors to coagulation factors in patients with gastrointestinal diseases. Eur J Gastroenterol Hepatol 2002;14:1383–7.
9. Broxson EH, Hathaway WE. Transplacental transfer of acquired factor VIII: C inhibitor. Thromb Haemost 1987; 57: 126.
10. Sahud MA, Pratt KP, Zhukov O, Qu K, Thompson AR. ELISA system for detection of immune responses to FVIII: A study of 246 samples and correlation with the Bethesda assay. Haemophilia 2007; 13: 317–22.
11. Franchini M. Rituximab in the treatment of adult acquired hemophilia A: A systematic review. Crit Rev Oncol Hematol 2007; 63: 47–52.
12. Wiestner A, Cho HJ, Asch AS, Michelis MA, Zeller JA, Peerschke EIB, et al. Rituximab in the treatment of acquired factor VIII inhibitors. Blood 2002; 100: 3426–8.
13. Franchini M, Veneri D, Lippi G, Stenner R. The efficacy of rituximab in the treatment of inhibitor-associated hemostatic disorders. Thromb Hemost 2006; 96: 119–25.
14. Oliveira B, Arkfeld DG, Weitz IC, Sihnada S, Ehresmann. Successful rituximab therapy of acquired factor VIII inhibitor in a patient with rheumatoid arthritis. J Clin Rheumatol 2007; 13: 89–91.
15. Sallah S, Wan JY. Efficacy of 2-chlorodeoxyadenosine in refractory factor VIII inhibitors in persons without hemophilia. Blood 2003; 101: 943–5.
16. Yamamoto K, Takamatsu J, Saito H. Intravenous immunoglobulin therapy for acquired coagulation inhibitors: A critical review. Int J Hematol 2007; 85: 287–93.
17. Franchini M, Lippi G. Acquired von Willebrand syndrome: an update. Am J Hematol 2007; 82: 368–75.
18. Savage WJ, Kickler TS, Takemoto CM. Acquired coagulation factor inhibitors in children after topical bovine thrombin exposure. Pediatr Blood Cancer 2007; 49: 1025–9.
19. Lawson JH, Lynn KA, Vanmatre RM, Domzalski BA, Klemp KF, Ortel TF, et al. Antihuman factor V antibodies after use of relatively pure bovine thrombin. Ann Thorac Surg 2005; 79: 1037–8.
20. Wiwanitkit V. Spectrum of bleeding in acquired factor V inhibitor: A summary of 33 cases. Clin Appl Thromb Hemost 2006; 12: 485–8.
21. Caers J, Reekmans A, Jochmans K, Naegels S, Mana F, Urbain D, et al. Factor V inhibitor after injection of human thrombin (tissucol) into a bleeding peptic ulcer. Endoscopy 2003; 35: 542–4.
22. Takahashi H, Fuse I, Abe T, Yoshino N, Aizawa Y. Acquired factor V inhibitor complicated by Hashimoto's thyroiditis, primary biliary cirrhosis and membranous nephropathy. Blood Coagul Fibrinolysis 2003; 14: 87–93.

Index